CRC HANDBOOK SERIES IN ZOONOSES

James H. Steele, D.V.M., M.P.H.
Editor-in Chief

SECTIONS AND SECTION EDITORS

SECTION A: BACTERIAL, RICKETTSIAL, AND MYCOTIC DISEASES

Section Editors
Herbert Stoenner, D.V.M.
    Director, Rocky Mountain Laboratory
    U.S. Public Health Service
    Hamilton, Montana

Michael Torten, D.V.M., Ph.D.
    Israel Institute for Biological Research
    Ness-Ziona
    Faculty of Medical Sciences
    Tel Aviv University School of Medicine
    Israel

William Kaplan, D.V.M., M.P.H.
    Mycology Division
    Center for Disease Control
    Atlanta, Georgia

SECTION B: VIRAL ZOONOSES

Section Editor
George W. Beran, D.V.M., Ph.D., L.H.D.
    Professor, Veterinary Microbiology
    and Preventive Medicine
    Iowa State University
    Ames, Iowa

SECTION C: PARASITIC ZOONOSES

Section Editor
Primo Arambulo, III, D.V.M.,
M.P.H., Dr. P.H.
    Public Health Veterinary Consultant
    PAHO/WHO
    Washington, D.C.

SECTION D: ANTIBIOTICS IN ZOONOSES CONTROL

Section Editors
George W. Beran, D.V.M., Ph.D.,
L.H.D.
    Professor, Veterinary Microbiology
    and Preventive Medicine
    Iowa State University
    Ames, Iowa

C. Don VanHouweling, D.V.M., M.S.
    Director, Bureau of Veterinary
    Medicine (Ret)
    Food and Drug Administration
    U.S. Public Health Service
    Rockville, Maryland

Herbert Dupont, M.D.
    School of Medicine
    University of Texas
    Houston, Tx 77025

Each section contains one or more volumes

CRC Handbook Series in Zoonoses

Zoonoses

James H. Steele, Editor-in-Chief

Assistant Surgeon General (Retired)
U.S. Public Health Service
Professor of Environmental Health
School of Public Health
University of Texas at Houston

Section A: Bacterial, Rickettsial, and Mycotic Diseases

Volume II

Section Editors

Herbert Stoenner
Director, Rocky Mountain Laboratory
U.S. Public Health Service
Hamilton, Montana

William Kaplan
Mycology Division
Center for Disease Control
Atlanta, Georgia

Michael Torten
Israel Institute for Biological Research
Ness-Ziona
Faculty of Medical Sciences
Tel Aviv University School of Medicine
Israel

CRC Press, Inc.
Boca Raton, Florida

Library of Congress Cataloging in Publication Data
Main entry under title:

Bacterial, rickettsial, and mycotic diseases.

 (CRC handbook series in zoonoses; section A,
V. 1-2)
 Includes bibliographies and indexes.
 1. Bacterial diseases. 2. Rickettsial diseases.
3. Mycoses. 4. Zoonoses. 5. Communicable diseases
in animals. I. Steele, James H. II. Series.
RC115.B3   616.9'2   78-10696
ISBN 0-8493-2907-8

Direct all inquiries to CRC Press, Inc. 2000 N.W. 24th Street, Boca Raton, Florida 33431.

© 1980 by CRC Press, Inc.

International Standard Book Number 0-8493-2900-0 (Complete Set)
International Standard Book Number 0-8493-2905-1 (Section A)
International Standard Book Number 0-8493-2906-X (Volume I)
International Standard Book Number 0-8493-2907-8 (Volume II)

Library of Congress Card Number 78-10696
Printed in the United States

PREFACE
CRC HANDBOOK SERIES IN ZOONOSES

The biological adventurousness of animal diseases is exceeded only by the insatiable adventuresomeness of man. The struggle of the infectious diseases of lower forms of life to adapt themselves to more highly developed hosts is unending. As these disease agents insure their continued existance by adapting themselves to a broader host spectrum, they become a greater threat to man's well-being. Man, in his most tenuous position on this earth, has been able to protect himself from this biological onslaught by his skill in developing the preventive medical practices that are the foundation of our present public health practices.

In this century, man has made greater progress in holding back or eliminating infectious diseases than since he appeared on earth. Progress in the control of host-specific human diseases, such as smallpox, diphtheria, cholera, poliomyelitis, and syphilis, has brought to the fore animal disease problems which in many areas of the world are major challenges to human health. The eradication of smallpox is one of the major health achievements of our times. One reason this was possible was that there is no animal reservoir of smallpox. The control of diphtheria, cholera, poliomyelitis, and other childhood diseases was possible because none of these diseases have an animal reservoir.

Animal diseases threaten man's health and well-being in many ways. To examine the importance of animal health to human health, it is well for us to consider the World Health Organization (WHO) definition of health as a guide. "Health is not the mere absence of disease or injury . . . it is a state of complete physical, mental, and social well-being." The contributions that veterinary medicine can make to reach the WHO objective are succinctly presented in the definition of veterinary public health: . . . "comprises all the community efforts influencing and influenced by the veterinary medical arts and science applied to the prevention of disease, protection of life, and promotion of the well-being and efficiency of man." The present epidemic of Rift Valley Fever in the Nile Vally is an example of how serious some zoonoses can be. The 1978 epidemic has effected thousands of persons and tens of thousands of cattle, sheep, and goats. Why Rift Valley Fever became so wide spread and virulent is unknown.

The definition of health, as established by WHO, provides a very broad framework upon which to develop our theme. How veterinary medicine will participate in protecting the public health and welfare is well expressed in the broad definition of veterinary public health, and the inter-relationship of disease and health in man and animals provides a challenge that tests the imagination, ingenuity, and knowledge of man.

James H. Steele
Editor-in-Chief

JAMES H. STEELE, EDITOR-IN-CHIEF
CRC HANDBOOK SERIES IN ZOONOSES

Dr. James H. Steele has held a broad and rewarding experience in veterinary medicine and public health. He entered the Michigan State Veterinary College in 1938 and completed his veterinary training in 1941 when he was awarded the D.V.M. degree. After an internship in veterinary medicine and the Michigan Public Health Laboratory, he was sent to Harvard School of Public Health on a U.S. Public Health Service Fellowship. On the completion of the M.P.H. degree in 1942, he was assigned to the Ohio Health Department as a sanitarian. In 1943, he was commissioned in the U.S. Public Health Service and assigned to Puerto Rico where he had his first opportunity to become acquainted with animal diseases in the tropics and received encouragement to develop a national and international program.

After world War II, he was called to the U.S. Public Health Service, Washington, D.C. to plan a program to deal with the zoonoses and veterinary public health. This was to be a part of the Communicable Disease Center in Atlanta, Georgia where it grew into a national program with an international influence. In addition to directing the CDC veterinary public health program, Dr. Steele was a consultant to U.S. government agencies and international organizations relating to the health of man and animals.

After the inauguration of the veterinary public health program in 1947, a category for veterinary officers was approved by the Surgeon General in 1948. In 1950 Dr. Steele was made Veterinary consultant to the Surgeon General and liaison to professional health organization. Later in 1967 he was to become the Assistant Surgeon General for Veterinary Affairs in the Public Health Service and Department of Health Education and Welfare. The first veterinary officer to be named to this post. He remained in this position until his retirement in 1971. During 1969 he was designated advisor to the White House office on Consumer Affairs.

Dr. Steele was a technical advisor to Surgeon General Thomas Parran when the United Nations organized the World Health Organization in 1946. Later he was appointed to the WHO Expert Committee on Zoonoses and served in varying roles. In 1966 he was elected Chairman. During 1946 the Food Agriculture Organization was having technical meetings at which he represented the United States. He has served as a consultant to the FAO on many occasions since. The Pan American Sanitary Bureau was the first to request his services in disease outbreaks in the Carribean and Panama during and after World War II. He has been a consultant to the Pan American Health Organization since 1945 and served as chairman of their Scientific Advisory Committee in 1970. In addition to serving as a consultant to international agencies, he has been an advisor to a number of countries and universities in developing veterinary public health programs.

He has received national and international recognition from numerous governments, agencies, and societies. The U.S. Public Health Service awarded him the Medal of Merit in 1963 and the Distinguished Service plaque on his retirement in 1971. The American Public Health Service presented Dr. Steele the prestigous Bronfman Award in 1971 and the Centennial medal in 1972. In 1966 the Conference of Public Health Veterinarians honored him the recipient of the K.F. Meyer Gold Headed Cane Award. These Handbooks of the Zoonoses are dedicated to K.F. Meyer. Dr. Steele has been made an honorary member of various scientific organizations in the Americas, Europe and Asia. In 1965 he was named president of the American Veterinary Epidemiology Society. He was instrumental in the estabblishment of the World Veterinary Epidemiology Society in 1972 which is affiliated with the World Veterinary Association. An award was established in his name by the WVES in 1976 which is presented to a young leader in international veterinary public health. He has been described by many of his colleagues as *Mister Veterinary Public Health.*

His publications span a period of almost 40 years and cover various subjects, especially the zoonoses of which there are more than 100 titles. He is a man of many interests.

PREFACE
SECTION A: BACTERIAL, RICKETTSIAL, AND MYCOTIC DISEASES
VOLUME II

Historically, zoonotic diseases have had a tremendous impact on the evolution of man, especially those cultures and societies that domesticated and bred animals for food and clothing. Early Biblical writers alluded to various associations between man and animals, particularly to those concerned with food habits and slaughtering practices. According to the Old Testament, cloven-hoofed ruminants and fish with scales were considered safe for human consumption while animals that died of natural causes and scavenger birds, presumably because they fed on animal carcasses, were disapproved of as a source of food. Likewise, blood and carcasses of animals that were not exsanguinated were unacceptable. Swine also were considered unfit for human consumption (unclean and abominable), partly because of their filthy habits and the offal and carrion they fed upon. In contrast, swine were eaten regularly by pre-Semitic inhabitants of Palestine and the Greeks often offered swine in sacrifice to their gods. Whether zoonotic diseases were even considered by early man in the development of attitudes toward various species of animals will remain conjecture. It may be assumed though that early Biblical translators and scholars focused on the religious aspects of practices and food habits and would have little reason to consider zoonotic diseases in their interpretation of scriptural writings.

The distribution of certain parasites in man and domestic and wild animals today suggests that these parasites had undergone adaptive processes to survive during the changes that man introduced in the parasite's ecosystem. For example, the speciation in the genus *Brucella* indicates that this organism made several adaptations designed to ensure its survival in independent cycles in wild and domestic animals. Although not highly host-specific, each of the major species — *abortus, suis,* and *melitensis* — is associated principally with one species of domestic animals. In Europe, there is a close epizootiologic relationship between leporine and porcine brucellosis, whereas in the U.S., *Brucella suis* occurs in *Lepus californicus* completely dissociated from swine. In Utah, *Br. neotomae* was found to occur only in *Neotoma lepida* despite the occurrence of many other species of wildlife hosts in its habitat. Very likely, all the species and biotypes of *Brucella* originated from a common ancestral parent from which variants become adapted to different ecological situations.

Because of the complex epizootiology of most zoonoses, responsibility for their control is often divided among health agencies, departments of agriculture, and organizations concerned with wildlife, including marine biologists. In some instances, none of the political subdivisions concerned assume responsibility, and the disease remains unchecked. Regardless of the structure of programs, control of zoonoses involves a large number of disciplines and occupational specialties in the fields of medicine, public health, regulatory veterinary medicine, and wildlife management. Hence, the primary purpose of preparing this Handbook is to provide a guide and comprehensive reference source for veterinarians, physicians, microbiologists, biologists, parasitologists, epidemiologists, health educators, and other health specialists engaged in research, control, and educational activities.

The major bacterial, rickettsial, and mycotic zoonoses are considered in Volumes I and II of this Section. Each contributor was asked to consider the following subject headings in the preparation of his chapter: the disease, etiologic agent, true and alternate hosts, distribution, disease in animals, disease in man, mode of spread, epidemiology, diagnosis, treatment, and prevention and control. Some contributors included extensive historical treatises, and some supplemented their chapters with detailed tabular information concerning various aspects of the disease. Sufficient detail is included so that the microbiologist can use the Handbook as a guide in the isolation and characterization of agents. Similarly, pertinent information presented on the clinical disease in man, diagnosis, and treatment should enable the practicing physician to use the Handbook as an aid in handling human infections. Finally, health and regulatory officials should find the Handbook helpful in the development and application of control measures.

Contributors were chosen on the basis of their expertise in various zoonotic diseases. As editors, we wish to express our sincere appreciation to contributors who spent long hours preparing chapters and, in many cases, compromised fulfilling other responsibilities to meet publication deadlines.

Herbert G. Stoenner
Michael Torten
William Kaplan

SECTION EDITORS

William Kaplan, is currently the Chief of the Developmental Mycology Branch, Center for Disease Control, Atlanta, Georgia. He received his B.S. and D.V.M. degrees from Cornell University in 1943 and 1946, respectively. He also received his M.P.H. degree in 1951 from the University of Minnesota. Following graduation from Cornell, Dr. Kaplan was employed as a clinical veterinarian by the United Nations Relief and Rehabilitation Administration and then was engaged in the private practice of veterinary medicine. During the period from 1948 to 1950, Dr. Kaplan was employed by the U.S. Department of Agriculture and assigned to Mexico where he was engaged in regulatory activities directed toward the eradication of foot and mouth disease in livestock. In 1951, Dr. Kaplan was employed by the Center for Disease Control, U.S. Public Health Service where he was engaged in studies on Q-fever, western equine encephalomyelitis, and chancroid disease. In 1955, he was assigned to the Mycology Division of the Center for Disease Control and has been a member of this division to the present time. His work in the area of medical mycology has been varied and has included investigations on dermatophytosis in animals and their public health importance, control of dermatophytosis in animal populations, research on the application of immunofluorescence to the diagnosis of mycotic diseases in man and animals, studies on dermatophilosis, protothecosis, and most of the subcutaneous and systemic mycoses in man and animals. He has also been involved in the presentation of courses and lectures on various aspects of medical mycology. Dr. Kaplan is an Adjunct Professor (Field), University of North Carolina, School of Public Health, Chapel Hill, North Carolina and an Adjunct Associate Professor of Microbiology, Georgia State University, Atlanta, Georgia. His society affiliations include membership on the International Society for Human and Animal Mycology, Medical Mycological Society of the Americas, American Veterinary Medical Association, American Society for Microbiology, American Public Health Association, and the Association of Military Surgeons of the United States. Dr. Kaplan is the author or co-author of close to 100 publications on various aspects of medical mycology.

Herbert G. Stoenner, is Director of the Rocky Mountain Laboratory, Hamilton, Montana which is one of the laboratories of the National Institute of Allergy and Infectious Diseases, National Institute of Health. Dr. Stoenner received his undergraduate training at William Jewel College, Liberty, Missouri and the University of Missouri, and he graduated in veterinary medicine from Iowa State University in 1943. Following graduation, he served for 3 years as a veterinarian in the U.S. Army and Air Force. Appointed as a commissioned officer to the Public Health Service in 1947, he was initially assigned to the Center for Disease Control, Atlanta, Georgia and attached to the Utah State Health Department where he conducted epidemiologic studies on human brucellosis and later discovered and described *Brucella neotomae,* one of the recognized species of *Brucella.* In 1949 he was assigned to the Rocky Mountain Laboratory to investigate the role of cattle in the epidemiology of Q fever. In 1953 he was attached to the Washington State Department of Agriculture to investigate bovine leptospirosis. He returned to the Rocky Mountain Laboratory in 1954 and has served as its Director since 1964. Although his career in the Public Health Service was largely administrative, he has authored more than 50 publications dealing with brucellosis, listeriosis, leptospirosis, relapsing fever, Q fever, and other rickettsial diseases. Since 1965 he has served on the Committee on Leptospirosis of the U.S. Animal Health Association.

Michael Torten, is Associate Professor of Medical and Veterinary Microbiology and Head of the Zoonoses Section, Faculty of Medical Sciences, Tel Aviv University, Tel Aviv, Israel and in the Department of Epidemiology, Israel Institute for Biological Research, Ness-Ziona, Israel. Dr. Torten graduated in 1963 from the University of California, Davis, with a D.V.M. and obtained his Ph.D. in Microbiology in 1968 from Hebrew University of Jerusalem, Israel. He is the Chief of the World Health Organization/Food and Agricultural Organization and National Leptospirosis Reference Laboratory and a member of the World Health Organization Expert Committee on Leptospirosis. Dr. Torten is a member of the Israel Veterinary Association, Israel and International Microbiological Associations, Israel and International Immunological Societies, and the Phi Zeta Honorary American Veterinary Society. Among other awards, he has received the "Zur" Award from the Ministry of Agriculture Veterinary Services for valuable contribution to veterinary medicine in Israel. He is also an Honorary Diplomate of the American Veterinary Epidemiology Society. Dr. Torten has published more than 70 scientific research papers. Since 1977, he has served as Editor-in-Chief of *Refuah Veterinarith, Israel Journal of Veterinary Medicine.*

FOREWORD

N. Sinai

The *CRC Handbook Series in Zoonoses* is especially timely. For years, scattered reports and writings have emphasized selected problems. Now, each volume in this series will serve as a compendium of modern knowledge and practice, a manual that expresses the ideals of preventive veterinary medicine applied on a global scale.

It is significant that the International Institute of Administrative Sciences (IIAS) chose three subjects for its studies of comparative public administration. The concern of this organization lay not in the structure of the laws of selected countries but rather in the actual application of these laws. The subjects chosen were (1) workmen's compensation, (2) river pollution by industrial enterprises, and (3) cattle diseases, particularly foot-and-mouth disease. A special report on cattle diseases was published in 1964.*

It is to the great credit of the veterinary profession that, almost since the beginning of the 18th century, prevention has played a predominant role in applied practice. This was the central purpose of the school of veterinary medicine established by royal decree in 1762 at Lyons, France. Steele** has written a vivid report on the economic devastation caused by cattle plague (*rinderpest*) when it invaded Italy in 1713 and spread throughout Europe. After nearly 50 years of "petitions, bickering, enormous economic losses, and subsequent social disturbances," the school at Lyons came into being, and the philosophy of prevention became firmly established.

The world need for protein foods and food products has been stressed and documented by numerous studies. Projections of needs are often made to the year 2000 (a mere 20 years away) when, according to demographers, the world population will be approximately six billion persons. The very massiveness of the data challenges the imagination and benumbs the feeling of impending disaster.

Byerly refers to ruminant livestock as one of man's most valuable "renewable resources."*** The key word is renewable, and he emphasizes six areas in which the need for research and development is both pressing and overdue. In summary, the following areas require a massive undertaking to achieve a projected 50% increase in productivity:

1. Pasture and range improvement, particularly in tropical regions
2. Genetic resistance and vector management, especially the arthropod-borne hematoprotozoal diseases and helminth parasites
3. Increased animal unit production through an improved conception rate and decreased fetal and perinatal mortality
4. Development and evaluation of systems — biological, ecological, engineering, economic, and social — for resource use, ruminant production, and product utilization
5. Development of new products such as meat protein concentrates, texturized products from trimmings and edible offals, and lactose-hydrolyzed milk for lactose-intolerant persons
6. Improvement of milk and meat production through genetic selection and feed-

---

* Anon., *Prevention of Cattle Diseases,* International Institute of Administrative Sciences, Brussels, 1964, 3.
** Steele, J. H., The socioeconomic responsibilities of veterinary medicine, *Public Health Rep.,* 79(7), 613, 1964.
***Byerly, T. C., Ruminant livestock: research and development, *Science,* 195, 450, 1977.

ing programs designed to satisfy energy, protein, mineral, and other nutrient requirements of pregnant and lactating animals

It is estimated that world financial support for research and development must approximate an increase of 45% during the next 25 years. As if this were not staggering enough in concept and magnitude, both veterinarians and agriculturists face other problems of applied science — the need for training not only in the broad aspects of public health but also in the field of anthropology. The importance of the latter is demonstrated too often by the failure of programs — public health, agricultural, educational, industrial — because of ignorance or inattention to cultural obstacles. No sophisticated nutritionist would make the mistake of suggesting an immediate utilization of beef or beef products for the population of India. However, there are many obstacles other than religious ones to changes in traditional tastes and food habits.

Cassava, the staple diet for millions of persons, is an example of the adjustment of agricultural research to food tradition. This food is notable for its high carbohydrate and extremely low protein content. Accepting the premise that it takes generations of time to shift from cassava to protein-rich soya, research is centered on producing a more balanced cassava through crossing wild strains, which have a much higher percentage of protein, with the product that is commonly grown. Predictions of a successful outcome range from 3 to 5 years.

Public health workers have learned many cultural lessons the hard way. Piping water to village huts in certain areas is a classic example. It was much more than a problem of developing a source, digging trenches, and providing pipe and hydrants. The resistance of the villages, despite the lengthy walk and the burden of carrying water, resulted from the fact that the well was the main social center of the community. At least temporarily, the cost of giving up the social center outweighed the benefit of piped water.

This series of Handbooks entails a program that presents huge potential. Its underlying foundation is biological science, but biological science cannot be applied as a completely independent entity. It must be buttressed by enormous input from the humanities and social sciences.

NATHAN SINAI

Nathan Sinai, D.V.M., M.S.P.H., Dr.P.H., professor emeritus of public health at the University of Michigan, one of the nation's most distinguished public health leaders and an internationally acclaimed medical care statesman, died November 28, 1977 at a hospital in South Laguna, California following a long illness. He was 83.

An inspired and inspiring teacher, Dr. Sinai originated and guided educational programs widely recognized and imitated. A noted health care pioneer, he became a world leader of the insurance movement. One of the founders and constant leaders in the field of medical care research, his pioneering work on group practice and on the organization and delivery of health services, dating from the early 1930s, is still followed by his students and other workers in the field.

Born November 28, 1894 in Stockton, California, Nathan Sinai attended San Francisco College where he received the Doctor of Veterinary Medicine degree in 1915. In 1924 he received the Master of Science in Public Health degree and two years later the Doctor of Public Health degree, both from the University of Michigan. He joined the University of Michigan faculty in 1924 as an instructor in public health and was appointed an assistant professor in 1927, associate professor in 1929, and full professor in 1932. Soon after his appointment to the Michigan faculty, he undertook a four-year assignment on the research staff of the Committee on the Costs of Medical Care, working with a talented group which provided leadership to American medical care research and action for the next half century.

In 1935, Dr. Sinai initiated a course in medical administration at Michigan, the first university to have such a program. He became secretary of the University of Michigan School of Public Health in 1941, the same year the school was officially designated as one of the colleges of the University, and held that position until 1952. Until 1959, Professor Sinai was director of the University's Bureau of Public Health Economics, which he established in 1943. He also worked as director of research of the Michigan State Medical Society (1932 to 1934) and was consultant to the Ann Arbor Health Department from 1941 to 1955.

Known internationally as well as nationally, Professor Sinai served as a consultant to the League of Nations and to the World Health Organization. Having taken a special interest in comparative studies of health care systems of other nations, he helped develop a health insurance plan in Windsor, Canada and was one of the earliest leading proponents of national health insurance in this country and remained so until his death. He made the most definitive study of the United States government's World War II program for Emergency Maternity and Infant Care (EMIC) and served as consultant to the U.S. Public Health Service (1936 to 1940), the Children's Bureau (1939 to 1947), the Manhattan Project, Oak Ridge, Tennessee (1944 to 1945), and many other national programs.

At the time he was named professor emeritus, in 1964 after 40 years of service to Michigan, U.M.'s regents said, "Keeping abreast of the rapid changes in the economic context of health services, Dr. Sinai became at once an expert in the field of medical insurance and a persuasive, popular exponent of the humane and sensible distribution of medical care. Within the School of Public Health, of which he was long the senior member of the faculty, he was esteemed for his superior teaching and his imaginative contributions to new instructional programs. He lent honor both to his School and to the University."

Professor Sinai remained very active throughout his retirement, maintaining his close ties to Michigan. In 1974, he returned to deliver the first annual Nathan Sinai Lecture, an honor bestowed upon him by the School of Public Health, and he returned again in 1976 to teach a course in the Department of Medical Care Organization. In all, his continuous association with medical care teaching and research at the University of Michigan spanned 54 years.

A member of the American Public Health Association for 53 years, Dr. Sinai served with generous spirit and notable effect in posts of leadership. In 1944, Dr. Sinai was one of the members of the newly formed Subcommittee on Medical Care (of the Committee on Administrative Practice) which played a leading role in the movement for a comprehensive national health program to bring adequate health care to all Americans. The Subcommittee, under a 1946 grant by the Rockefeller Foundation, carried out an ambitious program of studies of all aspects and problems of medical care. Their activities and interests eventually led to the movement to establish a Medical Care Section within APHA. In 1946, Dr. Sinai represented his state affiliate, Michigan, on the APHA Governing Council, and from 1952 to 1954 he served the Medical Care Section in the same capacity. He was a life member and fellow of APHA, a fellow and past president (1945) of the Michigan Public Health Association, and a member of Phi Kappa Phi and Delta Omega societies.

In 1974, on the occasion of his 80th birthday, the Medical Care Section of the Southern California Public Health Association invited many of his colleagues, former students, and friends to a symposium held in his honor. Many friends gathered to pay tribute to their teacher and friend; others who could not attend sent messages of remembrance to be read.

Dr. Paul Cornely, one of Professor Sinai's earliest doctoral students in medical care administration, has said that he remembers Nate Sinai "not only for his keen, well-disciplined mind of a reseacher, but much more for the grace, humor, charm, and sensitive consideration for each and all of his students, thus making him a long-remembered and most beloved teacher."

From *Am. J. Public Health,* 68(7), 701, 1978. With permission.

CONTRIBUTORS
SECTION A: BACTERIAL, RICKETTSIAL, AND MYCOTIC DISEASES
VOLUME II

Libero Ajello
Director, Mycology Division
Bureau of Laboratories
Center for Disease Control
Atlanta, Georgia

Benedict G. Archer
Assistant Professor
WOI Regional Program in
Veterinary Medicine
University of Idaho
Moscow, Idaho

J. Frederick Bell
Medical Director PHS (retired)
Rocky Mountain Laboratory
National Institute of Allergy and
Infectious Diseases
National Institutes of Health
Hamilton, Montana

Willy Burgdorfer
Head, Rickettsial Diseases Section
Rocky Mountain Laboratory
National Institute of Allergy and
Infectious Diseases
National Institutes of Health
Hamilton, Montana

Jay O. Cohen
Research Microbiologist
Biological Products Division
Bureau of Laboratories
Center for Disease Control
Atlanta, Georgia

E. Denis Erickson
Associate Professor
Department of Veterinary Science
University of Nebraska
Lincoln, Nebraska

A. Konrad Eugster
Head, Diagnostic Microbiology
Texas Veterinary Medical Diagnostic
Laboratory
College of Veterinary Medicine
Texas A & M University
College Station, Texas

B. D. Firehammer
Professor of Veterinary
Microbiology
Veterinary Research Laboratory
Agricultural Experiment Station
Montana State University
Bozeman, Montana

John Francis
Professor of Veterinary Preventive
Medicine and Public Health
Veterinary School
University of Queensland
St. Lucia, Queensland
Australia

Diana K. Goroff
Microbiologist
Department of Bacterial Diseases
Walter Reed Army Institute of
Research
Washington, D.C.

Elmer M. Himes
Veterinarian
National Veterinary Services
Laboratory
Ames, Iowa

S. S. Kalter
Director, Microbiology and
Infectious Diseases
Southwest Foundation for Research
and Education
San Antonio, Texas

William Kaplan
Assistant Director, Mycology
Division
Bureau of Laboratories
Center for Disease Control
Atlanta, Georgia

Dennis L. Kasper
Associate Professor of Medicine
Channing Laboratory
Harvard Medical School
Peter Bent Brigham Hospital
Boston, Massachusetts

L. D. Konyha
Chief Staff Veterinarian
Veterinary Services
Animal and Plant Health Inspection
Service
U.S. Department of Agriculture
Washington, D.C.

Robert A. MacLean
Deputy Director of Public Health
City of Houston Health Department
Houston, Texas

James A. McComb
Director (retired)
Biologic Laboratories
Commonwealth of Massachusetts
Instructor (retired)
Harvard School of Public Health
Boston, Massachusetts

Lyle L. Myers
Associate Professor of Veterinary
Biochemistry
Veterinary Research Laboratory
Agricultural Experiment Station
Montana State University
Bozeman, Montana

F. J. Mulhern
Administrator
Animal and Plant Health Inspection
Service
U.S. Department of Agriculture
Washington, D.C.

Arvind A. Padhye
Chief, Fungus Reference Branch
Mycology Division
Center for Disease Control
Atlanta, Georgia

Robert N. Philip
Assistant Director
Rocky Mountain Laboratory
National Institute of Allergy and
Infectious Diseases
National Institutes of Health
Hamilton, Montana

Allan C. Pier
Chief, Bacteriological and
Mycological Research Laboratory
Science and Education
Administration
National Animal Disease Center
Ames, Iowa

Julius Schachter
Professor of Epidemiology
George Williams Hooper Foundation
Acting Director
Karl Friedrich Meyer Laboratories
University of California
San Francisco, California

Emmett B. Shotts, Jr.
Professor of Medical Microbiology
College of Veterinary Medicine
University of Georgia
Athens, Georgia

Leo G. Staley
Major, U.S. Army
Deputy for Veterinary Activities
United States Military Academy
West Point, New York

James H. Steele
Professor of Environmental Health
School of Public Health
Health Science Center
University of Texas
Houston, Texas

Herbert Stoenner
   Director
   Rocky Mountain Laboratory
   National Institute of Allergy and
     Infectious Diseases
   National Institutes of Health
   Hamilton, Montana

Peter L. Stovell
   Animal Pathology Directorate
   Health of Animals Branch
   Agriculture Canada
   Pacific Area Laboratory
   Vancouver, British Columbia

Charles O. Thoen
   Professor of Microbiology
   Department of Microbiology and
     Preventive Medicine
   College of Veterinary Medicine
   Iowa State University
   Ames, Iowa

J. S. Walker
   Biological Safety Officer
   Plum Island Animal Disease Center
   USDA Science and Education
     Administration
   Greenport, New York

Leslie P. Williams, Jr.
   Public Health Veterinarian
   Office of Disease Monitoring and
     Control
   Oregon State Health Division
   Portland, Oregon

Boris Velimirovic
   Chief, Field Office/U.S.-Mexico
     Border
   Pan American Health Organization
   World Health Organization
   El Paso, Texas

ACKNOWLEDGMENTS

These zoonoses handbooks are an outgrowth of study, research, and experience covering almost 40 years. My introduction to the field began at the Michigan State College of Veterinary Medicine where I was a student, laboratory aide, and research assistant. Contact there with men who spoke of the veterinarian's contributions to public health stimulated an interest that led me to a lifelong career in that field. These men included Dean Ward Giltner and Professors H. J. Stafseth, W. L. Mallman, I. D. Huddleson, and W. T. S. Thorp among others too numerous to mention here. The opportunity to become a graduate student in public health came about through the efforts of Ward Giltner and C. C. Young, director of laboratories at the Michigan State Health Department, who arranged for my senior year to be spent in the public health laboratory so that I could be eligible for a U.S. Public Health Service fellowship upon graduation.

Harvard opened a whole new world in 1941. World issues were discussed and their effect upon the future of society was the daily fare. Many persons there encouraged the investigation of those animal diseases that affect man. Dean Cecil K. Drinker and his wife, Dr. Katherine Drinker, encouraged me to "fly under one flag" rather than remaining in school to obtain a medical degree (M.D.). Dr. Edward Huber, assistant dean, was a staunch supporter, as were Dr. Lloyd Aycock and Dr. John Gordon, epidemiologists, and Dr. John Enders, microbiologist. While at Harvard, I had frequent contact with Dr. C. A. Brandly, who was to become a lifelong friend and advisor and, later, dean of the College of Veterinary Medicine, University of Illinois, Urbana.

After spending 1 year in the Ohio Health Department and as a lecturer at the Ohio State University College of Veterinary Medicine, where I came to know and receive further encouragement from Dr. A. F. Schalk, Dr. R. E. Rebrassier, and Dean O. V. Brumley, I was commissioned in 1943 as a sanitarian in the U.S. Public Health Service. My first assignment, in Puerto Rico, brought me together with Dr. J. O. Dean, who was to have a profound influence on my career and the development of veterinary public health, particularly on the investigation and control of the zoonoses. During my tour of duty, I met Dr. Joe Mountin, assistant surgeon general, and Dr. Thomas Parran, surgeon general.

At the end of the war, Dr. Mountin brought me to Washington, D.C. to organize a veterinary public health program. There, Dr. Joe Dean, his wife, Amy, and her sister, Bessie Schaum, helped me to organize a review of the zoonoses in the U.S. and their public health implications. At this point in my career, I encountered many public health professionals who assisted me with their advice and encouragement. Among these were Charles Williams, Sr., assistant surgeon general; Louis Williams, director of international health; Eugene Dyer, director of the National Institutes of Health; and Dr. L. F. Badger, assistant to Dr. Dyer. Dr. Willard Wright, a veterinarian who directed the tropical medicine research program, was an invaluable resource person. At this time, Dr. Henry Holle was also very generous in helping to get the program off the ground, and Dr. C. L. Dunnahoo, chief of foreign quarantine, was another friend and supporter. Dr. Thomas Parran later became an advocate and good friend, as were all the surgeons general who succeeded him: Leonard Scheele, Lee Burney, Luther Terry, William Stewart, and Jesse Steinfeld. Also, a special word of thanks should be given to Dr. Phillip Lee, assistant secretary of health, whose support was most generous.

Outside of the U.S. Public Health Service, there were many professional colleagues and friends who offered me much technical and tactical advice. Many were distinguished public servants: William Hagen, dean of the New York Veterinary College and advisor to President Truman on veterinary affairs in Europe at Potsdam; Brigadier General Ray Kelser, chief of the U.S. Army Veterinary Corps and later dean of the University of Pennsylvania School of Veterinary Medicine; Brigadier General James McCallum, chief, U.S. Army Veterinary Corps and subsequently president of the American Veterinary Medical Association (AVMA); and Brigadier General Wayne Kester, assistant surgeon general for veterinary services, U.S. Air Force. The AVMA executive secretary, John G. Hardenburgh, and the staff of this organization gave generously of their time and technical resources, a practice that has continued throughout the years and the changes in leadership. The Bureau of Animal Industry chief, Dr. B. T. Simms, chief of pathology, Dr. Harry Schoening, and their staff were also very supportive.

After the establishment of the veterinary public health program in Washington, D.C., it was transferred to the then newly organized Communicable Disease Center (CDC) in Atlanta, which was concerned with the spread and control of such diseases in the U.S. CDC Director Raymond Vonderlehr and his deputy, Justin Andrews, gave me their complete support. Soon, zoonoses investigations became an important part of CDC's overall program, which included the study of many diseases in nature that had animal reservoirs. Here, I first met Dr. A. D. Langmuir, who became chief of epidemiology. This department was concerned with many of the veterinary public health activities, especially the investigation of zoonotic diseases. Later, these activities were to include surveillance, which provided hard data on the zoonoses and allowed control methods to be developed. Dr. Langmuir had a great positive influence on all veterinarians who were fortunate enough to come under his direction, and he provided many opportunities for them to further their development. His influence extended beyond the CDC and the U.S. Public Health Service, however. Today, nearly all veterinarians in the field of disease control receive training in epidemiology, developing a skill that is essential to their activities.

All of the past directors of CDC were interested in the success of zoonoses control activities. Two of them, Justin Andrews and T. J. Bauer, were good friends and supporters. Later, R. J. Anderson, C. A. Smith, James Goddard, and David Sencer threw the full weight of their support behind the zoonoses programs.

Many others at CDC should be mentioned, especially Dr. Philip Brachman, the current director of epidemiology, his staff, including Myron Schultz, and the many professionals with whom I worked for 28 years, especially Ernest Tierkel and other close friends and colleagues in the veterinary public health programs. Finally, I could not leave the subject of CDC without expressing my deepest appreciation for the person who typed innumerable manuscripts throughout the world — my secretary for almost 2 decades — Mrs. Betty Hooper.

Many persons at the University of Texas have given advice and support during the years in which the technical material for these handbooks was assembled, and I am duly appreciative of their support and encouragement: Dr. Charles Lemaistre, chancellor, Austin; Dr. Truman Blocker, acting president of the University of Texas Health Science Center, Houston; and Dean Reuel Stallones, dean of the School of Public Health, Houston.

For preparing the manuscripts and handling the voluminous correspondence, my special thanks is extended to Mrs. Mildred Hopper and Peggy Donnellan, who spent many hours organizing the chapters that comprise these volumes. Sylvia Ponce de Leon has been a great help in bringing the task to completion, and Miss Marcia Willis has been most generous of her time in reading and editing many chapters. It has been a pleasure to work with Sandy Pearlman, Pamela Woodcock, and Jodi Willoughby of CRC Press. They have been most cooperative.

To all of the consultants, editors, and associate editors — my sincerest thanks. You have been magnificent. My deepest appreciation is also extended to the handbook contributors, all recognized specialists within their respective fields. Without their cooperation, collaboration, and generosity, these volumes could never have been prepared. Thank you all.

It goes without saying that, too frequently, those closest to authors are not duly acknowledged. In the preparation and editing of these volumes, my wife, Brigitte Maria, has given invaluable advice and maintained a home in which it was a pleasure to work. Thanks, my love.

DEDICATION

KARL FRIEDRICH MEYER was born May 19, 1884 in Basel, Switzerland, the son of Theodor and Sophie (Lichtenhahn) Meyer, and was educated at the University of Zurich. He received the D.V.M. degree from the University of Zurich in 1905. The recipient of nine honorary degrees, "K.F." was most proud of an Honorary M.D. from the University of Zurich in 1937. After working in South Africa, he came to the U.S. in 1910 and taught at the University of Pennsylvania. He was naturalized in 1922.

In 1913, K.F. married Mary Elizabeth Lindsay of Philadelphia. She died in 1958. Surviving is their daughter, Charlotte, and four grandchildren with two great-grandchildren. In 1960, K.F. married Marion Lewis who is arranging his personal and professional papers.

K.F. came to the University of California in 1914 as Professor of Bacteriology and Experimental Pathology. He divided his time quite evenly between San Francisco, Berkeley, Davis, and the rest of the world. He became Director of the G.W. Hooper Foundation for Medical Research in 1924 and soon made it a center for study in world public health and epidemiology.

K.F. was a renowned and vigorous lecturer, sometimes lengthy, but never dull. His major contributions were in the control of botulism; the establishment of standards for the canning industry; the control of plague, encephalitis, and ornithosis; the development of public health standards and practices, and aid in many related research problems involving tropical diseases, mussel poisoning, dental caries, and disturbances of hearing. With over 300 publications, K.F. was the recipient of many honors. He was an avid philatelist with a unique collection of disinfected mail. The president of many scientific societies, K.F. was one of our most influential and distinguished scientific leaders.

K.F. was active until his 90th year. The May 1974 issue of *The Journal of Infectious Diseases* had a special supplement on plague that was dedicated to him. A longer biographical sketch is in the supplement. There are now plans for the editor and colleagues to edit his papers and publish a biography.

As this issue goes to press, the Editors have received the sad news of Dr. Meyer's death on April 27, 1979. The following is an excerpt from the lengthy obituary by Lawrence K. Altman that appeared in *The New York Times* on April 29:

Dr. Karl Friedrich Meyer was regarded as the most versatile microbe hunter since Louis Pasteur and a giant in public health.

As a youth in Basel, Switzerland, pictures of the Black Death, or plague, so fascinated him that he became an outdoor scientist instead of following in the aristocratic business world in which he grew up. He told friends that in choosing to become a veterinarian he could "be a universal man and study all diseases in all species."

Public health leaders yesterday called his contributions to medicine "monumental." His scientific work had such broad implications that it touched on virtually all fields of medicine.

Dr. Meyer is survived by his wife and daughter, to whom we extend our deep sympathy.

TABLE OF CONTENTS
SECTION A: BACTERIAL, RICKETTSIAL, AND MYCOTIC DISEASES
VOLUME I

TABLE OF CONTENTS
SECTION A: BACTERIAL, RICKETTSIAL, AND MYCOTIC DISEASES
VOLUME II

Bacterial Diseases

PNEUMONIA

J. H. Steele

There are many causes of pneumonia in man and animals, as have been discussed. An unusual occurrence in animals is *Streptococcus* pneumonia (formerly *Diplococcus* pneumonia), a common disease of man that occasionally affects calves and other ruminants, including sheep, goats, and other animals. The *Streptococcus pneumoniae* organism has been isolated from the upper respiratory tract of apparently healthy animals. At present, 70 serotypes are recognized. These are analogous to the Lancefield groups of streptococci and are differentiated chiefly on the basis of the Neufeld Quelling reaction, swelling of the capsule as induced by type-specific antisera.[1]

Human pneumonia is distributed world-wide, particularly in the very old and young; although in populations with adequate medical services, the disease is seen less frequently. It occurs in all climates and seasons. In the temperate zones, the incidence is highest in the winter and early spring. The disease is usually sporadic in the U.S., but epidemics may occur in institutions. In the tropics, pneumonia can be a serious disease in debilitated persons, especially in tropical highlands where night temperatures are chilly. In the mountains of New Guinea, pneumonia is often a fatal disease.

Occurrence of *S. pneumoniae* in animals was previously reported from western and northern Europe, especially in cattle and calves. Romer,[2] in an extensive review covering the period beginning in the late 19th century until 1960, arrived at the conclusions that follow.

PNEUMOCOCCUS INFECTIONS IN DIFFERENT ANIMAL SPECIES

It appears that some animal species are more or less resistant to pneumococcus* infections. Robertson and Sia (1927)[3] stated that dogs, cats, sheep, pigs, horses, chickens, and pigeons are resistant, whereas rabbits and guinea pigs are susceptible to pneumococci. These authors demonstrated that serum from resistant animals enables leukocytes from resistant as well as susceptible animals to phagocytize virulent pneumococci, whereas pneumococci treated with serum from susceptible animals are not phagocytized by leukocytes. Thus, the resistance is believed to be due to the fact that blood from resistant species normally contains a relatively high concentration of anti-pneumococcus opsonin.

The above facts are in accordance with the results of investigations that were begun in 1921 by Bull and McKee.[4] These researchers demonstrated, by mouse protection tests, that serum from chickens was able to protect mice against infection with the pneumococcus types known at that time. They stated that the protection referred to was type-specific so that a serum absorbed with one pneumococcus type still contained antibodies against the other types. The same conditions were demonstrated for serum from pigs by Sia[5] in 1929, who showed that unabsorbed serum from pigs protected mice against both type 1 and type 2 pneumococci, whereas serum absorbed with type 1 pneumococci continued to protect against type 2 infection.

Below, an account is given of the occurrence of pneumococcus infections in different species of animals. From this it will be evident that the above-mentioned resistance demonstrated in some species is not absolute. In some animals, even serious pneumococcus infections have occasionally been diagnosed.

---

* "Pneumococcus" is used in this chapter although current literature employs the term "streptococcus."

PNEUMOCOCCUS MASTITIS IN DAIRY COWS

Several cases of pneumococcus mastitis have been described in the literature, the first in 1931, with reports continuing until 1958. Some of these were acute mastitis in the affected cows while others were diagnosed on routine herd bacteriological examinations. Some acute cases became fatal septicemia. From available data, it appears that the great majority of cases were due to type 3 pneumococcus. The source of the infections was considered to be human carriers although the milking machine appears to have played a role. It is apparent that pneumococcus mastitis causes a considerable decline in milk production, chiefly in the acute phase of illness and probably in the remaining part of the lactation period. Romer[2] suggests the possibility that pneumococcus mastitis may be a cause of pneumococcus infections in calves. When these infections were more common than they are today, pasteurization and good milk hygiene practices were essential to prevent spread to calves.

Treatment with antibiotics eliminated the infection, and the decline of human carriers has probably been an important factor in the apparent disappearance of pneumococcal mastitis.

Pneumococcus infection in calves has been quite extensive, as measured by the comprehensive literature cited by Romer.[2] A review of the literature shows that the disease seems to be quite common in calves, especially during the first month of life, but it has also been seen in older calves of 1 to 3 months of age. Signs and symptoms of the disease vary according to the course, which may be peracute, acute, subacute, or chronic. A seasonal variation is recognized with the disease; it occurs more frequently during the winter months. It was common in northern and central Europe and is also described in papers from Russia, Poland, and the U.K. Outside of Europe, calf pneumococcal disease has only been reported in Canada. According to Romer, a broad spectrum of serotypes has been reported in Denmark. The 14 most frequent types in his findings constituted 85% of those isolated and included types 2, 6, 7, 8, 9, 10, 15, 17, 18, 19, 22, 23, 33, and 35.

Infection in pneumococcal disease in calves can occur by the umbilical, aerial, and alimentary routes. As late as 1954, umbilical infections (18%) were demonstrated in a study of 364 calves reported from Germany. The same report stated that aerial infections caused 73% of the cases, and about two thirds of these developed septicemia. Intestinal infection was the least important with less than 9% of the cases having arisen in that way. These latter intestinal cases and the umbilical infections were probably associated with poor hygiene. The aerosol route is most logically attributed to human carriers.

In experiments reported by Romer, it is seen that calves are susceptible to experimental infection with pneumococci and that the disease produced corresponds to that seen in spontaneous infection. Experimental calves given no colostrum have a somewhat higher mortality than calves given colostrum. This seems to suggest that normal colostrum provides some protection against the infection.

Pneumococcus infections in animals other than cattle were described by Romer and earlier investigators in guinea pigs, rabbits, monkeys, mink, horses, sheep, goats, and pigs. Some of these, e.g., horses, sheep, and pigs, seem to be relatively resistant to pneumococcus infections. However, under unusual conditions, pneumococci seem to be able to overcome the natural resistance of these animals and even cause diseases running a lethal course.

DISCUSSION

Of the above-mentioned species, guinea pigs are the most susceptible to pneumococcus infections, the disease having a enzootic character. The respiratory organs are particularly subject to attack with development of coryza, severe pleurisy and pneumonia (sometimes combined with peritonitis), and abortion and metritis in relation to pregnancy. The disease, caused almost exclusively by pneumococcus type 19 (in a few cases, other types are found), occurs most often in winter. Cold weather and vitamin deficiency therefore seem to be essential factors with regard to reducing the resistance of animals. For control of the disease, attention must be focused on precautions related to stable as well as nutritional hygiene. To combat already existing enzootic outbreaks, some researchers recommend, in addition to removal of sick animals, diagnosis of coryza and elimation of animals suffering from it because they seem particularly liable to maintain the infection. Others claim to have stopped enzootic outbreaks by vaccinating the healthy animals with a vaccine prepared from pneumococci isolated from the sick guinea pigs.

In monkeys, pneumococcus infections most often manifest themselves as pneumonia that may cause a considerable number of deaths among monkeys kept in limited premises, e.g., for laboratory use. Vaccination and treatment with antibiotics are stated to be effective with regard to controlling the disease.

Pneumococcal infections in mink — presumably of alimentary origin — may give rise to septicemia combined with pneumonia, pleurisy, muscular necrosis, and metritis (in pregnant animals). In the outbreaks described, a calf that died of pneumonia was fed to 135 mink, 91 of which died. Pneumococci type 23 was found to be responsible. The same type was recovered from the dead calf.

Pneumococcus infections in foals may produce septicemia that may either run a rapidly lethal course or be more protracted with a tendency towards development of such local diseases as pneumonia, pleurisy, arthritis, tendonitis, meningitis, and cerebral abscesses.

With regard to pneumococcus infection in sheep, it is worth mentioning that in an enzootic outbreak adult sheep as well as lambs were attacked. The disease ran a septicemic course in the puerperium, combined with metritis; in other cases it was associated with hemorrhagic inflammation of the upper air passage and sometimes also in pneumonia and pleurisy victims. In lambs, the septic conditions were usually combined with hemorrhagic enteritis. As described by Dhanda and Sekariah,[6] pneumococci also cause pneumonia in sheep and goats.

Pneumococcus infections in pigs do not seem to be important, but judging from cases described by Terpstra and Akkermans in Holland,[7] it appears that under special conditons pneumococcus infections may give rise to lethal disease in pigs, presumably transmitted from man. In this connection, mention may be made of the old custom whereby laymen performing castrations would spit into the castration wound at the conclusion of the operation, a practice that might have given rise to a large infection rate.

An unusual demonstration by a Danish investigator[9] of pneumococci in a sample of Argentine bones showed that insufficiently heat-treated meat-and-bone meal may be a source of pneumococci infection in domestic animals.

The disappearance of pneumococcal disease in animals parallels the decline of the disease in man. Benenson[8] refers to the disease as "previously very common." In a search of the literature of the last decade, there are few references to pneumococcal disease in animals, including farm, fur, laboratory, and pet animals. Sporadic cases are occasionally seen on autopsy of monkeys and other laboratory animals. Therefore, it can be assumed that environmental change and the wide use of antibiotics in man and animals have had a beneficial effect.

REFERENCES

1. **Bruner, D. W. and Gillespie, J. H.,** The lactobacillaceae: the genus *Diplococcus,* in *Hagan's Infectious Diseases of Domestic Animals,* 6th ed., Cornell University Press, Ithaca, N.Y., 1973.
2. **Romer, O.,** Pneumococcus infections in animals, *Commun. State Vet. Serum Lab.* (Copenhagen), 371, 1, 1962.
3. **Robertson, O. H. and Sia, R. H. P.,** as cited in Romer, O., Pneumococcus infections in animals, *Commun. State Vet. Serum Lab.* (Copenhagen), 371, 1, 1962.
4. **Bull, C. G. and McKee, C. M.,** as cited in Romer, O., Pneumococcus infections in animals, *Commun. State Vet. Serum Lab.* (Copenhagen), 371, 1, 1962.
5. **Sia, R. H. P.,** as cited in Romer, O., Pneumococcus infections in animals, *Commun. State Vet. Serum Lab.* (Copenhagen), 371, 1, 1962.
6. **Dhanda, M. R. and Chandra Sekariah, P.,** as cited in Romer, O., Pneumococcus infections in animals, *Commun. State Vet. Serum Lab.* (Copenhagen), 371, 1, 1962.
7. **Terpstra, J. I. and Akkermans, J. P.,** as cited in Romer, O., Pneumococcus infections in animals, *Commun. State Vet. Serum Lab.* (Copenhagen), 371, 1, 1962.
8. **Benenson, A. B.,** The pneumonias, in *Control of Communicable Diseases in Man,* 12th ed., American Public Health Association, Washington, D.C., 1975.
9. **Mueller, J. W.,** personal communication, 1953.

RAT-BITE FEVER

R. A. MacLean

Rat-bite fever is an acute illness in man caused by either *Streptobacillus moniliformis* or *Spirillum minus*. The illnesses share many clinical and epidemiologic features; however, there are enough differences to warrant separate discussions.

Illness following the bite of a rat was recorded in India at least 2300 years ago. Many observers believe that the disease originated in that country. Discrepancies in the early medical literature, both in the U.S. and abroad, resulted from failure to recognize the dual etiology of the disease. In 1908, Ogata described a syndrome in Japan that he called *sodoku* (*so* = rat; *doku* = poison) caused by what is know known as *S. minus*. The *Streptobacillus* was described by Schottmuller in 1914, who named the organism by its morphology and source: *Streptothrix morsus ratti* (filamentous thread from rate bite). In 1924, the spirochete was renamed *Spirillum minus* by Robertson, and in 1925 the bacillary organism was renamed *Streptobacillus moniliformis* by Levaditi. These names have been in general use ever since. For an excellent historical review of both diseases with extensive references, see the report of J. W. Roughgarden.[1]

STREPTOBACILLARY RAT-BITE (HAVERHILL) FEVER

Etiologic Agent

The etiologic agent of this disease is *S. moniliformis*, a Gram-negative pleomorphic bacterium, also known as *Streptothrix muris rattus*, *Actinomyces muris*, or *Haverhilla multiformis*.

Distribution

The organism is distributed world-wide, and there is no known significant reservoir other than the rat. It has been demonstrated that 50% of otherwise healthy laboratory as well as wild rats carry the streptobacillus among their normal flora.[2]

Disease in Man

In *S. moniliformis* disease, the bite site usually heals, followed by a latent period of 2 to 3 days (range: 1 to 22 days, but usually less than 10) before the abrupt onset of systemic symptoms. These consist of: (1) a high fever — septic, intermittent, or relapsing, (2) chills, (3) headache, (4) a morbilliform, petichial rash in 75%, commonly involving extensor surfaces of limbs near joints, (5) lymphadenitis (usually regional) in 25%, (6) polyarthritis in 40%, and (7) myalgia. Other symptoms that have been described include vomiting, sore throat, and backache. Differential diagnosis includes other bite-wound infections: tularemia, Rocky Mountain spotted fever, sodoku, and cat-scratch fever. Reported complications of untreated disease include bacterial endocarditis, pneumonia, pleural effusion, abscesses, and persistant severe arthritis. The fatality rate in reported cases from which organisms were isolated was 10.8%; 50% of these had bacterial endocarditis.[3]

Period of Communicability

None. There have been no reported cases of man-to-man transmission even though the occasional occurrence of pneumonia could theoretically result in airborne infection.

Diagnosis

Although the disease may be suspected by clinical history and findings, the diagnosis is confirmed by the isolation of *S. moniliformis* from blood, joint fluid, or pus on media enriched with 20% serum, preferably under microaerophilic conditions. Evidence of growth may be delayed several days. The organisms are Gram-negative and pleomorphic, and formation of filamentous chains with knobby excrescences is characteristic. Growth requirements and characteristic staining and morphology are considered sufficient for identification. Many strains spontaneously form microcolonies consisting of spheroplasts (L forms). Pathogenicity for mice consisting of septicemia and polyarthritis can be demonstrated, as can agglutinins in patient serum. A titer of 1:80 or greater is considered diagnostic; however, this test is not generally available.[4]

Treatment

The treatment of choice is parenteral penicillin. Although cures have been reported with as few as 24,000 units/day, 600,000 units administered twice daily for 7 days is usually prescribed for uncomplicated streptobacillary disease today.[1,5] In patients who are allergic to penicillin, chloramphenicol has been used successfully,[6] as has streptomycin and tetracycline.[1,7] Results of preantibiotic treatment with arsenicals were variable; this is probably therapeutic only in the spirillary form of the disease.[8,9]

Disease in Animals

Most infected rats show no sign of illness. The streptobacillus has been isolated from rats and mice having bronchopneumonia,[10] and epizootic incidents characterized by naturally occurring polyarthritis have occurred in laboratory mice. Isolations have also been made from the tendon sheath and sternal bursa of arthritic turkeys[11] and from cervical abscesses in guinea pigs. However, clinical disease in nonhuman hosts is rare. The organism's relative lack of pathogenicity in its natural host, the rat, insures its survival. Infection or isolation of the organism from other mammals may result from either a rat bite or, in the case of carnivores, passive transfer from the animal feeding on rats.

Mode of Spread

This form of the disease is spread almost exclusively by a rat bite. However, cases have been reported following the bite of other mammals, e.g., cat, dog, ferrett, weasel, and mouse.[8,9,12,13] In some cases, a bite has not been necessary. Disease has been reported in persons living in rat-infested buildings[14] and in persons in contact with dead rats or blood from an infected animal (dog).[9] Presence of the organism in oropharyngeal secretions accounts for these cases of infected droplet or contact transmission. An uncommon method of spread was documented as a result of an outbreak of 86 cases in Haverhill, Mass. in 1926. Disease was traced epidemiologically to the ingestion of raw milk distributed by one dairy, and the outbreak was abruptly halted when the firm was required to start pasteurizing its milk.[15] The role of rats was not suspected until the similarity between the organism isolated from some patients with the one known to cause rat-bite fever was recognized. Contamination of raw milk by the nasopharyngeal secretions of infected rats appeared to be the most likely explanation.

Epidemiology

Persons at risk are primarily those who have frequent contact with rats. The true incidence of the disease in man is unknown, but it is higher in urban areas where rat populations are high, particularly the inner cities. The disease is also an occupational hazard of laboratory workers.[5] In the U.S., 55% of reported cases have occurred in children less than 12 years of age. In Houston, a large metropolitan area, only two confirmed cases of *S. moniliformis* disease have been reported in 7 years: one a 9-year-old bitten by a white rate in a pet store, and the other in an adult laboratory worker. The only published study of the incidence of Haverhill fever reported that of 93 persons bitten by rats in a section of Baltimore adjacent to Johns Hopkins Hospital, 7 (10.7%) developed rat-bite fever.[16]

SODOKU

Etiologic Agent
The etiologic agent of sodoku is *Spirillum minus,* also known as *Sporozoa muris* or *Spirochaeta morsus muris.*

Distribution
Sodoku is found world-wide although reports are quite rare from North America.

Disease in Man
The distinctive features of spirillary rat-bite fever are a longer incubation period (1 to 30 days, usually more than 7); prompt initial healing at the bite site with the appearance of induration, ulceration, or eschar at the onset of fever; and a rash consisting of reddish or purplish plaques. In contrast to the bacillary form, arthritis is uncommon. Lymphadenitis, usually regional, is present in 50% of the cases, as is false-positive serologic test for syphilis. Mortality in untreated cases has been reported as 6.5%[1]

Period of Communicability
None. There is no evidence of man-to-man transmission.

Diagnosis
Confirmation depends upon the demonstration of spirilla in the patient by the inoculation of laboratory animals (usually uninfected guinea pigs or mice). Microscopic demonstration of *Spirillum minus* should also be attempted from blood, exudates, or cutaneous eruptions such as the bite site. Wet mounts should be examined by dark-field or phase-contrast microscopy. In inoculated animals, blood or peritoneal fluid should be examined in 2 weeks by dark-field microscopy and a Giemsa-stained film. Serologic testing by immobilizing live organisms with immune serum has been demonstrated, but the need to have a supply of infected animals makes the test impractical.[4]

Since it may be difficult to distinguish the spirillary and bacillary forms of rat-bite fever clinically, both bacterial culture and animal inoculations should be performed before treatment is initiated.

Treatment
Penicillin administered parenterally is the treatment of choice. Although the spirillary organism is more sensitive to penicillin, initial treatment should be directed toward the more resistant organism until laboratory confirmation is obtained. Patients allergic to penicillin may be treated with chloramphenicol.

Disease in Animals
The organism does not appear to cause significant illness in rats. It has been demonstrated most consistantly in blood and peritoneal fluid. Eye infections with keratitis and conjunctivitis occur occasionally. When a human case is traced to the bite of another mammal, it could be the result of passive contamination of the oropharynx from that animal having eaten rats.

Mode of Spread

Sodoku is spread directly — through the bite of an infected rat or, occasionally, another wild or domestic carnivore. Transmission among animals probably occurs most commonly as the result of a bite. Presence of the organism in conjunctival secretions could result in some instances of droplet transmission.

Epidemiology

As with the bacillary form, sodoku is primarily a risk for those having frequent contact with rats. The true incidence in man is unkown. Carrier rates among rats have been shown to vary widely according to geographic location.

Prevention and Control

Control of both diseases is aimed at reducing the rat population present in the human environment. Recognition of the disease as an occupational hazard of laboratory workers who handle rats should lead to earlier diagnosis and initiation of appropriate therapy. Rat elimination measures that place heavy emphasis on environmental control are most likely to achieve long-lasting results.

REFERENCES

1. **Roughgarden, J. W.**, Antimicrobial therapy of rat-bite fever, *Arch. Intern. Med.*, 116, 39, 1965.
2. **Strangeways, W. I.**, Rats as carriers of *Streptobacillus moniliformis*, *J. Pathol. Bacteriol.*, 37, 47, 1933.
3. **McGill, R. C., Martin, A. M., and Edwards, P. E.**, Ratbite fever due to *Streptobacillus moniliformis*, *Br. Med. J.*, 201, 703, 1966.
4. **Rogosa, M.**, *Streptobacillus moniliformis* and *Spirillum minor*, in *Manual of Clinical Microbiology*, 2nd ed., Lennette, E. H., Spaulding, E. H., and Truant, J. B., Eds., American Society for Microbiology, Washington, D.C., 1974, 326.
5. **Coll, J. S., Stoll, R. W., and Bulger, R. J.**, Rat-bite fever, report of three cases, *Arch. Intern. Med.*, 71, 979, 1969.
6. **Stokes, J. F., Gray, I. R., and Stokes, E. J.**, *Actinomyces muris* endocarditis treated with chloramphenicol, *Br. Heart J.*, 13, 247, 1951.
7. **Sprecher, M. and Copland, F.**, Haverhill fever due to *Streptobacillus moniliformis* treated with streptomycin, *JAMA*, 134, 1014, 1947.
8. **Mock, H. E. and Morrow, A. R.**, Ratbite fever transmitted by catbite, *Ill. Med. J.*, 61, 67, 1932.
9. **Ripley, H. S. and Vansant, H. M.**, Ratbite fever acquired from dog, *JAMA*, 102, 1917, 1934.
10. **Tunnicliff, R.**, Streptothrix in bronchopneumonia of rats similar to that of ratbite fever, *J. Infect. Dis.*, 19, 767, 1916.
11. **Yamamoto, R. and Clark, G. T.**, *Streptobacillus moniliformis* infection in turkeys, *Vet. Rec.*, 75, 95, 1966.
12. **Dick, G. E. and Tunnicliff, R.**, *Streptothrix* isolated from blood of patient bitten by weasel, *J. Infect. Dis.*, 23, 183, 1918.
13. **Farguhar, J. W., Edmunds, P. N., and Tilley, J. B.**, Sodoku in child: results of mousebite, *Lancet*, 2, 1211, 1958.
14. **Shwartzman, G., Florman, A., Bass, M. H., Karelitz, S., and Richtberg, D.**, Repeated recovery of a *Spirillum* by blood culture from two children with prolonged and recurrent fevers, *Pediatrics*, 8, 227, 1951.
15. **Place, E. H. and Sutton, L. E.**, Erythema arthriticum epidemicum (Haverhill fever), *Arch. Intern. Med.*, 54, 659, 1934.
16. **Richter, C. P.**, Incidence of rat bites and rat bite fever in Baltimore, *JAMA*, 128, 324, 1945.

SALMONELLOSIS

L. P. Williams, Jr.

INTRODUCTION

The most important zoonosis in developed countries is salmonellosis. It is in this principal position because of the number of cases (reported and unreported), the increasing frequency in man and animals during the last 3 decades, and our seeming inability to control its present movement in a huge animal reservoir.[1-6] It also causes immense economic loss.[4,7,8] In these developed countries, various animal products are a major source of protein; in order to meet the high demand for these foods, animals are fed formulated feeds while concentrated in great numbers.

These animals are commercially slaughtered (in numbers of thousands per hour or day), and food items are produced or packaged from them — often after several steps requiring handling and storage — and then widely distributed through a complex marketing system to domestic and foreign consumers.[7,9] If these products are properly handled, cooked, and served, even though contaminated with salmonellae during production, no cases or outbreaks will occur. If, contrary to the ideal situation, the animal-origin food product is mishandled during preparation, undercooked or served raw, or contaminated (or recontaminated) after cooking, one or more persons may become infected with the organism. If a large number of organisms are ingested, the victim will manifest gastroenteritis and possibly other symptoms of disease.

If the victim is either very young (less than 5 years) or old and very ill, medical help will be sought for relief of the symptoms; the attending physician may or may not submit a stool specimen for culture and report the disease. If the illness is mild, the victim will not seek medical help, and there is no chance that the episode will be reported.[9] Once reported, it is the duty (and opportunity) of the epidemiologist to analyze the serotypes or bacteriophage types and orient them in terms of time, place, and person in order to identify an outbreak, investigate the source, and if possible institute control measures to prevent recurrence.[10]

In developing countries, salmonellosis is also an important disease. However, it may be only one of a number of important causes of diarrhea[11] and one of several zoonoses that occur with regularity in the population — especially if these people maintain close contact with their animal populations and/or products that they garner from them. Cases that occur in developing populations may never be attended by medical personnel;[12] therefore, little will be known regarding the epidemiology of salmonellosis there. Animal-to-animal, animal-to-man, man-to-man, and environment-to-animal or man cycles continue uninterrupted except through herd die-off, natural disaster, nomadic movement, or industrialization.

With the latter comes the cycle with which we are best acquainted — and after 70 years, it is still just an acquaintance. This cycle consists of concentration of livestock, feeding of formulated feeds contaminated with salmonellae, slaughtering, carcass contamination, complex marketing practices that lead to widespread distribution of an unwholesome product, mishandling of it, and outbreaks or "sporadic cases." This cycle is an indicator of "development" or "progress." Attendant to it is the problem of sanitary disposal of several hundred thousand tons of animal waste[13] — a by-product of concentration (or confinement-rearing) — that has the capacity to contaminate the air, land, and water.

Approximately 1300[8,9] serotypes of salmonellae (one author states that there are 2000[14]) have been identified in the 90-year period since the type species, *Salmonella enteritis*, was identified. This first identification followed the occurrence of a food-borne outbreak, the source of which was an infected cow. Of this large and ubiquitous group, less than a dozen are completely or strongly host-adapted. These include *S. typhi, S. paratyphi A, B,* and *C* (man), *S. abortusovis* (sheep), *S. abortus-equi* (horse), and *S. gallinarum* (poultry); some investigators add to this list *S. dublin* (cattle), *S. cholera suis* (swine), and *S. pullorum* (poultry).[8,9,15] Others could be added, based on regional occurrences. Only the first seven are considered by this author not to have zoonotic pathways (one of these, *S. paratyphi B,* is questionable) and will not be considered in this presentation. Remaining serotypes have been (or eventually will be) isolated from animals and man, and some of the cycles between them have been identified.

DISEASE

The disease is called salmonellosis or *Salmonella* gastroenteritis. Occasionally, it is seen in the form of *Salmonella* enteric fever (or septic syndrome) or in focal infections.[9]

ETIOLOGIC AGENT

Salmonella is 1 of 11 genera of the tribe Enterobacteria. Within the genus are four numbered subgroups. Division into these groups is based on the differing biochemical reactions of the subgenera. Only two of these groups are of particular interest to the public health worker who deals with the zoonosis. Included in subgenera I are most of the serotypes that cause disease in animals and man — approximately 60% of the serotypes in the genus. Subgenera III — accounting for 23% of the species within the genus — are the so-called Arizona organisms carried by reptiles and mammals and capable of causing disease in any vertebrate if an infective dose is encountered and/or the host is experiencing some form of stress.[14]

All of these organisms are Gram-negative, nonspore-forming rods that are aerobic or facultatively anaerobic. Most strains are motile.[14,16] They are not highly resistant to physical or chemical agents and can be killed at 55°C in 1 hr or at 60°C in 15 to 20 min; therefore, they are destroyed by standard cooking procedures and pasteurization. Commonly available disinfectants will also kill them. The organisms grow in the presence of malachite or brilliant green dyes, whereas other enteric organisms are killed or inhibited by them. This characteristic is capitalized on in the laboratory with the latter dye commonly being incorporated into various selective media.[14] Freezing will decrease *Salmonella* numbers but will not kill them.[8,9]

The genus is divided into about 2000 serotypes based on various combinations of "O" or somatic antigens and "H" or flagellar antigens; the latter occur in two phases (a "Vi" antigen is also present in some strains but is of little importance in serotyping).[14] On the basis of the O antigens present, serotypes are grouped by use of the Kauffmann-White Schema. Approximately 40 of these groups or subgroups exist, identified by letter (i.e., A, B, C_1, C_2, D, etc.) or group-determining antigen (i.e., 50, 51, or 52). Several common serotypes have been further subdivided by bacteriophage-typing schemes.[14] The major (or possibly only) use of the serotype or bacteriophage type is to the epidemiologist while working through the maze from patient, to food product, to wholesaler, to processor, to slaughterer, to producer, to feed manufacturer or blender, and to animal protein supplier. If the involved serotype is a common one and no bacteriophage-typing scheme exists, epidemiologists may resort to the use of unusual cultural or biochemical reactions or an uncommon antibiotic-resistance pattern.[9]

While humans and animals build antibodies against O, H, or Vi antigens that can be identified and quantified, these are seldom protective for the host against a second contact with the organism, especially if the next encounter is with a differing sero-type.[16]

TRUE AND ALTERNATE HOSTS

The classification of hosts into true and alternate categories is very difficult and dependent upon the classifier, the area served, and the interests of investigators in that area or country. Based on isolations from animal carcasses examined in diagnostic laboratories and on surveys and animal disease reports (included in surveillance summaries published in the U.S.), an arbitrary list of true hosts would include domestic poultry, swine, cattle, and pets (referred to as companion animals, including the riding horse, in U.S. veterinary circles). All others are considered to be alternate hosts. This list would be acceptable to most investigators in the U.K.[3,17] and developed countries in Europe [4,5] although in some, swine would head the list. Some islands would begin their list with sheep because of intense husbandry of the species in a well-developed and carefully managed pasture ecosystem.

Salmonellae have been isolated from all wild and domesticated animals and birds, reptiles, confined fur-bearing species, laboratory primates and rodents, and many species of wild rodents.[9]

Salmonella in Poultry

Salmonella infection may cause disease and a high death rate in chicks of up to 3 weeks of age. Older birds are usually asymptomatic excretors that often carry their salmonellae to slaughter and are the source of widespread contamination of the processing plant environment and carcasses that enter the marketing chain. Some representative rates from surveys are as follows: the U.K. — turkeys (2.5%), geese (2%), ducks (1%), and chickens (0.4%); France — hens (12.5%); Germany — hens (15%) and ducks (3 to 55%); India — (1.7%); Georgia (U.S.) — hens (42%) and turkeys at slaughter (68%); Texas broilers at slaughter — (3.6%); the Netherlands — broilers at slaughter (18.7%) and hens (7.0%).[9,18]

Swine Isolations

In a review of *Salmonella* isolations from 1954 to 1965, the percentage of pigs excreting salmonellae on farms varied from 23% in Denmark to 0.5% in Louisiana with a median of 7.2% while the percentage of salmonellae excretors in the abbattoir holding pens varied from 0 to 94% with a median of 25%.[19] Since that time, the following rates of salmonella carriage or excretion have been reported: the U.K., 7%; Denmark, 3%; Australia, 22 and 8.4%;[9] the Netherlands, 30%;[1] and Northern Ireland, 3%.[20] In an extensive review, rates of 36% salmonellae carriage by swine slaughtered in Belgium and 25% of slaughter hogs presented to a British abattoir were reported.[21] The above figures were from fecal or cecal swab examinations. In some of the surveys, isolations from mesenteric lymph nodes were higher than the rates shown.

Salmonella in Cattle and Calves

In an extensive review of *Salmonella* in cattle, isolation rates varied from 13 to 15%. Only one survey conducted in Lebanon reported a rate as high as 21%. A very extensive survey of calves on 78 farms demonstrated only a 2.7% excretion rate.[9] In a beef-rearing unit in the U.K., 3.2% of calves arriving on the farm (1708 animals) were excreting salmonellae (range: 0 to 12%).[22] Investigations made at two different time periods in the Netherlands showed that 1 to 7% of calves coming to slaughter tested positive for salmonellae and 23% of abbatoir calves were excreting the pathogen.[21]

Salmonella in Sheep and Goats

Asymptomatic excretion rates varying from 4 to 15% of animals tested have been recorded.[9] In a recent survey conducted in India, 3.1% of 812 sheep and 3.8% of 683 goats were found to be salmonellae carriers.[23]

Salmonella in Dogs, Cats, and Other Pets

Between 1947 and 1965, there were 19 surveys of salmonellosis in dogs and cats reported in the literature. Average rates were 14% for dogs and 2% for cats.[24] A similar review of surveys of canine salmonellosis in four countries showed dogs culturally positive ranging from 0.5 to 27.6%.[25] In a 1976 survey in Iran of 672 adult dogs, the rate of excretion ranged from 4.4% for household dogs to 15.8% for strays.[26] Of 119 dogs in the Philippines, 19 (16.8%) were excreting one or more serotypes.[27] German investigators examined 320 cats on two animal farms and found that 9 (2.8%) were excreting one of five serotypes.[28] A recent review article cites rates in dogs ranging from 0.6 to 25.7% and a low rate of 0.7% for cats.[29] A rate of 6.9% has been shown for dogs tested in Brisbane, Australia.[3]

The highest rates of excretion or carriage in pet animals have been reported in turtles (terrapins) marketed in the U.S. as pets — 45 to 70%.[9,30] In addition to these commonly kept pets, salmonellae have been reported in guinea pigs, rabbits, monkeys, parakeets, and snakes.[9]

Salmonella in Other Animals

Laboratories in England list *Salmonella* infections occurring in the horse, mink, antelope, goat, cheetah, coypu, elephant, giraffe, lion, badger, camel, chinchilla, donkey, hedgehog, rat, lizard, tiger, and wallaby.[3] In a review of animal infections in Sweden, wild birds, pigeons, caged birds, hares, roes, foxes, ostriches, and seals were listed.[4] Various serotypes of *Salmonella* have been found in raccoons, snakes, white-tailed deer, opposums, starlings, 17 species of birds sampled in Canada, skunks, bats, rattlesnakes, tiger snakes, and common skinks.[9] Documented in recent reports are isolations from tortoises,[31-33] frogs,[31,34] constrictor species of snakes,[35] house sparrows, green finches, blackbirds, seagulls,[36-39] carabaos,[27] Adelie penguins and South Polar skuas,[39] heron species,[4] raccoons,[41] nonhuman primates,[42] a marsupial — the quokka,[43] mink,[44] cowbirds,[45] sparrows,[46] canaries,[47] and insects.[1] This extensive list is by no means complete. While many of the species listed above were examined because of their relationship to a human infection or outbreak, a number were examined in surveys and from specimens submitted to diagnostic laboratories, and their role in transmission to other animals or man is unknown. The high prevalence of salmonellae throughout the animal kingdom attests to the statement that salmonellae are ubiquitous, and one pales at the consideration of an eradication program.

DISTRIBUTION

Salmonellosis is a world-wide problem. It is reported wherever a search is initiated and there is a laboratory to support diagnostic procedures, animal or human surveys, or all of these. It has been found in such diverse places as the ghetto of a large city, a small sewage-contaminated stream in Kansas, rural watering holes (World War II bomb craters) in New Guinea, the Amazon jungle,[9] and in a recent report on the top of Stone Mountain in Georgia — a series of solid granite outcrops with extremely limited vegetation and seasonal pooling of rain water on their tops.[48] Although the

Table 1

A COMPARISON BY SEROTYPES
OF HUMAN *SALMONELLA*
INCIDENTS IN ENGLAND AND
WALES, 1960 TO 1971[9,53]

Serotype	Years		
	1960	1966	1971
S. typhimurium	2907	1407	2124
Other salmonellae[a]	1047	1089	3540
Totals	3954	2496	5664

[a]   Including human host-adapted types.

data are now a decade or more old, the most comprehensive coverage of the world *Salmonella* situation is in a book edited by Van Oye[49] concerning all continents and most regions of the world.

Importance of the disease in a given area or country is highly related to the occurrence of other diseases, the type and amount of animal agriculture, the availability of diagnostic services, whether or not the disease is reportable, and how animal protein foods are produced, marketed, and served.

There are approximately 20,000 salmonellae isolations reported each year to the U.S. Center for Disease Control, yielding an incidence rate of 10.5 cases per 100,000 persons. Based on investigations of several epidemics, it is estimated that two million human cases occur annually and that about 1% of them are reported.[2,8,50,51] The underreporting is further suggested by the findings of investigators conducting an intensive food-borne disease surveillance program in the state of Washington. In 1969, 69 outbreaks were reported there, an incidence rate of 23 outbreaks per million population. In the U.S. that same year, 371 outbreaks were reported for a rate of 1.9 per million population. If the Washington rate was applied to the country as a whole, the estimated number of outbreaks would be 4000. Since 49 (13%) of the 371 reported outbreaks were caused by salmonellae, the possible number of *Salmonella* outbreaks could have been 520.[52]

An interesting trend has been observed in England and Wales by comparing the number of incidents due to *S. typhimurium* since 1960 to the number of incidents due to other nonhost-adapted serotypes. These figures are shown in Table 1. The increase was due almost entirely to a marked increase in the number of incidents caused by seven serotypes that were associated with cycles of animal feedstuffs going to poultry or swine, to human foods, and to man.[53] McCoy[15] studied reports of the occurrences of human salmonellosis in England and Wales from 1941 to 1972 and was able to account for the increasing incidence by defining the following factors:

1. The importation of new foods during food rationing (1940 to 1953)
2. The derationing of feedstuffs and establishment of intensive animal-rearing units during the 1950s
3. Changes in the diet due to the relatively low price and ready availability of frozen, oven-ready food in the 1960s

The incidence of *Salmonella* infections in the Netherlands was shown graphically in two recent articles. There was a sharp increase in the number of infections from 1955, when less than 1000 cases were reported, to between 1959 and 1961, when about 9000

Table 2
RATES OF ASYMPTOMATIC *SALMONELLA* CARRIAGE REPORTED IN SEVERAL SURVEYS IN VARIOUS COUNTRIES[9]

Location	Age group	Persons tested	Number excreting	Percent excretors
Virginia (U.S.)	8 years	837	2	0.2
Panama	Infants	296	0	0.0
Japan				
City dwellers		15,096	3	0.02
Port area		7,980	10	0.12
England	Children less than 5 years of age	25,249	37	0.15

Table 3
RATES OF SALMONELLAE ISOLATION FROM PERSONS WITH DIARRHEA FROM SURVEYS IN VARIOUS COUNTRIES[9]

Area	Age group	Persons tested	Number excreting	Percent excreting
Virginia (U.S.)	8 years old	149	1	0.67
Canada	Infants	1103	15	1.36
Panama	Infants	1819	22	1.2
England	0—4 years	Unknown	Unknown	12.0
	7—5 years	Unknown	Unknown	3.0

cases were noted. The average number of cases approximated 7500/year for the next 10 years.[1,5] Of great interest is the number of serotypes identified in any given year. The average prior to 1961 was approximately 50, whereas in the succeeding decade it was approximately 75.[1] While the number of serotypes in humans increased threefold (1955 vs. 1971), in total number of isolates (mostly from feed and animals or their environment) during the same time period, the increase was fivefold.[1] The number of salmonellae isolations from persons in West Germany, Canada, Czechoslovakia, and Bulgaria has also been published.[9] The distribution by serotype and source of nonhuman isolates (incidence) for corresponding 5-year periods for England and Wales[3] and Sweden[4] has been published. In each of the countries, there was an increased number of serotypes identified in these sources during the period of examination.

Of great interest to the epidemiologist is the amount of asymptomatic carriage in various population groups. This has to be judged by results of various surveys. These carrier individuals move freely about a community and can be a special hazard in a close-knit family group, food-service establishment, or medical-care facility, especially if they are young children and/or have poor personal hygiene habits. Information on carrier rates is summarized in Table 2.

In persons with diarrheal disease, the rate of salmonellae isolation is higher. Table 3 lists the results of cultural surveys conducted in several areas of the world. An additional aspect of the distribution of *Salmonella* — the limitation of some serotypes to a specific area — is of interest to the epidemiologist. The differences seen were well illustrated in a review of *Salmonella* in seven eastern European countries where the following serotypes were either peculiar to the country listed or occurred there in great numbers: *S. abortus-equi* in Yugoslavian food animals (horses); *S. brandenburg* in

Bulgaria; *S. saint paul* and *S. barielly* in Hungary and Czechoslovakia; *S. newington* in Poland; *S. chester* in the U.S.S.R.; and *S. kottbus* and *S. manhattan* in Hungary.[9,49] Other serotypes peculiar to an area are *S. adelaide* in Australia; *S. miami* in Florida and Georgia; *S. dublin* in the western U.S. only; *S. javiana* in the Gulf Coast states of the U.S.; *S. loma-linda* in the Pacific and mountain states; *S. weltevreden* in Hawaii and the southwest Pacific; *S. atlanta* in Georgia; and *S. saphra* in Texas.[9] The usefulness of such information was illustrated by Christie.[17] When *S. irumu*, a "South African" type, was isolated from Lancashire patients with gastroenteritis contracted from ready-cooked ox heart, the serotype was further traced to the food handler who was also handling South African frozen eggs. A similar episode occurred in this country when an *S. miami* outbreak in Massachusetts was traced to Florida watermelon contaminated with the same isolate.[9]

DISEASE IN ANIMALS

Salmonellae can readily infect many animal hosts as discussed earlier. Asymptomatic carriage is commonly the result of infection. Gastroenteritis ("scours") or, depending upon the animal species or serotype (or both), a specific disease syndrome may result. Five clinical patterns have been described. The first, called primary salmonellosis, is due to a particular pathogen in a given species resulting in a recognized clinical picture. The serotype may be host-adapted or nearly so. Secondary salmonellosis is associated with another disease, physiological state, or other stress situation. The third form is that of the chronic carrier (usually convalescent) who, although now clinically well, excretes for weeks or occasionally months. The fourth is that of temporary carrier, often observed in slaughter animals. There are short periods of excertion that are reinforced by new lots of salmonellae-contaminated feed or, occasionally, a contaminated environment. The fifth form is designated a latent infection demonstrated by isolation of salmonellae from mesenteric lymph nodes at the time of slaughter.[9] This latter form may be part of the carrier-state syndrome resulting from repeated ingestion of contaminated feed.[19]

Poultry

If infection occurs during the first 3 days of life (some say up to the first 3 weeks), mortality due to salmonellosis may reach 80%.[9] Affected chicks or poultry exhibit anorexia, huddling, pasty vents, dehydration, droopy wings, somnolence, and sudden death. Of the nonhost-adapted serotypes, *S. typhimurium* is most commonly encountered;[3,4] however, numerous other serotypes can infect fowl and some will cause disease. In a 6-year period in England, 68 serotypes were reported from 1548 incidents in poultry.[3] Australian scientists reported an outbreak of *S. singapore* in broiler flocks, with a resultant high mortality. This serotype was isoltated from the breeder flock ration. In a follow-up survey, *S. typhimurium* was the predominant type, and its presence was traced to grain contamination during a rodent eruption.[54] English investigators reported an *S. california* outbreak in turkey poults and traced the source through contaminated pre-starter feed to meat and bone meal known to contain this serotype.[55]

Swine

Young pigs exhibit signs of gastroenteritis if infected by various *Salmonella* serotypes. "Scouring" pigs (1000 fecal samples) yielded 13 isolations of three serotypes in a survey in England. *S. dublin* and *S. typhimurium* were found in addition to *S. cholera suis*. *S. give* has been found in other clinical cases of pig salmonellosis.[20] Swedish workers reported 23 to 24 *Salmonella* outbreaks each year in swine in their country.

The three most common serotypes were *S. cholera suis, S. typhimurium,* and *S. derby.*[4] In a 6-year period in England, relatively few outbreaks of clinical disease were reported from six disease-investigation centers and veterinary diagnostic laboratories, suggesting that clinical salmonellosis was uncommon.[3]

Cattle

Calves less than 3 weeks of age are very susceptible to *Salmonella* infection and clinical disease. In a calf-rearing operation, morbidity could be as high as 85% and mortality 33%.[9] The most common serotypes in European countries are *S. dublin* and *S. typhimurium.* As noted previously, *S. dublin* in cattle is only found in the western U.S.[9] Adult cattle are often asymptomatic excretors, but they can show clinical disease, manifesting abortion, diarrhea, dehydration, and death.[9] Some cattle develop a septicemia, especially as a post parturient complication.[56]

Richardson[51] describes the clinical features of *S. dublin* in adult cattle as follows: depression, pyrexia, reduced milk yield for 24 to 36 hr, severe dysentery characterized by mucous in the feces, with a 7-day illness and often abortion. This same organism in calves 3 to 6 weeks of age may cause a "wasting syndrome" without diarrhea. Parentral antibiotics may decrease the mortality rate below the untreated level of 50 to 100%. With other serotypes in cattle there may be acute enteritis, pyrexia, and diarrhea; a few abortions may occur.[57] While *S. dublin* is often transmitted animal-to-animal (convalescent excretion may last 11 months or longer) or animal-environment-animal, herd outbreaks of other serotypes are often associated with contaminated feed.[57,58] An outbreak of *S. virchow* occurred in a herd of cattle in England. Nearly one half of the herd had severe diarrhea — some with blood and mucous — and one abortion occurred.[59]

Sheep and Goats

Salmonellae cause clinical disease in sheep and goats in all parts of the world. In England, *S. dublin* occurs in sheep in the same areas where it affects cattle.[9] Cattle were the source of a large outbreak of *S. typhimurium* in 1600 upland sheep with a high mortality rate in the flock.[60] In Britain, 5 to 13% mortality has been reported in *Salmonella* outbreaks in sheep,[21] and 10% mortality with 50 to 70% morbidity was observed in 1970 in a regional outbreak in feedlot sheep in Colorado.[61] Clinical signs were severe diarrhea, depression, anorexia, and death.[61]

Horses

Salmonellae are frequently isolated from horse meat produced for pet food or human consumption.[9] *S. typhimurium* is the most frequently isolated serotype from either carrier or diseased horses; however, others may be found.[4,27,62-65] In recent years, severe clinical disease often associated with treatment or surgery (or other stress) at large veterinary teaching hospitals has occurred in horses in many parts of the world. Within a few days after hospitalization or treatment, the animal develops diarrhea (may not occur), anorexia, congested mucous membranes, depression, and shock; septicemia may be present. Despite intensive antimicrobial and supportive therapy, the animals die following a short clinical course.[62-64] Treatment with tetracycline may enhance the development or increase the severity of the condition.[64,65] A 2% or greater carrier rate may exist in most horse populations and these animals will quickly manifest disease if stressed.[64] Since some of these horses show a neutropenia or decreased neutrophil count, it has been suggested that horses entering a clinic be checked for these signs before surgery or other stressful procedure is attempted.[62]

Dogs and Other Pets

Dogs, cats, and other pets can carry salmonellae and also manifest clinical disease, especially if they are young. The clinical picture is well described in a review by Morse and Duncan.[25] The signs do not differ from those seen in other animals with gastroenteritis; the death rate does not exceed 10% and abortion and stillbirths occur. Cats show the same clinical picture. Parakeets have diarrhea, ruffled feathers, anorexia, and depression, and they dehydrate rapidly. When a large shipment of canaries — 4400 — were moved from Holland to the U.S., a *Salmonella* epidemic due to *S. typhimurium* occurred during their first 3 weeks postentry; approximately 2000 died.[41]

DISEASE IN MAN

The most common clinical syndrome from *Salmonella* infection is gastroenteritis.[9,66,67] Fever (> 100°F), diarrhea, vomiting, abdominal cramps, and anorexia are commonly seen, and headache may be experienced in some cases. Although the acute stage lasts only 2 to 3 days, the patient is not well for several days.[9,68] In 117 children with gastroenteritis, Canadian researchers showed a mean duration of illness of 8.7 days (range: 1 to 60 days). This varied by age, and, in infants less than 3 months of age, averaged 19 days.[67] In an outbreak in which mostly adults were involved, duration of diarrhea was 6 days.[66]

While blood in the stool is not commonly associated with *Salmonella* gastroenteritis, in the Canadian series it was seen in 36% of the cases (children under 16). *Salmonella* bacteremia is also considered a rare finding. However, 24% of the above cases had positive blood cultures (various serotypes),[67] and in an *S. enteriditis* food-borne outbreak,[66] 3 of 17 villagers hospitalized (18%) had the organism in their blood. An interesting set of observations was made of convalescent excretion by the varying age groups of children in a Canadian hospital. Of those more than 3 months of age, 7% excreted salmonellae for 8 weeks and 2% for 6 months; however, in those less than 3 months of age, the comparable figures were 27% and 8%, respectively.[67]

The second most common clinical picture is enteric fever or septic syndrome.[9,16] It may follow a G.I. episode or be seen initially. The serotype isolated from these patients may be any of the nonhost-adapted types; however, *S. cholera suis* has been commonly reported.[9] Septicemia is common and blood cultures are positive. During a 4-year period, 31 persons who had salmonellosis and subsequently died had the enteric fever syndrome. The organism was isolated from the blood of 15 of these patients and the cerebrospinal fluid of 6 of them. Isolations were also made from various organs of the body.[68] *S. virchow* was the cause of 21 cases of salmonellosis in Manchester, England.[69] One third of them had enteric fever and septicemia indicating that this strain was highly invasive. Other serotypes or strains may also cause such a serious outbreak.

The third syndrome is that of localized infection. This may be secondary to bacteremia or it may be the first sign of *Salmonella* infection in the host. Any organ or tissue of the body can be affected by local inflammation or abcess formation. Salmonellae can cause bronchopneumonia, endocarditis, pyelonephritis, osteomyelitis, arthritis, or meningitis. The latter is most often seen in newborns and infants. Patients with localized infections usually have a striking leukocytosis — 20,000 to 30,000 polymorphonuclear cells per mℓ of blood.[9,70] When the offending serotype is *S. cholera suis*, the mortality rate may be as high as 20%.[9,70]

Investigators in New York studied the problem of nontyphoid septicemia over a 10-year period — 412 cases. More than one half of the cases had no underlying disease at the time the septicemia was diagnosed. However, one third of the patients over 60 years of age had lymphoma, leukemia, carcinoma, or liver disease. Examples of underlying conditions in the others were as follows: sickle cell anemia, leukemia, Hodgkin's disease, various liver diseases, diabetes mellitus, rheumatoid arthritis, bacterial pneumonia, meningitis, osteomyelitis, ulcerative colitis, systemic lupus erythematosis, and lymphosarcoma. The most common serotypes were *S. typhimurium, S. enteriditis, S. heidelberg,* and *S. oranienburg.* Of the patients with leukemia or lymphosarcoma, 70% had *S. typhimurium* septicemia whereas the pathogen in 50% of the sickle cell cases was *S. enteriditis. S. cholera suis* was not as common a secondary invader as it had been in the past. Children less than 5 years of age accounted for 40% of all patients, and patients more than 60 years old accounted for 17% of the total. The case fatality rate for these 412 patients was 13.3%. The part that *Salmonella* septicemia played in the death of the patient was difficult to discern.[71]

Salmonellae must enter the G.I. tract in large numbers for infection to occur — 400,000 to 16 million organisms could be required depending upon the serotype and host.[9] The organisms then multiply in the G.I. tract and cause inflammation of the mucosae. If they gain access to the blood, the organisms multiply and cause bacteremia and focal infections. Ordinarily, they are stopped by the mesenteric lymph nodes and any pathology is restricted to the G.I. tract. One of the major protective mechanisms is a healthy, normal intestinal flora. If this is altered by antibiotic therapy or gastric surgery, the host has greatly increased susceptibility.[70]

Rout and co-workers[72] studied the pathophysiology of *Salmonella* diarrhea (*S. typhimurium*) in the rhesus monkey. There were changes in ileal and jejunal transport, colonic water absorption, and net colonic secretion, and sodium chloride transport was altered. All infected monkeys had severe colitis. Bacterial invasion was never seen and morphological changes were minimal. These observations, coupled with the need for multiplication of the organism in the gut to produce symptoms, are compatible with the 8- to 48- hr incubation period observed in gastroenteritis in two thirds of the human cases. There is no direct action of a toxin on the host at the time of ingestion.[9,17]

GENERAL MODE OF SPREAD

The most common modes of spread are (1) from contaminated foods of animal origin to man and (2) from these foods to other nonanimal-origin foods to man. The contaminated item is usually left at room temperature or refrigerated in too large a quantity so that in several hours an infective dose of several hundred thousand to several million organisms is present. Often this will be poultry meat (especially large quantities of turkey), egg-containing products (i.e., ice cream, bakery goods, filled pastries), red meats or red meat-derived products, drugs or pharmaceuticals of animal origin, dried milk or eggs, water, or a host of miscellaneous food products.[2,9,17,50,68,73,74]

Salmonellae can be transmitted from animals directly to man. Often pets that are in very close contact with man are the source of infection. In addition to pet contact, persons are occasionally exposed through occupation — veterinarians, veterinary students, packing-house workers, dog kennel owners, rendering-plant workers, animal agriculture workers, laboratory personnel, and inspectors are all at increased risk depending upon their knowledge of the disease and precautions taken to prevent spread.[9]

The agent can also be transmitted from person to person[66,73,75,77] by (1) vertical transmission from mother to offspring or (2) horizontal transmission (in a hospital or other medical care facility) from patient to employee, or vice versa, or from patient to patient.[9,73] Because of their prolonged shedding period, infants may be a special hazard in the home or hospital nursery.[67] This seems to be a larger problem in institutions[73] although English investigators believe its importance can be overemphasized. Inadvertently, eight patients excreting salmonellae were admitted to a hospital over a period of time and no stool barrier controls were instituted. There was no secondary spread

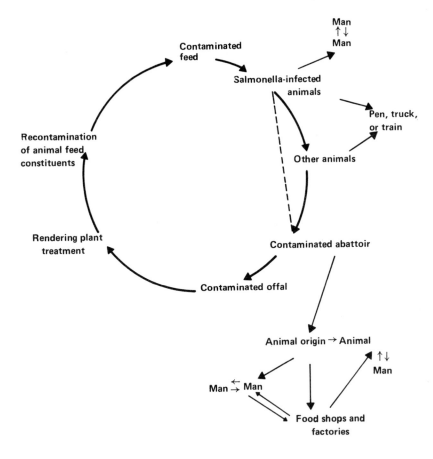

FIGURE 1.   *Salmonella* cycle. (From Williams, L. P., Jr. and Newell, K. W., *Am. J. Public Health*, 57, 466, 1967. With permission.)

to 265 patients or to hospital staff employees that could be documented (although some were not cultured until 21 days after exposure).[78]

Fomites or environment can be a source of infection for man; hospital equipment is often implicated. Included in a list of such sources are air, dust, delivery-room re-suscitators, bedside tables and cribs, a wood-mounted thermometer, a water bath for infant foods,[73] a contaminated suction machine,[6] and hand towels, scrub brushes, and bed linens.[9] Fomites can also play an important part in the cycle of food-borne disease wherein they are contaminated by a food item and in turn are the source of contamination for other foods (or the recontamination of the original item after it is cooked). Examples are contaminated meat blocks, a meat slicer,[79] dirty pans,[7] knives,[21] and cutting boards.[9]

EPIDEMIOLOGY

The epidemiology cycle of salmonellosis is shown in Figure 1.[80] It consists of a major portion that involves:

1. Contaminated animal protein meals being fed to domestic animals
2. Excretor animals infecting other animals directly or via the environment
3. These healthy animals going to slaughter and contaminating the abattoir (including pens)

4. The infected viscera being used to make animal protein meals that are contaminated after cooking
5. These meals being fed to other domestic livestock to begin the major cycle over again

Two subcycles naturally evolve from the above. One involves salmonellae from these excretor animals directly infecting other animals in the marketing chain (pens, trucks, trains, sales rings) or man. The second subcycle is the one with which man is most directly involved, especially in developed countries. Foods of animal origin that are contaminated with salmonellae enter the kitchen as is and can contaminate this area, or they can enter food processing plants, markets, or mass-feeding facilities where they contaminate other foods or are recontaminated themselves after cooking. These food products can also be fed directly to pets or be processed and fed to pets and *then* be the source of man's infection. At any part of the cycle when man becomes infected, he can transmit to other men or his animals. Implied by "other animals" in the cycle are wild birds and animals (including insects) that contract their infection from contaminated feed or feces and then contaminate new environments, other feed, rendered feed ingredients, or human food.[9]

The animal protein meals that are part of this perpetuating cycle are often meat, bone (or a combination of these two), fish, or feather meals.[9,18,21,53,81] These are incorporated as a protein and mineral source with grains, vegetable protein meals, and vitamin-mineral supplement to make a complete ration. The grains and vegetable proteins may also be contaminated with salmonellae.[9,18] Complete rations are then fed to domestic poultry, swine, cattle, and sheep although rations for the latter two species may not contain animal protein meals. A similar complete ration was also fed to breeding turtles (terrapins) in ponds in the southern U.S.[9,82]

All of these domestic animals are exposed to small numbers of salmonellae and develop a carrier state, often with infection of the mesenteric lymph nodes.[15] Excretion is low-level and intermittent unless livestock undergo some kind of stress, such as a disease outbreak, severe weather, very high protein ration, overcrowding, or transport.[9,19,21,55,56,58,59,61] Stress increases excretion, and salmonellae-bearing feces contaminate pens, watering troughs, hides and fleeces, and feeds.[9,61,80,83] These then are the source of infection for other animals entering the environment, e.g., birds,[46] rodents, or reptiles that may frequent the farm or abattoir pen.[9] Contaminated fleeces and hides as well as the infected intestinal contents become sources of contamination for carcasses and edible offal that then enter the marketing or food-processing chain.[9,18,80,83,84]

Numerous studies, reported in a previous review by the author and also by others, point out the problem of contaminated feed ingredients. Offal that bears salmonellae contaminates the receiving area and eventually other areas of the rendering plant. It also serves as a source of the organism after it is cooked to a salmonellae-free state and the oil is being expelled and the pressed cake ground into meal. Organisms have been found throughout the plant environment (including equipment and employees' clothing) and in rodents or birds that frequent that area.[5,9,85,86]

Not all investigators who work with salmonellosis agree with the concept that contaminated feed is the basis for much or most of the *Salmonella* outbreaks in this country. A group of workers in New York have studied their own data, that produced by the Center for Disease Control (CDC), and other published reports. Their analysis led to the conclusion that the major problems are human carriers and person-to-person spread, with occasional spread through foods causing spectacular outbreaks.[82,87] CDC investigators believe, however, that the same data and their experience support an animal feed-infected animal-contaminated food-man cycle, and that control should begin early in the cycle before animals are infected.[50]

Perhaps there is no better support for the feed-source side of the controversy than the international outbreak of *S. agona*. This serotype was first isolated by many countries from Peruvian fish-meal samples taken during routine surveillance of imported animal protein meals. It was then found in poultry and pigs consuming feed containing this meal. Within 2 or 3 years, it was among the top ten human serotypes in many of these countries;[4-6,15,53,74,77,88] no other source could be documented as a possible or probable source for the build-up. In a review of this problem, Clark et al.[88] stated that in 1970, 89 countries consumed three million tons of protein-rich (60 to 80%) fish meal valued at over 500 million dollars. The U.S. uses 600,000 tons of the product annually. About 300,000 tons of this is produced by domestic companies and the rest is imported, the majority of it from Peru. O. Grados[89] studied the occurrence of this serotype in Peru and found that it was one of the more common serotypes isolated from fish-meal samples collected between 1970 and 1973. He also noted that isolations from human carriers and cases increased steadily in that country during the 3-year period from 1971 to 1973.

Salmonellae can be transmitted from animals to man directly. This occurs most commonly between man (usually children) and domestic pets. It can also be transmitted through occupational contact with domestic livestock or contact with wildlife.[9] Episodes of pet turtle-associated salmonellosis are the best publicized and have occurred the most frequently. This problem is of greatest importance in the U.S. and has been reviewed by the author and others; epidemiological estimates suggest that 280,000 such cases may have occurred yearly.[6,9,30,90] Cases have occurred even though turtles were cultured in the state of origin and found to be "salmonellae-free."[6,91]

Studies of the source of infection for these animals showed that adult breeding turtles, the pond environment, pond water, and hatching materials were contaminated with salmonellae.[82] Terrapins have also been the source of human infection in England[29,92] and Germany.[32] Tortoises that may also carry salmonellae are sometimes kept as pets and displayed in zoos so that visitors can handle them.[9,29,31-33] Dogs and cats serve as a source of salmonellosis in man, who is often in close contact with these animals. Investigators have estimated that 20 to 25% of the dog population may be infected and transmission has been documented or shown epidemiologically.[9,24,25,29,93] Parakeets and "pet" Easter chicks and ducks may also be a source of infection for household members. Young children are most often affected.[9,94]

Infected wildlife may be the source of infection for man. New Zealand lizards, for the most part common skinks, were the source of *S. saint paul* outbreaks in man.[9] A marsupial (the quokka) found on Rottnest Island was the source of infection of *S. javiana* in an infant. Of the animals sampled on that island, 71% were excreting one or more *Salmonella* serotypes (including *S. javiana*).[43] MacDonald and Brown[95] found salmonellosis in humans who handled wild birds, the source of the infection. Florida raccoons living in state parks and rural and suburban areas were examined, and infection rates were found to vary between 13 and 22%. All 14 serotypes found in them have also been isolated from persons residing in Florida. However, no cases have ever been traced to raccoon exposure even though approximately 350 persons are bitten or scratched by the animal each year and, according to estimates, 158,000 raccoons are killed by man in every 2-year period.[41] Transmission of salmonellae from wildlife to man may be a rare event or simply an underreported one.

As noted before, salmonellae may be occupationally acquired. At risk are livestock handlers — especially those associated with calf-rearing operations — veterinarians and veterinary students, laboratory animal producers, and handlers of greyhound racing dogs.[9] In addition, pet shop and kennel owners may have an increased risk.[96,97] Two recent British outbreaks demonstrated that precautions should be taken by farm personnel when handling infected animals or their waste products. *S. typhimurium* caused high mortality in upland sheep, and cattle, a dog, and farm personnel associated with the sheep were also infected.[60] Of 41 farms in northwest England, 37 experienced outbreaks of salmonellosis in dairy cows during a single year. On 6 of these 41 farms (14%), humans experienced vomiting and diarrhea, and on 3 of these farms, the same serotype was found in residents and their cattle.[58] Veterinary personnel have experienced nongastrointestinal salmonellosis when treating cattle. Reports from England, Japan, and Canada have indicated that following obstetrical procedures, folloculitis of the arms occurred.[9,98]

Infected animals on the farm or in the marketing chain can infect other animals — usually via the environment.[1,99] Excretor sows and boars can spread the organism to their offspring, and cattle can transmit it between themselves. The extent of this problem depends upon housing, the type of environmental sanitation practiced, and other handling procedures.[9,56,57] Linton and co-workers[100] studied salmonellosis in calves on four farms during a 3-year period. The excretion rate among 2382 calves penned singly was 1.9% whereas the rate for 2062 animals penned in groups was 10.5%.

Concern has been expressed over a relatively recent problem associated with confinement-rearing — the use of slurry on fields.[38,101,102] Not only the contaminated field but the aerosols formed during distribution of the material can be a source of infection along with contaminated ground water from run-off.[38,60,103] One recent investigation indicated that slurry on fields was not such a problem. Twelve calves grazed on one eighth of an acre that had been dosed with *S. dublin*. During 420 calf days of observation and daily culturing, only one isolation of *S. dublin* was made (0.2%).[104]

Salmonellosis due to consumption of milk and eggs — two products that often are not further processed before consumption — should perhaps be included in this section. Eggs are found to be a source of salmonellosis in man, especially if they are less than Grade A or originate from ducks.[6,9,15] Raw milk-associated salmonellosis has occurred in man and in animals in England and the U.S. although it is much more common in the former.[6,15] The most common serotypes involved are *S. dublin* (usually transmitted cow-to-cow or cow-environment-cow) and *S. typhimurium*.[6,9,15,38,68,105]

Salmonella contamination of animal carcasses occurs in packing or processing plants when fecal matter settles on a carcass. This may occur when an animal is defeathered or dehaired because of equipment becoming contaminated from feces on the animal or from fecal leakage caused by a relaxed anal sphincter in the dead animal.[9,106,107] The carcass may also become contaminated during removal of the hide,[21,99] evisceration,[9] and, in the case of poultry, travel through the chill tank. Rates of contamination may be as high as 40%.[2,9,18,21,106-110]

In a recent survey, 40 of 221 pork carcasses yielded *Salmonella* and ten serotypes were found.[84] Once salmonellae are present on the carcass, they can then be passed via hands, knives, and various implements to other carcasses and edible offal.[9,21,111] Washing the carcasses, even with high-pressure or high-temperature water, does not remove salmonellae.[9,21] Chlorine (30 to 50 ppm) in chill tanks helps cut down salmonellae numbers,[112] and one group has advocated the use of 200 ppm.[106] Edible offal may have a high rate of *Salmonella* contamination in comparison with carcass sides.[21,51]

When the contaminated product moves into a production plant, home kitchen, institutional kitchen, or butcher shop, it contaminates equipment, hands, and other food, and it may cause diarrhea in food handlers.[5,7,9] The contaminated product may be cooked or processed in such a way that it is freed of its salmonellae but then be recontaminated when it comes into contact with man or the kitchen environment. In a South African study, rates were high — pork sausage, 40% and beef mince (ground beef), 64%.[110] In a survey of salmonellae isolations made in the Netherlands during an 8-year period,[6,116] *Salmonella* strains were isolated from foodstuffs consisting mainly of meat products, minced meat, venison, and poultry and egg products; a total of 95 serotypes were identified.[5]

A survey of federally inspected pork products (U.S. Department of Agriculture) gave high rates of contamination — 28% of 529 samples of pork trimmings and 28% of 56 samples of finished sausage.[113] A Public Health Laboratory Service research team examined 3309 samples of pork sausage from production plants and butcher shops of various sizes. While one large firm accounted for 95% of the 786 positives, another large manufacturer had less than 4% positives. Two medium-sized plants had isolation rates of 4 and 11%, but no isolations were made from samples from butcher shops.[114]

From such food contamination came outbreaks that involved small groups or were interstate or international. *S. new brunswick* occurred in several states and the source was the same in each — reconstituted powdered milk. The *S. javiana* interstate outbreak was associated with contaminated processed fish. One of the largest outbreaks on record occurred at a political rally where roast turkey was served.[9]

Food scientists assembled data necessary for an extensive review of food-borne disease associated with barbecued food. Of 62 episodes, 38 were due to salmonellae, and 32 of these occurred in the U.S. There were 2095 or more cases with a range per outbreak varying from 1 to 1350 cases.[115] Harvey[116] examined poultry carcasses coming into the kitchen of a South Wales hospital. They were frequently contaminated with salmonellae, and there was a correlation between the serotypes found in the fowl and those recovered from Moore's swabs placed in the sewer that serviced the pediatrics wing of the hospital. A Minnesota public health group investigated outbreaks that occurred at a picnic and a smorgasbord catered by the same firm. In both cases, the sources of infection were potato salad and chicken dressing, both of which were prepared in dirty pans where chickens had thawed. *S. schwarzengrund* was traced to a feed supplier who was selling poultry feed to the three farms where the chickens originated.[7]

An outbreak in the same state was traced epidemiologically to the consumption of rare or raw hamburger.[75] A small outbreak in an English resort hotel was traced to contaminated poultry and careless food handlers who had allowed salmonellae to multiply "mightily." Four serotypes were isolated from 11 vacationers, 3 of whom were clinically ill.[117] An analysis of the epidemiological investigation of food-borne disease in a 4-year period in England listed the following sources for general and family outbreaks: roast beef, 5; steak pies, 3; roast pork, 7; reheated pork, 1; cold ham, 8; luncheon meat, 1; roast chicken, 20; reheated chicken, 7; spit-roasted chicken, 7; roast turkey, 16; and reheated turkey, 9.[68]

DIAGNOSIS

The major method for isolation of salmonellae from man, animals, feedstuffs, food, or the environment is the placing of the sample in an enrichment medium, incubating overnight or longer, and streaking a small portion of it onto selective plating media. Characteristic *Salmonella*-like colonies (for the media in use) are then "picked" and placed in various biochemical media, confirmed as salmonellae, and then serotyped. Some dry or dehydrated products are more likely to yield the organism if they are pre-enriched with a broth for a short period of time. Many laboratories have adopted the fluorescent antibody (FA) technique for screening large numbers of samples, with varying success. An important aspect of diagnosis is collecting a proper sample. This has been reviewed extensively by the author, and it is recommended that this source[9] or a food microbiology textbook be consulted for details.

Pre-enrichment can be accomplished with lactose broth, buffered peptone, or nutrient broth.[9,118,119] Specimens are placed in the medium for 8 to 24 hr at 37°C, and a quantity (i.e., 1 to 10 mℓ) of the pre-enrichment broth is transferred to the enrichment medium (or media) of choice.[9,118] A method of pooling up to 25 preenrichment specimens into one enrichment-broth sample has been described for use in an industrial situation requiring examination of large samples, many of which might be negative. Small portions of the pre-enrichment broth cultures are retained while enrichment media are incubated and transferred to selective plate media. One or more of these can then be examined individually if a pool is positive. Such a scheme allows for examination of a great number of samples with a minimum use of expensive enrichment and plating media.[120]

A number of enrichment media are available. Those most commonly used are tetrathionate, Mueller-Kauffmann (M-K) modification of tetrathionate, selenite, selenite-F, selenite cystine, selenite brilliant-green (BG) sulfapyridine, and Rappaports.[9,21,121] Which of these should be chosen depends upon the experience of the user, type of product being sampled, and serotype to be isolated. Perhaps no aspect of salmonellosis has been more confusing to study in scientific literature of the past decade than variable findings by different investigators with the various enrichment media at differing temperatures. In the examination of frozen whole-liquid egg or whole-egg powder, German investigators found M-K tetrathionate incubated at 43°C for 48 hr superior to selenite cystine incubated at the same temperature and for the same amount of time.[118]

Investigators in the Netherlands compared M-K tetrathionate, potassium BG bile broth, selenite BG, and selenite-F in the examination of sewage effluents, sewer swabs, rinses of these swabs, and effluent filters. They recorded the greatest isolation rate from M-K tetrathionate at 43°C and also observed that pre-enrichment of effluent with buffered peptone was not useful.[122] German investigators, in surveying poultry for *Salmonella* infection, recommended the use of both selenite enrichment and tetrathionate incubated at 43°C for maximum yield since several rare serotypes were found after selenite enrichment that were not found in the other media.[123] Investigators examining frozen meat compared tetrathionate, M-K tetrathionate, selenite BG sulfapyridine, and selenite cystine enrichment broth at 35°C and 43°C. All yielded the greatest number of salmonellae at 43°C; ranked in order of effectiveness for these specimens, they were as follows: (1) selenite cystine, (2) selenite BG, (3) M-K tetrathionate, and (4) tetrathionate. These workers also recommended use of two enrichment broths.[119]

A number of researchers have found that the enrichment used has a relationship to the *Salmonella* serotype recovered. An example of such findings was given by a group examining frozen meat in an international collaborative study. Selenite BG favored the isolation of *S. schwarzengrund, S. typhimurium,* and *S. dublin* while selenite cystine was best for *S. senftenberg. S. newport* and *S. worthington* did equally well in tetrathionate or selenite BG sulfa broth.[124] Other researchers found that group C_1 salmonellae were isolated more readily from tetrathionate than selenite and that groups G, 35, and D were more readily isolated from selenite than tetrathionate.[125]

English investigators found selenite-F and BG broths inhibitory to *S. cholera suis* while this serotype was readily isolated from Rappaport's broth when sampling pig feces and mesenteric lymph glands.[20] One of the most extensive investigations of serotype differences in various enrichment media was reported from Massachusetts where 88 serotypes were test-grown in five enrichment broths at 37° and 43°C and subcultures were made at 24 and 48 hr to BG agar. Tetrathionates were generally better than selenites regardless of sample type and *Salmonella* serotype.[121]

Plating media used have included *Salmonella-shigellae,* MacConkey, BG (with or without sulfas added), bismuth sulfite of Wilson-Blair, desoxycholate citrate, XLD, and other agars, many of them modifications of the above.[9,14,16,126] To avoid an extensive discussion of the advantages and disadvantages of these numerous agars, the following quotation from the summary of an article on an international collaborative study to develop a method for the assay of salmonellae in raw meat follows. "Best results from selective agars were obtained when laboratories were allowed to choose their own, indicating that familiarity with a medium plays a significant role in its suitability for the isolation of *Salmonella*."[24]

FA has been used to detect salmonellae in foods, feeds, condiments, and environmental samples. Agreement with results from culture methods ranged from 56 to 97% depending upon the method used and the product tested.[127-131] Automated systems have been developed that may be useful in examining large numbers of samples.[132,133]

In addition to the isolation of salmonellae from feces, fecal swabs, or the suspected food vehicle or source (often requiring repeated sampling or use of multiple subsamples), salmonellae can be isolated from the blood if systemic signs indicate that a bacteremia might be present. They can also be isolated from pus, exudates, or cerebrospinal fluid if there is a focal infection. Specimens can be direct-plated to obtain an isolation as early as in 24 hr if it is suspected that the organism is present in large numbers. An aliquot of the specimen can also be put in an enrichment medium to afford an opportunity for recovery if salmonellae are in small numbers or in competition with large numbers of other bacteria.[9,70] Some patients will demonstrate a fourfold rise in titer (or a high titer if no acute specimen is available) against O, H, or Vi antigens if the serum is tested using agglutination tests.[16,70] While some researchers have used these tests in the investigation of outbreaks[66] or in serosurveys in man or animals,[134] the findings may be confusing and, therefore, these tests are not routinely used.

In addition to the laboratory methods used to make a diagnosis in the patient, the epidemiologist must make a diagnosis in an outbreak situation by determining the incubation period, analyzing signs and symptoms, and determining possible vehicles of infection. With experience and use of statistics, an epidemiological determination can be made as to the agent involved (i.e., *Clostridium, Staphylococcus,* etc.) and the probable vehicle; however, final "proof" is dependent upon recovery of the same agent from food items, the environment, and victims of the outbreak.[7,9,52,66,70,75]

PREVENTION AND CONTROL

Much of the *Salmonella* infection of animals and man could be prevented by elimination of the organism from animal protein meals and a subsequent cleanup of confinement-rearing facilities and animal holding areas. The most promising methods are heat treatment or irradiation of ingredients, pelleting, or high-temperature extrusion of the final product.[1-3,9,15,19,50,53,55,88,111,112,135,136] Investigators from the Netherlands showed that with pelleted food and careful sanitation, a group of nearly salmonellae-free pigs could be produced.[136] This type of control may require government regulation as is now practiced in some European countries and suggested for others.[8,15,53,58,88] These procedures will break the major cycle. Large quantities of material would be involved, and testing would be required to determine effectiveness and compliance.

The next type of defense is that of increasing resistance of the animals to infection. Vaccination of calves and lambs has been used with mixed results.[9] Vaccination was credited with stopping an outbreak of *S. typhimurium* in upland sheep, and in a clinical trial vaccinated sheep fared significantly better than controls.[60,137] Clinical trials in calves and the use of vaccines in a commercial beef unit in England gave little or no advantage to treated animals.[22,56]

Eggs have been treated with chemicals, antibiotics, or various washing techniques to rid them of contamination that could infect chicks. Gentamicin was effective in reducing *Salmonella* contamination (81% positive in untreated eggs vs. 2% in treated), and a ''commercial dip'' was more effective in preventing penetration of *S. typhimurium* than were five other chemicals.[138,139] Investigators applied Terramycin® and Chloromycetin® to turtle eggs to free them of *Salmonella* and Arizona infection. Turtles were found to be salmonellae-free if Terramycin® was applied at 1500 to 2000 μg/mℓ of solution on eggs laid early in the egg-laying season.[140] Copper sulfate at a level of 2 to 5 ppm was used in turtle ponds prior to egg laying to control salmonellosis in baby turtles. It was ineffective as there were as many infected turtles in the treated pond as the control pond.[82]

Since slurry, when dressed on a field, can be a source of infection for domestic species, experiments have been conducted to make it salmonellae-free. Minnesota investigators found that *S. typhimurium* survived 17 days postseeding in a model oxidation ditch at summer temperatures (20°C) and 47 days at winter temperatures (2°C); survival in a settling chamber connected to the system was as high as 87 days.[141]

Kampelmacher and Jansen[142] found that composting swine wastes in an aerated vat for 24 hr before discharge into an oxidation ditch reduced salmonellae to negligible numbers if the level in the slurry was less than 10^2 organisms per milliliter of waste and water (combined to facilitate movement of the waste). When infection levels of confined swine reached the point where *Salmonella* counts exceeded 10^2/mℓ of slurry, the 100-fold reduction in the composting vat allowed viable salmonellae to reach the oxidation ditch where they could be a source of environmental contamination. These investigators recommended chlorination of the effluent before discharge into the ditch until, through sanitation controls on hog-fattening farms, Netherlands pigs are relatively free of salmonellae.

One approach to the control of transmission by slurry is to avoid its use on pastures.[38,102,103] A recommendation has been made that a minimum of 6 months should elapse between the application of slurry to pasture and the grazing of animals.[21] Related to this aspect of transmission is the contamination by abbatoir effluents of areas where livestock are held. This should be carefully guarded against, and livestock watering places should certainly be protected.[3,21,97] General sanitation of barns, pens, and isolation and treatment areas and disinfection whenever possible are also highly recommended.[9,28,56]

Within packing and processing plants, control involves education of the workers, proper cleanup and sanitizing of equipment, and the change of some practices. The change from scalding water to live steam for feather removal has been shown to decrease salmonellae on poultry carcasses, the use of chlorine in chill tanks has been shown to be beneficial, thorough plant cleaning (even twice a day) is advocated, proper evisceration techniques and careful handling of the hide or fleece are important, and clean hands and small equipment are essential. Even the veterinary inspector must exercise care so as not to transmit salmonellae in the process of inspection.[1,9,15,21,50,80,106,108,111,112,143] Rapid chilling and sanitary storage after a thorough carcass washing are also necessary parts of proper plant practice.[1,9,19,21,80]

The final level of prevention and control of salmonellosis in man is the proper handling and preparation of animal-origin foods in the house or institutional kitchen coupled with proper sanitation practices within the facility. This requires an education program for persons who prepare food in the home and for professional foodhandlers. Food must be kept below 45 or above 140°F and be refrigerated in small quantities. Utensils must be clean, hands must be washed after bowel movements or handling of raw products, sick workers must be excused from work (without loss of compensation) until well, insects and rodents must be eliminated from food preparation areas, and raw products must be separated from cooked or finished ones.[1,3,9,15,17,21,50,70,72,73,144]

Person-to-person and direct animal-to-person spread are controlled in much the same manner. Hands should be thoroughly cleansed after handling a patient or animal or single-use disposable gloves worn. Human and pet animal wastes should be disposed of in the toilet, including contaminated turtle water. Workers with diarrhea should not handle or contact patients, and animals with diarrhea should be isolated (especially from children) until well.[8,9,17,70,73]

In some situations, governments may need to enact legislation to control the spread of salmonellae. Importation of feedstuffs has been regulated,[2,50] and liquid egg products must be pasteurized.[9,15] Sale of domestic poultry for pets has been banned.[9] The most recent action by a government has been a ban on the interstate sale of pet turtles and importation of turtles or tortoises except for scientific purposes.[9]

There are no internationally required measures to control salmonellosis. International reporting of isolations and outbreaks has been advocated as a means of better understanding the movement of the organisms and eventually controlling them.[9]

EDITORIAL COMMENT*

An outbreak of gastroenteritis occurred in February 1976 at Whyalla, a city with a population of 33,000, situated 250 miles north of Adelaide, the capital of South Australia. The outbreak was sudden. Forty patients, mainly infants and children, were seen at the hospital on the first day of the outbreak with symptoms of vomiting, abdominal pain, and diarrhea. Many other patients with similar symptoms were treated by private medical practitioners in the city. More than 500 cases of gastroenteritis were recorded during the outbreak, most occurring during the first 3 days.

Although the age range of affected persons was from 1 month to 70 years, 90% of patients were under 15 years of age, and two thirds were under 10. *Salmonella typhimurium* phage type 9 was isolated from 78 of the 273 persons investigated. The characteristics of the outbreak suggested a common source, probably milk, and 95% of the patients gave a history of consumption of raw milk. The rest of the cases were in family contacts.

At the time of the outbreak, Whyalla had two milk suppliers — one providing pasteurized, homogenized milk sold in cartons, the other a local dairy selling bottled, unpasteurized milk. *S. typhimurium* phage type 9 was isolated from ten samples of unpasteurized milk, both bulk and bottled, collected early in the outbreak. Investigation of the dairy herd of 193 cows showed that two of the animals were excreting *S. typhimurium* type 9. One of the employees also was found to be excreting the same organism.

Distribution of the unpasteurized milk was stopped, and the outbreak quickly abated. The raw milk supply has since been discontinued in the city.

CDC editorial note — Pasteurization has essentially eliminated milk-borne enteric diseases in the U.S. Since 1966, pasteurized milk has been suspected as the vehicle of transmission in only two outbreaks in the U.S. — one caused by *Shigella flexneri*[145] and the other by *S. newport*.[146] Several *Salmonella* outbreaks have been traced to certified raw milk,[147] and in 1976 an outbreak of yersiniosis was caused by milk to which chocolate syrup had been added after pasteurization.[148]

*   Seglenieks, Z. and Dixon, S., Outbreak of milk-borne *Salmonella* gastroenteritis — South Australia, Morbidity and Mortality Weekly Report, Vol. 26, Issue No. 15, U.S. Department of Health, Education, and Welfare, Public Health Service, Center for Disease Control, Atlanta, 1977.

REFERENCES

1. **Edel, W., Guinée, P. A. M., van Schothorst, M., and Kampelmacher, E. H.,** *Salmonella* cycles in foods with special reference to the effects of environmental factors, including feeds, *Can. Inst. Food Sci. Technol. J.,* 6, 64, 1973.
2. **Christopher, P. J., Claxton, P. D., Dorman, D. C., O'Connor, B. F., Proudford, R. W., and Sutton, R. G. A.,** Salmonellosis: an increasing health hazard, *Med. J. Aust.,* 1, 337, 1974.
3. **Sojka, W. J., Wray, C., Hudson, E. B., and Benson, J. A.,** Incidence of Salmonella infection in animals in England and Wales, 1968-73, *Vet. Rec.,* 96, 280, 1975.
4. **Gunnarsson, A., Hurvell, B., Nordblom, B., Rutqvist, L., and Thal, E.,** *Salmonella* isolated from animals and feedstuffs in Sweden over the period 1968-72, *Nord. Veterinaermed.,* 26, 499, 1974.
5. **Guinée, P. A. M. and Valkenburg, J.,** *Salmonella* isolations in the Netherlands, 1966-1973, *Zentralbl. Bacteriol. Parasitenkd. Infektionskr. Hyg. Abt. 1: Orig. Reihe A,* 231, 97, 1975.
6. **Fox, M. D.,** Recent trends in salmonellosis epidemiology, *J. Am. Vet. Med. Assoc.,* 165, 990, 1974.
7. **Levy, B. S., McIntire, W., Damsky, L., Lashbrook, R., Hawk, J., Jacobsen, G. S., and Newton, B.,** The Middleton outbreak: 125 cases of foodborne salmonellosis resulting from cross contaminated food items served at a picnic and a smorgasbord, *Am. J. Epidemiol.,* 101, 502, 1975.
8. **Morse, E. V. and Duncan, M. A.,** Salmonellosis — an environmental problem affecting animals and man, *Proc. 78th Annu. Meet. U. S. Animal Health Assoc.,* Spencer, Richmond, Va., 1974, 288.
9. **Williams, L. P., Jr. and Hobbs, B. C.,** Enterobacteriaceae infections, in *Diseases Transmitted from Animals to Man,* 6th ed., Hubbert, W. T., McCulloch, W. F., and Schnurrenberger, P. R., Eds., Charles C Thomas, Springfield, Ill., 1975, 33.
10. **Williams, L. P., Jr.,** The surveillance of foodborne diseases in man and animals, *Proc. 74th Annu. Meet. U. S. Animal Health Assoc.,* Spencer, Richmond, Va., 1970, 336.
11. **Baker, W. H.,** Perspectives on acute enteric disease epidemiology and control, *Pan. Am. Health Organ. Bull.,* 9, 148, 1975.
12. **Anon.,** World health situation, *JAMA,* 212, 1970, 1970.
13. **Chanlett, E. T.,** *Environmental Protection,* McGraw-Hill, New York, 1973, 305.
14. **Wilson, G. S. and Miles, A. A.,** *Topley and Wilson's Principles of Bacteriology, Virology and Immunity,* 6th ed., Williams & Wilkins, Baltimore, 1975, 839 and 918.
15. **McCoy, J. H.,** Trends in *Salmonella* food poisoning in England and Wales 1941-72, *J. Hyg. (Cambridge),* 74, 271, 1975.
16. **Jawetz, E., Melnick, J. L., and Adelberg, E. A.,** *Review of Medical Microbiology,* 10th ed., Lange Medical Publications, Los Altos, Calif., 1972, 199.
17. **Christie, A. B.,** *Infectious Diseases,* Churchill, Livingstone, Edinburgh, 1974, 3.
18. **Vaughn, J. B., Williams. L. P., Jr., LeBlanc, D. R., Helsdon, H. L., and Taylor, D.,** *Salmonella* in a modern broiler operation: a longitudinal study, *Am. J. Vet. Res.,* 35, 737, 1974.
19. **Newell, K. W. and Williams, L. P., Jr.,** The control of salmonellae affecting swine and man, *J. Am. Vet. Med. Assoc.,* 158, 89, 1971.
20. **McCaughey, W. J., McClelland, T. G., and Roddy, R. M.,** *Salmonella* isolations in pigs, *Vet. Rec.,* 92, 191, 1973.
21. **Meara, R. J.,** Salmonellosis in slaughter animals as a source of human food poisoning, *J. S. Afr. Vet. Assoc.,* 44, 215, 1973.
22. **Osborne, A. D., Linton, A. H., and Pethiyagoda, S.,** Epidemiology of *Salmonella* infection in calves. II. Detailed study in a large beef rearing unit, *Vet. Rec.,* 94, 604, 1974.
23. **Kumar, S., Saxena, S. P., and Gupta, B. K.,** Carrier rate of salmonellosis in sheep and goats and its public health significance, *J. Hyg.* (Cambridge), 71, 43, 1973.
24. **Williams, L. P., Jr.,** Bacterial contamination of pet foods in Proc. 18th Annu. Food Hygiene Symp., U. S. Department of Agriculture, APHIS, 1977, 123.
25. **Morse, E. V. and Duncan, M. A.,** Canine salmonellosis: prevalence, epizootiology, signs, and public health significance, *J. Am. Vet. Med. Assoc.,* 167, 817, 1975.
26. **Shimi, A., Keyhani, M., and Bolurchi, M.,** Salmonellosis in apparently healthy dogs, *Vet. Rec.,* 98, 110, 1976.
27. **Tacal, J. V., Jr. and Menez, C. F.,** *Salmonella* studies in the Philippines. XIV. *Salmonella* isolations from carabaos, horses, pigeons, dogs, and cats, *Philipp. J. Vet. Med.,* 13, 46, 1975.
28. **Stoll, L. and Kohl, V.,** Isolation of *Salmonella* from cats, *Berl. Muench. Tieraerztl. Wochenschr.,* 88, 455, 1975.
29. **Borland, E. D.,** *Salmonella* infection in dogs, cats, tortoises, and terrapins, *Vet. Rec.,* 96, 401, 1975.
30. **Lamm, S. H., Taylor, A., Jr., Gangarosa, E. J., Anderson, H. W., Young, W., Clark, M. H., and Bruce, A. R.,** Turtle-associated salmonellosis. I. Magnitude of the problem in the United States 1970-1971, *Am. J. Epidemiol.,* 95, 511, 1972.

31. **Ang, O., Ozek, O., Cetin, E. T., and Toreci, K.,** *Salmonella* serotypes isolated from tortoises and frogs in Istanbul, *J. Hyg.* (Cambridge), 71, 85, 1973.

32. **Weber, A. and Pietzsh, O.,** Occurrence of *Salmonella* infections in tortoises from pet stores and private homes, *Berl. Muench. Tieraerztl. Wochenschr.,* 87, 257, 1974.

33. **Jackson, C. G., Jr. and Jackson, M. M.,** The frequency of *Salmonella* and Arizona microorganisms in zoo turtles, *J. Wildl. Dis.,* 7, 130, 1971.

34. **Sharma, V. K., Kaura, Y. K., and Singh, I. P.,** Frogs as carriers of *Salmonella* and *Edwardsiella,* *Antonie van Leeuwenhoek; J. Microbiol. Serol.,* 40, 171, 1974.

35. **Kennedy, M. E.,** *Salmonella* isolations from snakes and other reptiles, *Can. J. Comp. Med.,* 37, 325, 1973.

36. **Wuth, H. H.,** *Salmonella* in a breeding colony of black-headed sea gulls, *Berl. Muench. Tieraerztl. Wochenschr.,* 86, 255, 1973.

37. **Berg, R. W. and Anderson, A. W.,** Salmonellae and *Edwardsiella tarda,* in gull feces: a source of contamination in fish processing plants, *Appl. Microbiol.,* 24, 501, 1972.

38. **Williams, B. M., Richards, D. W., and Lewis, J.,** *Salmonella* infections in the herring gull (*Lans argentatus*), *Vet. Rec.,* 98, 51, 1976.

39. **Oelke, H. and Steiniger, F.,** *Salmonella* in Adelie penguins (*Pygoscelis adeliae*) and South Polar skuas (*Catharacta maccormicki*) on Ross Island, Antarctica, *Avian Dis.,* 17, 568, 1973.

40. **Locke, L. N., Ohlendorf, H. M., Shillinger, R. B., and Jareed, T.,** Salmonellosis in a captive heron colony, *J. Wildl. Dis.,* 10, 143, 1974.

41. **Bigler, W. J., Hoff, G. L., Jasmin, A. M., and White, F. H.,** *Salmonella* infections in Florida raccoons, *Procyon lotor, Arch. Environ. Health,* 28, 261, 1974.

42. **Ford, A. C., Speltie, T. M., and Hendricks, W. D. H.,** Studies on the prevalence of *Salmonella* serotypes in non-human primates, *Lab. Anim. Sci.,* 23, 649, 1973.

43. **Iveson, J. B. and Bradshaw, S. D.,** *Salmonella javiana* infection in an infant associated with a marsupial, the quokka, *Setonix brachyurus* in western Australia, *J. Hyg.* (Cambridge), 71, 423, 1973.

44. **Williams, D. R. and Bellhouse, R.,** The prevalence of salmonellae in mink, *J. Hyg.* (Cambridge), 72, 71, 1974.

45. **Radevan, A. J. and Lampky, J. R.,** *Enterobacteriaceae* isolated from cowbirds (*Molothrus ater*) and other species of wild birds in Michigan, *Avian Dis.,* 16, 343, 1972.

46. **Quevedo, F., Lord, R. S., Dobosch, D., Granier, I., and Michanie, S. C.,** Isolation of *Salmonella* from sparrows captured in horse corrals, *Am. J. Trop. Med. Hyg.,* 22, 672, 1973.

47. **Harrington, R., Jr., Blackburn, B. O., and Cassidy, D. R.,** Salmonellosis in canaries, *Avian Dis.,* 19, 827, 1975.

48. **Thomason, B. M., Biddle, J. W., and Cherry, W. B.,** Detection of salmonellae in the environment, *Appl. Microbiol.,* 30, 764, 1975.

49. **Van Oye, E.,** *The World Problem of Salmonellosis,* W. Junk, The Hague, 1964.

50. **Gangarosa, E. J., Baker, W. H., Jr., Baine, W. B., Morris, G. K., and Rice, P. A.,** Man vs. animal feeds as the source of human salmonellosis (letter to the editor), *Lancet,* 1, 878, 1973.

51. **Gould, K. L., Gooch, J. M., and Ching, G. Q. L.,** Epidemiologic aspects of salmonellosis in Hawaii, *Am. J. Public Health,* 62, 1216, 1972.

52. **Baker, W. H., Jr., Sagerser, J. C., Hall, C. V. H., Anderson, H. W., and Francis, B. J.,** Foodborne disease surveillance — Washington state, *Am. J. Public Health,* 64, 854, 1974.

53. **Lee, J. A.,** Recent trends in human salmonellosis in England and Wales: the epidemiology of prevalent serotypes other than *Salmonella typhimurium, J. Hyg.* (Cambridge), 72, 185, 1974.

54. **Bains, B. S. and MacKenzie, M. A.,** Transmission of *Salmonella* through an integrated poultry organization, *Poult. Sci.,* 53, 114, 1974.

55. **Hugh-Jones, M. E., Harvey, R. W. S., and McCoy, J. H.,** A *Salmonella california* contamination of turkey feed concentrate, *Br. Vet. J.,* 131, 673, 1975.

56. **Getty, G. M., Coy, C. H., Ellis, D. J., Krehbiel, J. D., Carter, J. R., and McAllister, H.,** Salmonellosis in dry lot and hospitalized dairy cattle, *Vet. Med. Small Anim. Clin.,* 71, 1599, 1976.

57. **Richardson, A.,** Salmonellosis in cattle, *Vet. Rec.,* 96, 329, 1975.

58. **Richardson, A. and Fawcett, A. R.,** *Salmonella dublin* infection in calves: the value of rectal swabs in diagnosis and epidemiological studies, *Br. Vet. J.,* 129, 151, 1973.

59. **Whiteford, R. B.,** An acute outbreak of salmonellosis in a dairy herd, *Vet. Rec.,* 93, 422, 1973.

60. **Hunter, A. G., Corrigall, W., Mathieson, O., and Scott, J. A.,** An outbreak of *S. typhimurium* in sheep and its consequences, *Vet. Rec.,* 98, 126, 1976.

61. **Pierson, R. E., Poduska, P. J., Cholas, G., and Brown, G.,** Relationship of management and nutrition to salmonellosis in feedlot sheep, *J. Am. Vet. Med. Assoc.,* 161, 1217, 1972.

62. **Dorn, C. R., Coffman, J. R., Schmidt, D. A., Garner, H. E., Addison, J. B., and McCune, E. L.,** Neutropenia and salmonellosis in hospitalized horses, *J. Am. Vet. Med. Assoc.,* 166, 65, 1975.

63. **Wenkoff, M. S.**, A review and case report. *Salmonella typhimurium* septicemia in foals, *Can. Vet. J.*, 14, 284, 1973.
64. **Owen, R. ap R.**, Post-stress diarrhea in the horse, *Vet. Rec.*, 96, 267, 1975.
65. **Morse, E. V., Duncan, M. A., Fessler, J. F., and Page, E. H.**, The treatment of salmonellosis in *Equidae*, *Mod. Vet. Pract.*, 57, 47, 1976.
66. **Bender, T. R., Jones, T. S., DeWitt, W. E., Kaplan, G. J., Saslow, A. R., Nevius, S. E., Clark, P. S., and Gangarosa, E. J.**, Salmonellosis associated with whale meat in an Eskimo community, *Am. J. Epidemiol.*, 96, 153, 1972.
67. **Kazemi, M., Gumpert, G., and Marks, M. I.**, Clinical spectrum and carrier of non-typhoidal *Salmonella* infections in infants and children, *Can. Med. Assoc. J.*, 110, 1253, 1974.
68. **Vernon, E. and Tillett, H. E.**, Food poisoning and *Salmonella* infection in England and Wales, 1969-1972. An analysis of reports to the Public Health Laboratory Service, *Public Health* (London), 88, 225, 1974.
69. **Mani, V., Brennard, J., and Mandal, B. K.**, Invasive illness with *Salmonella virchow* infection, *Br. Med. J.*, 2, 143, 1974.
70. **Hook, E. W.**, Diseases caused by *Salmonella*, in *Cecil-Loeb Textbook of Medicine*, 13th ed., W. B. Saunders, Philadelphia, 1971, 574.
71. **Cherubin, C. E., Neu, H. C., Imperato, P. J., Harvey, R. P., and Bellen, N.**, Septicemia with non-typhoid *Salmonella*, *Medicine* (Baltimore), 53, 365, 1974.
72. **Rout, W. R., Formal, S. B., Dammin, G. J., and Giannella, R. A.**, Pathaphysiology of *Salmonella* diarrhea in the Rhesus monkey: intestinal transport, morphological and bacteriological studies, *Gastroenterology*, 67, 59, 1974.
73. **Baine, W. B., Gangarosa, E. J., Bennett, J. V., and Baker, W. H., Jr.**, Institutional salmonellosis, *J. Infect. Dis.*, 128, 357, 1973.
74. **Glencross, E. J. G.**, Pancreatin as a source of hospital-acquired salmonellosis, *Br. Med. J.*, 2, 376, 1972.
75. **Fleming, D. S., Papra, J., Stoffels, M. A., and Havir, R.**, *Salmonella typhimurium* gastroenteritis. Statewide outbreak, *Minn. Med.*, 56, 722, 1973.
76. **Lowenstein, M. S.**, An outbreak of salmonellosis propagated by person to person transmission on an Indian reservation, *Am. J. Epidemiol.*, 102, 257, 1975.
77. **Anon.**, Salmonellosis (editorial), *Med. J. Aust.*, 1, 333, 1974.
78. **MacGregor, R. R. and Reinhart, J.**, Person-to-person spread of *Salmonella*: a problem in hospitals?, *Lancet*, 2, 100, 1973.
79. **Jordan, M. C., Powell, K. E., Corothers, T. E., and Murray, R. J.**, Salmonellosis among restaurant patrons: the incisive role of a meat slicer, *Am. J. Public Health*, 63, 982, 1973.
80. **Williams, L. P., Jr. and Newell, K. W.**, Patterns of *Salmonella* excretion in market swine, *Am. J. Public Health*, 57, 466, 1967.
81. **Novilla, M. N., Menez, C. F., and Eustaquio, A. O.**, Studies on salmonellosis in animals and man in the Philippines. I. Isolation of *Salmonellae* from animal feed ingredients in the Philippines, *Philipp. J. Vet. Med.*, 13, 33, 1975.
82. **Kauffmann, A. F., Fox, M. D., Morris, G. K., Wood, B. T., Feeley, J. C., and Frix, M. K.**, Turtle-associated salmonellosis. The effects of environmental *Salmonellae* in commercial turtle breeding ponds, *Am. J. Epidemiol.*, 95, 521, 1972.
83. **Grau, F. H. and Smith, M. G.**, *Salmonella* contamination of sheep and mutton carcasses related to pre-slaughter holding conditions, *J. Appl. Bacteriol.*, 37, 111, 1974.
84. **Carpenter, J. A., Elliot, J. G., and Reynolds, A. E.**, Isolation of salmonellae from pork carcasses, *Appl. Microbiol.*, 25, 731, 1973.
85. **Tittiger, F.**, Studies on the contamination of products produced by rendering plants, *Can. J. Comp. Med.*, 35, 167, 1971.
86. **Tittiger, F. and Alexander, D. C.**, Recontamination of products with salmonellae after rendering in Canadian plants, *Can. Vet. J.*, 12, 200, 1971.
87. **Cherubin, C. E.**, Salmonellosis in livestock and man, *Lancet*, 2, 377, 1972.
88. **Clark, G. M., Kaufmann, A. F., Gangarosa, E. J., and Thompson, M. A.**, Epidemiology of an international outbreak of *Salmonella agona*, *Lancet*, 2, 490, 1973.
89. **Grados, O.**, Presence of *Salmonella enteriditis, serotype agona*, in Peru, *Pan Am. Health Organ. Bull.*, 8, 228, 1974.
90. **Altman, R., Gorman, J. C., Bernhardt, L. L., and Goldfield, M.**, Turtle associated salmonellosis. II. The relationship of pet turtles to salmonellosis in children in New Jersey, *Am. J. Epidemiol.*, 95, 578, 1972.
91. **Polk, L. D.**, Salmonellosis in children from turtles certified *Salmonella*-free, *Clin. Pediatr.* (Philadelphia), 13, 719, 1974.

92. **Clegg, F. C. and Heath, P. J.,** *Salmonella* excretion by terrapins and the associated hazard to human health, *Vet. Rec.,* 96, 90, 1975.

93. **Forster, D., Holland, U., and Tesfamariam, H.,** Occurrence of canine *Salmonellae* infection, *Zentralbl. Veterinaermed. Reihe B,* 21, 124, 1974.

94. **Madewell, B. R. and McChesney, A. E.,** Salmonellosis in a human infant, a cat, and two parakeets in the same household, *J. Am. Vet. Med. Assoc.,* 167, 1089, 1975.

95. **MacDonald, J. W. and Brown, D. D.,** *Salmonella* infection in wild birds in Britain, *Vet. Rec.,* 94, 321, 1974.

96. **Anderson, H. W., Peterson., D. R., and Watkins, R. B.,** Shigellosis and salmonellosis from a spider monkey, Morbidity and Mortality Weekly Report, Vol. 20, U. S. Department of Health, Education and Welfare, Public Health Service, Center for Disease Control, Atlanta, 1971, 291.

97. **Reynolds, P. J.,** Salmonellosis in British Columbia, Salmonella Surveillance Report, Vol. 122, U.S. Department of Health, Education, and Welfare, Public Health Service, Center for Disease Control, Atlanta, 1975, 5.

98. **Pantekoek, J. F., Rhodes, C. S., and Saunders, J. R.,** *Salmonella* folliculitis in veterinarians infected during obstetrical manipulation of a cow, *Can. Vet. J.,* 15, 123, 1974.

99. **Smith, M. G. and Grau, F. H.,** Occurrence of salmonellosis in the hides and fleeces of cattle and sheep at slaughter, *Aust. Vet. J.,* 49, 218, 1973.

100. **Linton, A. A., Howe, K., Pethiyagoda, S., and Osborne, A. D.,** Epidemiology of *Salmonella* infection in calves. I. Its relation to their husbandry and management, *Vet. Rec.,* 94, 581, 1974.

101. **Jones, P. W. and Hall, G. A.,** Detection of *Salmonella* infection in pig herds by examination of slurry, *Vet. Rec.,* 97, 351, 1975.

102. **Findlay, C. R.,** Salmonellae in sewage sludge. I. Occurrence, *Vet. Rec.,* 93, 100, 1973.

103. **Robertson, J. S.,** Salmonellosis in livestock, *Lancet,* 1, 1334, 1972.

104. **Taylor, R. J.,** A further assessment of the potential hazard for calves allowed to graze pasture contaminated with *S. dublin* in slurry, *Br. Vet. J.,* 129, 354, 1973.

105. **MacLachlan, J.,** Salmonellosis in Midlothian and Peeblesshire, *Public Health* (London), 88, 79, 1974.

106. **Nivas, S. C., Kumar, M. C., York, M. D., and Pomeroy, B. S.,** *Salmonella* recovery from three turkey-processing plants in Minnesota, *Avian Dis.,* 17, 605, 1973.

107. **Schuler, G. A. and Badenhop, A. F.,** Microbiology survey of equipment in selected poultry processing plants, *Poult. Sci.,* 51, 830, 1972.

108. **Dougherty, T. J.,** *Salmonella* contamination in a commercial poultry (broiler) processing operation, *Poult. Sci.,* 53, 814, 1974.

109. **Radan, M., Fuchs, V., and Bejerano, S.,** A ten year survey of *Salmonella* isolation from food products of animal origin, *Refu. Vet.,* 29, 67, 1972.

110. **Prior, B. A. and Badenhorst, L.,** Incidence of *Salmonella* in some meat products, *S. Afr. Med. J.,* 48, 2532, 1974.

111. **Watson, W. A.,** Salmonellosis and meat hygiene: red meat, *Vet. Rec.,* 96, 374, 1975.

112. **Watson, W. A. and Brown, J. M.,** *Salmonella* infection and meat hygiene: poultry meat, *Vet. Rec.,* 96, 351, 1975.

113. **Surkiewiez, B. F., Johnston, R. W., Elliott, P. R., and Simmons, E. R.,** Bacteriological survey of fresh pork sausage produced at establishments under federal inspection, *Appl. Microbiol.,* 23, 515, 1972.

114. **Anon.,** *Salmonellas* in sausages, *Br. Med. J.* (editorial), 4, 669, 1975.

115. **Todd, E. and Pivnick, H.,** Public health problems associated with barbecued food. A review, *J. Milk Food Technol.,* 36, 1, 1973.

116. **Harvey, R. W. S.,** Proceedings: three studies of salmonellae in South Wales, *J. Clin. Pathol.,* 27, 931, 1974.

117. **Cavanagh, P.,** Salmonellosis in livestock and man, *Lancet,* 2, 377, 1972.

118. **Pietzsch, O., Kreschmer, F. J., and Bulling, E.,** Comparative studies of methods of *Salmonella* enrichment, *Zentralbl. Bakteriol. Parasitenkd. Infektionskr. Hyg. Abt. 2: Orig. Reihe A,* 232, 232, 1975.

119. **Silliker, J. H. and Gabis, D. A.,** ICMSF metbods studies. V. The influence of selective enrichment media and incubation temperatures on the detection of salmonellae in raw frozen meats, *Can. J. Microbiol.,* 20, 813, 1974.

120. **Price, W. R., Olsen, R. A., and Hunter, J. E.,** *Salmonella* testing of pooled pre-enrichment broth cultures for screening multiple food samples, *Appl. Microbiol.,* 23, 679, 1972.

121. **Carlson, V. L. and Snoeyenbos, G. H.,** Comparative efficacies of selenite of tetrathionate enrichment broths for the isolation of *Salmonella* serotypes, *Am. J. Vet. Res.,* 35, 711, 1974.

122. **Kampelmacher, E. H. and Jansen, L. M. v. N.,** Comparative studies on the isolation of *Salmonella* from effluents, *Zentralbl. Bacteriol. Parasitenkd. Infektionskr. Hyg. Abt. 1: Orig. Reihe B,* 157, 71, 1973.

123. **Siems, H., Hildebrandt, G., Inal, T., and Sinell, H. J.,** Official inquiry into the presence of *Salmonella* in frozen slaughtered poultry on the German market, *Zentralbl. Bakteriol. Parasitenkd. Infektionskr. Hyg. Abt. 1: Orig. Reihe B,* 160, 84, 1975.

124. **Erdman, I. E.,** ICMSF methods studies. IV. International collaborative assay for the detection of *Salmonella* in raw meat, *Can. J. Microbiol.,* 20, 715, 1974.

125. **Huhtanen, C. N. and Naghski, J.,** Effect of type of enrichment and duration of incubation on *Salmonella* recovery from meat-and-bone meal, *Appl. Microbiol.,* 23, 578, 1972.

126. **Tompkin, R. B. and Kueper, T. V.,** Factors influencing detection of salmonellae in rendered animal by-products, *Appl. Microbiol.,* 25, 485, 1973.

127. **Insalata, N. F., Mahnke, C. W., and Durlap, W. G.,** Rapid direct fluorescent-antibody-method for the detection of salmonellae in foods and feeds, *Appl. Microbiol.,* 24, 645, 1972.

128. **Insalata, N. F., Mahnke, C. W., and Dunlap, W. G.,** Direct fluorescent-antibody technique for the microbiological examination of food and environmental swab samples for salmonellae, *Appl. Microbiol.,* 26, 268, 1973.

129. **Hilker, J. S. and Solberg, M.,** Evaluation of a fluorescent antibody-enrichment serology combination procedure for the detection of salmonellae in condiments, food products, food by-products, and animal feeds, *Appl. Microbiol.,* 26, 751, 1973.

130. **Smyser, C. F. and Snoeyenbos, G. H.,** Fluorescent-antibody methods for detecting salmonellae in animal by-products, *Avian Dis.,* 17, 99, 1973.

131. **Karlsson, K. A. and Thal, E.,** Studies on the detection of salmonellae in fishmeal by the direct and indirect immunofluorescent method, *Nord. Veterinaermed.,* 26, 492, 1974.

132. **Thomason, B. M., Herbert, G. A., and Cherry, W. Z.,** Evaluation of a semiautomated system for direct fluorescent antibody detection of salmonellae, *Appl. Microbiol.,* 30, 557, 1975.

133. **Insalata, N. F., Dunlap, W. G., and Mahnke, C. W.,** Evaluation of the salmonellae fluoro-kit for fluorescent-antibody staining, *Appl. Microbiol.,* 25, 202, 1973.

134. **Singh, I. P., Kaura, Y. K., and Sharma, V. K.,** Sero-survey of *Salmonella* infection in man and animals by indirect haemagglutination test, *Zentralbl. Bakteriol. Parasitenkd. Infektionskr. Hyg. Abt. 1: Orig. Reihe A,* 226, 55, 1974.

135. **Edel, W., van Schothorst, M., Guineé, P. A. M., and Kampelmacher, E. H.,** *Salmonella* in pigs on farms feeding pellets and on farms feeding meal, *Zentralbl. Bakteriol. Parasitenkd Infektionskr. Hyg. Abt. 1: Orig. Reihe A,* 226, 314, 1974.

136. **Edel, W., van Schothorst, M., Guineé, P. A. M., and Kampelmacher, E. H.,** Preventive measures to obtain *Salmonella*-free slaughter pigs, *Zentralbl. Bacteriol. Parasitenkd. Infektionskr. Hyg. Abt. 1: Orig. Reihe B,* 158, 568, 1974.

137. **Cooper, B. S. and MacFarlane, D. J.,** Single and double vaccination schedules in sheep against experimental infection with *Salmonella typhimurium* or *Salmonella bovismorbificans,* N. Z. Vet. J., 22, 95, 1974.

138. **Saif, Y. M. and Shelley, S. M.,** Effect of gentamicin sulfate dip on *Salmonella* organisms in experimentally infected turkey eggs, *Avian Dis.,* 17, 574, 1973.

139. **Williams, J. E. and Dillard, L. H.,** The effect of external shell treatments on *Salmonella* penetration of chicken eggs, *Poultr. Sci.,* 52, 1084, 1973.

140. **Siebeling, R. J., Neal, P. M., and Granberry, W. D.,** Evaluation of methods for the isolation of *Salmonella* and Arizona organisms from pet turtles treated with antimicrobial agents, *Appl. Microbiol.,* 29, 240, 1975.

141. **Will, L. A., Diesch, S. L., and Pomeroy, B. S.,** Survival of *Salmonellae typhimurium* in animal manure disposal in a model oxidation ditch, *Am. J. Public Health,* 63, 322, 1973.

142. **Kampelmacher, E. H., Jansen, L. M. v. N.,** Reduction of *Salmonella* in compost in a hog-fattening farm oxidation vat, *J. Water Pollut. Control Fed.,* 43, 1541, 1971.

143. **Patrick, T. E., Collins, J. A., and Goodwin, T. L.,** Isolation of *Salmonella* from carcasses of steam and water scalded poultry, *J. Milk Food Technol.,* 36, 34, 1973.

144. **Noah, N. D.,** Cooking the Christmas dinner, *Br. Med. J.,* 4, 714, 1975.

145. **Center for Disease Control,** Morbidity and Mortality Weekly Report, Vol. 15, Issue No. 51, U.S. Department of Health, Education, and Welfare, Public Health Service, Atlanta, 1966, 442.

146. **Center for Disease Control,** Morbidity and Mortality Weekly Report, Vol. 24, Issue No. 49, U.S. Department of Health, Education, and Welfare, Public Health Service, Atlanta, 1975, 413.

147. **Center for Disease Control,** Morbidity and Mortality Weekly Report, Vol. 23, Issue No. 19, U.S. Department of Health, Education, and Welfare, Public Health Service, Atlanta, 1974, 175.

148. **Center for Disease Control,** Morbidity and Mortality Weekly Report, Vol. 26, Issue No. 7, U.S. Department of Health, Education, and Welfare, Public Health Service, Atlanta, 1977, 53.

APPENDIX 1*

Edwardsiella tarda was isolated from the large intestine of 7 (17%) of 42 raccoons from Florida. The rate varied from 12% in southern Florida to 25% in northern Florida. In addition, 52% of the raccoons examined were carrying *Salmonella*, with numerous serotypes represented (*Arch. Environ. Health*, 30, 602, 1975).

Based on 37 isolates submitted for identification between 1959 and 1965, Ewing et al.[1] described a new genus and species, *Edwardsilla tarda,* to be included in the family Enterobacteriaceae. Most of these isolates were from man; however, one isolate was from a cow, and two were unidentified as to animal source.

E. tarda has been isolated from snakes,[2] turtles,[3] fish (*Ictalurus punctatus, Micropterus salmoides*),[4,5] alligators (*Alligator mississippiensis*),[5,6] and a sea lion (*Zalophus californianus*).[6]

Except for an earlier isolation from a sick ostrich,[7] *E. tarda* has only recently been found in avian species, specifically large aquatic birds.[5] Also, *E. tarda* has been found in surface freshwater specimens in Florida.[5]

In man, *E. tarda* has been incriminated as a cause of wound infection,[8] abscesses,[8,9] meningitis,[10,11] and *Salmonella*-like intestinal infections.[8,12-14]

There are only a few reports of *E. tarda* isolations from domestic or wild mammals. In the Philippines, *E. tarda* was found in the bile of 3 of 1000 apparently healthy pigs at slaughter.[15] Recently, *E. tarda* was isolated from the intestinal tract of a pig in the U.S.[16] D'empaire reported using two isolants from cattle, one isolant from a pig, and one from a panther in growth studies of *E. tarda.*[17]

The present report records the isolation of *E. tarda* from raccoons (*Procyon lotor*) from two widely separated regions of Florida, and extends the numbers of *Salmonella* serotypes previously reported from raccoons in Florida.[18]

RESULTS

Of the 42 raccoons examined, 7 (17%) were carrying *E. tarda* in the large intestine. Of the 24 raccoons from Collier County, 3 (12%) were carrying *E. tarda.* Of the 16 raccoons from Duval County, 4 (25%) were carrying this enteric pathogen. Two raccoons from Indian River County were free of *E. tarda.*

In addition to infection with *E. tarda, Salmonella* was isolated from the large intestine of 52% of all raccoons cultured.

In Collier County, *Salmonella* was isolated from 13 (54%) of 24 raccoons with 2 raccoons each carrying two serotypes and another raccoon carrying three serotypes. Serotypes isolated consisted of *S. tallahassee, S. bareilly, S. anatum, S. hartford, S. oranienberg, S. newport, S. carran, S. litchfield, S. javiana, S. st. paul, S. infantis,* and two unidentified serotypes.

In Duval County, *Salmonella* was isolated from 8 (50%) of 16 raccoons with 1 animal carrying two serotypes. Another raccoon carried both *Salmonella* and *E. tarda.* The serotypes isolated were *S. muenchen, S. miami, S. manhattan, S. oranienberg,* and *S. hartford.*

S. hartford was isolated from the large intestine of one of two raccoons from Indian River County.

Gross lesions were not observed in the raccoons at necropsy, and bacteria were not recovered from cultures of liver.

---

*   White, F. H., Watson, J. J., Hoff, G. L., and Bigler, W. J., *Edwardsiella tarda* infections in Florida raccoons, *Procyon lotor, Arch. Environ. Health,* 30, 602, 1975. Copyright 1975, American Medical Association. With permission.

COMMENT

The description of *E. tarda* in 1965[1] was based largely on isolates from man. New isolates from man have been reported frequently and have been described as the causative agents in both intestinal and extraintestinal infections.[8-14]

Associaton of *E. tarda* with definite infections in domestic or wild species has not been as firmly established. The organism was associated with bovine diarrhea in one report[1] and was considered the cause of hemorrhagic disease in a large-mouth bass.[5] It produced "emphysematous putrefactive disease" in channel catfish[4] and was associated with enteric infection in an ostrich.[7] *E. tarda* was associated with hemorrhagic enteritis in brown pelicans and common loons but could not be definitely incriminated as the causative agent.[5]

Jordan and Hadley[8] believe that *E. tarda* can produce disease patterns in man similar to those caused by *Salmonella*, probably including enteric fever, and that the asymptomatic carrier state can exist. This seems to be a reasonable assessment with current knowledge of the organisms.

In the present study, the raccoons were carrying both *E. tarda* and various *Salmonella* serotypes. It seems likely that under favorable conditions either organism could demonstrate its pathogenic nature to man or animals.

In a previous study 14 *Salmonella* serotypes were found in Florida raccoons.[18] In the present survey, five additional serotypes were found. In the previous study the infection rate was 17% while in the present study it was 52%. The increased isolation rate may have been due to the different methods used. Contents of the small intestine were cultured in the former study, and contents of the large intestine in the present. This also may explain why *E. tarda* was not isolated in the previous study of Florida raccoons.*

NOTE

This study was supported by research grant 1270 from the Florida Game and Fresh Water Fish Commission. This is a contribution of the Federal Aid to Wildlife Restoration Program, Florida Pittman Robertson Project No. W-41.

REFERENCES

1. Ewing, W. H., McWhorter, A. C., Iscobar, M. R., et al., *Edwardsiella*, a new genus of Enterobacteriaceae based on a new species, *E. tarda*, *Int. Bull. Bact. Nomen. Taxon.*, 15, 33, 1965.
2. Sakazaki, R., Studies on the Asakusa group of Enterobacteriaceae (*Edwardsiella tarda*), *Jpn. J. Med. Sci. Biol.*, 20, 205, 1967.
3. Jackson, M. M., Jackson, C. G., and Fulton, M., Investigation of the enteric bacteria of the *Testudinata*. I. Occurrence of the genera *Arizona*, *Citrobacter*, *Edwardsiella* and *Salmonella*, *Bull. Wildl. Dis. Assoc.*, 5, 328, 1969.
4. Meyer, F. P. and Bullock, G. L., *Edwardsiella tarda*, a new pathogen of channel catfish (*Ictalurus punctatus*), *Appl. Microbiol.*, 25, 155, 1973.
5. White, F. H., Simpson, C. F., and Williams, L. E., Isolation of *Edwardsiella tarda* from aquatic animal species and surface waters in Florida, *J. Wildl. Dis.*, 9, 204, 1973.

*   Address reprint requests to the Veterinary Science Department, University of Florida, Institute of Food and Agricultural Science, Gainesville, Fla. 32601.

6. Wallace, L. J., White, F. H., and Gore, H. L., Isolation of *Edwardsiella tarda* from a sea lion and two alligators, *J. Am. Vet. Med. Assoc.*, 149, 881, 1966.

7. White, F. H., Neal, F. C., Simpson, C. F., et al., Isolation of *Edwardsiella tarda* from an ostrich and an Australian skunk, *J. Am. Vet. Med. Assoc.*, 155, 1057, 1969.

8. Jordan, G. W. and Hadley, W. K., Human infection with *Edwardsiella tarda*, *Ann. Intern. Med.*, 70, 283, 1969.

9. Gonzalez, A. B. and Ruffolo, E. H., *Edwardsiella tarda*: etiologic agent in a post-traumatic subgaleal abscess, *South. Med. J.*, 59, 340, 1966.

10. Okubadejo, O. A. and Alausa, K. O., Neonatal meningitis caused by *Edwardsiella tarda*, *Br. Med. J.*, 3, 357, 1968.

11. Sonnenwirth, A. C. and Kallus, B. A., Meningitis due to *Edwardsiella tarda*, *Am. J. Clin. Pathol.*, 49, 92, 1968.

12. Bhat, P. and Meyers, R. M., *Edwardsiella tarda* in a study of juvenile diarrhoea, *J. Hyg.* (Cambridge), 65, 293, 1967.

13. Bockemuhl, J., Pan-Urai, R., and Burkhardt, F., *Edwardsiella tarda* associated with human disease, *Pathol. Microbiol.*, 37, 393, 1971.

14. King, B. M. and Adler, D. L., A previously undescribed group of Enterobacteriaceae, *Am. J. Clin. Pathol.*, 41, 230, 1964.

15. Arambulo, P. V., Westerlund, N. C., Sarmiento, R. V., et al., Isolation of *Edwardsiella tarda*: a new genus of Enterobacteriaceae from pig bile in the Philippines, *Far East Med. J.*, 3, 385, 1967.

16. Owens, D. R., Nelson, S. L., and Addison, J. B., Isolation of *Edwardsiella tarda* from swine, *Appl. Microbiol.*, 27, 703, 1974.

17. D'empaire, M., Les facteurs de croissance des *Edwardsiella tarda*, *Ann. Inst. Pasteur*, 116, 63, 1969.

18. Bigler, W. J., Hoff, G. L., Jasmin, A. M., et al., Salmonella infections in Florida raccoons, *Procyon lotor*, *Arch. Environ. Health*, 28, 261, 1974.

19. Edwards, P. R. and Ewing, W. H., *Identification of Enterobacteriaceae*, 3rd ed., Burgess, Minneapolis, 1972.

APPENDIX 2

ZOONOTIC POTENTIAL OF ANIMAL STRAINS OF *ESCHERICHIA COLI*

L. L. Myers

INTRODUCTION

During the past 10 years, it has become increasingly clear that enteropathogenic *E. coli* (EEC) are responsible for a significant portion of the diarrheal disease problem in both animals and man. As more information is gained regarding enteric colibacillosis (diarrheal disease caused by *E. coli*), it appears there are several forms of the disease and that the characteristics of enteric colibacillosis in animals and man are similar.

The prevalence of colibacillosis in food animals and man varies greatly between different geographic areas of the world. The potential for transmission of disease causing *E. coli* from animals to man may be influenced by:

- The locally prevalent strains of *E. coli* in animals
- The density and general health of the human population
- Mobility of the population
- Cultural and sanitation practices.

There appears to be considerable variation in the serotypes of EEC involved in animal and human diarrhea from various parts of the world. Different serotypes of *E. coli* may have markedly different zoonotic potential.

Some characteristics of enteric colibacillosis in animals and man that may relate to the zoonotic potential of animal *E. coli* are discussed herein. Also discussed is the direct evidence regarding transmission of *E. coli* from animals to man. Irrefutable evidence showing that *E. coli* enteropathogenic in humans is transmitted from animals is lacking. However, the available information suggests that diarrheal disease in humans caused by *E. coli* transmitted from animals occurs under some conditions.

PATHOGENESIS AND EPIDEMIOLOGICAL ASPECTS OF ENTERIC COLIBACILLOSIS

It is clear that EEC can cause diarrheal disease in animals and man with clinical signs ranging from a profuse watery diarrhea, dehydration, electrolyte imbalance, and shock, to mild diarrheas of short duration. The mechanism of diarrheal disease caused by *E. coli* can be placed in the following three categories:

1. Disease caused by enterotoxigenic *E. coli* (ETEC) following colonization of the small bowel and production of heat-labile (LT) and/or heat-stable (ST) enterotoxin
2. Disease caused by invasion of the mucosa of the large intestine with local-invasive strains of *E. coli*
3. Disease caused by EEC via mechanisms not yet understood[1-3]

The pathogenesis of diarrheal disease caused by ETEC is similar in man and young animals. Oral inoculation of the susceptible host with 10^9 to 10^{10} viable cells results in colonization of the small and large intestine. ETEC adhere to villous epithelial cells and produce enterotoxin that causes an alteration in the metabolism of the mucosal epithelial cells resulting in a net movement of water and electrolytes from the blood into the lumen of the small intestine. ETEC are generally not invasive and do not cause marked pathologic lesions. For unknown reasons, the infection is self-limiting and other bacteria become predominant in the intestines usually within 2 to 4 days. The disease is most severe among the young of animals and man. Oral inoculation of young colostrum-fed pigs or calves with 10^{10} viable cells of ETEC often results in profuse diarrhea, severe dehydration, and morbidity within 2 to 3 days after inoculation.[4-9] A similar acute diarrheal syndrome caused by ETEC occurs in human infants (especially institutionalized infants) under 2 years of age.[10-12] Calves more than 2 days of age are relatively insensitive to oral challenge inoculation with 10^{10} viable cells of ETEC.[4] Piglets lose some sensitivity to ETEC by the time they reach 1 week of age and are relatively insensitive to ETEC when they reach the weanling period.[13,14] The disease is not recognized as a problem in mature animals. In contrast, it has recently become clear that adult human beings often develop acute diarrheal disease caused by ETEC, especially when traveling abroad.[15-18] The serotypes of ETEC responsible for traveler's diarrhea generally differ from those causing diarrhea in infants.[19]

Studies with human strains of *E. coli* in animals (monkey, guinea pigs, and rabbits) have shown that local-invasive strains of *E. coli* can cause disease resembling shigellosis by invasion of the epithelial cells of the large bowel.[2,20] These *E. coli* do not produce classical *E. coli* enterotoxin or invade the blood or extraintestinal tissues of the host, but they do give a positive Sereny test by induction of keratoconjunctivitis in the guinea pig.[21] Local-invasive strains of EEC have not been recognized as causes of diarrheal disease in food animals.[1] A commonly occurring condition in calves about 1 to 2 weeks of age is a catarrhal, mucopurulent, or hemorrhagic enteritis associated with large numbers of predominately one strain of *E. coli* in the intestinal tract. The etiology of this condition is not understood and may be caused in part by the local-invasive type of EEC.

Recently, another possible pathogenic mechanism for colibacillosis in animals and man has been described. It has been shown that acute diarrhea and deaths in laboratory rabbits can be caused by a rabbit strain of *E. coli* with pili but lacking both invasive ability and classical enterotoxin-producing ability.[22,23] While the pathogenesis of this type of diarrheal disease is not well understood, it appears that diarrhea is caused by *E. coli* capable of attachment to the denuded surface of intestinal epithelial cells and production of small amounts of *Shigella dysenteriae*-like enterotoxin. This type of colibacillosis appears to be an important cause of naturally occurring diarrhea in laboratory rabbits.[70] Further study, including the development of a sensitive toxin assay system, is needed to establish the importance of this type of colibacillosis in food animals and man.

Little work has been done to directly assess the enteropathogenicity of animal strains of EEC in human beings and vice versa. In one study, strain 263 that is enteropathogenic for pigs was shown to cause a mild diarrhea in one of four adult volunteers who were given oral challenge inoculation with 10^{10} viable cells.[2] It was concluded that strain 263 could induce illness in the human host although at a reduced level of pathogenicity. In another study of the pathogenicity of animal EEC in humans, two adult volunteers were orally challenged with 10^9 and 10^{10} viable cells of a strain of *E. coli* (09:K35, K99) enteropathogenic for calves, pigs, and lambs. No clinical signs of disease were caused in the two volunteers by this EEC.[71]

The recent recognition of ETEC as a frequent cause of diarrhea in adult humans, especially travelers, presents an opportunity to examine the zoonotic potential of *E. coli*.[17,24-27] In most geographical areas where traveler's diarrhea commonly occurs, little is known about the serotypes of EEC in animals. Victims of traveler's diarrhea apparently receive a large oral challenge with *E. coli* by consumption of contaminated food or water. *E. coli* capable of causing traveler's diarrhea may be inhabitants of the intestinal tract of both man and animals in endemic areas. The human population native to the endemic area is resistant to *E. coli* responsible for traveler's diarrhea.[28]

A noninvasive, ST-producing strain of *E. coli* (214-4) was isolated from an adult with traveler's diarrhea and was found to be enteropathogenic when given orally to adult volunteers.[29] This strain gave positive results in the lamb ligated intestinal loop test (the lamb test gives results similar to or identical with those of the calf ligated intestinal loop test).[30] Strain 214-4 was given orally (10^{10} viable cells) to an 8-hr-old colostrum-fed calf.[71] Clinical signs of disease included labored breathing, apathy, mild diarrhea, and the presence of blood-tinged stools containing mucus. The rectal temperature was normal. The calf was killed *in extremis* 18 hr after inoculation. The intestinal tract of the calf was colonized with the challenge strain, but *E. coli* was absent from the blood and tissues. Widespread lesions of congestion, edema, and hemorrhage with vascular thrombosis (perhaps initiated by endotoxin) were observed. The clinical syndrome in this calf was not typical of that caused by calf strains of ETEC.

The likelihood of humans becoming infected with ETEC of animal origin via contaminated food was demonstrated by a study done in the U.S. in which 19 of 240 strains of *E. coli* obtained from food of animal origin (sausage, hamburger, and cheese) were producers of LT or ST and LT.[31] These strains of ETEC represented a variety of serotypes including serotype 0149:H19 that caused diarrheal disease in calves and pigs.[32,33] Although the origin of the *E. coli* in this study was not determined, it suggests that certain foods may be potentially important vehicles in the transmission of animal strains of *E. coli* to man.

ENTEROTOXINS AND COLONIZATION FACTORS OF *E. COLI* FROM ANIMALS AND MAN

Strains of ETEC of animal and human origin produce a proteinaceous enterotoxin and/or a low-molecular-weight, polypeptide type of enterotoxin.[10,28,34] Enterotoxins produced by strains of *E. coli* of animal or human origin are plasmid mediated and similar in structure and function. The intestinal epithelial cells of human beings and food animals are susceptible to the effects of both ST and LT. Enterotoxins elaborated by *E. coli* can be detected in the pig, calf, lamb, and rabbit intestinal loop models, the infant mouse gastric test, and various tissue-culture tests.[4,30,35-40] While the various animal intestinal loop models detect both LT and ST, results in each test are not identical for all strains of *E. coli*.[30,41] A number of strains of ETEC isolated from humans in Bangladesh caused fluid accumulation in the calf and lamb ileal-loop test comparable with that produced by calf strains of ETEC.[30,37] One would expect that some of these strains would also cause colibacillosis in the intact calf or lamb. Reactions in animal ligated intestinal loop models may give an indication of the enteropathogenicity of *E. coli* isolates in various hosts. Most strains of ETEC isolated from calves produce only ST.[32,42,43] Strains of ETEC isolated from pigs and human beings produce ST and/ or LT. There are no apparent structural, functional, or antigenic differences between enterotoxins produced by animal or human strains of ETEC. There is also no apparent quantitative difference in enterotoxigenicity of human compared with animal strains of ETEC.

On the surface of many strains of ETEC is found the fimbrial or pilus type of structure that apparently is a virulence factor that facilitates adherence to villous epithelial cells and thus colonization of the small intestine.[44] These structures are plasmid determined, proteinaceous, appear to differ antigenically but not morphologically between animal and human strains of *E. coli*, and may confer some properties of host specificity on *E. coli*.[45,46] Evidence indicates that only a limited number of serotypes of EEC exist, indicating that perhaps unique surface characteristics of different strains of *E. coli* determine their ability to accept and retain enterotoxin and colonization factor plasmids.[13,47-50] Most ETEC carrying the K88 fimbrial antigen are of pig origin although pig strains of ETEC without K88 antigen are common.[51] ETEC of calf and lamb origin usually have the K99 fimbrial antigen.[48,52] The K99 antigen has also been found in a few pig strains of ETEC.[53] Many human strains of ETEC possess an as yet unidentified fimbrial type of colonization factor(s) that is antigenically different from K88 or K99 antigens.[46,49,54]

SEROTYPES OF *E. COLI* THAT INFECT MAN AND ANIMALS

Knowledge regarding the serotypes of *E. coli* that infect man and animals is incomplete due partially to the presence of numerous strains in which the complete serotype (O, K, and H antigens) is undetermined.[55] In general, serotypes of *E coli* identified in animals differ from those identified in man.[55,56] Historically, serotypes of *E. coli* frequently associated with episodes of diarrhea in man or animals have been referred to as "enteropathogenic serotypes" without prior determination of their true pathogenic potential.[57] Most of these strains were subsequently found incapable of enterotoxin production although it is possible that they are enteropathogenic by some as yet unrecognized mechanism.[47,55,58,59] Since animal and human "enteropathogenic serotypes" are generally different, routine serological procedures would miss human infections with EEC of animal origin.

While *E. coli* serotypes of animal origin generally differ from those found in human beings, there are reports indicating that some strains of *E. coli* are able to infect, but not necessarily cause disease, in both animals and man. In a study conducted in England, 103 different O types of *E. coli* were found in calves and 78 of those 103 types were isolated from human beings.[60,61] In a study using 600 *E. coli* strains of human origin and 264 strains isolated from calves, no significant differences in serotypes based on O antigen determination could be found.[61] Strains of *E. coli* with O antigens 8, 9, and 101 were frequently found in both humans and animals. Other studies have found strains of *E. coli* with these O antigens to be enterotoxigenic and/or enteropathogenic for calves and pigs.[32,47,48,62]

There are several reports describing strains of *E. coli* pathogenic in both animals and man. *E. coli* serotype 078:K80:H12 that produced ST caused an outbreak of infantile diarrhea in a hospital special-care nursery.[10] This strain apparently also caused diarrhea in adults in Bangladesh and in India and was isolated from swine in England.[19,27,63] Serotype 055:B5 was shown to produce gastroenteritis in man and in young colostrum-deprived pigs.[64,65] Serotype 0149:H10, suspected of having caused a foodborne infection in humans, had the K88 antigen and belonged to a serotype considered enteropathogenic in piglets.[49] Serotype 026:B6 is recognized as a cause of neonatal diarrhea in humans and this serotype was isolated from an infant, a calf, and a bull on the same farm in Switzerland.[66] Strain 026:B6 has also been isolated from newborn calves with diarrhea in England, several European countries, and the U.S.[67,68]

SUMMARY

The need for additional research in the area of zoonotic potential of animal strains of *E. coli* was mentioned in an earlier review of human enteric colibacillosis and is equally true today.[69] A more complete assessment of the zoonotic potential of *E. coli* would be facilitated by additional information regarding:

- The various forms of enteric colibacillosis in animals and man
- The antigenic components of *E. coli* with emphasis on the capsular K antigens and the colonization factor antigens
- Epidemiologic information including the source of *E. coli* in enteric colibacillosis of adult humans

The few reported attempts to directly assess the enteropathogenicity of animal strains of EEC by oral inoculation of human volunteers with 10^9 to 10^{10} viable cells indicated that animal strains are not pathogenic or only mildly pathogenic in humans. However, studies of this type have the important shortcoming that adult human beings are inappropriate subjects for evaluation of the enteropathogenicity of an *E. coli* that is pathogenic in young, but not in mature, animals. Human infants may be more susceptible than adults to strains of *E. coli* that cause diarrheal disease only in young animals.

It would be of interest to evaluate the enteropathogenicity for animals of strains of *E. coli* that cause traveler's diarrhea. This could be done in various ages and species of animals. Useful information regarding the zoonotic potental of *E. coli* may also be gained through an epidemiological study of the sources of infection and the serotypes of *E. coli* in animals and man in geographical areas where enteric colibacillosis in adult humans is prevalent.

Human beings and animals are sometimes infected with *E. coli* of the same serotype and a few strains of *E. coli* appear to be enteropathogenic for both animals and man. The commonly used diagnostic procedures would not identify human infection with most strains of EEC from animals. Based upon the similarities between EEC of human and animal origin, it appears likely that additional strains of *E. coli* will be shown to be enteropathogenic in both animals and man.

In many cases, human beings under natural conditions may receive far more than 10^{10} viable cells, the dosage normally used as the upper limit for challenge inoculation in experimental studies of the enteropathogenicity of *E. coli*. When a sufficient amount of the proper strain of animal *E. coli* gains access to the intestinal tract of the susceptible human host, diarrheal disease would be expected to occur. It is likely that in the past these conditions have been met many times, resulting in various forms of diarrheal disease.

REFERENCES

1. **Moon, H. W.**, Pathogenesis of enteric disease caused by *Escherichia coli*, *Advances in Veterinary Science and Comparative Medicine*, Vol. 18, Academic Press, New York, 1974, 179.
2. **DuPont, H. L., Formal, S. B., Hornick, R. B., Snyder, M. J., Libonati, J. P., Sheahan, D. G., LaBrec, E. H., and Kalas, J. P.**, Pathogenesis of *Escherichia coli* diarrhea, *N. Engl. J. Med.*, 285, 1, 1971.
3. **Gurwith, M. C., Wiseman, D. A., and Chow, P.**, Clinical and laboratory assessment of the pathogenicity of serotyped enteropathogenic *Escherichia coli*, *J. Infect. Dis.*, 135, 736, 1977.
4. **Smith, H. W. and Halls, S.**, Observations by the ligated intestinal segment and oral inoculation methods on *Escherichia coli* infections in pigs, calves, lambs, and rabbits, *J. Pathol. Bacteriol.*, 93, 499, 1967.
5. **Newman, F. S., Myers, L. L., Firehammer, B. D., and Catlin, J. E.**, Prevention of experimentally induced enteric colibacillosis in newborn calves, *Infect. Immun.*, 8, 540, 1973.
6. **Kohler, E. M., Cross, R. F., and Bohl, E. H.**, Protection against neonatal enteric colibacillosis in pigs suckling orally vaccinated sows, *Am. J. Vet. Res.*, 36, 757, 1975.

7. **Logan, E. F., Pearson, G. R., and McNulty, M. S.,** Studies on the immunity of the calf to colibacillosis. VII. The experimental reproduction of enteric colibacillosis in colostrum-fed calves, *Vet. Rec.,* 101, 443, 1977.

8. **Myers, L. L., Newman, F. S., Wilson, R. A., and Catlin, J. E.,** Passive immunization of calves against experimentally induced enteric colibacillosis by vaccination of dams, *Am. J. Vet. Res.,* 34, 29, 1973.

9. **Bywater, R. J. and Logan, E. F.,** The site and characteristics of intestinal water and electrolyte loss in *Escherichia coli*-induced diarrhea in calves, *J. Comp. Pathol.,* 84, 599, 1974.

10. **Ryder, R. W., Wachsmuth, I. K., Buxton, A. E., Evans, D. G., DuPont, H. L., Mason, E., and Barrett, F. F.,** Infantile diarrhea produced by heat-stable enterotoxigenic *Escherichia coli, N. Engl. J. Med.,* 295, 849, 1976.

11. **Gorbach, S. L. and Khurana, C. M.,** Toxigenic *Escherichia coli.* A cause of infantile diarrhea in Chicago, *N. Engl. J. Med.,* 287, 791, 1972.

12. **Gordon, J. E.,** Neonatal enteric infections caused by *Escherichia coli, Ann. N. Y. Acad. Sci.,* 176, 9, 1971.

13. **Lariviere, S. and Lallier, R.,** *Escherichia coli* strains isolated from diarrheic piglets in the province of Quebec, *Can. J. Comp. Med.,* 40, 190, 1976.

14. **Stevens, J. B., Gyles, C. L., and Barnum, D. A.,** Production of diarrhea in pigs in response to *Escherichia coli* enterotoxin, *Am. J. Vet. Res.,* 33, 2511, 1972.

15. **Morris, G. K., Merson, M. H., Sack, D. A., Wells, J. G., Martin, W. T., Dewitt, W. E., Feeley, J. C., Sack, R. B., and Bessudo, D. M.,** Laboratory investigation of diarrhea in travelers to Mexico: evaluation of methods for detecting enterotoxigenic *Escherichia coli, J. Clin. Microbiol.,* 3, 486, 1976.

16. **Rowe, B., Taylor, J., and Bettelheim, K. A.,** An investigation of traveler's diarrhea, *Lancet,* 1, 1, 1970.

17. **Sack, D. A., McLaughlin, J. C., Sack, R. B., Orskov, F., and Orskov, I.,** Enterotoxigenic *Escherichia coli* isolated from patients at a hospital in Dacca, *J. Infect. Dis.,* 135, 275, 1977.

18. **Shore, E. G., Dean, A. G., Holik, K. J., and Davis, B. R.,** Enterotoxin-producing *Escherichia coli* and diarrheal disease in adult travelers: a prospective study, *J. Infect. Dis.,* 129, 577, 1974.

19. **Orskov, F., Orskov, I., Evans, D. J., Sack, R. B., Sack, D. A., and Wadstrom, T.,** Special *Escherichia coli* serotypes among enterotoxigenic strains from diarrhea in adults and children, *Med. Microbiol. Immunol.,* 162, 73, 1976.

20. **Cantey, J. R., O'Hanley, P. D., and Blake, R. K.,** A rabbit model of diarrhea due to invasive *Escherichia coli, J. Infect. Dis.,* 136, 640, 1977.

21. **Serény, B.,** Experimental keratoconjunctivitis shigellosa, *Acta Microbiol. Acad. Sci. Hung.,* 4, 367, 1957.

22. **Takeuchi, A., Inman, L. R., O'Hanley, P. D., Cantey, J. R., and Lushbaugh, W. B.,** Scanning and transmission electron microscopic study of *Escherichia coli* 015 (RDEC-1) enteric infection in rabbits, *Infect. Immun.,* 19, 686, 1978.

23. **Cantey, J. R. and Blake, R. K.,** Diarrhea due to *Escherichia coli* in the rabbit: a novel mechanism, *J. Infect. Dis.,* 135, 454, 1977.

24. **Sack, D. A., Merson, M. H., Wells, J. G., Sack, R. B., and Morris, G. K.,** Diarrhea associated with heat-stable enterotoxin-producing strains of *Escherichia coli,* Lancet, 2, 239, 1975.

25. **Merson, M. H., Morris, G. K., Sack, D. A., Wells, J. G., Feeley, J. C., Sack, R. B., Creech, W. B., Kapikian, A. Z., and Gangarosa, E. J.,** Traveler's diarrhea in Mexico: a prospective study of physician and family members attending a congress, *N. Engl. J. Med.,* 294, 1299, 1976.

26. **Gorbach, S. L., Kean, B. H., Evans, D. G., Evans, D. J., and Bessudo, D.,** Traveler's diarrhea and toxigenic *Escherichia coli, N. Engl. J. Med.,* 292, 933, 1975.

27. **Sack, R. B., Gorbach, S. L., and Banwell, J. G.,** Enterotoxigenic *Escherichia coli* isolated from patients with severe cholera-like disease, *J. Infect. Dis.,* 123, 378, 1971.

28. **DuPont, H. L., Olarte, J., Evans, D. G., Pickering, L. K., Galindo, E., and Evans, D. J.,** Comparative susceptibility of Latin American and United States students to enteric pathogens, *N. Engl. J. Med.,* 295, 1520, 1976.

29. **Levine, M. M., Caplan, E. S., Waterman, D., Cash, R. A., Hornick, R. B., and Snyder, M. J.,** Diarrhea caused by *Escherichia coli* that produce only heat-stable enterotoxin, *Infect. Immun.,* 17, 78, 1977.

30. **Ansari, M. M. and Myers, L. L.,** Use of the ovine ligated intestinal segment procedure to test for enterotoxigenic *Escherichia coli,* 58th Annu. Conf. Res. Workers Anim. Dis., November 28 to 29, 1977, 46(Abstr.), 8, 1977.

31. **Sack, R. B., Sack, D. A., Mehlman, I. J., Orskov, F., and Orskov, I.,** Enterotoxigenic *Escherichia coli* isolated from food, *J. Infect. Dis.,* 135, 313, 1977.

32. **Ellis, R. P. and Kienholz, J. C.,** Heat-labile enterotoxin produced by *Escherichia coli* serogroup 0149 isolated from diarrheic calves, *Infect. Immun.,* 1, 1002, 1977.

33. **Ellis, R. P.,** A two year survey of *Escherichia coli* serogroups associated with colibacillosis in pigs and calves, *Proc. 17th Annu. Meeting,* American Association of Veterinary Laboratory Diagnosticians, Madison, Wis., 1974, 133.

34. **Alderete, J. F. and Robertson, D. C.,** Purification and chemical characterization of the heat-stable enterotoxin produced by porcine strains of enterotoxigenic *Escherichia coli, Infect. Immun.,* 19, 1021, 1978.

35. **Donta, S. T., Moon, H. W., and Whipp, S. C.,** Detection of enterotoxigenic *E. coli* with the use of adrenal cells in tissue culture, *Science,* 183, 334, 1974.

36. **Guerrant, R. L., Brunton, L. L., Schnaitman, T. C., Rebhun, I., and Gilman, A. G.,** Cyclic adenosine monophosphate and alteration of Chinese hamster ovary cell morphology: a rapid, sensitive *in vitro* assay for the enterotoxins of *Vibrio cholerae* and *Escherichia coli, Infect. Immun.,* 10, 320, 1974.

37. **Myers, L. L., Newman, F. S., Warren, G. R., Catlin, J. E., and Anderson, C. K.,** Calf ligated intestinal segment test to detect enterotoxigenic *Escherichia coli, Infect. Immun.,* 11, 588, 1975.

38. **Speirs, J. I., Stavric, S., and Konowalchuk, J.,** Assay of *Escherichia coli* heat-labile enterotoxin with vero cells, *Infect. Immun.,* 16, 617, 1977.

39. **Acres, S. D., Laing, C. J., Saunders, J. R., and Radostits, O. M.,** Acute undifferentiated neonatal diarrhea in beef calves. I. Occurrence and distribution of infectious agents, *Can. J. Comp. Med.,* 39, 116, 1975.

40. **Dean, A. G., Ching, Y. C., Williams, R. G., and Harden, L. B.,** Test for *Escherichia coli* enterotoxin using infant mice: application in a study of diarrhea in children in Honolulu, *J. Infect. Dis.,* 125, 407, 1972.

41. **Sivaswamy, G. and Gyles, C. L.,** The prevalence of enterotoxigenic *Escherichia coli* in the feces of calves with diarrhea, *Can. J. Comp. Med.,* 40, 241, 1976.

42. **Moon, H. W., Whipp, S. C., and Skartvedt, S. M.,** Etiologic diagnosis of diarrheal diseases of calves: frequency and methods for detecting enterotoxin and K99 antigen production by *Escherichia coli, Am. J. Vet. Res.,* 37, 1025, 1976.

43. **Myers, L. L.,** Enteric colibacillosis in calves: immunogenicity and antigenicity of *Escherichia coli* antigens, *Am. J. Vet. Res.,* 39, 761, 1978.

44. **Bertschinger, H. U., Moon, H. W., and Whipp, S. C.,** Association of *Escherichia coli* with the small intestinal epithelium. I. Comparison of enteropathogenic and nonenteropathogenic porcine strains in pigs, *Infect. Immun.,* 5, 595, 1972.

45. **Evans, D. G., Evans, D. J., Jr., and Tjoa, W.,** Hemagglutination of human group A erythrocytes by enterotoxigenic *Escherichia coli* isolated from adults with diarrhea: correlation with colonization factor, *Infect. Immun.,* 18, 330, 1977.

46. **Evans, D. G., Evans D. J., Jr., Tjoa, W. S., and DuPont, H. L.,** Detection and characterization of colonization factor of enterotoxigenic *Escherichia coli* isolated from adults with diarrhea, *Infect. Immun.,* 19, 727, 1978.

47. **Guinée, P. A. M., Agterberg, C. M., Jansen, W. H., and Frik, J. F.,** Serological identification of pig enterotoxigenic *Escherichia coli* strains not belonging to the classical serotypes, *Infect. Immun.,* 15, 549, 1977.

48. **Myers, L. L. and Guinee, P. A. M.,** Occurrence and characteristics of enterotoxigenic *Escherichia coli* isolated from calves with diarrhea, *Infect. Immun.,* 13, 1117, 1976.

49. **Orskov, I. and Orskov, F.,** Special O:K:H: serotypes among enterotoxigenic *E. coli* strains from diarrhea in adults and children. Occurrence of the CF (colonization factor) antigen and of hemagglutinating abilities, *Med. Microbiol. Immunol.,* 163, 99, 1977.

50. **Finkelstein, R. A., Vasil, M. L., Jones, J. R., Anderson, R. A., and Barnard, T.,** Clinical cholera caused by enterotoxigenic *Escherichia coli, J. Clin. Microbiol.,* 3, 382, 1976.

51. **Moon, H. W., Nagy, B., and Isaacson, R. E.,** Intestinal colonization and adhesion by enterotoxigenic *Escherichia coli:* ultrastructural observations on adherence to ileal epithelium of the pig, *J. Infect. Dis.,* 136, 5124, 1977.

52. **Orskov, I., Orskov, F., Smith, H. W., and Sojka, W. J.,** The establishment of K99, a thermolabile, transmissible *Escherichia coli* K antigen, previously called "K co," possessed by calf and lamb enteropathogenic strains, *Acta Pathol. Microbiol. Scand. Sect. B,* 83, 31, 1975.

53. **Moon, H. W., Nagy, B., Isaacson, R. E., and Orskov, I.,** Occurrence of K99 antigen on *Escherichia coli* isolated from pigs and colonization of pig ileum by K99+ enterotoxigenic *E. coli* from calves and pigs, *Infect. Immun.,* 15, 614, 1977.

54. **Evans, D. G., Silver, R. P., Evans, D. J., Jr., Chase, D. G., and Gorbach, S. L.,** Plasmid-controlled colonization factor associated with virulence in *Escherichia coli* enterotoxigenic for humans, *Infect. Immun.,* 12, 656, 1975.

55. **Orskov, I., Orskov, F., Jann, B., and Jann, K.,** Serology, chemistry, and genetics of O and K antigens of *Escherichia coli, Bacteriol. Rev.,* 41, 667, 1977.

56. Bettelheim, K. A., Bushrod, F. M., Chandler, M. E., Cooke, E. M., O'Farrell, S., and Shooter, R. A., *Escherichia coli* serotype distribution in man and animals, *J. Hyg.*, 73, 467, 1974.

57. Sack, R. B., Enterotoxigenic *Escherichia coli* — an emerging pathogen, *N. Engl. J. Med.*, 295, 893, 1976.

58. Donta, S. T., Wallace, R. B., Whipp, S. C., and Olarte, J., Enterotoxigenic *Escherichia coli* and diarrheal disease in Mexican children, *J. Infect. Dis.*, 135, 482, 1977.

59. Goldschmidt, M. C. and DuPont, H. L., Enteropathogenic *Escherichia coli.* Lack of correlation of serotype with pathogenicity, *J. Infect. Dis.*, 133, 153, 1976.

60. Howe, K. and Linton, A. H., A longitudinal study of *Escherichia coli* in cows and calves with special reference to the distribution of O-antigen types and antibiotic resistance, *J. Appl. Bacteriol.*, 40, 331, 1976.

61. Hartley, C. L., Howe, K., Linton, A. H., Linton, K. B., and Richmond, M. H., Distribution of R plasmids among the O-antigen types of *Escherichia coli* isolated from human and animal sources, *Antimicrob. Agents Chemother.*, 8, 122, 1975.

62. Moon, H. W., Sorenson, D. K., and Sautter, J. H., *Escherichia coli* infection of the ligated intestinal loop of the newborn pig, *Am. J. Vet. Res.*, 27, 1317, 1966.

63. Ryder, R. W., Sack, D. A., Kapikian, A. Z., McLaughlin, J. C., Chakraborty, J., Rehman, A. S. M., Merson, M. H., and Wells, J. G., Enterotoxigenic *Escherichia coli* and reovirus-like agent in rural Bangladesh, *Lancet*, 1, 659, 1976.

64. Sakazaki, R., Tamura, I., and Saito, M., Enteropathogenic *Escherichia coli* associated with diarrhea in children and adults, *Jpn. J. Med. Sci. Biol.*, 20, 387, 1967.

65. Corley, L. D., Staley, T. E., and Jones, E. W., Uptake and pathogenesis of *Escherichia coli* 055:B5 in the young gnotobiotic pig, *Res. Vet. Sci.*, 14, 69, 1973.

66. Fey, H. and Margadant, A., Pathogenesis of coli septicemia in calves, *Zentralb. Bakteriol. Parasitenkd. Infektionskr. Hyg. Abt. 1: Orig.*, 182, 465, 1961.

67. Wood, P. C., The epidemiology of white scours among calves kept under experimental conditions, *J. Pathol. Bacteriol.*, 70, 179, 1955.

68. Glantz, P. J. and Dunne, H. W., Isolation of anaerogenic *E. coli* 026:B6 serotype from a case of calf scours, *Science*, 121, 902, 1955.

69. Sack, R. B., Human diarrheal disease caused by enterotoxigenic *Escherichia coli*, *Annual Review of Microbiology*, Vol. 29, Annual Reviews, Palo Alto, Calif., 1975, 333.

70. Cantey, J. R., personal communication.

71. Myers, L. L., unpublished data.

APPENDIX 3*

Abstract — In September 1974, the largest outbreak of food-borne salmonellosis ever reported to the Center for Disease Control — affecting an estimated 3400 persons — occurred on the Navajo Nation Indian Reservation. The responsible agent was *Salmonella newport,* and the vehicle of transmission was potato salad served to an estimated 11,000 persons at a free barbecue. The cooked ingredients of the potato salad had been stored up to 16 hr at improper holding temperatures.

The magnitude of the outbreak allowed us to study secondary transmission by calculating the rates of diarrheal illness during the 2 weeks following the outbreak in persons who did not attend the barbecue and by examining the results of stool cultures obtained after the outbreak. We found no secondary transmission.

We conclude that a health official should monitor food preparation and service at large social gatherings and that person-to-person transmission of salmonellosis probably does not normally occur even in settings considered highly conducive to cross-infection.

*   Horwitz, M. A., Pollard, R. A., Merson, M. H., and Martin, S. M., A large outbreak of foodborne salmonellosis on the Navajo Nation Indian Reservation, epidemiology and secondary transmission (abstract), *Am. J. Public Health,* 67(11), 1071, 1977. With permission.

STAPHYLOCOCCAL DISEASES

J. O. Cohen

The relationship of staphylococci to disease in humans ranges from that of a harmless or commensal one to a severe, life-threatening disease. Serious chronic infections of the bone, muscles, heart, and other organs also occur. Staphylococci may invade any organ in the body of a patient debilitated by such diseases as cancer, influenza, or diabetes. Correct antibiotic treatment initiated at the earliest sign of staphylococcal invasion is necessary to save the patient's life.[1,2]

A similar range in infectivity occurs in animals. Chronic staphylococcal infection is exemplified in bovine and ovine mastitis. The bovine udder is especially susceptible to both chronic and acute infection because of its disproportionate size and the nutrient nature of its secretions. Some animals rarely have infections due to staphylococci although they may carry staphylococci peculiar to their species.[3,4]

Research during the last 50 years has identified several toxins and enzymes as pathogenicity factors in staphylococci, yet the concept of virulence has best been realized in retrospect through epidemiological analysis by marker systems such as phage typing or serotyping. Indiscriminate use of antibiotics may select epidemic strains.

Host factors that invite staphylococcal infection are better understood. Both young, immunologically immature, and elderly, infirm humans and animals may be quite susceptible to staphylococcal infection. Also, any underlying illness that tends to compromise the immune system or reticuloendothelial system predisposes both groups to infection by staphylococci or other opportunistic bacteria, such as *Streptococcus viridans*, *Escherichia coli*, and *Pseudomonas aeruginosa*, either singly or in combination.

STAPHYLOCOCCAL DISEASES OF ANIMALS (OTHER THAN MASTITIS AND TICK PYEMIA)

Identification

Pyogenic lesions in animals may be caused by infectious agents other than staphylococci. For example, infections in pets that produce lesions analogous to furuncles and boils in humans are frequently caused by organisms such as *Pasteurella multicoda*. Therefore, identification of *Staphylococcus* as the source of infection depends upon its cultivation, isolation, and confirmatory tests such as for coagulase production.

Serious infections, such as osteomyelitis, discospondylitis, pyelonephritis, and septicemia, have been reported in dogs.[5-8] In addition, infections due to staphylococci in laboratory mice have been described in several reports, most of which deal with laboratory-induced infections.[9-11] A specific staphylococcal infection of the apocrine gland[5] in four dogs was recently reported by Schwartzman and Maguire.[12] Staphylococci often colonize the animal as well as the human upper respiratory tract, an area in which the potential as a reservoir for infection varies according to host animal, strain being carried, and environmental conditions.

Occurrence

Staphylococci are ubiquitous in warm-blooded animals as well as man. For example, staphylococcal colonization and disease were recently reported in porpoises.[13] It is important to distinguish between the carrier and disease states because staphylococcal carriage in some species seldom leads to infection.[14] In addition to carrying animal strains, pets may carry human strains of staphylococci that may be transmitted to humans.[15,16] The dominant staphylococcal infection in farm animals is mastitis, which will be discussed separately as will be tick pyemia. In order to diagnose a disease as being of staphylococcal origin, laboratory isolation and identification are necessary to rule out other microorganisms capable of causing similar symptoms.

Infectious Agent

Staphylococci are Gram-positive, catalase-positive cocci about 0.5 to 0.8 μm in diameter that occur in irregular clusters. Both coagulase-positive (*S. aureus*) and coagulase-negative (*S. epidermidis*) staphylococci cause disease, but it is important to distinguish between the two species. *S. aureus* is usually more virulent and more often the cause of epidemics or epizootics, whereas *S. epidermidis* is usually a commensal microorganism but may cause infection when the host is compromised. *S. aureus* causes both acute and chronic infections, while *S. epidermidis* is implicated in chronic infections.

Animal strains of *S. aureus* generally produce beta hemolysin and do not elaborate fibrinolysin.[14] Human strains usually produce alpha hemolysin and occasionally cause infections in domestic animals and pets.[15-19] There are other observed differences between animal and human strains to be discussed later.

The coagulase test is the best procedure for determining species and potential pathogenicity. Rabbit plasma is suitable for demonstration of the clotting effect of human *S. aureus* strains as well as of many animal strains. Its use obviates the precautions necessary when pooled human plasma is used in the laboratory. Animal strains may exhibit the coagulase reaction more readily in plasma from one animal species than from another.[18,20] Isolates from dogs did coagulate bovine plasma but coagulated human plasma only irregularly.[18,21] Pigeons yielded staphylococcal strains that lacked the clumping factor and exhibited a more intense coagulase reaction in human plasma than in bovine plasma.[21] The pigeon and dog strains were isolated from the nasal passages of healthy animals.

Grossgebauer and associates[22] recently studied the ability of staphylococci to produce lysozyme and found that *S. aureus* produced it but *S. epidermidis* did not. They therefore suggest that lysozyme production rather than coagulase production be used as a taxonomic criterion for determining the species.[22,23]

Staphylococci can usually be isolated on ordinary laboratory culture media such as tryptic soy agar or blood agar; however, media with a high salt content (approximately 7.5%) such as mannitol salt agar are useful for isolating staphylococci from highly contaminated samples.[24]

Such so-called pathogenicity factors as alpha, beta, and delta hemolysins,[25] coagulase,[26] and leukocidin[27] have been studied in great detail. Jeljaszewicz[25] found that strains from infections were positive for the production of more of these pathogenicity factors than strains from carriers. Virulence appears to be due to the interaction of several toxins and factors. Although many papers on bovine mastitis refer to hemolytic streptococci, hemolysis is a rough criterion for separating pathogenic cocci from nonpathogens. Coagulase-negative staphylococci may produce hemolysins, so one must depend upon the coagulase test for separating the two species. If performed under anaerobic conditions, testing for mannitol fermentation is useful in identification of *S. aureus* and correlates well with coagulase production.[24]

Differences between animal and human staphylococci have been demonstrated by phage susceptibilities and serology. The phage-typing system[28] widely used for epidemiological tracing of staphylococci in human disease does not delineate most epizootic strains because the phages in the International Set fail to lyse most animal strains.[29] A number of collections of phages have been developed for typing animal strains of staphylococci. A collaborative investigation of phages for typing bovine staphylococci was reported by Davidson.[30] Antigenic differences between human and animal strains of staphylococci have been observed by serotyping[31-36] and by differences in precipitinogens.[35-39]

Until recently, staphylococci from both human and animal sources had been subdivided taxonomically into two species: *S. aureus* and *S. epidermidis*. *S. aureus* was then subdivided into serotypes or phage types and *S. epidermidis* into biotypes[40] or, occasionally, phage types.[41] More intense study of the biochemical and morphological characteristics of human staphylococci has led to proposals to subdivide staphylococci into several new species.[42-44] Staphylococci from various animal species have been investigated biochemically and antigenically in a systematic manner.[18,36-39,45-49] We can expect an effort to subdivide the species *S. aureus* according to biochemical and antigenic differences of strains from different animal species. This may result either in acceptance of new species of coagulase-positive staphylococci or subdivisions such as types or subspecies.

According to L'Ecuyer,[50] Sompolinsky first reported an exudative dermatitis in young pigs caused by a Gram-positive coccus that he designated *Micrococcus hyicus*. Because the disease is often epizootic, it is important economically.[50-53] Underdahl et al.[54] suggested that the primary infectious agent might be a virus and that the severity of the disease relates to secondary invasion by the staphylococci. The name *Staphylococcus hyicus* has been suggested.[50-53]

Porcine strains of *S. aureus* from nasal passages of healthy pigs have been studied recently at several different laboratories.[36,46,55] Such strains usually produce beta and delta hemolysins but not fibrinolysin. Oeding et al.[36] found that porcine strains in phage group II usually show the type-A reaction on crystal violet agar and are serotype c_1. Another group of porcine strains by contrast was lysed by phages of groups other than II, and most were serotype h_2. All three studies showed that more than half of the isolates were resistant to tetracycline but penicillin resistance in porcine *S. aureus* strains was uncommon. The authors attributed the tetracycline resistance to the use of antibiotics in feeds. Further work is necessary to discover whether these narrow parameters apply to porcine *S. aureus* cultures in general or whether they are merely characteristic of the herds studied thus far.

In a recent study, Devriese and Oeding[56] tested bovine, poultry, and porcine strains of staphylococci. The porcine strains were isolated from exudative epidermidis cases. Despite the fact that all strains produced a heat-stable deoxyribonuclease (DNase) and most coagulated rabbit plasma, other biochemical properties resembled those of *S. epidermidis* biotype 2 of Baird-Parker.[24] Serum-gel diffusion experiments indicated these strains had poly A_1 or poly A_1C cell-wall teichoic acids. No other cell-wall teichoic acids were detected. All cultures were refractory to the International Set of Typing Phages at routine test dilution (RTD), but two strains were lysed by phage 187 at $100 \times$ RTD. Of the strains tested, 26% were serologically typable. When only one serum reacted (i.e., h_2), it would be interesting to know whether the authors tested to see if the positive strains could remove the h_2 antibody from the factor serum using a human *S. aureus* strain known to possess the h_2 antigen as an indicator of h_2 antibody. It is important to show that the factor antisera are truly monovalent when testing staphylococci of widely divergent sources.

With a wider range of tests and taxonomic criteria, results on animal staphylococci indicate that there are distinct differences between animal and human strains. Furthermore, subgroups can be demonstrated among both human and animal staphylococci that have epidemiological if not taxonomic importance. Interest in exploiting these differences for diagnostic, epidemiological, and taxonomic purposes should increase.

Reservoir

Staphylococci can be isolated from the nasopharynx and skin of animals and humans. Occasionally, humans may be a source of infection to domestic animals and pets, but animals appear to be colonized by varieties of staphylococci peculiar to each species.

Mode of Transmission

Domestic animals, wild animals, and humans often carry coagulase-positive or -negative staphylococci in the nose and throat.[18-21] Skin carriage seems to be important in sheep,[57] whereas chronic udder infection is an important reservoir for spread of bovine or ovine mastitis. Nasal carriage in some animals does not appear to predispose them to disease. A draining, purulent lesion can be the source of epizootic spread of staphylococcal disease. Even though pets themselves appear to be refractory to disease, they can carry human strains of staphylococci and act as reservoirs for human infection.[15,16] Direct contamination by animal-to-animal contact or self-infection by contaminating one's skin with nasal secretions appear to be important means of spreading staphylococcal infections. Although staphylococci have been frequently isolated from fomites, the spread of infection by inanimate objects seems infrequent except in the case of milking machinery implicated in the spread of mastitis.

Incubation Period

In the American Public Health Association's book *"Control of Communicable Diseases in Man,"* the incubation period for human staphylococcal disease is listed as "indefinite, commonly 4 to 10 days."[58] This incubation period is also appropriate for staphylococcal disease in animals. Since staphylococci are frequently carried by animals with no apparent ill effects, it is often impossible to know when a traumatic event, immunologic malfunction, or intrusion of a new strain initiates infection. After initiation, such an infection may not incubate as a viral infection but develops steadily. What is called the incubation period delineates the time that it takes for an infection to become apparent. Staphylococci are often the cause of focal infections, i.e., boils. A small boil on the leg of an animal may not be recognized as a disease at all. If it does not spread, it may go through a self-healing process without being noticed. Under the right circumstances, however, a boil can spread to other tissue and lead to a serious disease. This capacity of staphylococci to interact with a host as a commensal, a cause of focal infection, or a life-threatening invasion of the blood stream or lungs makes it impossible to define accurately "a period of incubation."

Period of Communicability

An animal is capable of infecting other animals as long as it sheds staphylococci. A draining lesion is particularly hazardous to other animals.[1] Communicability is affected by virulence of the staphylococci and susceptibility of the host.

Susceptibility and Resistance

Patterns of susceptibility and resistance to staphylococcal infections play an important role in determining which individuals become ill and whether the infection remains localized or becomes more general. Although epizootics due to staphylococci have been occasionally observed in wild animals,[37] too few attempts have been made to study staphylococci in wild animals in their natural habitats. Wild animals often carry staphylococci but are not usually infected. Antibiotic treatment of pets promotes their harboring antibiotic-resistant human strains that appear to be more hazardous to humans than to the animals.[15-17] Furthermore, the selection of antibiotic-resistant, virulent strains of staphylococci is often the result of antibiotic treatment in humans.[17]

Methods of Control

Preventive Measures

Farm animals should be kept under hygienic conditions with a good diet and enough space per animal. Pets should be kept in a clean environment and dogs periodically bathed and groomed.

Care should be taken in antibiotic treatment of farm animals and pets. Indiscriminate use of antibiotics leads to the emergence of resistant strains of microorganisms. Viral ailments should not be treated with antibiotics unless there is good evidence of secondary infection.

Control of Infected Animals, Contacts, and the Immediate Environment

There is no requirement for reporting individual cases. Human cases are class 4 reports. Epizootics should be reported to local public health and agricultural officials. Infected animals should be penned, housed, and fed separately from other animals where it is practical.

Areas contaminated by infected animals should be disinfected with phenolic solutions or quarterinary ammonium disinfectants. Care should be taken to follow instructions closely on the proper dilution and use of disinfectants. Mercuric chloride solutions should not be used because mercury is a cumulative poison in humans and animals.

No specific quarantine instructions apply. Animals from herds in which staphylococcal infections are prevalent should not be sold or transferred to herds relatively free of infection. Milk from animals with mastitis or those being treated with antibiotics should not be sold or mixed with milk from healthy cattle.

Immunization of contacts is not practical. Some experiments involving immunization of cattle have been performed. Veterinarians in small animal practice have occasionally used autogeneous vaccines (prepared from the infecting strain) to treat recurring staphylococcal infections with moderate success.

To investigate contacts, animals should be examined for draining lesions. In epizootic situations, search for carriers of staphylococci in which the phage type or serotype is identical to that of isolates from infections within the herd.

Systemic antibiotics are not indicated in localized infections.[58] Such infections often respond to topical preparations or may heal spontaneously. If systemic treatment is used, it is important that an appropriate antibiotic be chosen; this is best determined by sensitivity testing. If there is no opportunity to do sensitivity testing, use methicillin or other penicillinase-resistant penicillin. When penicillin allergy is present, use a cephalosporin, erythromycin, clindamycin, gentamicin, or Vancomycin®.[58]

Epizootic Measures

Staphylococci have presented a challenge to physician, veterinarian, and epidemiologist alike. The relationships between these microorganisms and their hosts have been greatly influenced by the introduction of antibiotics into medicine. Staphylococci readily develop a resistance to penicillin, producing penicillinase, an enzyme that inactivates penicillin; they have also developed resistance to many other antibiotics. Selected strains of more virulent or epizootic staphylococci can be traced by their antibiotic-resistant patterns, as well as by phage type or serotype. A result of these changes in the relationship of staphylococci to infection in humans has been increased incidence of hospital-acquired infections. Serious, often life-threatening infections have been observed, especially in burn patients or other debilitated patients. The identification of carriers of an epidemic strain depends upon our ability to recognize the strain against a background of normally present staphylococci. This is usually done by phage typing and occasionally serotyping although antibiotic-resistance patterns are also useful. Phage typing of animal strains requires a set of phages different from those used in the identification of human strains.[29]

Epizootics in wild animals can seldom be influenced by man and usually burn themselves out by elimination of susceptible animals. Epizootics among pets are uncommon. However, carriage of antibiotic-resistant strains of staphylococci occurs in pets in veterinary hospitals.[14,31,32] Feeding antibiotics to swine to help increase their rate of weight gain can result in their carrying staphylococci that are resistant to the antibiotic being fed (usually one of the tetracyclines).[36,46,55]

Individual studies of epizootics in sentry dogs have been reported by Blouse and Meekins,[59] among laboratory animals by Blackmore and Francis,[60] and in subhuman primates by Blouse et al.[61] Other studies include a survey by Hughes and associates[62] of perinatal lamb mortality, an experimental epidemiology report by Devriese et al.,[63] in which *S. aureus* was sprayed above chickens to establish colonization, and a study by Ash[64] of chronic skin ulceration in rats.

In the study of sentry dogs, staphylococcal carriage was similar in dogs with respiratory trouble and normal controls, suggesting a problem of viral rather than staphylococcal origin. In the laboratory animal study, staphylococcal infections were found in 34 mice, 7 rats, 4 guinea pigs, and 28 rabbits.[60] Only rabbits seemed particularly susceptible to staphylococci. The study of lambs was a survey of various bacterial pathogens. *S. aureus* was not a major cause of perinatal mortality in lambs;[62] *Pasteurella haemolytica* and anaerobic bacteria were isolated far more frequently.

In the experiments in which *S. aureus* was deliberately sprayed on chickens, high colonization levels persisted 6 weeks later.[63] When two or three strains were sprayed simultaneously, one strain dominated in most chickens. Colonization with one strain generally prevented superinfection with a second strain.[63] The study of postoperative staphylococcal infections in subhuman primates resembled similar studies in humans. The epizootic appeared to be caused by a strain of phage group II, type 3A/55/71, the source being the apes themselves rather than the handlers (although an earlier human source cannot be ruled out).[61]

These studies reinforce the picture given earlier of an opportunistic microorganism often having a commensal relationship with its host. To this it must be added that *S. aureus* is a microorganism that may give rise to particularly virulent or epizootic clones. Finally, there is the role of man as the manipulator in his use and abuse of antibiotics. With the gradual increase of methicillin-resistant staphylococci, it seems only a matter of time before new antibiotics will be needed.[2] A change in the pattern of sensitivity, giving way to resistance, requires a more cautious approach to the use of antibiotics.

TICK PYEMIA IN LAMBS

Identification

Tick pyemia in lambs is usually caused by staphylococci. The symptoms are lameness, joint abscesses, bacteremia, and death.[65]

Occurrence

The disease occurs throughout tick-infested areas of the British Isles.[66,67] This author has not found reference to tick pyemia as a specific disease in other geographic areas.

Infectious agent

Strains of staphylococci with or without concurrent infection with the virus of tick-borne fever.[65,67]

Reservoir

S. aureus appears to reside on the skin of the lambs.

Mode of Transmission

Infection develops when the lamb receives tick bites that break the skin and force in staphylococci. Tick-borne fever can infect lambs without staphylococcal superinfection. Tick pyemia can occur in the absence of the virus of tick-borne fever. Frequently, all three elements are present when tick pyemia infects a herd of sheep.[68] The tick *Ixodes ricinus* has been implicated.[66]

Incubation Period

The exact period is unknown. Several days are probably required from the time tick bites occur until obvious infection can be observed.

Period of Communicability

Cross-colonization of lambs by a virulent strain of staphylococcus renders them susceptible, if ticks are present to initiate the disease. The interrelationship of coccus, tick, virus, and host is complex. Duration of communicability cannot be defined since absence of any one element may lead to absence of infections. Lambs are still at some level of risk as long as viable staphylococci are shed into the environment.

Susceptibility and Resistance

Lambs are usually susceptible and become infected when both ticks and *S. aureus* are present. Tick pyemia is seldom a problem when tick infestation is light. Strains of tick-borne fever virus that are alike immunologically but differ in virulence have been observed.[67]

Methods of Control

Preventive Measures

1. Treatment with antibiotics such as procaine penicillin or erythromycin has little effect on the mortality caused by tick pyemia. Treatment does hasten the recovery of surviving animals.[65]
2. No vaccines or antisera are available either for the staphylococci or the virus of tick-borne fever.[67]
3. Dipping lambs in chlorphenvinphos 0.05% greatly reduces the level of tick infestation and thereby the amount of tick pyemia and staphylococcal infection.[67]
4. Quarantine. Avoid transferring lambs from infected herds to herds that have been free of infection.
5. Immunization of contacts: no method has been developed for immunizing lambs against tick pyemia.
6. Investigation of contacts: although strictly speaking, tick pyemia does not appear to be vector borne, control methods center around reducing the tick infestation level rather than preventing the spread of the staphylococci.
7. Specific treatment: antibiotic treatment hastens the recovery of lambs that survive tick pyemia even though the overall death rate in the herd seems to be unchanged by treatment.[65]

Epizootic Measures

1. Keep down tick infestation by dipping sheep.
2. Avoid bringing lambs from infected herds into those where tick pyemia has been absent.
3. Treat infected lambs with appropriate antibiotics.

STAPHYLOCOCCAL BOVINE AND OVINE MASTITIS

Identification

Mastitis in cattle and sheep can be either acute or chronic. When Little and Plastridge[69] wrote their monograph on bovine mastitis in 1946, they listed the major cause as *Streptococcus agalactiae* with some chronic mastitis caused by staphylococci, *Streptococcus dysgalactiae,* and *Streptococcus uberis.* The use of penicillin in the treatment of mastitis has resulted in streptococcal mastitis being eradicated in some herds. Concurrently, staphylococcal mastitis, now frequently caused by penicillin-resistant strains, has become the predominant form.[70]

Both acute and chronic mastitis are caused by *S. aureus.* Staphylococcal mastitis may vary in intensity from inapparent infection, only detectable by culturing foremilk, to fulminating infection that destroys the infected quarter. Economic loss due to mastitis is great. Much time and money have been spent treating infected cows; therefore, losses in cattle, milk, and productivity continue to occur. Annual toll to the U.S. dairy industry from bovine mastitis has been placed between $225 and $500 million.[71] Considerable research is being done on epizootiology and means to prevent, treat, and control mastitis.

Occurrence

Distribution of bovine mastitis of staphylococcal origin is world-wide. Similarly, wherever sheep and goats are raised, mastitis due to *S. aureus* is common.

Infectious Agent
S. aureus
Bovine strains predominate with occasional severe infection due to a human strain.

S. epidermidis
Coagulase-negative staphylococci cause chronic udder infections ranging from inapparent to serious.

Inflammatory Response in Mastitis
Procedures that measure the degree of inflammation as indicated by the leukocyte count or California Mastitis Test reaction correlate well with bacteriological identification.[72] Naidu and Newbould[73] found beta hemolysin, common to animal staphylococci, to be a potent inflammatory agent when infused into the bovine udder. Kronvall et al.[74] found that strains of *S. aureus* with high levels of protein A were more likely to be isolated from acute mastitis, whereas those low in protein A were more likely to be isolated from chronic mastitis.

Differentiation of Staphylococci from Mastitis
Markham and Markham[75] compared carriage of staphylococci by humans and animals, including cattle. Bovine strains produced beta hemolysin and yielded different phage types than human strains.[75,76] Brown et al.[77] investigated means of differentiat-

ing strains of *S. epidermidis* from bovine udders by comparing results of physiological and biochemical tests, serological typing of extracellular proteolytic enzymes by colony morphology, and the spectrophotometric analysis of methanol-extracted pigments. Approximately 75% of the cultures reacting with antisera for the first four proteinase groups could be placed in one of Baird-Parker's biochemical groups.[24]

Phage Typing (S. aureus)

Human strains of staphylococci are usually typed on the basis of their susceptibilities to specific bacteriophages. These phage types are useful in epidemiological tracing. Animal strains, however, are seldom subject to lysis by phages of the International Set.[78] Different sets of phages developed for use with bovine strains have been reported.[30,77-84] Thorne and Hallander[83] tried with some success a system combining phages of the International Set and some of the phages of Davidson.[30] Nyhan and Archer[85] demonstrated the usefulness of phage typing in studying several mastitis outbreaks in a single herd. In a recent study, Rose and McDonald[86] isolated phages from *S. epidermidis,* probably in anticipation of developing means to phage-type coagulase-negative staphylococci.

Reservoir

The reservoir of staphylococci in bovine mastitis is the infected udder itself.[87] Extramammary reservoirs for *S. aureus* are the skin of the teats and the teat cups of the milking machine.[87] Staphylococci are occasionally isolated from other sites in the cattle but not often in large numbers.

Mode of Transmission

Mastitis is transmitted primarily during the milking process.[87] Staphylococci have been shown to survive on teat cups and wash cloths despite the use of disinfectants.[87]

Incubation Period

The incubation period is 1 to 2 days when cows are deliberately inoculated with *S. aureus* via the teat canal.[88] When the inoculum concentration is low, dry quarters do not exhibit infection before 7 to 9 days.[88]

Period of Communicability

Cattle that are shedding staphylococci are infectious to other cattle. Any cow must be considered a potential source of infection as long as *S. aureus* can be cultivated from its foremilk.

Susceptibility and Resistance

Infection process in the cow has been studied in detail. The integrity of the teat duct itself is important. Prasad and Newbould[89] studied the relationship of teat duct length to susceptibility to *S. aureus* infection and found a higher infection rate following inoculation as far as 4 mm up the teat ducts rather than 3 mm. The authors questioned whether there might be critical anatomical differences in this region (4 mm). They also found that high milking rates (0.40 kg/min) favored infection after inoculation of staphylococci to 4.0 mm. Chandler et al.[90] studied the ultrastructure of the bovine teat duct and concluded that the mesh-like nature of the keratin reduced the rate of movement of staphylococci from teat opening to mammary gland. Their work did not rule out other defense methods such as antibacterial substances. Harmon et al.[91] proposed that lactoferrin, an iron-binding protein of milk, may have an important role in protecting the mammary gland from infection.

Reiter and Oram[92] found that the numbers of leukocytes in milk were important in the defense against staphylococcal or streptococcal mastitis. Thomas and associates[93] studied the effect of milking vs. drying-off when the teats of cows were deliberately dipped in a suspension of staphylococci and streptococci. There was a lower incidence of new infection in the milked quarters that the researchers attributed to the fact that many bacteria entering the teat duct milking would be flushed out with the milk.

El Etreby and Abdel-Hamid[94] studied deliberately induced ovine mastitis and concluded that mastitis due to *S. aureus* in sheep was similar to bovine mastitis in that both chronic and acute mastitis occur. Factors such as the general health of the sheep, whether the sheep has been dried off or is lactating, numbers of invading bacteria, and the strain of *S. aureus* affect the severity of the infection.

Methods of Control
Preventive Measures

Stopping cross-infections — The objective is to prevent spread from cow to cow. Washing hands between the milking of different cows, hot-water pasteurizing of the teat cups of the milking machine, and using separate, disposable towels to wipe the teats before and after each milking are useful measures for preventing the spread of staphylococci.[87] Mechanical milking machines should be in good condition. Milking should not be too fast, and the process should be monitored to avoid damage to the udder or teat canal and to prevent cross-contamination.[89]

Prompt treatment — Edwards and Smith[95] used procaine penicillin to treat cows early in the dry period. Although it was effective in preventing mastitis due to *Corynebacterium pyogenes,* this antibiotic did not reduce the incidence of *S. aureus* infections. They suggested retrospective treatment of *S. aureus* and other infections. However, other investigators report various degrees of success with treatment of dry cows and recommend early treatment of mastitis both for therapy and control.[96-99] Smith et al.[100] had considerable success using sodium cloxacillin in 3% aluminum monostearate base. These authors agree that antibiotic treatment of cows must be combined with other preventive measures in order to provide significant control of staphylococcal mastitis.

Control of Mastitis

Regulations — Staphylococcal mastitis is widespread and not controlled by quarantine or a system of reporting. However, regulations have been applied to commercially marketed milk to prevent contaminated lots from being sold or mixed with acceptable milk. Also, after a cow has received antibiotic therapy, a specified period of time must elapse before its milk can be marketed in order to prevent the antibiotics from being consumed by humans.[101] In the early years of penicillin therapy, such restrictions often went unheeded; this resulted in people inadvertently becoming sensitized to penicillin. Thus, rapid milking, unsanitary handling of cows, and irresponsible use of antibiotics may yield short-term economic benefits, but such poor management practices will result in a chronic mastitis problem.

Etiologic factors — Jasper[102] explained the interrelationship of therapy and dairy management in a review article on etiologic factors in bovine mastitis. He spoke of the reinfection of treated cattle with another pathogen and asked that this be remembered: "The noninfected herd is a highly susceptible herd."

Herd management — Significant reduction in the amount of staphylococcal mastitis in two herds was obtained by (1) culling the herds of chronically infected animals and (2) milking cows in such an order that those shedding staphylococci were milked last.[103] Brander[104] gave a detailed description of efforts to improve the hygiene of cattle and their environment in order to prevent infection with Gram-negative bacteria and coagulase-negative staphylococci. White and Rattray[105] studied the frequency of milking and the role of white cells in the management of clinical mastitis. They concluded it was advantageous to milk dairy cows three times per day.

Evaluation of methods to prevent cross-infection — In a study of bovine mastitis in New South Wales, Johnston and Lepherd[106] found that herds in which the udders were washed with running water instead of water from buckets had fewer staphylococci. Experiments in which disinfectant solutions are applied after milking indicate that such solutions reduce the numbers of staphylococci. Pearson et al.[107] used a germicidal iodophor teat spray, whereas Forse et al.[108] evaluated a polymeric biguanide germicide. Kirkbride and Erhart[71] studied the effects of different milking machines and vacuum settings on udder damage and subsequent mastitis but found these parameters difficult to quantify. Munch-Petersen[109] attempted to determine time onset of an udder infection by taking frequent samples of foremilk over the entire period of lactation. His results suggested that the use of slow release antibiotics during the dry period might be advantageous. Edwards and Smith[110] questioned the effectiveness of disinfectants in their study of various methods of avoiding cross-infection.

Diagnosis of infected cattle is important in any mastitis control program. Spooner and Miller[111] developed a rapid method for detecting hemoglobin-reactive protein of cattle that they found in those animals suffering from acute inflammation. Others have made numerical comparisons between various mastitis tests, such as the relationship between Wisconsin Mastitis Test scores and leukocyte counts[112] or among California Mastitis Test Scores, catalase test results, and milk samples from individual quarters.[113]

Mastitis control: public and private programs — In 1969, Dahl[114] described a program for evaluating all aspects of the dairy operation in an attempt to reduce udder infections. This included methods for testing milk and environment. At the same time, Smith[115] described the Wisconsin Mastitis Control program. The program was voluntary at first but, in late 1967, written regulations were compiled. Dairy milk quality is checked by the catalase test and leukocyte counts. If one million leukocytes are present per ml of milk, if pathogenic organisms are isolated, or if the milk is from a dairy where one or more cows have clinical mastitis, it is illegal to sell the milk or otherwise offer it for human consumption.

Immunization to prevent mastitis — Despite numerous experiments to develop vaccines, no immunization method can be recommended. Nevertheless, these studies indicate that the natural resistance of the udder to infection can be enhanced by vaccination. The usefulness of any method will depend upon its feasibility in a cost-benefit analysis. These approaches are of some scientific interest and are, therefore, discussed below.

Using sheep and goats, Plommet and Le Gall[116,117] experimented with both parental and local (udder) immunization with hemolysins and killed staphylococci as immunogens. Vaccinated sheep did become infected when challenged, but the disease was milder than that seen in unvaccinated controls. Derbyshire and Smith[118] immunized goats with a staphylococcal cell-toxoid vaccine with results similar to those of Plommet and Le Gall. Fujikura[119] did similar experiments with goats. The virulence of his staphylococcal strain was demonstrated by its ability to cause severe infections in unvaccinated goats. Four udders vaccinated with formalin-killed staphylococcal vaccine were protected from challenge with his strain S 63231. According to Fujikura, "several problems must be settled before a vaccine can be used effectively against mastitis in the field, but the future is not without hope." In other caprine experiments, Singleton et al.[120] immunized goats with purified cell wall of staphylococci with very limited success. McDowell and Watson[121] immunized ewes and observed some protection against challenge with 1 mℓ of broth containing 10^6 staphylococci.

Slanetz et al.,[122] using an uninoculated group of cattle as controls, studied the effect of intramuscular injection of staphylococcal toxoid and bacterin-toxoid on the incidence of mastitis. New cases occurred among the uninoculated cows but not among those vaccinated. The paper discusses earlier reports of Richou and associates and lists references.[122] In contrast, Oehme and Coles[123] used a commercially available vaccine and saw no decrease in clinical incidence of mastitis. They concluded that "vaccination was of limited value for controlling *S. aureus* mastitis." In a more recent review, Norcross and Stark[124] attributed the difficulty of preparing vaccines to induce immunity to staphylococcal mastitis to the diversity of types and strains. They inferred that vaccines, when successful, tend to protect against only a few strains. The diverse types of staphylococci, however, carry group-specific antigens as well as those determining type. Theoretically, vaccines could be prepared that would evoke a general response against most *S. aureus* strains. However, all antibodies evoked are not necessarily protective.

Williams et al.[125,126] experimented with a lysed-cell polyvalent bacterin developed by Greenberg.[127] They reported success in preventing mastitis[125] and developing resistance to direct challenge.[126] Brock et al.[128] vaccinated cows with killed *S. aureus* cells by simultaneous intramammary and intramuscular inoculation, but they found no reliable protection against infection even with very low numbers of challenge organisms. Willoughby[129] reported experiments in pathology and immunology of staphylococcal mastitis. He injected a heifer with commercial bacterin toxoid subcutaneously on the left side of the mammary gland and recommended that "vaccine should be injected to prime the regional lymph nodes of the mammary gland." Despite the occasional successful experiment in immunization against staphylococcal mastitis, no practical procedure based upon immunization can be recommended to help prevent or control mastitis.

Specific treatment — Antibiotic treatment of infected animals should be part of a continuous program for control of mastitis.[96,102] Treatment of infected cows during the dry period is recommended as a routine measure.[96,97,99] The choice of antibiotic has changed over the years. Penicillin treatment reduced the incidence of streptococcal mastitis and was also effective against most bovine staphylococci when introduced into veterinary use. Most *S. aureus* isolates from mastitis today, however, are resistant to penicillin.

Swarbrick[130] successfully used parental erythromycin to treat mastitis but found that intramammary infusion was not effective. By udder infusion, Daniel and Steffert[98] tested several combinations of antibiotics, including sodium cloxacillin alone, with considerable success. Langley et al.[131] found both sodium cloxacillin and a penicillin-novobiocin combination to be effective when given as an udder infusion. Hamdy and co-workers[132] tested 87 strains of *S. aureus* for sensitivity to penicillin, novobiocin, and to a combination of the two. The combination was most effective.

In human medicine, methicillin and related penicillinase-resistant penicillins have become the means for treating disease caused by penicillin-resistant staphylococci. Devreise et al.[133] and Devreise and Hommez[134] studied methicillin (cloxacillin)-resistant staphylococci from dairy cattle. Although Devreise et al.[133] originally classified these as animal strains, he finally concluded that the staphylococci resistant to methicillin were of human origin.[134] Thus far, the problem of methicillin-resistant staphylococci as a cause of bovine mastitis is limited to certain geographical areas. Cloxacillin, therefore, seems to be a drug of choice for treating staphylococcal mastitis with the proviso that sensitivity checks be performed on the staphylococcus if the animal does not respond to treatment.

Ziv and associates[135] of the Israeli Kimron Veterinary Institute recently announced the development of a new drug, Quinaldofur®, for the treatment of bovine mastitis. It is a chemotherapeutic agent related both to the nitrofurans and quinoline. The activity of Quinaldofur® against mastitis streptococci and *S. aureus* was compared in vitro to that of penicillin, streptomycin, erythromycin, and other antibiotics. Quinaldofur® was more active on a per weight basis than the established therapeutic agents. However, it was not sufficiently active in vitro in milk against *Escherichia coli* and *Pseudomonas aeruginosa*. The drug has been tested in cattle by infusion into the udder via the teat canal.[136] The absorption, distribution, and excretion of Quinaldofur® after intramammary treatment were investigated in four cows. These preliminary experiments indicated that it is well tolerated and probably useful for the treatment of bovine mastitis. Furthermore, Quinaldofur® is rapidly excreted from the udder (undetectable after 72 hr) and would be used only for treatment of mastitis.[136]

REFERENCES

1. Shulman, J. A. and Nahmias, A. J., Staphylococcal infections: clinical aspects, in *The Staphylococci*, Cohen, J. O., Ed., John Wiley & Sons, New York, 1972, 457.
2. Eickhoff, T. C., Therapy of staphylococcal infection, in *The Staphylococci*, Cohen, J. O., Ed., John Wiley & Sons, New York, 1972, 517.
3. Hearst, B. R., Low incidence of staphylococcal dermatitides in animals with high incidence of *Staphylococcus aureus*. I. Preliminary study of cats, *Vet. Med. Small Anim. Clin.*, 62, 475, 1967.
4. Hearst, B. R., Low incidence of staphylococcal dermatides in animals with high incidence of *Staphylococcus aureus*. II. Preliminary study of dogs, *Vet. Med. Small Anim. Clin.*, 62, 541, 1967.
5. Clark, W. T., Staphylococcal infection of the urinary tract and its relation to urolithiasis in dogs, *Vet. Rec.*, 95, 204, 1974.
6. Gage, E. D., Treatment of discospondylitis in the dog, *J. Am. Vet. Med. Assoc.*, 116, 1164, 1975.
7. Madewell, B. R., Creed, J. E., and Hopkins, J. R., Hydronephrosis and pyelonephritis in a dog, *J. Am. Vet. Med. Assoc.*, 167, 377, 1975.
8. Olson, P. S., Staphylococcal septicemia in puppies (a case report), *Vet. Med. Small Anim. Clin.*, 70, 1159, 1975.
9. Easmon, C. S. F. and Glynn, A. A., The role of humoral immunity and acute inflammation in protection against staphylococcal dermonecrosis, *Immunology*, 29, 67, 1975.
10. Easmon, C. S. F. and Glynn, A. A., Cell-mediated immune responses in *Staphylococcus aureus* infections in mice, *Immunology*, 29, 75, 1975.
11. Rhoden, C. H., Leeper, D. B., Smith, I. M., Evans, T. C., and Duling, B. R., Blood pressure changes in mice after lethal staphylococcal infection and endotoxin challenge, *Proc. Soc. Exp. Biol. Med.*, 149, 622, 1975.
12. Schwartzman, A. M. and Maguire, H. C., Staphylococcal apocrine gland infections in the dog (canine hidradenitis suppurativa), *Br. Vet. J.*, 125, 121, 1969.
13. Streitfeld, M. M. and Chapman, C. G., *Staphylococcus aureus* infections of captive dolphins *(Tursiops truncatus)* and oceanarium personnel, *Am. J. Vet. Res.*, 37, 303, 1976.
14. Marandon, J.-L. and Oeding, P., Investigations on animal *Staphylococcus aureus* strains. I. Biochemical characteristics and phage typing, *Acta Pathol. Microbiol. Scand.*, 67, 149, 1966.
15. Live, I. and Nichols, A. C., The animal hospital as a source of antibiotic resistant staphylococci, *J. Infect. Dis.*, 108, 195, 1961.
16. Live, I., Differentiation of *Staphylococcus aureus* of human and of canine origins: coagulation of human and of canine plasma, fibrinolysin activity, and serologic reaction, *Am. J. Vet. Res.*, 33, 385, 1972.
17. Blouse, L., Husted, P., McKee, A., and Gonzalez, J., Epizootiology of staphylococci in dogs, *Am. J. Vet. Res.*, 25, 1195, 1964.
18. Hajek, V. and Marsalek, E., A study of staphylococci isolated from the upper respiratory tract of different animal species. I. Biological properties of *Staphylococcus aureus* strains of canine origin. II. Biochemical properties of *Staphylococcus aureus* strains of pigeon origin, *Zentralbl. Bakteriol. Parasitenkd. Infektionskr. Hyg. Abt. 1: Orig.*, 212, 60, 1970.
19. Poole, P. M. and Baker, J. R., An outbreak of infection due to *Staphylococcus aureus* phage type 80/81 in a veterinary school, *Mon. Bull. Minist. Health Public Health Lab.*, 25, 116, 1966.
20. Hajek, V. and Marsalek, E., A study of staphylococci of bovine origin, *Staphylococcus aureus* var. *bovis*, *Zentralbl. Bakteriol. Parasitenkd. Infektionskr. Hyg. Abt. 1: Orig.*, 209, 154, 1969.

21. Oeding, P., Marandon, J.-L., Hajek, V., and Marsalek, E., Comparison of antigenic structure and phage pattern with biochemical properties of *Staphylococcus aureus* strains isolated from dogs and pigeons, *Acta Pathol. Microbiol. Scand. Sect. B*, 78, 414, 1970.

22. Grossgebauer, K., Schmidt, B., and Langmaack, H., Lysozyme production as an aid for identification of potentially pathogenic strains of staphylococci, *Appl. Microbiol.*, 16, 1745, 1968.

23. Hussels, H., Langmaack, H., Grossgebauer, K., and Forster, D., Uber die Lysozym- und Toxinbildung von Tierstaphylokokken, *Zentralbl. Bakteriol. Parasitenkd. Infektionskr. Hyg. Abt. 1: Orig.*, 214, 203, 1970.

24. Baird-Parker, A. C., Classification and identification of staphylococci and their resistance to physical agents, in *The Staphylococci*, Cohen, J. O., Ed., John Wiley & Sons, New York, 1972, 1.

25. Jeljaszewicz, J., Toxins (hemolysins), in *The Staphylococci*, Cohen, J. O., Ed., John Wiley & Sons, New York, 1972, 249.

26. Tager, M., Current views on the mechanism of coagulase action on blood clotting, *Ann. N.Y. Acad. Sci.*, 236, 277, 1974.

27. Woodin, A. M., Staphylococcal leucocidin, in *The Staphylococci*, Cohen, J. O., Ed., John Wiley & Sons, New York, 1972, 281.

28. Blair, J. E. and Williams, R. E. O., Phage typing of staphylococci, *Bull. W.H.O.*, 24, 771, 1961.

29. Giesecke, W. H., Van Den Heever, L. W., and DuToit, I. J., Staphylococcal mastitis: phage types and patterns of *S. aureus*, *Onderstepoort J. Vet. Res.*, 39, 87, 1972.

30. Davidson, I., A collaborative investigation of phages for typing bovine staphylococci, *Bull. W.H.O.*, 46, 81, 1972.

31. Marandon, J.-L. and Oeding, P., Investigations on animal *Staphylococcus aureus* strains. II. Antigens, *Acta Pathol. Microbiol. Scand.*, 70, 300, 1967.

32. Live, I. and Nichols, A. C., Serological typing of staphylococci as an aid in epidemiological studies, *J. Infect. Dis.*, 115, 197, 1965.

33. Live, I., Staphylococci in animals: differentiation and relationship to human staphylococcosis, in *The Staphylococci*, Cohen, J. O., Ed., John Wiley & Sons, New York, 1972, 443.

34. Malik, B. S. and Singh, C. A., Studies on staphylococci with particular reference to strains from bovine udder, *J. Infect. Dis.*, 106, 256, 1960.

35. Oeding, P., Marandon, J.-L., Hajek, V., and Marsalek, E., A comparison of phage pattern and antigenic structure with biochemical properties of *Staphylococcus aureus* strains isolated from cattle, *Acta Pathol. Microbiol. Scand. Sect. B*, 79, 357, 1971.

36. Oeding, P., Marandon, J.-L., Meyer, W., Hajek, V., and Marsalek, E., A comparison of phage pattern and antigenic structure with biochemical properties of *Staphylococcus aureus* strains isolated from swine, *Acta Pathol. Microbiol. Scand. Sect. B*, 80, 525, 1972.

37. Oeding, P., Hajek, V., and Masalek, E., A comparison of antigenic structure and phage pattern with biochemical properties of *Staphylococcus aureus* strains isolated from hares and mink, *Acta Pathol. Microbiol. Scand. Sect. B*, 81, 567, 1973.

38. Oeding, P., Hajek, V., and Marsalek, E., A comparison of antigenic structure and phage pattern with biochemical properties of *Staphylococcus aureus* strains isolated from horses, *Acta Pathol. Microbiol. Scand. Sect. B*, 82, 899, 1974.

39. Oeding, P., Hajek, V., and Marsalek, E., A comparison of antigenic structure and phage pattern with biochemical properties of *Staphylococcus aureus* strains isolated from sheep, *Acta Pathol. Microbiol. Scand. Sect. B*, 84, 1976.

40. Baird-Parker, A. C., A classification of micrococci and staphylococci based on physiological and biochemical tests, *J. Gen. Microbiol.*, 30, 409, 1963.

41. Verhoef, J., Van Boven, C. P. A., and Winkler, K. C., Characters of phages from coagulase-negative staphylococci, *J. Med. Microbiol.*, 4, 413, 1971.

42. Schleifer, K. H. and Kloos, W. E., Isolation and characteristics of staphylococci from human skin. I. Amended description of *Staphylococcus epidermidis* and *Staphylococcus saprophyticus*, and descriptions of three new species: *Staphylococcus cohnii*, *Staphylococcus haemolyticus*, and *Staphylococcus xylosus*, *Int. J. Syst. Bacteriol.*, 25, 50, 1975.

43. Kloos, W. E. and Schliefer, K. H., Isolation and characterization of staphylococci from human skin. II. Descriptions of four new species: *Staphylococcus warneri*, *Staphylococcus capitis*, *Staphylococcus hominis*, and *Staphylococcus simulans*, *Int. J. Syst. Bacteriol.*, 25, 62, 1975.

44. Kloos, W. E. and Schleifer, K. H., Simplified scheme for routine identification of human *Staphylococcus* species, *J. Clin. Microbiol.*, 1, 82, 1975.

45. Hajek, V. and Marsalek, E., The differentiation of pathogenic staphylococci and a suggestion for their taxonomic classification, *Zentralbl. Bakteriol. Parasitenkd. Infektionskr. Hyg. Abt. 1: Orig. Reihe A*, 217, 176, 1971.

46. **Hajek, V. and Marsalek, E.**, A study of staphylococci isolated from the upper respiratory tract of different animal species. III. Physiological properties of *Staphylococcus aureus* strains of porcine origin, *Zentralbl. Bakteriol. Parasitenkd. Infektionskr. Hyg. Abt. 1: Orig.*, 215, 68, 1970.

47. **Hajek, V., Marsalek, E., and Hubacek, J.**, A study of staphylococci isolated from the upper respiratory tract of different animal species. V. Communication: physiological properties of *Staphylococcus aureus* strains from mink, *Zentralbl. Bakteriol. Parasitenkd. Infektionskr. Hyg. Abt. 1: Orig. Reihe A*, 222, 194, 1972.

48. **Hajek, V. and Marsalek, E.**, Staphylococci outside the hospital, *Staphylococcus aureus* in sheep, *Zentralbl. Bakteriol. Parasitenkd. Infektionskr. Hyg. Abt. 1: Orig. Reihe B*, 161, 455, 1976.

49. **Hajek, V., Marsalek, E., and Harna, V.**, A study of staphylococci isolated from the upper respiratory tract of different animal species. VI. Physiological properties of *Staphylococcus aureus* strains from horses, *Zentralbl. Bakteriol. Parasitenkd. Infektionskr. Hyg. Abt. 1: Orig. Reihe A*, 229, 429, 1974.

50. **L'Ecuyer, C.**, Exudative epidermitis in pigs. Bacteriological studies on the causative agent *Staphylococcus hyicus*, *Can. J. Comp. Med. Vet. Sci.*, 31, 243, 1967.

51. **Amtsberg, V. G., Bollwohn, W., Hazem, S., Jordan, B., and Schmidt, U.**, Bakteriologische, serologische, und tierexperimentelle Untersuchungen zur atiologischen Bedeutung von *Staphylococcus hyicus* beim Nassenden Ekzem, *Dtsch. Tieraerztl. Wochenschr.*, 80, 521, 1974.

52. **Amtsberg, V. G., Bollwohn, W., Hazem, S., Jordan, B., and Schmidt, U.**, Bakteriologische, serologische und tierexperimentelle Untersuchungen zur antiologischen Bedeutung von *Staphylococcus hyicus* beim Nassenden Ekzem des Schweines, *Dtsch. Tieraerztl. Wochenschr.*, 80, 496, 1974.

53. **Schultz, W.**, Untersuchungen zur Atiologie der exsudativen Epidermitis der Ferkel unter besonderer Berucksichtigung des *Staphylococcus hyicus*, *Arch. Exp. Veterinaermed.*, 23, 415, 1969.

54. **Underdahl, N. R., Grace, D. D., and Twihaus, M. J.**, Porcine exudative epidermitis: characterization of bacterial agent, *Am. J. Vet. Res.*, 26, 617, 1965.

55. **Kusch, D. and Siems, H.**, A contribution to the characteristics of staphylococci recovered from swine, *Zentralbl. Bakteriol. Parasitenkd. Infektionskr. Hyg. Abt. 1: Orig. Reihe B*, 159, 95, 1974.

56. **Devriese, L. A. and Oeding, P.**, Coagulase and heat-resistant nuclease producing *Staphylococcus epidermidis* strains from animals, *J. Appl. Bacteriol.*, 39, 197, 1975.

57. **Williams Smith, H.**, Staphylococcal diseases, in *Infectious Diseases of Animals*, Vol. 2, Stableworth, A. W. and Galloway, I. A., Eds., Butterworth, London, 1959, 572.

58. **Benenson, A. S., Ed.**, Staphylococcal disease, in *Control of Communicable Diseases in Man*, 12th ed., American Public Health Association, Washington, D.C., 1975, 298.

59. **Blouse, L. and Meekins, W. E.**, Isolation and use of experimental phages for typing *Staphylococcus aureus* isolates from sentry dogs, *Am. J. Vet. Res.*, 29, 1817, 1968.

60. **Blackmore, D. K. and Francis, R. A.**, The apparent transmission of staphylococci of human origin to laboratory animals, *J. Comp. Pathol.*, 60, 645, 1970.

61. **Blouse, L. E., Brockett, R. M., Homme, P. J., and Jones, E. F.**, Epizootic staphylococcal infections in subhuman primates after surgical operations, *Am. J. Vet. Res.*, 37, 731, 1976.

62. **Hughes, K. L., Haughey, K. G., and Hartley, W. J.**, Perinatal lamb mortality: infections occurring among lambs dying after parturition, *Aust. Vet. J.*, 47, 472, 1971.

63. **Devriese, L. A., Devos, A. H., and Beumer, J.**, *Staphylococcus aureus* colonization on poultry after spray inoculations, *Avian Dis.*, 16, 656, 1972.

64. **Ash, G. W.**, An epidemic of chronic skin ulceration in rats, *Lab. Anim.*, 5, 115, 1971.

65. **Foggie, A.**, Further experimentation on the treatment of tick pyaemia of lambs with antibiotics, *Vet. Rec.*, 66, 690, 1954.

66. **Watson, W. A.**, Studies on the distribution of the sheep tick *(Ixodes ricinus,* L.) and the occurrence of enzootic staphylococcal infection of lambs in north-west Yorkshire and north-east Lancashire, *Vet. Rec.*, 76, 743, 1964.

67. **Watson, W. A., Brown, P. R. M., and Wood, J. C.**, The control of staphylococcal infection (tick pyaemia) in lambs by dipping, *Vet. Rec.*, 79, 101, 1966.

68. **Foster, W. N. M. and Cameron, A. E.**, Observations on ovine strains of tick-borne fever, *J. Comp. Pathol.*, 80, 429, 1970.

69. **Little, R. B. and Plastridge, W. H.**, *Bovine Mastitis, A Symposium*, McGraw-Hill, New York, 1946, 1.

70. **Wilton, J. W., Van Vleck, L. D., Everett, R. W., Guthrie, R. S., and Roberts, S. J.**, Genetic and environmental aspects of udder infections, *J. Dairy Sci.*, 55, 183, 1972.

71. **Kirkbride, C. A. and Erhart, A. B.**, The effect of milking machine function on udder health, *J. Am. Vet. Med. Assoc.*, 155, 1499, 1969.

72. **Wesen, D. P., Luedecke, L. D., and Forster, T. L.**, Relationship between California Mastitis Test reaction and bacteriological analyses of stripping samples, *J. Dairy Sci.*, 51, 679, 1968.

73. **Naidu, T. G. and Newbould, F. H. S.**, Significance of beta-hemolytic *Staph. aureus* as a pathogen to the bovine mammary gland, *Zentralbl. Veterinaermed. Reihe B*, 22, 308, 1975.

74. **Kronvall, G., Holmberg, O., and Ripa, T.,** Protein A in *Staphylococcus aureus* strains of human and bovine origin, *Acta Pathol. Microbiol. Scand. Sect. B,* 80, 735, 1972.

75. **Markham, N. P. and Markham, J. G.,** Staphylococci in man and animals, Distribution and characteristics of strains, *J. Comp. Pathol.,* 76, 49, 1966.

76. **Meyer, W.,** Der Kristallviolett-Test, ein Hilfsmittel zur Auslese von *Staphylococcus-aureus*-Stammen der var. bovis und der Lysogruppe IV, *Z. Gesamte Hyg. Ihre Grenzgeb.,* 12, 907, 1967

77. **Brown, R. W., Sandvik, O., Scherer, R. K., and Rose, D. L.,** Differentiation of strains of *Staphylococcus epidermidis* isolated from bovine udders, *J. Gen. Microbiol.,* 47, 273, 1967.

78. **Meyer, W.,** *Staphylococcus aureus* strains of phage-group IV, *J. Hyg.,* 65, 430, 1967.

79. **Nakagawa, M.,** Studies on bacteriophage typing of staphylococci isolated from bovine milk. III. Typing by means of a new phage set, *Jpn. J. Vet. Res.,* 8, 331, 1960.

80. **Nakagawa, M.,** Studies on bacteriophage typing of staphylococci isolated from bovine milk. II. Some observations on the lysogenic strains, *Jpn. J. Vet. Res.,* 8, 279, 1960.

81. **Frost, A. J.,** Phage typing of *Staphylococcus aureus* from dairy cattle in Australia, *J. Hyg.,* 65, 311, 1967.

82. **Frost, A. J.,** The assessment of a selected set of bacteriophages in the typing of *Staphylococcus aureus* of bovine origin in Australia, *Aust. J. Exp. Biol. Med. Sci.,* 48, 651, 1970.

83. **Thorne, H. and Hallander, H. O.,** Phage typing of *Staphylococcus aureus* from bovine mastitis, A comparison of phages according to Davidson to the conventional phage set, *Acta Pathol. Microbiol. Scand. Sect. B,* 78, 425, 1970.

84. **Matejovska, V. and Bastar, M.,** Occurrence of staphylococci in cases of bovine mastitis, *J. Hyg. Epidemiol. Microbiol. Immunol.,* 13, 90, 1969.

85. **Nyhan, J. F. and Archer, G. T. L.,** Phage types of *Staphylococcus aureus* in herd bulk milk and in quarter samples, *Vet. Rec.,* 81, 202, 1966.

86. **Rose, D. L. and McDonald, J. S.,** Isolation and host range studies of *Staphylococcus epidermidis* and *Micrococcus* spp. bacteriophage, *Am. J. Vet. Res.,* 34, 1973.

87. **Newbould, F. H. S.,** Epizootiology of mastitis due to *Staphylococcus aureus,* *J. Am. Vet. Med. Assoc.,* 153, 1683, 1968.

88. **Reiter, B., Sharpe, M. E., and Higgs, T. M.,** Experimental infection on the non-lactating bovine udder with *Staphylococcus aureus* and *Streptococcus uberis,* *Res. Vet. Sci.,* 19, 18, 1970.

89. **Prasad, L. B. M. and Newbould, F. H. S.,** Inoculation of the bovine teat duct with *Staph. aureus:* the relationship of teat duct length, milk yield and milking rate to development of intramammary infection, *Can. Vet. J.,* 9, 107, 1968.

90. **Chandler, R. L., Lepper, A. W. D., and Wilcox, J.,** Ultrastructural observations on the bovine teat duct, *J. Comp. Pathol.,* 79, 315, 1969.

91. **Harmon, J., Schanbacher, F. L., Ferguson, L. C., and Smith, K. L.,** Concentration of lactoferrin in milk of normal lactating cows and changes occurring during mastitis, *Am. J. Vet. Res.,* 36, 1001, 1975.

92. **Reiter, B. and Oram, J. D.,** Bacterial inhibitors in milk and other biological fluids, *Nature* (London), 216, 328, 1967.

93. **Thomas, C. L., Neave, F. K., Dodd, F. H., and Higgs, T. M.,** The susceptibility of milked and unmilked quarters to intra-mammary infection, *J. Dairy Res.,* 39, 113, 1972.

94. **El Etreby, M. F. and Abdel-Hamid, Y. M.,** Experimental ovine mastitis, a pathologic study, *Pathol. Vet.,* 7, 246, 1970.

95. **Edwards, S. J. and Smith, G. S.,** An experiment to test the value of hygienic measures in the control of staphylococcal infection of the dairy cow, *Br. Vet. J.,* 126, 106, 1970.

96. **Natzke, R. P.,** Therapy: one component in a mastitis control system, *J. Dairy Sci.,* 54, 1895, 1971.

97. **Rosenzuaig, A. and Mayer, E.,** A note on dry cow therapy in an Israeli dairy herd, *Vet. Rec.,* 87, 409, 1970.

98. **Daniel, R. C. W. and Steffert, I. J.,** A comparison of four types of bovine mastitis therapy at drying off, *Aust. Vet. J.,* 45, 530, 1969.

99. **Uvarov, O.,** Drugs against mastitis, *Vet. Rec.,* 88, 674, 1971.

100. **Smith, A., Neave, F. K., Dodd, F. H., and Brander, G. C.,** Methods of reducing the incidence of udder infection in dry cows, *Vet. Rec.,* 79, 233, 1966.

101. **Olsen, C. D.,** United States Public Health Service program for the control of abnormal milk, *J. Am. Vet. Med. Assoc.,* 155, 1978, 1969.

102. **Jasper, D. E.,** Interrelationships of etiologic factors in bovine mastitis, *J. Am. Vet. Med. Assoc.,* 155, 1969, 1969.

103. **White, G.,** An attempt to control the spread of staphylococcal mastitis in two herds by segregation and culling, *Vet. Rec.,* 77, 1384, 1965.

104. **Brander, G. C.,** Dairy herd environment and the control of mastitis, *Vet. Rec.,* 92, 501, 1973.

105. **White, F. and Rattray, E. A. S.**, The role of white cells and frequency of milking in the control of staphylococcal mastitis, *J. Comp. Pathol.*, 77, 143, 1967.

106. **Johnston, K. G., Lepherd, E. E., and Lutz, P.**, Bovine mastitis in the Camden district of New South Wales, *Aust. Vet. J.*, 42, 405, 1966.

107. **Pearson, J. K. L., Greer, D. D., Poole, N., Gordon, F. J., and Acheson, M. D.**, Evaluation of an iodophor teat spray in the control of infections and cellular reactions in the udder, *Vet. Rec.*, 96, 423, 1975.

108. **Forse, S. F., Hall, R., Jackson, P. S., and Sandoe, A. J.**, Evaluation of teat-dipping formulations containing a germicidal polymeric biguanide, *Vet. Rec.*, 86, 506, 1970.

109. **Munch-Petersen, E.**, Incidence of udder infections arising at various stages of lactation of cows, *Aust. Vet. J.*, 44, 543, 1968.

110. **Edwards, S. J. and Smith, G. S.**, An experiment to test the value of hygienic measures in the control of staphylococcal infection of the dairy cow, *Br. Vet. J.*, 126, 106, 1970.

111. **Spooner, R. L. and Miller, J. K.**, The measurement of haemoglobin reactive protein in ruminants as an aid to diagnosis of acute inflammation, *Vet. Rec.*, 88, 2, 1971.

112. **Kroger, D. and Jasper, D. E.**, Relationships between Wisconsin Mastitis Test scores and cell counts in milk, *J. Dairy Sci.*, 50, 1226, 1967.

113. **Raby, C. T., Hubbard, P. L., and Cobbins, R. H.**, Comparison of the California mastitis test, catalase test, and pH readings on quarter milk samples, *J. Dairy Sci.*, 50, 1234, 1967.

114. **Dahl, J. C.**, Mastitis control program in dairyherds, *J. Am. Vet. Med. Assoc.*, 155, 1974, 1969.

115. **Smith, A. R.**, Wisconsin mastitis control program, *J. Am. Vet. Med. Assoc.*, 115, 1982, 1969.

116. **Plommet, M. and LeGall, A.**, Mammite staphylococcique de la brebis. III. Recherches sur l'immunite antitoxique and antimicrobienne, *Ann. Inst. Pasteur*, 104, 770, 1963.

117. **Plommet, M. and LeGall, A.**, Mammite staphylococcique de la brebis. IV. Vaccination locale, *Ann. Inst. Pasteur Paris*, 105, 535, 1963.

118. **Derbyshire, J. B. and Smith, G. S.**, Immunization against experimental staphylococcal mastitis in the goat by the intramammary infusion of cell-toxoid vaccine, *Res. Vet. Sci.*, 10, 559, 1969.

119. **Fujikura, T.**, Studies on experimental mastitis in goats: staphylococcal infection in the mammary glands of experimental goats and a protection test with formalized staphylococcal vaccine, *Natl. Inst. Anim. Health Q.*, 6, 1, 1966.

120. **Singleton, L., Ross, G. W., Stedman, R. A., and Chanter, K. V.**, Immunization with staphylococcal cell walls against mastitis, *J. Comp. Pathol.*, 77, 279, 1967.

121. **McDowell, G. H. and Watson, D. L.**, Immunity to experimental staphylococcal mastitis: comparison of local and systemic immunization, *Aust. Vet. J.*, 50, 533, 1974.

122. **Slanetz, L. W., Bartley, C. H., and Allen, F. E.**, The immunization of dairy cattle against staphylococcal mastitis, *J. Am. Vet. Med. Assoc.*, 134, 155, 1959.

123. **Oehme, F. W. and Coles, E. H.**, Field use and evaluation of a vaccine for bovine staphylococcic mastitis, *J. Dairy Sci.*, 50, 1792, 1967.

124. **Norcross, N. L. and Stark, D. M.**, Immunity to mastitis, a review, *J. Dairy Sci.*, 53, 387, 1970.

125. **Williams, J. M., Mayerhofer, H. J., and Brown, R. W.**, Clinical evaluation of a *Staphylococcus aureus* bacterin (polyvalent somatic antigen), *Vet. Med. Small Anim. Clin.*, 61, 789, 1966.

126. **Williams, J. M., Shipley, G. R., Smith, G. L., and Gerber, D. L.**, A clinical evaluation of *Staphylococcus aureus* bacterin in the control of staphylococcal mastitis in cows, *Vet. Med. Small Anim. Clin.*, 70, 587, 1975.

127. **Greenberg, L.**, Staphylococcus vaccines, *Bull. N.Y. Acad. Med.*, 44, 1222, 1968.

128. **Brock, J. H., Steel, E. D., and Reiter, B.**, The effect of intramuscular and intramammary vaccination of cows on antibody levels and resistance to intramammary infection by *Staphylococcus aureus*, *Res. Vet. Sci.*, 19, 152, 1975.

129. **Willoughby, R. A.**, Bovine staphylococcic mastitis: an immunohistochemical study of the cellular sites of antibody formation, *Am. J. Vet. Res.*, 27, 522, 1966.

130. **Swarbrick, O.**, The use of parental erythromycin in the treatment of bovine mastitis, *Vet. Rec.*, 79, 508, 1966.

131. **Langley, O. H., Meaney, W. J., Cullen, N. P., and Cunningham, J. F.**, The control of mastitis, *Vet. Rec.*, 89, 315, 1971.

132. **Hamdy, A. H., Olds, N. L., and Roberts, B. J.**, Activity of penicillin and novobiocin against mastitis pathogens, *Am. J. Vet. Res.*, 36, 259, 1975.

133. **Devriese, L. A., Van Damme, L. R., and Fameree, L.**, Methicillin (cloxacillin)-resistant *Staphylococcus aureus* strains isolated from bovine mastitis cases, *Zentralbl. Veterinaermed. Reihe B*, 19, 598, 1972.

134. **Devriese, A. and Hommez, J.**, Epidemiology of methicillin-resistant *Staphylococcus aureus* in dairy herds, *Res. Vet. Sci.*, 19, 23, 1975.

135. **Ziv, G., Saran, A., and Schoenberger, E.,** Quinaldofur — a new synthetic drug for treatment of mastitis. I. In vitro characteristics, *Zentralbl. Veterinaermed. Reihe B,* 23, 301, 1976.
136. **Ziv, G. and Saran, A.,** Quinaldofur — a new synthetic drug for the treatment of mastitis. II. Pharmacology, residues, udder irritation and clinical efficacy, *Zentralbl. Veterinaermed. Reihe Med. B,* 23, 310, 1976

STREPTOCOCCOSIS

E. D. Erickson

INTRODUCTION

This chapter considers the zoonotic aspects of streptococcal infections. The volume of printed information on pathogenic streptococci is such that a complete bibliography has not been attempted. Instead, reference is made both to those articles that pertain directly to the zoonotic aspects of the subject and to those that provide further helpful bibliographic sources.* The choice of organizing the paper around Lancefield's serological groupings was prompted by the popularity of this classification and the characteristic host association patterns of organisms in certain groups.

In spite of the abundance of relevant literature, points of taxonomy, pathogenicity, and epizootiology within the various streptococcal groups remain unclear. Reliance on a limited number of standard laboratory tests has caused some errors in identification of isolates that thereby resulted in underestimation of the full prevalence or host range of some beta-hemolytic streptococci. These and other aspects of the ecology of pathogenic streptococci will be discussed in the appropriate sections.

GROUP A

Etiologic Agent

Streptococcus pyogenes, the only species in Lancefield's serogroup A, is predominantly a pathogen of man.[1,2] In addition to the group-specific determinant *N*-acetyl glucosamine, this organism has several cell-wall proteins.[3] Two of these, designated M and T, are used for serotyping, and at least 65 types based on the M protein have been described.[4,5] Recent reviews and monographs have dealt with the bacteriology, pathogenicity, and epidemiology of this streptococcus.[2,6-8]

Hosts

While man is the primary host of group A streptococci, *S. pyogenes* type 50 is rarely a problem in humans. It does produce a naturally occurring infection in commercially reared and wild mice.[9,10] Scattered reports of group A infections in primates and swine are available.[10-12] In the preantibiotic era, the occurrence of epidemic sore throat associated with milk consumption initiated searches for *S. pyogenes* in market milk, and the species was isolated in certain outbreaks.[10]

Distribution

Group A streptococcoses in humans occur throughout most populations of the world.[8] Nutrition, hygiene, and antibiotics have helped to reduce the prevalence, but the acute and chronic forms of group A streptococcal infections still occur.[13] Endemicity of the acute syndrome is difficult to estimate because of variations in description of disease states, methods of detection, and reporting.[8]

Disease in Animals

Spontaneous *S. pyogenes* type 50 infection in reared mice occurs as a chronic contagious lymphadenitis, pneumonia, or bacteremia.[10] In wild mice, swelling of the extremities has led to the name "big foot" for a cellulitis caused by a group A strepto-

* The literature review for this chapter was ended in the fall of 1976.

Table 1
SUPPURATIVE AND NONSUPPURATIVE CLINICAL MANIFESTATIONS OF GROUP A STREPTOCOCCAL INFECTIONS IN MAN[13, 16-18]

Suppurative phase	Nonsuppurative phase
Cervical adenitis	Arthralgia
Empyema	Chorea
Erysipelas	Erythema marginata
Impetigo	Glomerulonephritis
Infections of trauma sites	Rheumatic carditis
Otitis	Subcutaneous nodules
Pectoral abscess	
Perianal cellulitis	
Peritonsillar abscess	
Pharyngitis	
Puerperal fever	
Pneumonia	
Polyarthritis	
Scarlet fever	
Septicemia	

coccus of uncertain type. These foot lesions also occur in type 50-infected mice raised on wire-floored cages.[10]

Group A streptococci have been isolated from a variety of other sources including bovine mastitis.[10,14,15] The occasional infections of captive primates are seen as erysipelas and abscesses.[10,11] Sporadic reports of isolates from swine have been associated with generalized infections, abortions, and endocarditis.[12]

Disease in Man

In man, the variety of clinical manifestations of group A streptococcoses is considerable. Table 1 lists most of these suppurative and nonsuppurative diseases.

Epidemiology

The contagion of group A streptococcal disease is primarily dependent upon direct or close contact.[17] Transfer via inanimate objects is insignificant due to the rapid loss of infectivity following environmental exposure.[19] Pharyngeal infections spread by aerosolized droplets over short distances and vaginal colonization of the mother result in spread by direct contact to the neonate at birth.[13]

Transmission of group A streptococci to animals, when it does occur, is likely from human carriers. Transmission of epidemic streptococcal sore throat by bovine milk represents at least one example of a cyclic transmission pattern in which a milker, acting as a carrier, is the source for udder infection that in turn is the source for pharyngitis in raw milk drinkers.[10,15]

Since close association between carrier and recipient host is required, pharyngitis is most common in close living situations such as military barracks and winter housing. Conversely, impetigo is more frequent during summer months and in warmer climates where exposure of the skin is more frequent.[17] Perpetuation of infections in the community is facilitated by the number of nonsymptomatic cases and carrier individuals.[7] Table 2 gives some indication of the dichotomous nature of the two syndromes.

The attack rates and frequency of poststreptococcal complications in Europe and North America have diminished considerably since the 1920s.[17] Reported prevalence varies with geographical regions, economic status, and the clinical syndrome as it relates to seasons.[17,20-22]

Diagnosis

Determination of the presence and the status of a group A streptococcal infection is achieved by clinical and laboratory examinations coordinated to evaluate the significance of positive and negative results. Laboratory tests rely on the cultural, biochemical, and serological features of the organism and have been reviewed recently.[23] The conventional features of beta-hemolysis, particularly in reduced oxygen, and sensitivity to bacitracin have been supported more diligently in recent years by serogrouping and serotyping.[24-26] These tests have been modified or adapted to utilize such phenomena as coagglutination, immunofluorescence, immunoelectroosmophoresis, and the detection of serum opacity factor.[27-31] Tests that detect antibody specific for cell-wall and extracellular products include the streptozyme, hemagglutination, and complement-fixation tests.[32-36] The extremely sensitive, enzyme-linked immunosorbent assay (ELISA) has been adapted for detecting streptococcal M protein antibodies.[37]

Prevention and Control

Improvement of socioeconomic conditions is the best preventive measure against rheumatic fever and pyoderma-associated nephritis.[17,38,39] Long-acting penicillin is the preferred treatment for acute streptococcal pharyngitis and prevention of subsequent rheumatic fever while erythromycin is recommended in penicillin-sensitive patients.[13] Development of an effective immunizing product has met with problems, but immunity has been demonstrated following use of recently described preparations of M protein.[40]

GROUP B

Etiologic Agent

S. agalactiae, the only species in group B, contains galactose, *N*-acetyl glucosamine, and rhamnose as components of its serogroup determinant.[41] The type-specific antigens have been described for type I (Ia, Ib, Ic) and type III isolates.[42,43] Cultural characteristics include variable degrees of hemolysis on 5% blood agar and a positive CAMP reaction.[44] Hydrolysis of hippurate but not esculin is characteristic of this organism.[45,46] Lactose is fermented by bovine but not human isolates, and bacitracin sensitivity (0.02 unit discs) is common.[47-49]

Hosts

Although *S. agalactiae* is primarily a pathogen of the ruminant mammary gland, it has been isolated with increasing frequency from humans.[14,41,50,51] Group B streptococci have also been isolated from swine, dogs, and other species.[12,48,52,53] The known host range of this and other streptococci may expand as accurate surveillance data from a variety of species become available.

Distribution

World-wide distribution of this streptococcus forms a background for the regional prevalence of certain serotypes.[51,52,54-56] The frequency of isolation of group B streptococci is not well defined. A recent report indicates it may be 1.5% of all streptococcal isolates from the bovine udder.[57] Another author reported *S. agalactiae* was found in 0.4 to 6.9% of all udder samples examined and in 23 to 85% of all streptococcal isolates from the bovine udder.[58] Endemicity rates in humans have been reviewed and vary considerably between reports.[59]

Table 2
CHARACTERISTICS OF THE PHARYNGITIS AND PYODERMA SYNDROMES IN MAN CAUSED BY *STREPTOCOCCUS PYOGENES*

	Characteristic	
Factors	Pharyngitis	Pyoderma
Season	Winter	Summer
Climatic regions	Temperate	Tropical
Sequelae	Rheumatic fever, AGN[a]	AGN
Nephritogenic serotypes	1, 3, 4, 12, 25, 49	2, 31, 49, 52, 55, 56, 59, 60, 61
Latency of AGN	Short	Long
Age	School	Preschool

[a] Acute glomerulonephritis.

From Wannamaker, L. W., *Dis. Mon.*, 10, 3, 1975. With permission.

Disease in Animals

Bovine mastitis is the best known syndrome caused by *S. agalactiae* and occurs as a peracute, acute, or chronic mammary infection.[50] Penetration of the ductular epithelium results in severe edema, inflammation, and cellular infiltration.[60] Acute phase damage is followed by fibrosis in chronic cases, and the resulting milk yield is proportionally reduced. Group B streptococcal mastitis is seldom fatal in cattle but may be in ewes or does.[50] Leukocyte count of the lacteal secretion is elevated during the acute and chronic stages of infection, and this has provided a means of detecting inflammation on a single gland or herd basis.[14] Clinical problems in other domestic species are less noteworthy.[61]

Diease in Man

While there has been evidence for *S. agalactiae* infections in man since 1938, extent of the colonization and infection has only recently been appreciated.[51,62,63] Group B streptococci cause sepsis in neonates, puerperal infections, and a variety of more sporadic clinical syndromes.[51,64] Colonization of adults may be asymptomatic or symptomatic and includes wound, respiratory tract, osseous, and urogenital tract infections.[59,65] Neonates may develop an early- or late-onset septicemia with or without meningitis.[66] The acute stage is typically a respiratory distress syndrome.[67,68] While certain features may distinguish group B infection from hyaline membrane disease, the typical history, clinical signs, and radiographic findings are virtually the same.[67] Hyaline membrane formation is a feature of both, and Gram-positive cocci can be found within this membrane in group B infections.[68] Meningitis may develop subsequent to early-onset septicemias but more commonly follows late-onset infections.[69,70]

Epidemiology

The reservoirs and methods of spread for group B streptococci are being defined more completely. Until recently, the bovine udder was considered to be the only significant source of *S. agalactiae*.[61,71] Milking equipment and dairy personnel are probably the most common vehicles for spread of infection to other cows, and consumption of raw milk may account for transfer to humans.[58] Accumulated evidence now indicates that humans are frequent carriers.[51,71] Colonization of the neonate occurs during delivery through the infected birth canal or by contact with adults or other infected infants in the post-partum period.[59,70] Dissemination between adult humans probably occurs through aerosols and direct contact including sexual activity.[59,73]

In dairy cows, the prevalence of *S. agalactiae* mastitis may be as high as 25% in untreated herds and higher if asymptomatic colonization rates are included.[50] Recent surveys found recovery rates of group B streptococci from bovine milk to be less, which may reflect the use of antibiotics and good dairy management.[50,57,58,74] Serotypes most commonly associated with bovine mastitis are Ia, II, and III.[47,48] They usually ferment lactose and are CAMP-test positive.[47] The ability of *S. agalactiae* to adhere to bovine mammary ductular cells is undoubtedly exploited by the organism in this host-parasite relationship and may be a factor in its colonization and persistence in other species as well.[75-77]

Isolates of group B streptococci from humans are predominantly serotypes Ia, II, and III.[47,48,52] A correlation between serotypes and clinical syndromes exists, showing that Ia is most commonly associated with sepsis, whereas type III is more frequently recovered from blood and cerebrospinal fluid of neonates with late-onset meningitis and sepsis. This distribution is not found uniformly by all researchers and may be due to variations in culture and identification techniques. The apparent higher virulence of Ia isolates may be caused by lack of a particular non-type-specific opsonin in most children.[56] The colonization rates and prevalence of clinically apparent disease vary considerably between reports. Vaginal carrier rates vary from 2.3 to 35.9%, and these women may be concurrent fecal carriers.[59,78] The reported colonization rates of infants born to carrier women range from 12 to greater than 50% of live births.[59] Clinical disease in the neonate may be strongly influenced by the specific immune status of the mother and the maternally derived passive protection it receives.[79] Mortality rates are reported to be 1% or less, but case-fatality rates are much higher.[71,80] High risk factors for neonatal sepsis include low birth weight, prematurity, and prolonged membrane-rupture-to-delivery interval.[51]

Animal reservoirs of this organism have not been considered a threat to human health.[48,51,81,82] A recent study found some biochemical differences between human and bovine isolates, but the serotypes and their frequency of isolation were similar in the two species.[47] It is of interest to note that the human population in this study was mainly university students, who may have represented a variety of racial, national, and even international communities. While certain differences can be found in group B streptococci from these two sources, the potential for transmission is suggested by the fact that (1) human isolates can produce bovine mastitis and (2) raw-milk consumers have a high colonization rate.[48,58] It is likely that the organism has become established in and has adapted to these separate hosts, persistence within each being independent of the other; nevertheless, the potential for cross infection remains. Continued examination of epidemiological aspects of the infection, including the potential for venereal transmission, seems imperative.

Diagnosis

Diagnostic techniques for group B streptococci were included in the previously cited review.[23] Isolations can be maximized by addition of selective enrichment broths.[78] Blood agar containing esculin and ferric chloride is also useful in dairy bacteriology for isolation and identification of *S. agalactiae*.[46] Serological classification using a monospecific group antiserum is the method of final identification, but hippurate hydrolysis and CAMP reaction are used more frequently for presumptive identification.[25,44,45,83]

Prevention and Control

Group B streptococcal infections were a major concern to the dairy industry and veterinarians long before the current level of interest in human infections. Bovine infections have been the focus of attack for mastitis control programs that have sought to reduce the level of infection and increase dairy milk production through improved milking hygiene and antibiotic therapy.[74] In recently infected glands, penicillin continues to be effective in eliminating infection.[84]

Concentrated attention has only recently been given to human infections with *S. agalactiae,* and control programs are not well established. Continued acquisition of epidemiological data is required to accurately define reservoirs, carriers, and colonization rates. Standardization of laboratory tests and sampling procedures would expedite this task. The immediate need is for routine, accurate, and rapid identification of carrier women in the immediate pre-partum and parturition stages when known predisposing factors are present.[51] Similarly, the predisposition of immunologically deficient children requires that rapid analysis of specific immunity be available.[56,79] More bacteriological and immunological data would provide much needed information for management of the disease in both animals and man.

GROUP C

Etiologic Agent

Four recognized streptococcal species carry the unifying cell-wall determinant *N*-acetyl galactosamine.[3] These organisms are pathogens of a variety of animal species and man. Cultural, serological, and epidemiological features serve as the basis for species differentiation.[61,85,86] Trypsin-labile cell-wall antigens are responsible for type specificity; based on this, *S. equi, S. dysgalactiae, S. equisimilis,* and *S. zooepidemicus* have 1, 2, 4, and 15 serotypes, respectively.[88,91] The role of the M protein-like antigen in development of type-specific immune protection has been confirmed, at least for *S. equi* and *S. equisimulis.*[88,90,92] A hyaluronic acid capsule was identified in early studies of some beta-hemolytic streptococci and, in the case of *S. equi,* it was recently described in detail.[93,94] As a result, most isolates of *S. equi* develop large mucoid colonies, but atypical colony varieties have been described.[95]

Hosts

The host range of group C streptococci is considerable and varies among members of the species. *S. equi* is restricted to equids; reports of isolations from man lack confirming evidence.[96-98] *S. dysgalactiae* is a pathogen of the ruminant mammary gland although reports of infection in other animals are available.[14,99] The remaining species of this group have multiple hosts. *S. equisimilis* is primarily isolated from pigs and man,[12,25] and *S. zooepidemicus* is probably the most frequent streptococcal isolate from horses but has also been found in sheep, pigs, cattle, guinea pigs, and man.[12,89,101-103]

Distribution

Group C streptococcal infection in man and animals has been reported from most latitudes and geographical areas.[8,87,104,105] Current levels of endemicity in man or animals are not well defined.

Diseases in Animals
Swine

The majority of the streptococci isolated from swine are Lancefield's group C, and of these *S. equisimilis* is the most common.[106,107] It may be associated with a variety of clinico-pathological conditions including meningitis, septicemia, pneumonia, endocarditis, arthritis, mastitis, endometritis, and other suppurative lesions.[12,108]

Table 3
CULTURAL CHARACTERISTICS OF GROUP C STREPTOCOCCI[1,61]

Species	Hemolysis	Fermentation		
		Lactose	Trehalose	Sorbitol
S. dysgalactiae	v[a]	v	+	v
S. equi	Beta	−	−	−
S. equisimilis	Beta	v	+	−
S. zooepidemicus	Beta	v	−	+

[a] Variable.

Isolations of *S. zooepidemicus* and *S. dysgalactiae* have also been made from swine. These were found either on routine bacteriological surveys or associated with a variety of suppurative conditions such as endocarditis, encephalitis, and pneumonia.[12,99]

Ruminants

S. dysgalactiae is a cause of bovine mastitis.[14] *S. zooepidemicus* and *S. equisimilis* have also been isolated from clinical mastitis, respiratory disease, and metritis.[86,89,103,107] *S. zooepidemicus* infection of lambs causes acute sepsis, pneumonia, polyserositis, and death.[101]

Horses

Beta-hemolytic streptococci are the most frequent bacterial isolates from horses.[109] Infections of the respiratory and genital tracts predominate, but abscesses, wound infections, and neonatal septicemias also occur.[50,61] *S. equi* is the cause of strangles, a suppurative lymphadenopathy primarily affecting the equine head and neck.[110] Urogenital infections and respiratory infections other than strangles commonly yield *S. zooepidemicus*.[111-114] Reports of *S. equisimilis* isolations from horses are rare.[85,86]

Other Species

S. equisimilis is a frequent group C isolate from the respiratory and urogenital tracts of dogs and cats[107,115] and has also been found in enzootic streptococcal infections of poultry.[116] Colonies of laboratory guinea pigs frequently harbor *S. zooepidemicus*, and the resulting enzootics of cervical lymphadenitis are common.[93,102,103,117,118] Myocarditis and polyserositis of guinea pigs have also been associated with this infection.[119,120]

Diseases in Man

Group C streptococci are not considered highly virulent pathogens for man; nevertheless, several reported isolations of members of this group are available.[25,49,73,81,96-98,103-105,121-128]

An early report of group C infections recorded isolations from patients with wounds, septicemias, and empyema,[122] and a recent review and report of group C streptococcal endocarditis lists four previous cases.[98] Arteriosclerotic aneurysm of the abdominal aorta secondarily infected with a group C streptococcus has also been reported.[123] Glomerulonephritis following an epidemic of milk-borne *S. zooepidemicus* infection indicates that at least some group C organism may be capable of initiating nonsuppurative sequelae.[103] The possibility of nongroup A streptococci playing a significant role in postinfection glomerulonephritis has been considered.[104,128]

Epidemiology

S. equi can be dispensed with as a zoonotic problem, but the rest of the group C species have multiple hosts with a potential for transmission to humans. *S. dysgalactiae* may cause infections other than bovine mastitis, but the epidemiology of these infections has not been described.

S. equisimilis is a frequent isolate from swine and humans. Carrier sows are probably the most significant source of infection for young pigs. However, a more complete epidemiological picture is dependent upon a study of the distribution of particular serotypes.[90,106] Existing evidence indicates that swine and human isolates are of different serotypes.[90]

S. zooepidemicus has the broadest host range of the group C streptococci and perhaps the greatest capacity for interspecies transmission. The frequency with which the bacterium may be isolated from equine tonsils and cervicovaginal mucosa is indicative of the capacity of horses to act as reservoirs of infection.[100,111,114] It is not known whether they are sources of infection for other species. There is evidence that bovine mastitis may be the source of *S. zooepidemicus* infection in epidemics of human pharyngitis;[103] the organism was isolated from dairymen, milk samples, and throat swabs of consumers.[103] While bacitracin sensitivity has been a useful screening procedure, its specificity is such as to allow the misidentification of some nongroup A organisms.[49] As methods of group, species, and serotype identification are utilized more extensively, epidemiological patterns such as this may be realized more frequently.

There is a tendency for some investigators to assume a certain homogeneity within a serological group when referring to diseases in man and animals caused by group members.[98,129] To suggest that some group C streptococci cause strangles in horses and have been isolated from a variety of suppurative infections in man overlooks the fact that *S. equi* infects equids only and *S. equisimilis,* the most frequent isolate from humans, is seldom associated with disease in horses. Even the same species of streptococcus, identified in divergent locations, may consist of different serotypes, the antigenic nature of which directly influences their ability to colonize and invade the respective host.[75,130,131]

Diagnosis

Laboratory procedures reviewed recently are applicable to the identification of members of this group.[23] The fermentation reactions in trehalose, sorbitol, and lactose in addition to a serogroup C specific reaction are the basis for classifying equine isolates.[87] Additional sources for identification procedures are readily available.[1,46,57,61]

Prevention and Control

Few effective prevention and control measures relate directly to group C streptococcal infections in man or animals. Most isolates are quite sensitive to penicillin and other common antibiotics.

OTHER STREPTOCOCCI

The remaining streptococci of medical interest are less well classified but contain organisms that have been isolated from suppurative lesions of man, animals, or both. With one or two notable exceptions, the zoonotic aspects of these infections are not defined, but the apparent potential for transmission would seem to justify their inclusion in this survey.

Group D

Group D streptococci include *S. faecalis* and enterococci indigenous to the human digestive tract.[1,13,132] *S. bovis* and *S. equinus,* common to the digestive tract of their respective animal hosts, are considered nonenterococcal streptococci when isolated from humans.[13] The distinction has considerable significance in that nonenterococcal group D streptococci are presently much more responsive to routine antibiotic therapy, yet both enterococci and nonenterococci are the predominant isolates from endocarditis and meningitis lesions as well as urogenital tract colonizations in humans.[49,73,133,134]

A particular isolate from piglets in England gains access through the palatine tonsils and causes epidemic arthritis and meningitis.[135-137] There appears to be some confusion in the serological classification of these isolates and others from The Netherlands; however, the species name *S. suis,* containing two serotypes, has been recognized provisionally.[1,12,137] A report of canine urolithiasis indicates that group D streptococci may be associated with the development of this syndrome.[138]

Group E

Organisms belonging to Lancefield's group E have been obtained from bovine mastitis and porcine jowl abscesses.[12,25,139] *S. mutans* type e, one of the viridan streptococci that is cariogenic in man and laboratory animals, cross-reacts with group E antisera.[129] Zoonotic relationships between group E infections in man and animals have not been considered. Swine isolates colonize the tonsilar tissue and persist there in carrier animals, while the human cariogenic type is resident in the human oral cavity, particularly on the teeth.[131,140]

Group F

Humans, pigs, monkeys, and guinea pigs have been the source of serogroup F streptococci.[141-144] The species name *S. anginosus* is used in reference to this group, but members are quite heterogeneous with regard to source and cultural characteristics.[141,145] In man, group F streptococci have been isolated from suppurative foci in various locations including postoperative abdominal sites, the perineum, respiratory tract, and meninges.[97,133,141,145-147] No reports of significant disease problems in animals associated with group F streptococci are available.

Group G

Members of group G streptococci are without species names although *S. anginosus* has been used to designate serotype I isolates.[1,148] The confusion immediately arises with group F organisms bearing the same name.[1] While these bacteria have a group-specific cell-wall determinant, there is a potential for cross-reaction with serogroup B due to chemical similarities in the carbohydrate complex.[149] Cross-reactions have also been found between group G isolates from humans in Trinidad and type 12 M protein of *S. pyogenes* (group A).[150] Both of these cross reactivities can be a source of confusion in differentiating beta-hemolytic streptococcosis for purposes of therapy and epidemiological study.

Sources of isolates of group G streptococci include neonatal sepsis, endocarditis, and pharyngitis in man.[81,148,151] In animals, group G streptococci have been isolated from cases of bovine mastitis,[152,153] necrotic dermatitis of laboratory mice, and routine culturing of the throat and urogenital tracts, as well as suppurative lesions of dogs.[115,152-155]

Groups H and K

Streptococci belonging to groups H and K are infrequent isolates from animals.[142] In humans, they have been found associated with cases of septicemia, endocarditis, and other deep suppurative lesions.[122,128] A series of cases of pericarditis was the source of group K isolates.[97]

Groups L and M

These serogroups have been isolated from a variety of sources. Group L isolates from pigs have been associated with septicemias, arthritis, meningitis, and endocarditis.[12,156,157] They may also cause bovine mastitis, and some authors suspect that one source for udder infections may be infected swine.[157,158] The dog is a frequently cited host.[61,128] Cultures from humans have also yielded group L streptococci in association with infectious disease processes.[125,159] One reported case, involving a wound acquired while handling pork and other meats, may be an example of the zoonotic potential of some members of this group.[128]

Group M streptococci are commonly thought of as canine streptococci, but they have also been isolated from cattle, swine, and sheep.[61,142] In humans, isolations from cases of respiratory disease, endocarditis, and surgical wounds are on record.[125,159]

Groups N, O, P, and Q

Reports of isolates belonging to these groups are available, but there are insufficient data to determine their host range and epidemiological patterns.[12,125,128,159]

Groups R, S, T, U, and V

Streptococci in these groups have not stimulated a great deal of medical interest. The exception, members of group R, may be the best example of a zoonotic streptococcal infection.[160] Beta-hemolytic streptococci were implicated in meningitis and septicemia of pigs in England. From a similar syndrome in The Netherlands, streptococci were isolated that were classified in groups R, S, and T.[161,162] The serological relationship between these isolates and those from outbreaks in Britain have been reviewed.[137] Within the last 10 years, several cases of group R streptococcal meningitis and septicemia in humans have been described.[160,163-165] Almost all cases of group R streptococcosis have been in swine raisers or meat handlers, in whom wound contamination was a common finding.[163] Major source of the remaining serogroups has been swine with septicemia and lymphadenopathy.[162,166] With examples such as this, the medical community should be encouraged to identify streptococci of potential zoonotic interest.

Nongroupable Streptococci

Nongroupable streptococci are included in surveys of streptococcal isolates from man and animals. Whether they represent mutable forms of classified streptococci or serologically undefined pathogens is unclear. Their role in zoonoses is, therefore, even more obscure.   One of these, *S. pneumoniae* (*Diplococcus pneumoniae*), is an extensively studied pathogen of man.[2] Respiratory disease, otitis media, and other suppurative lesions from which it is isolated continue to occur.[167] In animals, *S. pneumoniae* has been isolated from cases of pneumonia and mastitis in ruminants.[168] Guinea pigs and other laboratory animals may carry virulent pneumococci and suffer from fibrinopurulent infections of the lungs and serosal surfaces caused by this organism.[117] The source of these infections and, in turn, the potential for transmission to other species (including man) have not been defined.

Bacteriologists, encouraged to search for anaerobic pathogens, have located *Peptostreptococcus* species in a variety of deep suppurative lesions.[1] The epidemiological and zoonotic aspects of these infections are unknown.

SUMMARY

A vast amount of information about pathogenic streptococci has been acquired, and yet relevant epidemiological information, except in selected cases, is limited. Wherever this information is available, it has been acquired by accurate bacteriological and serological identifications. Such is the case in group A streptococcoses of humans, as well as septicemia and meningitis syndromes caused by members of Lancefield's group B and R streptococci. Clinical and laboratory personnel in all branches of medicine should be encouraged to continue their efforts toward the furthering of descriptions of streptococcal diseases.

REFERENCES

1. **Buchanan, R. E. and Gibbons, N. E.,** *Bergey's Manual of Determinative Bacteriology*, 8th ed., Williams & Wilkins, Baltimore, 1974, 490.
2. **Wilson, G. S. and Miles, A.,** The streptococci, in *Topley and Wilson's Principles of Bacteriology and Immunity*, Vol. 1, 6th ed., Williams & Wilkins, Baltimore, 1975, 712.
3. **Krause, R. M.,** The streptococcal cell: relationship of structure to function and pathogenesis, in *Streptococci and Streptococcal Diseases*, Wannamaker, L. W. and Matsen, J. M., Eds., Academic Press, New York, 1972, 4.
4. **Dillon, H. C., Jr., Derrick, C. W., and Gooch, P. E.,** A new M-type of group A streptococcus of clinical importance in pyoderma and pharyngitis, *J. Gen. Microbiol.*, 91, 119, 1975.
5. **Ludwicka, A.,** T antigen of *Streptococcus pyogenes:* isolation and purification, *Infect. Immun.*, 13, 993, 1976.
6. **Heymer, B.,** Pathogenitatsfaktoren β-hamolysierender streptokokken, *Zentralbl. Bakteriol. Parasitenkd. Infektionskr. Hyg. Abt. 1: Orig. Reihe A*, 227, 150, 1974.
7. **Wannamaker, L. W.,** The streptococcal siren, *Infect. Dis. Rev.*, 3, 167, 1974.
8. **Haverkorn, M. J., Valkenberg, H. A., and Goslings, W. R. O.,** Epidemiology of streptococcal acquisition, in *Streptococci Disease and the Community*, Haverkorn, M. J., Ed., Excerpta Medica, Amsterdam, 1974, 227.
9. **Wildfeuer, A., Heymer, B., Schachenmayr, W., and Haferkamp, O.,** Morphological and immunological characteristics of *Streptococcus pyogenes*, group A, type 50, *Med. Microbiol. Immunol.*, 161, 193, 1975.
10. **Lancefield, R. C.,** Group A streptococcal infections in animals — natural and experimental, in *Streptococci and Streptococcal Diseases*, Wannamaker, L. W. and Matson, J. M., Eds., Academic Press, New York, 1972, 313.
11. **Krushak, D. H., Zimmerman, R. A., and Murphy, B. L.,** Induced group A beta-hemolytic streptotocci infection in chimpanzees, *J. Am. Vet. Med. Assoc.*, 157, 742, 1970.
12. **Shuman, Richard D. and Ross, R. F.,** Streptococcosis, in *Diseases of Swine*, 4th ed., Dunne, H. W. and Leman, A. D., Eds., Iowa State University Press, Ames, 1975, 630.
13. **Wannamaker, L. W.,** Streptococcal infections — updated, *Dis. Mon.*, 10, 3, 1975.
14. **Schalm, O. W., Carroll, E. J., and Jain, N. C.,** *Bovine Mastitis*, Lea & Febiger, Philadelphia, 1971,128.
15. **Brown, J. H.,** The streptococci of milk with special references to human health, *Cornell Vet.*, 23, 110, 1933.
16. **Stollerman, G. H.,** Streptococcal diseases, in *Textbook of Medicine*, 4th ed., Beeson, P. B. and McDermott, W., Eds., W. B. Saunders, Philadelphia, 1975, 290.
17. **Stollerman, G. H.,** *Rheumatic Fever and Streptococcal Infection*, Grune & Stratton, New York, 1975.
18. **Amren, D. P.,** Unusual forms of streptococcal disease, in *Streptococci and Streptococcal Diseases*, Wannamaker, L. W. and Matsen, J. M., Eds., Academic Press, New York, 1972, 545.
19. **Srisuparbh, K. and Sawyer, W. D.,** Effect of exposure to the atmosphere on the infectivity of group A streptococci, *Infect. Immun.*, 5, 176, 1972.
20. **Zimmerman, R. A., Bender, J. S., Edelen, J. S., and Knostman, J. D.,** Streptococcal surveillance and control in Alaskan natives, in *Streptococcal Disease and the Community*, Haverkorn, M. J., Ed., Exerpta Medica, Amsterdam, 1974, 189.

21. **Kaplan, E. L.,** Unresolved problems in diagnosis and epidemiology of streptococcal infection, in *Streptococci and Streptococcal Diseases,* Wannamaker, L. W. and Matsen, J. M., Eds., Academic Press, New York, 1972, 558.

22. **Dillon, H. C., Jr. and Derrick, C. W., Jr.,** Recent studies of streptococcal skin and throat infections in Alabama, in *Streptococci Disease and the Community,* Haverkorn, M. J., Ed., Excerpta Medica, Amsterdam, 1974, 226.

23. **Facklam, R. R.,** A review of the microbiological techniques for the isolation and identification of streptococci, *CRC Crit. Rev. Clin. Lab. Sci.,* 6(4), 287, 1975.

24. **Murray, P. R., Wold, A. D., Schreck, C. A., and Washington, J. A.,** Effects of selective media and atmosphere of incubation on the isolation of group A streptococci, *J. Clin. Microbiol.,* 4, 54, 1976.

25. **Lancefield, R. C.,** A serological differentiation of human and other groups of hemolytic streptococci, *J. Exp. Med.,* 57, 571, 1933.

26. **Lancefield, R. C.,** The antigenic complex of *Streptococcus hemolyticus.* I. Demonstration of a type-specific substance in extracts of *Streptococcus hemolyticus, J. Exp. Med.,* 47, 91, 1928.

27. **Maxted, W. R. and Widdowson, J. P.,** The protein antigens of group A streptococci, in *Streptococci and Streptococcal Diseases,* Wannamaker, L. W. and Matsen, J. M., Eds., Academic Press, New York, 1972, 251.

28. **Christensen, P.,** Agglutinability of some selected streptococci by immune complexes, *Acta Pathol. Microbiol. Scand. Sect. B,* 83, 28, 1975.

29. **Edwards, E. A. and Larson, G. L.,** New method of grouping beta-hemolytic streptococci directly on sheep blood agar plates by coagglutination of specifically sensitized protein A-containing staphylococci, *Appl. Microbiol.,* 28, 972, 1974.

30. **Cars, O., Forsum, U., and Hjelm, E.,** New immunofluorescence method for the identification of group A, B, C, E, F, and G streptococci, *Acta Pathol. Microbiol. Scand. Sect. B,* 83, 148, 1975.

31. **Wadstrom, T., Nord, C. E., Lindberg, A. A., and Mollby, R.,** Rapid grouping of streptococci

32. **Bisno, A. L. and Ofek, I.,** Serologic diagnosis of streptococcal infection, *Am. J. Dis. Child.,* 127, 676, 1974.

33. **Berger-Rabinowitz, S., Fleiderman, S., Ferne, M., Rabinowitz, K., and Ginsberg, I.,** The new streptozyme test for streptococcal antibodies, *Clin. Pediatr.* (Philadelphia), 14, 804, 1975.

34. **El Kholy, A., Hafez, K., and Krause, R. M.,** Specificity and sensitivity of the streptozyme test for the detection of streptococcal antibodies, *Appl. Microbiol.,* 27, 748, 1974.

35. **Beachey, E. H., Ofek, I., and Bisno, A. L.,** Studies of antibodies to non-type-specific antigens associated with streptococcal M protein in the sera of patients with rheumatic fever, *J. Immunol.,* 111, 1361, 1973.

36. **Wittner, M. K. and Fox, E. N.,** Micro complement fixation assay for type-specific group A streptococcal antibody, *Infect. Immun.,* 4, 441, 1971.

37. **Russell, H., Facklam, R. R., and Edwards, L. R.,** Enzyme-linked immunosorbent assay for streptococcal M protein antibodies, *J. Clin. Microbiol.,* 3, 501, 1976.

38. **Gordis, L. and Markowitz, M.,** Environmental determinants in rheumatic fever prevention, in *Streptococci and Streptococcal Diseases,* Wannamaker, L. W. and Matsen, J. M., Eds., Academic Press, New York, 1972, 572.

39. **Dillon, H. C.,** Streptococcal infections of the skin and their complication: impetigo and nephritis, in *Streptococci and Streptococcal Diseases,* Wannamaker, L. W. and Matsen, J. M., Eds., Academic Press, New York, 1972, 572.

40. **Fox, E. M.,** M proteins of group A streptococci, *Bacteriol. Rev.,* 38, 57, 1974.

41. **Lancefield, R. C.,** Cellular antigens of group B streptococci, in *Streptococci and Streptococcal Diseases,* Wannamaker, L. W. and Matsen, J. M., Eds., Academic Press, New York, 1972, 57.

42. **Wilkinson, H. W.,** Immunochemistry of purified polysaccharide type antigens of group B streptococcal type Ia, Ib, and Ic, *Infect. Immun.,* 11, 845, 1976.

43. **Russell, H. and Norcross, N. L.,** The isolation and some physiochemical and biologic properties of the type III antigen of group B streptococci, *J. Immunol.,* 109, 90, 1972.

44. **Darling, C. L.,** Standardization and evaluation of the CAMP reaction for the prompt, presumptive identification of *Streptococcus agalactiae* (Lancefield Group B) in clinical material, *J. Clin. Microbiol.,* 1, 171, 1975.

45. **Edberg, S. C. and Samuels, S.,** Rapid, colorimetric test for the determination of hippurate hydrolysis by group B streptococcus, *J. Clin. Microbiol.,* 3, 49, 1976.

46. **Brown, R. W., Morse, G. E., Newbould, F. H. S., and Slantez, L. W.,** *Microbiological Procedures for the Diagnosis of Bovine Mastitis,* National Mastitis Council, University of New Hampshire Press, Durham, 1969, 10.

47. **Norcross, N. L.,** The distribution and characterization of group B streptococci in New York State, *Cornell Vet.,* 66, 240, 1976.
48. **Butter, M. N. W. and de Moor, C. E.,** *Streptococcus agalactiae* as a cause of meningitis in the newborn, and of bacteraemia in adults, *Antonie van Leeuwenhoek J. Microbiol. Serol.,* 33, 439, 1967.
49. **Feingold, M. D., Stagg, N. L., and Kunz, L. J.,** Extrarespiratory streptococcal infections, *N. Engl. J. Med.,* 275, 356, 1966.
50. **Blood, D. C. and Henderson, J. A.,** *Veterinary Medicine,* 4th ed., Bailliere Tindall, London, 1974, 257.
51. **Eickhoff, T. C.,** Group B streptococci in human infection, in *Streptococci and Streptococcal Diseases,* Wannamaker, L. W. and Matsen, J. M., Eds., Academic Press, New York, 1972, 533.
52. **Wilkinson, H. W., Facklam, R. R., and Wortham, E. C.,** Distribution by serological type of group B streptococci isolated from a variety of clinical material over a five-year period (with special reference to neonatal sepsis and meningitis), *Infect. Immun.,* 8, 228, 1973.
53. **Riising, H. J.,** Streptococcal infections in pigs. I. Serological and biochemical examinations, *Nord. Veterinaermed.,* 28, 80, 1976.
54. **Dodd, F. H., Griffin, T. K., and Kingwill, R. G., Eds.,** *Proc. Seminar on Mastitis Control,* International Dairy Federation, Reading, England, 1975.
55. **Jelinkova, J., Rotta, J., and Duben, J.,** Long-term study of the prevalence of different groups of streptococci in the general population, in *Streptococcal Disease and the Community,* Haverkorn, M. J., Ed., Excerpta Medica, Amsterdam, 1974, 198.
56. **Mathews, J. H., Klesius, P. H., and Zimmerman, R. A.,** Opsonin system of the group B streptococci, *Infect. Immun.,* 10, 1315, 1974.
57. **McDonald, T. J.,** Streptococci isolated from bovine intramammary infections, *Am. J. Vet. Res.,* 37, 377, 1976.
58. **Tolle, A.,** Mastitis — the disease in relation to control methods, in *Proc. Seminar on Mastitis Control,* Dodd, F. H., Griffin, T. K., and Kingwill, R. G., Eds., International Dairy Federation, Reading, England, 1975, 3.
59. **Patterson, M. J. and Hafeez, A. E. B.,** Group B streptococci in human disease, *Bacteriol. Rev.,* 40, 774, 1976.
60. **Jubb, K. V. F. and Kennedy, P. C.,** *Pathology of Domestic Animals,* 2nd ed., Academic Press, New York, 1970, 552.
61. **Bruner, D. W. and Gillespie, J. H.,** *Hagan's Infectious Diseases of Domestic Animals,* 6th ed., Cornell University Press, Ithaca, N.Y., 1973, 283.
62. **Fry, R. M.,** Fatal infections by haemolytic streptococcus group B, *Lancet,* 1, 199, 1938.
63. **Finn, P. D. and Holden, F. A.,** Observations and comments concerning the isolation of group B β-hemolytic streptococci from human sources, *Can. Med. Assoc. J.,* 103, 249, 1970.
64. **Howard, J. B. and McCracken, G. H., Jr.,** The spectrum of group B streptococcal infections in infancy, *Am. J. Dis. Child.,* 128, 815, 1974.
65. **Hutto, J. H. and Ayoub, E. M.,** Streptococcal osteomyelitis and arthritis in a neonate, *Am. J. Dis. Child.,* 129, 1449, 1975.
66. **Hood, J., Janney, A., and Dameron, G.,** Beta-hemolytic streptococcus group B associated with problems of the perinatal period, *Am. J. Obstet. Gynecol.,* 82, 809, 1961.
67. **Ablow, R. C., Driscoll, G., Effmann, E. L., Gross, I., Jolles, C. J., Uauy, R., and Warshaw, J. B.,** A comparison of early-onset group B streptococcal neonatal infection and the respiratory-distress syndrome of the newborn, *N. Engl. J. Med.,* 294, 65, 1976.
68. **Katzenstein, A., Davis, C., and Braude, A.,** Pulmonary changes in neonatal sepsis due to group B β-hemolytic streptococcus: relation to hyaline membrane disease, *J. Infect. Dis.,* 4, 430, 1976.
69. **Wilkinson, H. W.,** Radioimmunoassay for measuring antibody specific for group B streptococcal types Ia, Ib, Ic, II and III, *J. Clin. Microbiol.,* 3, 480, 1976.
70. **Baker, C. J. and Barrett, F. F.,** Group B streptococcal infections in infants, *JAMA,* 230, 1158, 1974.
71. **Reid, R. M. S.,** Emergence of group B streptococci in obstetric and perinatal infections, *Br. Med. J.,* 2, 533, 1975.
72. **Hemming, V. G., Overall, J. C., and Britt, M. R.,** Nosocomial infections in a newborn intensive-care unit, *N. Engl. J. Med.,* 294, 1310, 1976.
73. **Christensen, K. K., Christensen, P., Flamholc, L., and Ripa, T.,** Frequencies of streptococci of groups A, B, C, D, and G in uretha and cervix swab specimens from patients with suspected gonococcal infection, *Acta Pathol. Microbiol. Scand. Sect. B,* 82, 470, 1974.
74. **Kingwill, R. G., Neave, F. K., Dodd, F. H., Griffin, T. K., and Westgarth, D. R.,** The effect of mastitis control system on levels of subclinical and clinical mastitis in two years, *Vet. Rec.,* 87, 94, 1970.

75. **Frost, A. J.,** Selective adhesion of microorganisms to the ductular epithelium of the bovine mammary gland, *Infect. Immun.,* 12, 1154, 1975.
76. **Furatado, D.,** Experimental group B streptococcal infections in mice: heterogenous virulence and mucosal colonization, *Infect. Immun.,* 13, 1315, 1976.
77. **Mardh, P. A. and Westrom, L.,** Adherence of bacteria to vaginal epithelial cells, *Infect. Immun.,* 13, 661, 1976.
78. **Baker, C. J., Goroff, D. K., Alpert, S. L., Hayes, C., and McCormack, W. M.,** Comparison of bacteriological methods for the isolation of group B streptococcus from vaginal cultures, *J. Clin. Microbiol.,* 4, 46, 1976.
79. **Baker, C. J. and Kasper, D. L.,** Correlation of material antibody deficiency with susceptibility to neonatal group B streptococcal infection, *N. Engl. J. Med.,* 294, 753, 1976.
80. **Franciosi, R. A., Knostman, J. D., and Zimmerman, R. A.,** Group B streptococcal neonatal and infant infections, *J. Pediatr.,* 82, 707, 1973.
81. **Simmons, R. T. and Keogh, E. V.,** Physiological characters and serological types of haemolytic streptococci of groups B, C and G from human sources, *Aust. J. Exp. Biol. Med. Sci.,* 18, 151, 1940.
82. **El Ghoroury, A. A.,** Comparative studies of group B streptococci of human and bovine origin: serological characters, *Am. J. Public Health,* 40, 1278, 1950.
83. **Facklam, R. R., Padula, J. F., Thacker, L. G., Wortham, E. C., and Sconyers, B. J.,** Presumptive identification of group A, B and D streptococci, *Appl. Microbiol.,* 27, 207, 1974.
84. **McDonald, J. S., McDonald, T. J., and Stark, D. R.,** Antibiograms of streptococci isolated from bovine intramammary infections, *Am. J. Vet. Res.,* 37, 1185, 1976.
85. **Dimock, W. W. and Edwards, P. R.,** Hemolytic streptococci of horses and other animals, and their relation to the streptococci of man, *K. Agric. Exp. Stn. Bull.,* 338, 25, 1933.
86. **Edwards, P. R.,** The differentiation of hemolytic streptococci of human and animal origin by group precipitan tests, *J. Bacteriol.,* 27, 527, 1934.
87. **Bazeley, P. L. and Battle, J.,** Studies with equine streptococci. I. A survey of beta-hemolytic streptococci in equine infections, *Aust. Vet. J.,* 16, 140, 1940.
88. **Woolcock, J. B.,** Purification and antigenicity of an M-like protein of *Streptococcus equi, Infect. Immun.,* 10, 116, 1974.
89. **Bakshi, S. N. and Singh, C. M.,** Antigenic relationship between mastitis streptococci belonging to group-C, *J. Comp. Pathol.,* 74, 398, 1974.
90. **Khan, M. W. and Ross, R. F.,** Antigenic type-specificity of swine isolates of *Streptococcus equisimilis, Can. J. Comp. Med.,* 36, 256, 1972.
91. **Moore, B. O. and Bryand, J. T.,** Type-specific antigenicity of group C streptococci from diseases of the horse, in *Proc. 2nd Int. Conf. Equine Infect. Dis.* S. Karger, New York, 1970, 231.
92. **Erickson, E. D. and Norcross, N. L.,** The cell surface antigens of *Streptococcus equi, Can. J. Comp. Med.,* 39, 110, 1975.
93. **Seastone, C. V.,** Hemolytic streptococcus lymphadenitis in guinea pigs, *J. Exp. Med.,* 70, 347, 1939.
94. **Woolcock, J. B.,** The capsule of *Streptococcus equi, J. Gen. Microbiol.,* 85, 372, 1974.
95. **Woolcock, J. B.,** Studies in atypical *Streptococcus equi, Res. Vet. Sci.,* 19, 115, 1975.
96. **Drusin, L. M., Ribble, J. C., and Topf, B.,** Group C streptococcal colonization in a newborn nursery, *Am. J. Dis. Child.,* 125, 820, 1973.
97. **Braunstein, H., Tucker, E., and Gibson, B. C.,** Infections caused by unusual beta-hemolytic streptococci, *Am. J. Clin. Pathol.,* 55, 424, 1971.
98. **Finnegan, P., Fitzgerald, M. X. M., Cumming, G., and Geddes, A. M.,** Lancefield group C streptococcal endocarditis, *Thorax,* 29, 245, 1974.
99. **Solberg, I.,** *Streptococcus dysgalactiae:* a possible disease producing agent in various animal species, *Nord. Veterinaermed.,* 20, 26, 1968.
100. **Woolcock, J. B.,** Epidemiology of equine streptococci, *Res. Vet. Sci.,* 18, 113, 1975.
101. **Stevenson, R. G.,** *Streptococcus zooepidemicus* infection in sheep, *Can. J. Comp. Med.,* 38, 243, 1974.
102. **Kunstyv, I. and Matthiesen, T.,** Two forms of streptococcal infection (serologic group C) in guinea pigs, *Z. Versuchstierkd.,* 15, 348, 1973.
103. **Duca, E.,** A new nephritogenic streptococcus, *J. Hyg.,* 67, 691, 1969.
104. **Belcher, D. W., Afoakwa, S. N., Osei-Tutu, E., Wurapa, F. K., and Osfi, L.,** Non-group-A streptococci in Ghanaian patients with pyoderma, *Lancet,* 2, 1032, 1975.
105. **Bengtsson, S., Cars, O., and Forsum, U.,** A retrospective study of the occurrence of beta-haemolytic streptococci of various Lancefield groups in routine cultures from the county of Uppsala, *Scand. J. Infect. Dis.,* 8, 83, 1976.
106. **Riising, H. J., Nielsen, N. C., Bille, N., and Svendsen, J.,** Streptococcal infections in sucking pigs. I. Epidemiological investigations, *Nord. Veterinaermed.,* 5, 835, 1953.

107. **Thal, V. E. and Moberg, K.,** Serologische Gruppenbestimmung der bei Tieren vorkommenden β-haemolytischen Streptokokken, *Nord. Veterinaermed.,* 5, 835, 1953.
108. **Ross, R. F.,** Streptococcal infection in swine, in *Streptococci and Streptococcal Diseases,* Wannamaker, L. W. and Matsen, J. M., Eds., Academic Press, New York, 1972, 339.
109. **Bryans, J. T. and Moore, B. O.,** Group C streptococcal infections of the horse, in *Streptococci and Streptococcal Diseases,* Wannamaker, L. W. and Matsen, J. M., Eds., Academic Press, New York, 1972, 327.
110. **Van Dorssen, C. A.,** On the aetiology of strangles, *Tijdschr. Diergeneeskd.,* 83, 852, 1958.
111. **Kamada, M. and Akiyama, Y.,** Studies on the distribution of *Streptococcus zooepidemicus* in equine respiratory tracts, *Exp. Rep. Equine Health Lab.,* 12, 53, 1975.
112. **Van Bonengel, H., Schels, H., and Reissinger, H.,** β-hamolysierende streptokokken in puerperalgeschenhen bei der Stute, *Berl. Muench. Tieraerztl. Wochenschr.,* 87, 445, 1974.
113. **Millar, R. and Francis, J.,** The relation of clinical and bacteriological findings to fertility in thoroughbred mares, *Aust. Vet. J.,* 50, 351, 1974.
114. **Hughes, J. P. and Loy, R. G.,** The relation of infection to infertility in the mare and stallion, *Br. Equine Vet. Assoc. J.,* 7, 155, 1975.
115. **Erickson, E. D.,** unpublished data, 1976.
116. **Milanov, M., Chiler, D., Pacher, S. T., and Reginka, G.,** Streptococcosis in chickens. II. Cultural, morphologic, and biochemical studies of streptococcus strains, *Vet. Med. Nauki,* 13, 73, 1976.
117. **Ganaway, J. R.,** Bacterial, mycoplasma and rickettsial diseases, in *The Biology of the Guinea Pig,* Wagner, J. E. and Manning, P. J., Eds., Academic Press, New York, 121, 1976.
118. **Sebesteny, A.,** Disease of guinea pigs, *Vet. Rec.,* 98, 418, 1976.
119. **Fraunfelter, F. C., Schmidt, R. E., Beattie, R. J., and Garner, F. M.,** Lancefield Type C streptococcal infections in strain 2 guinea pigs, *Lab. Anim.,* 5, 1, 1971.
120. **Rae, M. V.,** Epizootic streptococcic myocarditis in guinea pigs, *J. Infect. Dis.,* 59, 236, 1936.
121. **Ogumbi, O., Lasi, Q., and Lawal, S. F.,** An epidemiological study of β-hemolytic streptococcal infections in a Nigerian (Lagos) urgan population, in *Streptococcal Disease and the Community,* Haverkorn, M. J., Ed., Excerpta Medica, Amsterdam, 1974, 282.
122. **Foley, G. E.,** Further observations on the occurrence of streptococci of groups other than A in human infection, *N. Engl. J. Med.,* 237, 809, 1947.
123. **Perkins, D. E. and McRae, R. P.,** An arteriosclerotic aneurysm of the abdominal aorta secondarily infected with group C, beta-hemolytic streptococci, *Am. J. Clin. Pathol.,* 62, 646, 1974.
124. **Sanders, V.,** Bacterial endocarditis due to a group C beta-hemolytic streptococcus, *Ann. Intern. Med.,* 58, 858, 1963.
125. **Nordlander, I., Thal, E., and Tunevall, G.,** Occurrence and significance of hemolytic streptococci groups B-U in human infectious disease, *Scand. J. Infect. Dis.,* 7, 35, 1975.
126. **Mogabgab, W. J.,** Beta-hemolytic streptococcal and concurrent infections in adults and children with respiratory disease, 1958 to 1969, *Am. Rev. Respir. Dis.,* 102, 23, 1970.
127. **Benjamin, J. T. and Periello, V. A.,** Pharyngitis due to group C hemolytic streptococci in children, *J. Pediatr.,* 89, 254, 1976.
128. **Duma, R. J., Weinberg, A. N., Medrek, T. F., and Kunz, L. J.,** Streptococcal infections. A bacteriologic and clinical study of streptococcal bacteremia, *Medicine* (Baltimore), 48, 87, 1969.
129. **Hamada, L. and Slade, H. D.,** Purification and immunochemical characterization of type e polysaccharide antigen of *Streptococcus mutans, Infect. Immun.,* 14, 68, 1976.
130. **Ellen, R. P. and Gibbons, R. J.,** M protein associated adherence of *Streptococcus pyogenes* to epithelial surfaces: prerequisite for virulence, *Infect. Immun.,* 5, 826, 1972.
131. **Gibbons, R. J. and Van Houte, J.,** Bacterial adherence in oral microbial ecology, in *Annual Review of Microbiology,* Vol. 29, Mortimer, P. S., Ingraham, L., and Raffel, S., Eds., Annual Reviews, Palo Alto, Calif., 1975, 19.
132. **Krause, R. M.,** The antigens of group D streptococci, in *Streptococci and Streptococcal Diseases,* Wannamaker, L. W. and Matsen, J. M., Eds., Academic Press, New York, 1972, 67.
133. **Lerner, P. I.,** Meningitis caused by streptococcus in adults, *J. Infect. Dis.,* 131(Suppl. S9), 1975.
134. **Toala, P., McDonald, A., Wilcox, C., and Finland, M.,** Susceptibility of group D streptococcus (enterococcus) to 21 antibiotics in vitro, with special reference to species differences, *Am. J. Med. Sci.,* 258, 416, 1969.
135. **Elliott, S. D.,** Streptococcal infections in young pigs. I. An immunochemical study of the causative agent (PM streptococcus), *J. Hyg.,* 64, 205, 1966.
136. **Williams, D. M., Lawson, G. H. K., and Rowland, A. C.,** Streptococcal infection in piglets: the palatine tonsils as portals of entry for *Streptococcus suis, Res. Vet. Sci.,* 15, 352, 1973.
137. **Windsor, R. S. and Elliott, S. D.,** Streptococcal infection in young pigs. IV. An outbreak of streptococcal meningitis in weaned pigs, *J. Hyg.,* 75, 69, 1975.
138. **Weaver, A. D.,** Relationship of bacterial infection in urine and calculi to canine urolithiasis, *Vet. Rec.,* 97, 48, 1975.

139. **Cullen, G. A.,** *Streptococcus uberis* — a review, *Vet. Bull.* (London), 39, 155, 1969.
140. **Riley, G. I., Morehoure, L. G., and Olson, L. D.,** Detection of tonsillar and nasal colonization of group E streptococcus in swine, *Am. J. Vet. Res.,* 34, 1167, 1973.
141. **Wort, A. J.,** Observations on group F streptococci from human sources, *J. Med. Microbiol.,* 8, 455, 1975.
142. **Krantz, G. E. and Dunne, H. W.,** An attempt to classify streptococcic isolates from domestic animals, *Am. J. Vet. Res.,* 26, 951, 1965.
143. **Seegal, B. C., Heller, G., and Jablonowitz, J.,** Incidence of hemolytic streptococci and pneumococci in the pharyngeal flora of normal rhesus monkeys, *Proc. Soc. Exp. Biol. Med.,* 34, 812, 1936.
144. **Berger, U. and Hahn, G.,** Group F streptococci in guinea pigs, *Zentralbl. Bakteriol. Parasitenkd. Infektionskr. Hyg. Abt. 1: Orig. Reihe A,* 299, 436, 1974.
145. **Poole, P. M. and Wilson, G.,** Infection with minute-colony-forming β-haemolytic streptococci, *J. Clin. Pathol.,* 29, 740, 1976.
146. **Koepke, J. A.,** Meningitis due to *Streptococcus anginosus* (Lancefield group F), *JAMA,* 193, 115, 1965.
147. **Koshi, G.,** Lancefield group F streptococci causing liver abscess and empyema, *Indian J. Med. Res.,* 59, 45, 1971.
148. **Baker, C. J.,** Unusual occurrence of neonatal septicemia due to group G streptococcus, *Pediatrics,* 53, 568, 1974.
149. **Curtis, S. N. and Krause, R. M.,** Antigenic relationships between groups B and G streptococci, *J. Exp. Med.,* 120, 629, 1964.
150. **Maxted, W. R.,** Occurrence of the M substance of type 28, group A in streptococci of Lancefield groups B, C, and G, *J. Gen. Microbiol.,* 2, 1, 1948.
151. **Hill, H. R.,** Epidemic of pharyngitis due to streptococci of Lancefield group G, *Lancet,* 2, 371, 1969.
152. **Barnum, D. A.,** Report on an outbreak of chronic mastitis in cattle caused by a streptococcus of Lancefield's group G, *Can. J. Comp. Med.,* 17, 465, 1953.
153. **Hamilton, C. A. and Stark, D. M.,** Occurrence and characterization of Lancefield group G streptococci in bovine mastitis, *Am. J. Vet. Res.,* 31, 397, 1970.
154. **Stewart, D. D., Buck, G. E., McConnell, E. E., and Amster, R. L.,** An epizootic of necrotic dermatitis in laboratory mice caused by Lancefield group G streptococci, *Lab. Anim. Sci.,* 25, 296, 1975.
155. **Laughton, N.,** Canine β-hemolytic streptococci, *J. Pathol. Bacteriol.,* 60, 471, 1948.
156. **Jones, J. E. T.,** The serological classification of streptococci isolated from diseased pigs, *Br. Vet. J.,* 132, 163, 1976.
157. **Jones, J. E. T.,** The carriage of beta-hemolytic streptococci by healthy pigs, *Br. Vet. J.,* 132, 276, 1976.
158. **Van Den Berg, J. and Grootenhuis, G.,** Mastitis and streptococci of the L group, *Tijdschr. Diergeneeskd.,* 1975.
159. **Broome, C. V., Moellering, R. C., and Watson, B. K.,** Clinical significance of Lancefield groups L-T streptococci isolated from blood and cerebrospinal fluid, *J. Infect. Dis.,* 133, 382, 1976.
160. **Perch, B. and Kjems, E.,** Group R streptococci in man, *Acta Pathol. Microbiol. Scand. Sect. B,* 79, 549, 1971.
161. **Field, H. I., Buntain, D., and Done, J. T.,** Studies on piglet mortality. I. Streptococcal meningitis and arthritis, *Vet. Rec.,* 66, 452, 1954.
162. **de Moor, C. E.,** Septicaemic infections in pigs, caused by haemolytic streptococci of new Lancefield groups designated R, S and T, *Antonie van Leeuwenhoek J. Microbiol. Serol.,* 29, 272, 1963.
163. **Hickling, P.,** Meningitis caused by group R haemolytic streptococci, *Br. Med. J.,* 2, 1299, 1976.
164. **Zanen, H. C. and Engel, H. W. B.,** Porcine streptococci causing meningitis and septicemia in man, *Lancet,* 1, 1286, 1975.
165. **Kloppenburg, M.,** Septicemia due to porcine streptococci, *Lancet,* 2, 1218, 1975.
166. **Jelinkova, J. and Kubin, V.,** Proposal of a new serological group ("V") of hemolytic streptococci isolated from swine lymph nodes, *Int. J. Syst. Bacteriol.,* 13, 434, 1974.
167. **Sullivan, R. J., Dowdle, W. R., Marine, W. M., and Hierholzer, J. C.,** Adult pneumonia in a general hospital, *Arch. Intern. Med.,* 129, 935, 1972.
168. **Romer, O.,** Bovine mastitis due to *Streptococcus pneumoniae, Nord. Veterinaermed.,* 11, 361, 1959.

APPENDIX 1*

Summary

Twenty-five strains of *Streptococcus agalactiae* (SA) of human origin were injected into mammary glands of 30 dairy cows. Of 98 glands inoculated, 78.6% became infected. The disease was more acute in dairy cows than that produced by bovine SA strains, and most infections were eliminated by the cow without the use of antibiotics.

Based on our studies, we have concluded that SA of human origin are more pathogenic than SA of bovine origin and are different biotypes. Therefore, there is no basis to suspect that bovine strains are involved in human disease.

Discussion

There are only a few differences between human and bovine SA strains. Human SA strains are nearly always lactose negative, and we were unable to convert four cultures to utilize lactose. One bovine vaginal strain was identical to the human strains. Human SA strains are resistant to both bacitracin and nitrofurazone, whereas bovine strains are sensitive to these two antibiotics. We cannot explain these differences in antibiotic sensitivity.

Although there are differences in biochemical tests and in antibiotic sensitivity between human and bovine isolates, serologically, all are Lancefield group B test positive. This finding is not unexpected because there are different biotypes in other Lancefield serological groups.

When 100 to 500 CFU of a SA of human origin were injected into a bovine mammary gland, most glands became infected. Infection was more acute and severe than infection by bovine SA strains. Nearly all human SA infections in the bovine mammary gland were eliminated by the cow, whereas bovine SA infections nearly always have to be treated with antibiotics before they can be eliminated.

If these human SA isolates originate from the bovine and are carried in contaminated dairy products,[6] one would expect to see more throat problems, e.g., tonsillitis and pharyngitis. Possibly, consumption of contaminated dairy products could result in tonsillitis or pharyngitis. Even though these two diseases do occur in humans and are related to SA, most human disease caused by SA is related to the genitourinary tract and subsequent contamination of the neonate during delivery.[2,3,5]

From our studies and those of others,[4] we have concluded that SA of human origin are more pathogenic than SA of bovine origin and are different biotypes. Also, in some human and bovine vaginal canals, there are lactose-negative SA strains. The carrier rate may be lower in the bovine than in the human population. However, bovine strains of SA are not likely to be involved in human disease.

Infection of the bovine mammary gland is a disease that affects the dairyman economically. The main effect of this infection is a decrease in milk production by the infected gland. Infection by SA is an eradicable disease, and the organism is sensitive to penicillin. SA should be eradicated from the national dairy herd.

*   McDonald, J. S., McDonald, T. J., and Anderson, A. J., Characterization of Bovine Intramammary Infection by Group B *Streptococcus agalactiae* of Human Origin, Proc. U. S. Animal Health Assoc., 1977, U. S. Department of Agriculture, Agricultural Research Service, National Animal Disease Center, North Central Region, Ames, Iowa.

REFERENCES

1. **Anon.**, Standardized disc susceptibility test directions for use, *Fed. Regist.*, 37, 20527, 1972.
2. **Baker, C. J. and Barrett, F. W.**, Transmission of group B streptococci among parturient women and their neonates, *J. Pediatr.*, 83, 919, 1973.
3. **Eickhoff, T. C.**, Group B. streptococci in human infection, in *Streptococci and Streptococcal Diseases*, Wannamaker, L. W. and Matsen, J. M., Eds., Academic Press, New York, 1972.
4. **Ghoroury, A. A. E.**, Comparative studies of group B streptococci of human and bovine origin. I. Cultural and biochemical characters, *Am. J. Public Health*, 40, 1273, 1950.
5. **Grossman, J. and Thompkins, R. I.**, Group B beta-hemolytic streptococcal meningitis in mother and infant, *N. Engl. J. Med.*, 290, 387, 1974.
6. **Jelinkova, J., Neubauer, M., and Duben, J.**, Group B streptococci in human pathology, *Zentralbl. Bakteriol.*, 214, 450, 1970.
7. **McDonald, T. J. and McDonald, J. S.**, Streptococci isolated from bovine intramammary infections, *Am. J. Vet. Res.*, April 1976.
8. **Svartz, N.**, The primary cause of rheumatoid arthritis is an infection: the agent exists in milk, *Acta Med. Scand.*, 192, 231, 1972.

Appendix 2*

Nineteen instances of wound sepsis occurred among 59 employees of a Vermont abattoir from November 1976 through February 1977. Group A streptococcus was isolated from eight of nine wounds cultured. Contact with contaminated meat may have been the source of infection of some workers.

The abattoir began operation on Oct. 29, 1976. It employed many inexperienced workers who consequently suffered frequent abrasions and cuts. Two weeks after the abattoir opened, ten persons reported wounds that had become acutely inflamed; several had lymphangitis and cellulitis (Figure 1). A total of 19 such cases occurred during the next 3 months. One such infection was reported in the same time period in two comparable Vermont abattoirs that were surveyed.

From nine wounds, eight of which were cultured by practitioners in the community, group A β-hemolytic streptococcus was isolated in eight; *Pasteurella multocida* was recovered from one atypical wound that resulted from a boar bite on the kill line. The rate of infections per man-month of employment was significantly greater in those who worked in meat-handling areas (kill floor, holding cooler and cutting and pork rooms) (17 infections per 92 man-months) compared to other areas of the plant (2/69). The frequencies of infection in each meat-handling area were similar.

During the initial investigation on Dec. 14, 1976, group A streptococcus M41 T3/13 SOR− was cultured from 1 of 30 meat cultures, from the healing wound of a man who worked in the cutting room distal to the holding cooler, and from the throats of three meat handlers. Two other group A strains were isolated from throat cultures of three employees: T13 MNT SOR + (two isolates) and T28 MNT SOR + (one isolate). The frequency of positive cultures or serologic evidence of infection with any one or all of these three strains (using bactericidal or SOR-inhibition assays) was similar in those who worked in meat-handling and other areas and in cases and well persons. Anterior nares and anus cultures were negative for group A streptococci.

Transmission of infection to workers may have occurred by person-to-person spread or by contact with fomites. The initial ten cases occurred shortly after a man with a chronic impetiginous infection began work on the kill floor November 14. The earliest cases may have become infected by contact with him or the meat he handled; however, only two cases had culture-proven or serologic evidence of infection with the strain isolated from meat in December.

The outbreak subsided after recommendations were instituted for prompt local care of all wounds, culture of all infected wounds, and exclusion from work of persons with infected wounds until cultures became negative.

CDC Editorial Note — The natural reservoir of group A β-hemolytic streptococcus is man; however, rarely, animals may become infected through contact with ill persons. The mode of transmission in this outbreak is unclear; however, culture of a single streptococcal strain from both meat and a healing wound suggests that after introduction of the organism into the plant, meat may have served as a fomite in subsequent transmission to some cases.

Although this is the first reported outbreak of group A streptococcal wound infection among abattoir workers in the U.S., eight such outbreaks have occurred in Great

---

* Allen, J., Froins, J., Laitinen, D., McBean, M., and Watson, W., Group A streptococcal wound infections in an abattoir — Vermont, Morbidity and Mortality Weekly Report, Vol. 26, Issue 15, U. S. Department of Health, Education and Welfare, Public Health Service, Center for Disease Control, Atlanta, 1977.

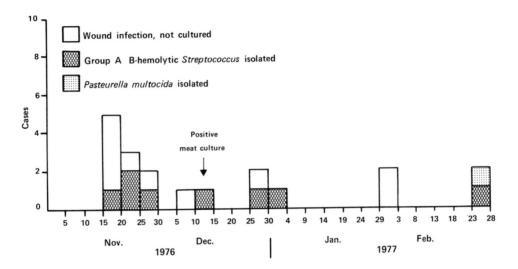

FIGURE 1.   Wound infections at a Vermont abattoir, November 1976 to February 1977.

Britain since 1974.* Group A streptococcal wound sepsis is an occupational hazard of abbattoir workers that may be underestimated.

---

*   Fraser, C. A. M., Morris, C. A., Ball, L. C., and Noah, A. D., Serological characterization of group A streptococci associated with skin sepsis in meat handlers, *J. Hyg.* (Cambridge), in press.

CURRENT STATUS OF GROUP B STREPTOCOCCAL INFECTIONS IN MAN

D. K. Goroff and D. L. Kasper

The role of group B streptococci (GBS) as the cause of serious neonatal infection has been well established during the last 10 years.[1,2] Based on the age at onset of the disease, two clinical syndromes have been described for neonates with GBS infections.[2] The early-onset type of infection occurs in neonates 5 days of age or less and is characterized by septicemia with pulmonary inflammatory response and "atypical" hyaline membranes. This syndrome is associated with a high rate of maternal obstetric complications and results from intrapartum transmission of organisms from the maternal genital tract. The late-onset type of infection is characterized by onset beyond the tenth day of life and is infrequently associated with purulent leptomeningitis and modes of transmission, in addition to the mother-to-infant route. Early-onset disease results in a case-fatality rate in excess of 50%, whereas the mortality rates in the late-onset syndrome are considerably lower. Although frequency and severity of infections due to GBS decreases after infancy, the organism has been reported to be the etiological agent in a variety of human pathological conditions, e.g., post-partum infection, gangrene, cellulitis, endocarditis, and osteomyelitis.[3]

Lancefield's serologic classification of GBS is based on two cell wall antigenic determinants: (1) the group B polysaccharide (Bsss) common to all strains and (2) the type-specific sss, that is specific for type Ia, Ib, II, and III organisms.[4,5] A fifth serotype, type Ic, has been defined by Wilkinson as containing an sss antigen identical to Ia and a protein antigen, the Ibc protein, that is common to all type Ib and Ic strains.[6] The distribution of these organisms, based on serotype among asymptomatic mothers and neonates with early-onset disease, is nearly identical. Approximately 33 to 37% are type III, 35 to 44% are type II, and 18 to 28% are type Ia, Ib, and Ic. However, more than 90% of the strains isolated from infants with late-onset-type disease are type III.

A variety of extraction procedures have been employed to isolate and examine the specific sss antigens present on these organisms. The earliest method, using a hot acid-extraction procedure, successfully isolates the group and type antigens and has been useful in the serotyping of these organisms. However, this procedure results in an incomplete, small, molecular-sized preparation that is chemically impure. A number of investigators have purified this HCl-extracted antigen using alcohol fractionation or ion-exchange chromatography, thus separating the group and type components.[7,8] These HCl-treated antigens have been reported to contain varying amounts of glucose, galactose, and glucosamine. Extraction of GBS with cold tri-chloroacetic acid results in the isolation of a more complete molecule that has been described to contain sialic acid in addition to the sugars mentioned above. Isolation of a large molecular-sized pure sss antigen from the type III GBS has been accomplished using a gentle neutral-buffer wash of the organisms.[9] This method allows for purification of the antigens in their most native form. Analysis of this preparation has shown the presence of sialic acid, galactose, heptose, glucose, glucosamine, and mannose.

A radioactive antigen binding assay (RABA) has been employed to examine the role of antibody in neonatal GBS infection.[10] Using the RABA, the development of antibody in response to invasive infection with type III strains of GBS was studied in sera from 31 infants and 4 adults. Low concentrations of antibody were consistently found in the acute sera of patients who developed clinical illness. Although adults with puerperal sepsis and infants with bone or joint infection uniformly demonstrated significant rises in serum antibody concentration after recovery, much lower levels of antibody were detected in convalescent sera from infants recovering from meningitis or sepsis.

These studies have also demonstrated that the mean concentration in sera from 42 parturients with type III strains of GBS isolated from vaginal cultures whose neonates failed to develop symptomatic disease was significantly greater than that in sera from 29 mothers of infants with invasive type III GBS infection. Studies of paired maternal and cord sera demonstrated a significant correlation between the antibody concentration in a mothers serum and that in her neonate. These data thus suggest that transplacental transfer of maternal antibody protects infants from invasive GBS infection with type III strains. Therefore, a reasonable means of preventing these life-threatening infections among neonates may be immunization of women documented to be antibody-deficient with a sss vaccine.

REFERENCES

1. **Baker, C. J., Barnett, F. F., Gordon, R. C., and Yow, M. D.,** Suppurative meningitis due to streptococci of Lancefield's group B: a study of 33 infants, *J. Pediatr.,* 82, 724, 1973.
2. **Franciosi, R. A., Knostman, J. D., and Zimmerman, R. A.,** Group B streptococcal neonatal and infant infections, *J. Pediatr.,* 82, 707, 1973.
3. **Patterson, M. J. and Hafeez, A. B.,** Group B streptococci in human disease, *Bacteriol. Rev.,* 40, 774, 1976.
4. **Lancefield, R. C.,** A serologic differentiation of specific types of bovine hemolytic streptococci (group B), *J. Exp. Med.,* 59, 441, 1934.
5. **Lancefield, R. C.,** Two serologic types of group B hemolytic streptococci with related but not identical type-specific substances, *J. Exp. Med.,* 67, 25, 1938.
6. **Wilkinson, H. W. and Eagon, R.,** Type-specific antigens of group B type Ic streptococci, *Infect. Immun.,* 4, 596, 1971.
7. **Wilkinson, H. W.,** Immunochemistry of purified polysaccharide type antigens of group B streptococcal types Ia, Ib and Ic, *Infect. Immun.,* 11, 845, 1975.
8. **Russell, H. and Norcross, N. L.,** The isolation and some physiochemical and biologic properties of the type III antigen of group B streptococci, *J. Immunol.,* 109, 90, 1972.
9. **Baker, C. J., Kasper, D. L., and Davis, C. E.,** Immunochemical characterization of the "native" type III polysaccharide of Group B *Streptococcus, J. Exp. Med.,* 143, 258, 1976.
10. **Baker, C. J., Kasper, D. L., Tager, I. B., Parades, A., Alpert, S., McCormack, W. M., and Goroff, D. K.,** Quantitative determination of antibody to capsular polysaccharide in infection with type III strains of group B *Streptococcus, J. Clin. Invest.,* 59, 810, 1977.

EDITORIAL COMMENT — SUMMARY OF THE NATIONAL INSTITUTE OF HEALTH (NIH) WORKSHOP ON PERINATAL INFECTIONS DUE TO GROUP B *STREPTOCOCCUS**

The reason for the rise of the group B *Streptococcus* as a frequent pathogen associated with serious neonatal infections in this decade is unknown. Although this microorganism has been linked causally to human disease since 1938, it is now the leading cause of meningitis during the first 2 months of life in several geographic regions.[12] Since attack rates for serious infection attributed to other bacteria have not diminished in recent years, the appearance of group B stretococcal disease has resulted in an absolute increase in the incidence of neonatal bacterial infection in the U.S.[3] From the reported attack rates for group B streptococcal disease among neonates and young infants,[1,4,5] one can conservatively estimate that between 12,000 and 15,000 babies will develop this disease during the next year; approximately 50% of these infants will die, and up to 50% of the survivors with meningeal invation will develop neurological sequelae.[6] Although safe and effective antimicrobial agents are available for the treatment of group B streptococcal infection, even when administered early in the course of this illness, these agents are frequently unable to arrest the fatal progression of the disease.

The magnitude and severity of infection due to group B *Streptococcus* prompted the convening of this workshop. The purpose of the workshop was to present information regarding the biology of the organism, including host-parasite interactions, as well as information regarding the epidemiology, pathogenesis, and clinical features of these infections. One objective identified by consensus was that a search for preventive rather than therapeutic intervention should be given high priority. The immunological aspects relevant to disease control were believed to be of particular importance to future investigation. Specific areas for further research were identified, and cogent questions were posed.

HISTORICAL BACKGROUND

Out of the numerous investigations regarding the agents associated with epidemics among American military personnel during World War I arose the serological classification of hemolytic streptococci into several groups. This classification scheme of Lancefield was based upon precipitin reactions that occur when group-specific polysaccharide antigens (C substances) are combined with group-specific rabbit antisera. These group-specific antigens are isolated from whole organisms exposed to dilute acid (HCI) and heat. Although the majority of isolates obtained from humans since this classification was reported in 1933 have been strains designated group A, group B streptococci were reported in association with perinatal infection as early as 1938. Early studies of both asymptomatic and acutely ill parturients reported the isolation of group B streptococci from vaginal cultures, but the majority of women with group B streptococcal infection were asymptomatic. A few of these women had fatal uterine infections, and strains designated group B rather than group A *Streptococcus* were isolated from both vaginal and blood cultures.[7]

During the preantibiotic era, however, group A strepococci were the most common agents associated with puerperal fever. From 1940 to 1970 sporadic cases of group B streptoccal disease were reported to occur in both parturients and neonates. Because the group B *Streptococcus*, or *Streptococcus agalactiae*, was known best by its histor-

* From *J. Infect. Dis.*, 136(1), 137, 1977. With permission.

ical association with bovine mastitis rather than for perinatal infection, it was not widely appreciated as a potential human pathogen until 1964.[8] However, with the beginning of this decade, group B *Streptococcus* became a frequent agent associated with serious infections among neonates and young infants. In some geographic regions, it is now the most frequent cause of serious neonatal infection. Reasons for this apparent upsurge in the incidence of invasive disease due to group B *Streptococcus* remain obscure.

EPIDEMIOLOGY

Incidence of Disease

There is no longer any doubt that an increase in the number of symptomatic group B streptococcal infections among neonates and young infants has occurred throughout the U.S. Investigators from Denver,[1] St. Louis,[5] Houston,[10] and Los Angeles[9] have stated that this microorganism is the most frequent agent associated with serious infection during the first 3 months of life. Recent data from the Neonatal Meningitis Cooperative Study involving 12 institutions in this country identified a total of 131 cases of bacterial meningitis, of which 31% were attributed to group B *Streptococcus* and 38% to *Eschericia coli.*[3] Although there have been some discrepancies in the reported rates for asymptomatic neonatal group B streptococcal colonization, striking uniformity in the attack rates for the early-onset type of infection has been observed. This rate has varied from 3.0 to 4.2/1000 live births.[1,4,25] Attack rates for late-onset infections are not known but have been estimated to be approximately 0.5 to 1.0/1000 live births.

There is no indication that any of the individuals that have been found to be infected had contact with animals that may have been shedding group B *Streptococcus* which is a common cause of mastitis in milk cows. There is much speculation on the relationship of animal group B *Streptococcus* and human group B *Streptococcus*, but from the data available at the workshop, there is no epidemiological relation.

There is no evidence that the animal group B *Streptococcus* are a cause of human disease. It should be pointed out (see previous Editorial Comment) that human group B *Streptococcus* produces an acute transitory inflammatory action in the udder cows.

REFERENCES

1. **Franciosi, R. A., Knostman, J. D., Zimmerman, R. A.,** Group B streptococcal neonatal and infant infections, *J. Pediatr.,* 82, 707, 1973.
2. **Baker, C. J., Barrett, F. F., Gordon, R. C., and Yow, M. D.,** Supportive meningitis due to streptococci of Lancefield group B: a study in 33 infants, *J. Pediatr.,* 82, 724, 1973.
3. **McCracken, G. H., Jr.,** Editorial comment, *J. Pediatr.,* 89, 203, 1976.
4. **Baker, C. J. and Barrett, F. F.,** Transmission of group B streptococci among parturient women and their neonates, *J. Pediatr.,* 83, 919, 1973.
5. **Feigin, R. D.,** The perinatal group B streptococcal problem: more questions than answers, *N. Engl. J. Med.,* 294, 106, 1976.
6. **Horn, K. A., Zimmerman, R. A., Knostman, J. D., and Meyer, W. T.,** Neurological sequelae of group B streptococcal neonatal infections, *Pediatrics,* 53, 501, 1974.
7. **Fry, R. M.,** Fatal infections by haemolytic streptococcus group B, *Lancet,* 1, 199, 1938.
8. **Eickhoff, T. C., Klein , J. O., Daly, A., Ingall, D., and Finland, M.,** Neonatal sepsis and other infections due to group B beta-hemolytic streptococci, *N. Engl. J. Med.,* 271, 1221, 1964.
9. **Anthony, B. F. and Concepcion, N. F.,** Group B Streptococcus in a general hospital, *J. Infect. Dis.,* 132, 561, 1975.
10. **Baker, C. J. and Barrett, F. F.,** Group B streptococcal infections in infants: the importance of the various serotypes, *JAMA,* 230, 1158, 1974.
11. **Paredes, A., Wong, P., Mason, E. O., Clark, D., Yow, M. D., and Barrett, F. F.,** Nosocomial colonization of pregnant females and their neonates, *Pediatrics,* 59(5), 679, 1977.

TETANUS (LOCKJAW)

J. A. McComb

Tetanus is an acute infectious disease resulting from intoxication of the nervous system. It is characterized by persisting spasmodic contractions of the entire body musculature or of a single group of muscles without impairment of the consciousness. It is caused by a spore-forming organism, *Clostridium tetani*, growing anaerobically at the site of injury.

HISTORY

Hippocrates first described this disease in about 360 B.C. In 1884, Carle and Rattone[2] inoculated pus from a human case into rabbits, thus determining its transmissability. Although Nicolaier[3] described the organism in the same year, it remained for Kitasato[4] to isolate it in pure culture in 1889. Inoculation into animals of these pure cultures was successful in reproducing the disease (Table 1).

ETIOLOGIC AGENT

C. tetani is a large, Gram-positive, actively motile bacillus that forms spores on one or both ends (Figures 1A and 1B). While it is usually stated to be a strict anaerobe, the best strain of the organism that is now used around the world for toxin production was isolated by J. Howard Mueller of the Harvard Medical School. This strain is not particular as to its anaerobic requirements nor does it easily form spores.

The clostridia grow well on laboratory media at 37°C. Vegetative bacilli are readily killed, but spores are highly resistant. Although direct sunlight will kill spores in due time, they are resistant to ordinary boiling but are readily killed by steam under pressure in a properly packed (not overloaded) autoclave. Dry-heated ovens are less dependable.

The organism exists in the digestive tracts of warm-blooded animals including man. The heat-labile tetanus exotoxin that it produces under proper conditions has two components: (1) tetanospasmin, the neurotoxin that produces the muscle spasms and (2) tetanolysin that hemolyses blood agar plates. The exotoxin is extremely stable when dried while toxin in solution is quite labile. It is one of the most powerful poisons known — 0.000001 (10^{-6}) g of dried toxin is fatal for a mouse. Tetanus toxin is fixed by nervous tissue. According to Mellanby and van Heyningen,[11] fixation is due to the ganglioside content of the tissue.

Because the disease can be produced by only a few organisms, direct examination of pus from a lesion is too often negative. Cultural methods require repeated platings to obtain pure cultures. All types of the organism produce a common toxin that is neutralized by a common antitoxin. The test for toxin production requires a specific toxic reaction on laboratory animals, such as local or general tetanus in a mouse, using mice that have received protective doses of tetanus antitoxin as controls. Fluorescent-labeled antisera may be found useful in the laboratory for identification of the organism in cultures or tissues. Also, hemagglutination tests are useful for determining rapid, inexpensive, relative values for antitoxin in sera. Toxin is effective when injected subcutaneously, intramuscularly, intraperitoneally, intravenously, or intracerebrally; it is harmless when given orally.

Table 1
MILESTONES IN THE HISTORY OF TETANUS

			Ref.
Second century	—	Aretaeus, the Cappadocian, described tetanus.	1
1884	—	Carle demonstrated the transmissibility of tetanus by inoculation into rabbits of pus from a human case.	2
1884	—	Nicolaier described the tetanus bacillus. He was, however, unable to isolate the organism in pure culture.	3
1889	—	Kitasato obtained the pure culture of *C. tetani*.	4
1890	—	von Behring and Kitasato described antitoxins and their immunizing powers.	5
1927 and 1933	—	Ramon and Zoeller discussed the use of tetanus toxoid in active immunization of humans.	6, 7
1942	—	U.S. military establishment effectively used the emergency medical identification device.	
1946	—	Cohn and co-workers fractionated human plasma so that TIG(H) became available.	8
1966	—	McComb, Levine, Dwyer, and Latham established 250 units as the routine prophylactic dose for TIG(H).	9, 10

From Furste, W. and Wheeler, W. L., in *Curr. Probl. Surg.*, October 1972. Copyright 1972 by Yearbook Medical Publishers, Inc., Chicago. With permission.

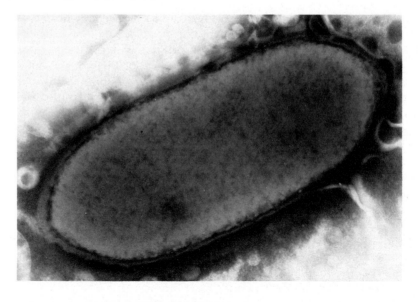

FIGURE 1A.   Surface of *Clostridium* tetanus; negatively stained with phosphotungstic acid. Courtesy of A. K. Eugster.

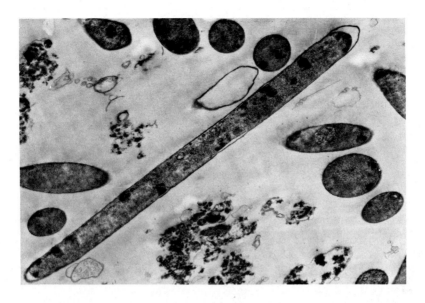

FIGURE 1B.   Cross sections of *Clostridium tetanus*, stained with lead citrate-uranyl acetate. Courtesy of A. K. Eugster.

TRUE AND ALTERNATE HOSTS

The tetanus organism has been found in the digestive tracts of man and most warm-blooded domestic animals as well as a few animals only occasionally domesticated, such as monkeys and rabbits. Investigators have found feces positive for the organism in percentages varying from 16 to 18% in the horse, 0 to 20 % in cattle, 25% in sheep, more than 50% in dogs, 30% in rats, and about 15% in poultry. A possible explanation for the high percentage found in dogs could be their habit of eating horse manure and hoof trimmings. There can be little reason to doubt that other warm-blooded animals have tetanus organisms in their digestive tracts, both domesticated and wild, Carnivora and Herbivora. For instance, an extremely high incidence of tetanus in New Guinea exists in areas where there are no domestic animals except swine and dogs.

In man, the organism has been found in a great number of fecal samples but in a very wide range of percentages that might indicate that it was not always a natural inhabitant of the human intestine but an organism of passage only. If this premise is true, *C. tetani* would be found more often in persons having contact with animals or farms or living in areas of the world where vegetables and raw food grow in soil that receives heavy applications of animal manure and nightsoil.

On the basis of the above reasoning, an "educated" guess would designate the warm-blooded, domestic, herbiverous animals as the true hosts and all others as accidental hosts.

DISTRIBUTION

Figure 2 shows the geographic distribution of human cases in the U.S. This figure covers the then new Tetanus Surveillance Program of the U.S. Public Health Service, Center for Disease Control (CDC), Atlanta. Thus, it shows basic environmental factors and represents the reported cases for the year 1967. It is doubtful that a better picture of soil contamination could be obtained until a survey of soils in various parts

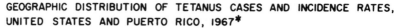

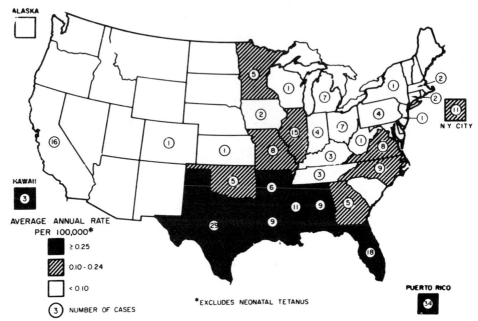

FIGURE 2.   Geographic distribution of tetanus cases and incidence rates, U.S. and Puerto Rico, 1967. (From Center for Disease Control, Tetanus Surveillance, No. 2, U.S. Department of Health, Education, and Welfare, Atlanta, April 1, 1969, 5.)

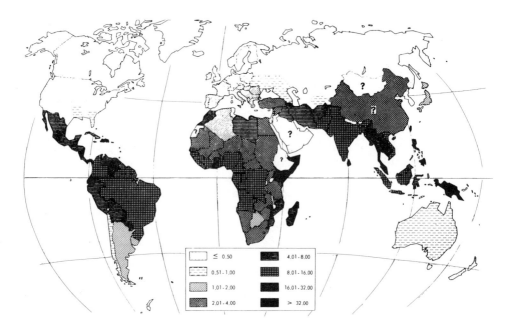

FIGURE 3.   Incidence of tetanus, 1951 to 1960. (From Bytchenko, B., *Principles on Tetanus,* Hans Huber, Bern, 1967, 31. With permission.)

of the U.S. has been made. Similar figures for later surveys show fewer cases. This chiefly reflects better immunization of the population; the number of horses is increasing, so there is little reason to believe that environmental conditions have improved.

Figure 3 gives a world picture of the incidence of tetanus for the years 1951 to 1960 as estimated by Bytchenko.[12] He also estimates that during this period, 1,600,000 persons world-wide could have died from the disease. The underdeveloped countries bear the greatest burden, mainly due to lack of sufficient active immunization. In the rapidly changing scene in Africa, it is difficult to choose a typical geographical area in the equatorial region. A recent report from Uganda indicates a rapid population growth (2.5 to 3%/year) with an increasing tetanus case load in Mulago Hospital, rising from 4 cases per 1000 admissions in 1963 to 6.9 cases per 1000 admissions in 1967.[13] More cases occurred during the wet season, but otherwise there were no seasonal differences. The hospital is equipped to care for tetanus patients. Curiously, during the recent strife in Uganda, no increase in tetanus cases was noticed.

In the U.S., the incidence has been slowly declining and, at least until recently, the average age of those contracting the disease has been slowly rising. Increased age seems to produce a declining interest in preventive medicine.

As a general rule, mortality figures are much more accurate than morbidity statistics. The first tetanus records in Massachusetts began in 1907 with eight cases reported and 31 deaths. For the first 9 years of record-keeping, more cases than deaths were reported only in 2 years. It was not until the 1940s that morbidity figures became more believable.

Sakurai[14] of Japan reported on an area of 5034 km² near Tokyo with a record of land use going back 800 to 2000 years. This area was agricultural during its early history but now has a population of almost three million persons. His own investigation began with records dating back to 1872. He was able to closely relate the human cases with the high incidence of veterinary tetanus in several old livestock farms and areas around rivers. Listed in order of the number of deaths, the animals mentioned were swine, horses, cattle, sheep, goats, rabbits, dogs, and monkeys. Also of interest were the most common locations of entry for the organisms: swine, castration; horses, hoof injury; cattle, castration; sheep, tail docking; goats, dehorning; rabbits, dogs, and monkeys, injury. Surprisingly, only 53 of a total of 342 deaths are listed as "cause unknown;" this would seem to indicate a diligent search for lesions.

In some areas of the U.S., the incidence has been high enough on some farms for it to be economically worthwhile to give prophylactic antitoxin to animals about to undergo such surgery as castrations, dehornings, dockings, etc. On one such farm (to this author's knowledge), the farmer himself had tetanus and recovered.

Man, warm-blooded animals, and poultry are symptomless carriers of this organism in their digestive tracts and, together with most types of soils, constitute the known reservoirs. Sergeeva and Matveev[15] have done extensive work in investigating more than 5000 soil samples in various climatic and geographical zones in the U.S.S.R. They found the distribution of tetanus organisms to be uneven with the highest concentration in southern regions having fertile black soil and long periods for plants and soil organisms to vegetate. The highest rate of soil contamination occurred in places overcrowded with both humans and animals. It should be pointed out that the inclusion of tetanus in a series on zoonoses does not mean that it is transmissible from animals to man, man to man, or man to animals; any transmission would be passive. There is no period of communicability. There are no epidemics in the ordinary sense, but historically, infected sutures, plaster of paris casts, and breakdowns in sterilization often resulted in several simultaneous cases.

DISEASE IN ANIMALS

In animals, the first noticeable symptoms are usually the careful chewing of food, slow swallowing, and stiffness of the legs. In the horse, a prolapse of the membrana nictitans in the inner corner of the eye is an early symptom. The nostrils become greatly expanded. Because it is the most highly susceptible domestic animal, early symptoms are usually quickly followed by trismus (lockjaw), stiff neck, and extreme sensitivity to sound. Urine is more concentrated and micturition is delayed.

Symptoms vary only slightly in other domestic animals. In cattle, there is a suppression of rumination and distention of the left flank. Sheep and goats show stiffness and opisthotonos usually occurs with moderate bloating. In swine, stiffness of the legs and rigid ears are the first symptoms, followed by generalized tetanus. Dogs do not commonly contract tetanus and, when they do, the disease is less likely to become severe. The occurrence of tetanus is unusual in poultry.

Pathogenesis

If death occurs, it usually comes within 10 days. Growth of the organisms is confined to the local anaerobic area, usually a wound; however, in a varying percentage of the cases, no wound is found. The debate over how the toxin spreads has been long and heated, but apparently it both travels up the interstitial spaces of the peripheral nerves and is distributed by the blood and lymph. The fact that trismus is one of the earliest symptoms in both the horse and man could possibly be explained by the greater ability of the trigeminal nerves to bind toxin.

Necropsy reveals no gross or histological findings that are diagnostic. Hyperemia of the gray matter, fatty changes in the heart muscle, and vertebral fractures are commonly found. Tetanolysin is considered by van Heyningen[16] to be cardiotoxic, causing cardiac damage in the clinical disease. Other complications include degenerative changes of respiratory muscles with subsequent pulmonary changes.

The incubation period in animals may be deceptive, but it apparently can be as short as 24 hr in young animals. This is especially true for horses, in which the incubation period is usually 1 to 2 weeks. Although considerably longer incubation periods have been reported, it is difficult to be certain that the disease was caused by the suspected injury. Long incubation periods usually indicate a milder form of the disease, and the converse is also true. Susceptibility of different animal species to tetanus toxin varies greatly. Man and horses are at approximately the same level, followed by the guinea pig, monkey, mouse, goat, rabbit, dog, and cat. Poultry are enormously resistant.

DISEASE IN MAN

Unimmunized Persons

Contracting tetanus does not confer immunity. There are records of individuals having had the disease as many as three times. Usually, diagnosis presents few difficulties when the disease appears in the general form that is characterized by convulsive tonic contractions of the voluntary muscles. The first symptom is often a burning sensation or muscular spasms in the region of the local infection, followed by trismus, stiff neck, opisthotonos, risus sardonicas, and sensitivity to sounds and light. Fever may or may not be present. Local tetanus that does not develop general symptoms sometimes may not be diagnosed.[17]

Cole et al.[18] have published a rare subjective report on a patient who showed symptoms 1 week after cutting his finger:

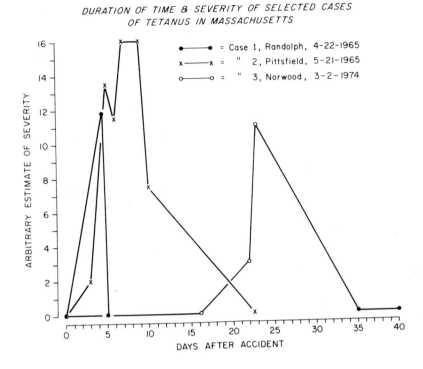

FIGURE 4.   Duration of time and severity of selected cases of tetanus in Massachusetts.

Sudden tightening around the throat, difficult breathing and swallowing. Spasms of the throat usually appeared at rest, lasting about 10 min in early stages, later more prolonged and 2 days after hospital admission seemed continuous. About this time voice reduced to a whisper and jaw felt stiff. The symptoms from then on are only snatches of memory. I felt like snarling, my upper lip involuntarily drawing back over teeth (ricus sardonicus) and a peculiar twitch was vaguely present in my limbs.

The patient had no acute pain except for joint cramps. He had double vision and discomfort from lying in one position. Turning him every 2 hr offered great relief. Great discomfort was felt at night when the patient was awakening, and there were effects that he attributed to medication. He noted other things, such as the fact that the ceiling looked only 18 in. away when lying on his back, and that, while his hearing was acute, the worst times were when there was nothing to hear!

Partially Immunized Persons

In countries with active immunization programs, it is unfortunate but true that many individuals never complete basic immunization and many more do not receive boosters, especially in the upper age groups, unless they receive an injury that requires professional attention. The clinician is therefore required to be alert to the possibility of modified forms of tetanus that can be confounding or perhaps entirely overlooked. In Figure 4, cases 1 and 2 had previous immunization while case 3 may have had one toxoid injection. All available blood samples of these three cases were tested for circulating antitoxin. Without attempting a complete analysis of Figure 4, it seems obvious that case 1 was mild but atypical and case 2 was quite severe. While case 3 had a longer incubation period, every effort was made—without success—to find an injury other than the trivial one occurring on day zero. The high blood titer of case 2 (self-produced homologous antitoxin) at day 5 or possibly before failed to prevent serious disease.

Tetanus toxin is, however, an excellent antigen if enough basic circulating protection to prevent death exists. Stated in another way, it is quite probable that most of the toxin value is in hyperimmunization. In case 2, this happened "naturally" but did not prevent a close brush with death. There is little question but that excellent clinical medicine was the principle lifesaving factor in the treatment of case 2. Blood samples taken at the time of hospital entry were not available for antitoxin studies. Cases 1 and 2 had normal gamma globulin; their immune blood titers are discussed elsewhere.[19] In the rare event that tetanus occurs in the previously immunized, every effort should be made to get blood antitoxin titers at the time of hospital entry, and gamma globulin studies for the detection of abnormalities should be made.[19a]

Pathogenesis is essentially the same as in animals. The incubation period in completely susceptible individuals has a median of 7 to 8 days, and most cases occur 14 days or less after injury. A short incubation period usually indicates a severe case. While textbooks quote short and long periods of incubation, one should at least consider the possibility of another injury that was missed or appeared too trivial to be blamed. The military in World War I was so convinced of a great possibility of activation of tetanus spores in old, healed wounds that they gave a prophylactic dose of antitoxin before any attempt at late wound revision, even though months had elapsed since the original injury. Bonney et al.[20] described one case in which tetanus bacilli were isolated from uterine tissue 10 years after an operation that had been followed by tetanus with recovery.

GENERAL MODE OF SPREAD

Manure from herbivorous domestic animals must be considered the greatest factor in the spread of the disease, either through movement of herds of animals or transportation of their manure for agricultural purposes. Street- and room-dust specimens also yield the organisms on occasion.

EPIDEMIOLOGY

The epidemiologic cycle most often resulting in tetanus cases is manure from herbivorous domestic animals to soil to broken skin or to a more severe injury such as a laceration, deep puncture, crush, or injection. Septic abortion, circumcision, excision, gangrene, frostbite necrosis, puerperal conditions, and otorrhea also act as portals of entry (Table 2). It is reported that in India only 40% of human tetanus cases are due to traumatic injuries. In some areas of the world, such diseases as molluscum contagiosum and the various trematodes and nematodes are a problem.

Principle reservoirs are the feces of herbivorous animals and soil of agricultural fields and pastures. Not much is known regarding the best type of soil for harboring the organisms. Fertile black soil with a high humus content would be expected to harbor more infection than very sandy soil with high drainage capabilities. As evidence, tropical and subtropical areas have been shown to be more dangerous than temperate zones.

A factor perpetrating endemicity is land use in relation to animals. Other conditions being equal, animal feedlots used for that purpose throughout the year would probably have the highest level of danger. In the tropics, the practice of accumulating huge mounds of vegetative and animal humus because of the porosity of the soil makes the vegetables produced thereon (many of them eaten uncooked) contaminated in a more or less continuous cycle.

Table 2
SELECTED SPECIFIC WOUNDS AND
CONDITIONS ASSOCIATED WITH
TETANUS—U.S. 1968 AND 1969

Wound or condition	Total number of cases	Fatal cases	Unknown outcome
Drug addiction	27	17	5
Lawnmower injury to extremity	12	5	1
Burn	10	5	1
Abortion or attempted abortion	5	3	—
Surgical			
Amputation of extremity	3	1	—
Incarcerated umbilical hernia with perforation of small bowel	1	1	—
Automobile accident	3	2	—
Gunshot	2	2	—
Dog bite or scratch	2	1	—
Insect bite	2	2	—
Compound fracture	3	1	1
Gangrenous extremity	2	2	—
Decubitus ulcer	1	1	—
Foot blister	2	—	—
Tornado related	1	—	—

From Center for Disease Control, Tetanus Surveillance, No. 2, U.S. Department of Health, Education, and Welfare, Public Health Service, Atlanta, March 31, 1970.

DIAGNOSIS

Animals

In horses, it is difficult to mistake tetanus for any other disease. Strychnine poisoning closely simulates tetanus in both man and animals, and diagnosis is made from clinical symptoms. Because of the great danger to man, rabies must be ruled out at once. The scar formed at point of bite (most often lips, nostrils, and front extremities) shows increased sensitiveness. The animal may gnaw at the site of the bite or rub it against objects and show fright, unrest, and aggressive behavior; it will not drink.

Cattle rabies is primarily aggressive, as is the rabies of sheep and goats. Swine show early symptoms of irritation, run in all directions, drink only with difficulty, and salivate abundantly. In both horses and cattle, there may be genital excitement.

Dogs have a low incidence of tetanus. Clinically, dog rabies occurs in two forms: dumb and furious. Because of the intimacy dogs share in most households, any dog that shows behavior or voice changes should immediately be placed under the care of a veterinarian for quarantine and observation unless it has been repeatedly vaccinated against rabies. If a rabid dog (or possibly fox or wolf) with the furious form of rabies crosses the path of a herd of grazing domestic animals, it bites anything moving that crosses its path and may attack several animals rather than one. Thus, several animals of a herd may come down with rabies within a short period of time.

The prognosis for tetanus in animals is never good, especially in horses. If the point of entry is known, the incubation period long, and the spasms mild, there is increased hope of survival. Because horses are the most susceptible animals and puncture wounds of the hooves are so dangerous and cause immediate lameness, prompt drainage of the wound is imperative. Prompt drainage of any wound using debridement and prophylactic antitoxin is also important if no symptoms are recognized. Veterinary equine antitoxin in therapeutic doses may be given intravenously according to the manufacturers recommendations, but its value has never been fully established. Just how elaborate any further treatment should be depends upon the value of the animal as a breeding, racing, sporting, or pet animal. Good nursing care includes quiet darkened quarters. If the horse is capable of drinking and eating, this should be aided by holding pails high enough to compensate for its stiff neck. Slings — if deemed necessary — can be used and should be carefully observed 24 hr a day. Muscle relaxants, a tracheostomy, and feces and urine elimination may be helpful.

Man

Where the incidence of tetanus is high (as is found in tropical countries), adults are familiar with the terror of this disease. Hysterical lockjaw and convulsions rank at the top of the list of diagnostic errors. Abscess or fracture of the jaw, tonsilitis, and pharyngitis may be confused with trismus and the dysphagia of tetanus. Infectious diseases such as rabies and meningitis must be ruled out. Abdominal rigidity of undiagnosed origin without other evidence can present a diagnostic problem. Strychnine poisoning must also be considered a possibility.

Prognosis

Much can be said for the view—best expressed by Creech et al.[21]—that the outcome of a case of tetanus is largely determined by the time treatment is instituted. In areas of the world where active immunization has been vigorously pursued, a careful history should be obtained whenever possible to learn if any toxoid was given early enough to be of some help. This might include neonatal tetanus in a baby born to a partially immune mother. Even a small amount of passive maternal antitoxin might be lifesaving in this group that usually has the highest mortality rate. In determining prognosis, many workers rely upon the time between onset of the first symptom and the first spasm as an indicator. Patel et al.[22] found that in 3929 cases in which the onset occurred in less than 48 hr there was a death rate of 63.1%, whereas in cases with an onset of more than 48 hr the death rate was reduced to 22.4%. Here again, tetanus toxoid is such an effective antigen that even partial immunization should improve these figures.

Treatment

Tetanus remains a discouraging disease to treat. Furste and Wheeler[23] consider the management of a human case a truly emergency **team** effort if the terrifying symptoms are to be controlled; constant nursing care is required. Meticulous debridement of any wound and proper nutrition are important, and analgesics, sedatives, muscle relaxants, and antibiotics should be administered in a darkened, private, quiet room. In the more extreme cases, a tracheostomy, feces and urine elimination, and decubital ulcer care involve enough decisions to challenge any "team." Tetanus immune globulin (human) (TIG[H]) occupies a place in therapy, but its value has been difficult to assess thus far, although it has been proven to be of value in prophylaxis following injuries.* TIG(H) must be given intramuscularly. Globulin-modified equine tetanus antitoxin may be given to patients who are negative to sensitivity tests by the intravenous route.

_____

* Editorial comment.

In both human and veterinary practice, tetanus toxoid should be given and followed up on after recovery to complete the basic immunization; booster shots should be included.

PREVENTION AND CONTROL

Man

Surgical care of wounds — The advice of the Committee on Trauma of the American College of Surgeons and the American Public Health Association's "Control of Communicable Diseases" should be consulted for the most complete coverage. This information is in booklet form and is updated from time to time. Surgical procedures include early care, aseptic technique, adequate help, gentle handling, complete debridement, and wound irrigation. *If in doubt about a wound providing anaerobic conditions, it should be left open for drainage.*

Immunization following injury — Here again, one should refer to the advice of the American Public Health Association and the Committee on Trauma. Classified briefly:

1. Satisfactory history of immunization during the past 5 to 10 years
    a. 0.5 cc adsorbed tetanus toxoid
    b. Severe, neglected, or old (more than 24-hr) tetanus-prone wounds. TIG(H): 250 units separate syringe, separate location, plus 0.5 cc adsorbed tetanus toxoid
2. When patient has been actively immunized more than 10 years previously.
    a. See above
    b. See above
    c. Consider providing antibiotics
3. Unimmunized or partially immunized patient
    a. See b. above and follow up with basic immunization described elsewhere as well as booster doses at proper intervals.

Other methods of prevention — These include:

1. Education, e.g., teaching midwives about hygiene and discouraging tribal customs and rites such as the application of cobwebs, manure, or ashes for the treatment of wounds and umbilical cords
2. Active immunization, especially in pregnant women
3. Providing medical identification on the wrist, necktag, or in the billfold, or at least making pertinent information available in the patients medical history
4. Active immunization for international travelers
5. Methods of prevention outside the medical field include making highways, machinery, work areas, and playgrounds safe from trauma.

An interesting and early successful attempt at reducing tetanus was a 1943 Massachusetts law prohibiting the sale of fireworks in the state. There was an immediate drop in the July 4th-holiday incidence of tetanus. A curious sidelight of that period was a local fireworks factory that actually used horse manure for wadding in their products! Deaths were down 38% for the 5 years immediately following enactment of the law, compared with the 5 years preceding 1943. While tetanus toxoid was barely available for the civilian population during the earlier part of this 11-year period, it was not distributed by the state laboratories until 1949. The impact of this free distribution may be gleaned from the following: (1) for the period 1944 to 1948 inclusive, 18 deaths were reported, (2) 1949 to 1953 inclusive, 12 deaths, and (3) 1954 to 1958 inclusive, 7 deaths. By this time, there was a better reporting of cases than in the earlier days of reporting: 1944 to 1948, 62 cases; 1949 to 1953, 28 cases; 1954 to 1958, 30 cases.

Active immunization of the entire population — Again, the best advice other than following the manufacturer's recommendations is that noted under prophylaxis. The American Academy of Pediatrics fits tetanus immunization in with the other childhood immunizations, and these are constantly being updated. It should be emphasized that basic immunization consists of two doses of adsorbed tetanus toxoid 4 weeks apart and one dose 6 months to 1 year later. Most researchers recommend that children 2 months to 6 years of age should get diphtheria and tetanus toxoids with pertussis vaccine. They also advise that routine booster doses be given 5 to 10 years apart. This includes booster doses of tetanus toxoid following injury whenever necessary. There is a preparation of diphtheria and tetanus toxoid with a low dose of each for use in the adult years.

PREVENTION AND CONTROL

Animals
Surgical Care of Wounds

In the horse, the most dangerous injury is a penetrating wound in the hoof; lameness quickly becomes apparent. Hoof forceps should be used to locate the injury through moderate pressure, and the hoof must be cleaned before operating. Use a hoof knife and cut a hole the size of a nickle through the outer sole. Using a scalpel, make a hole the size of a lead pencil through the wall. Apply antiseptic pack for a few hours. Give a prophylactic dose of veterinary tetanus antitoxin and 0.5 cc adsorbed tetanus toxoid using separate syringes and locations. Recommend the completion of basic immunization to the owner of the horse: 0.5 cc toxoid at 4 weeks and again at 6 months to 1 year. Consider antibiotics.

Saddle and harness sores should be prevented, if possible, and treated when they do occur. Wire cuts in the fetlock region, barbed wire cuts, and all trauma should receive surgical attention. To prevent tetanus neonatorum, careful treatment of the umbilical cord and prophylactic antitoxin should be given. In a separate syringe and at a separate location, 0.5 cc of adsorbed tetanus toxoid should also be administered.

In areas where tetanus is a problem, "springtime surgery" in other animals should be preceded by the administration of prophylactic antitoxin and toxoid (as described), and the surgery should be performed in as aseptic a manner as possible. Most wounds should be left open to provide adequate drainage.

Immunization

Horses should receive basic tetanus immunization and booster doses. The value of an individual animal determines whether or not it actually does receive it. Tetanus toxoid is now combined with trivalent equine encephalomyelitis vaccine, and a great many horses only receive this at the time of threatened outbreaks of encephalitis.

If tetanus is a problem on individual farms, other classes of livestock can be immunized. This would probably be confined to valuable breeding animals. Unless economically feasible, it would be difficult to encourage immunization of swine, sheep, and cattle destined for the feedlot and slaughter at an early age.

Man

Reactions to Tetanus Toxoid

Much credit should be given to Dr. J. Howard Mueller of the Department of Bacteriology, Harvard Medical School, for his development of a high-potency, purified, and low-reactive tetanus toxoid. It is impossible to assess how much his work has promoted the general acceptance by the public of tetanus immunization.The present tetanus toxoid is a far cry from that used by the armed services during World War II.

Nevertheless, by the late 1950s it was noted that reactions could be a problem in certain persons after repeated injections. In a study of this problem, it was concluded that these reactions occurred in previously immunized persons and that they were age-dependent, increasing in frequency after the 25th year but practically insignificant at less than 20 years of age.[24] McComb and Levine[25] established that a dose as low as 0.2 flocculating units (Lf)* afforded an acceptable booster response. The following four reactions occurred in Massachusetts National Guardsmen who had extensive immunization histories:

Case 1 — J. G. Z., a 28-year-old man, had basic immunization at 20, a reinforcing dose at 22, and a booster dose at 25 years of age; 5 Lf of tetanus toxoid was followed by severe abdominal pain and diarrhea for 3 days, during which time he was confined to bed, with no appetite. He had persistent joint pains in one leg that was placed in a cast to afford sleep. He was unable to work for 1 week, and symptoms persisted for several weeks. The blood titer was 20 units of tetanus antitoxin per milliliter.

Case 2 — B. C. A., a 34-year-old man with a history of hay fever, treated yearly, had basic immunization at 28, a reinforcing dose at 29, and a booster dose between 30 and 32 years of age; 5 Lf was followed by a large local swelling, temperature of 102°F for 2 or 3 days, chills, and an upset stomach. He was unable to work for 1 week. The blood titer was 20 units of tetanus antitoxin per milliliter.

Case 3 — G. L., a 26-year-old man, had basic immunization at 19, a reinforcing dose at 20, and a booster dose at 23 years of age. There was a history of some reaction to each of the preceding injections; 1 Lf of tetanus toxoid (1 Lf of diphtheria) produced a small local reaction and a temperature of 101°F for 25 hr. The blood titer 3 weeks after injection showed 20 units of tetanus antitoxin per milliliter.

Case 4 — N. J. M., a 31-year-old man, had basic immunization at 17, a reinforcing dose at 24 (followed by a severe reaction), and a booster dose at 29 years of age; 1 Lf of tetanus toxoid was followed by slight fever for 48 hr and general weakness. The blood titer was 20 units of tetanus antitoxin per milliliter.

Although all four cases reached the same extremely high antitoxin level — 20 units (0.01 unit is deemed protective) — cases 1 and 2 received 5 Lf with severe reactions while cases 3 and 4 had more moderate reaction responses with 1 Lf. Note Tables 3, 4, and 5. Although there is no record of Lf strength in Tables 3 and 4, in Table 5 there is obviously a huge overdose of both tetanus and diphtheria toxoids as far as Lf content is concerned. Lack of ample purification of the toxoids can also contribute to reactions.

Homologous vs. Heterologous Antitoxin

This important subject should be discussed in some depth, principally because of its importance in human medicine. The many years during which horse antitoxin was depended upon because there was no other readily available antitoxin have left their "scars" both on prophylaxis and treatment. Very early after the discovery of tetanus antitoxin in the late 1800s, its value for prophylaxis in the horse was firmly established;

---

* 1.0 Lf is the amount of toxoid that will flocculate most rapidly with 1 unit of antitoxin.

Table 3
REACTIONS OF A MALE TO TETANUS TOXOID WITH REPEATED DOSES

Year	Age	Type of toxoid given subcutaneously	Reason	Reaction
1949	2	DPT	Initial series	0
1949	2	DPT	Initial series	0
1951	4	Pptd. T	Injury	0
1952	5	DPT	Booster	0
1953	6	Pptd. T	Injury	0
1955	8	Pptd. T	Injury	Redness and induration greater than anticipated
1963	16	Pptd. T	Injury	Redness and induration of half of upper arm
1964	17	Pptd. T	Injury	Redness and induration from elbow to shoulder: "almost double in size"

Note: September 1965; serum tetanus antitoxin titer: 3 units per mℓ.

From Furste, W. and Wheeler, W. L., *Curr. Probl. Surg.,* October 1972. Copyright 1972 by Yearbook Medical Publishers, Inc., Chicago. With permission.

Table 4
TOTAL NUMBER OF REPORTED SYSTEMIC REACTIONS TO MONOVALENT TETANUS TOXOID IN DENMARK, 1951 TO 1970 (2.5 MILLION INJECTIONS)

	Number of cases	Injection number
Deleterious		
Death	0	
Survival with:		
Neurologic sequelae	1	$\geqslant 4$
Glomerulonephritis	1	2
No permanent damage		
Acute collapse	2	1, 1
Late allergy		
Urticaria, arthralgia, lymphadenitis (8th day)	3	1, 1, 1
Urticaria persisting longer than 1 month	2	$\geqslant 4, 6$
Polyradiculitis	1	4

From Christensen, P., Side Reactions to Tetanus Toxoid, paper presented at the Third International Conference on Tetanus, Sao Paulo, 1970. With permission.

Table 5
DEATHS WITHIN 3 DAYS AFTER VACCINE INJECTION IN RELATION TO TOTAL NUMBER OF INJECTIONS, DENMARK

Composition of vaccine

Period	12 Lf tetanus		12 Lf tetanus 50 Lf diphtheria		12 Lf tetanus 12 Lf diphtheria		7 Lf tetanus 30 Lf diphtheria 16 × 10⁹ pertussis organisms	
	Number of injections	Deaths	Number of injections	Deaths	Number of injections	Deaths	Number of injections	Deaths
1947—1951	68,000	0	570,000	3	73,000	0		
1952—1960	620,000	0	2,000,000	0	550,000	0		
1961—1970	1,850,000	0	670,000	0	610,000	0	2,500,000	10

From Christensen, P., Reactions to Tetanus Toxoid, paper presented at the Third International Conference on Tetanus, Sao Paulo, 1970. With permission.

by 1920, its 1500-unit dose for prophylaxis in the horse was widely accepted. This is still true today. While it was soon used in other dosages for other domestic animals and found valuable, failures were reported. Again, this is still true today when the same veterinary preparation is used.

In animals other than the horse, the antitoxin is a foreign protein and is therefore eliminated more quickly from the body. While reactions to it can be expected to occur in animals other than the horse, this has never become the problem that it is in humans.

Because of these reactions, various methods were used to modify the antitoxin in such a manner as to eliminate — as much as possible — the untoward reactions and, at the same time, preserve its antitoxic qualities. As early as 1951, Hartley[26] learned that this modification, sometimes called despeciation, was done at the expense of its longevity in the body (Figure 5). In this experiment, digested horse antitoxin had practically disappeared after 2 weeks, whereas the unmodified antitoxin lasted above the same level for 6 weeks. The greater antigenicity of adsorbed over fluid toxoid is also shown in Figure 5.

The use of 1500 units prophylactively by the British Army during World War I established its value for many workers in the field. However, at this time there was no essential difference between the human and the veterinary product. Today, dosages at least as high as 10,000 units have been recommended and used for prophylaxis in humans, and thousands of failures have been reported in the world medical literature. The only advantage the modified horse antitoxin has over TIG(H) in humans is that it can be given intravenously if it seems advisable to have it in the general circulation as soon as possible. This cannot be done with the human product. Because the incubation period for tetanus can be short, and when several hours have elapsed before medical care has been sought, the 250-unit dose could be doubled and given in separate locations. Depending upon the location of the wound, it might be feasible to infiltrate intramuscularly around it. Since reactions to TIG(H) are extremely rare, the only objections to larger doses are that other areas of the world are still in need, and its usefulness in natural and man-made disasters is beyond estimation.

All that has been said for serum prophylaxis can be repeated for serum therapy except that its value in therapy is not established and may never be. If one could be sure that 250 units TIG(H) could be distributed in the body before any toxin was

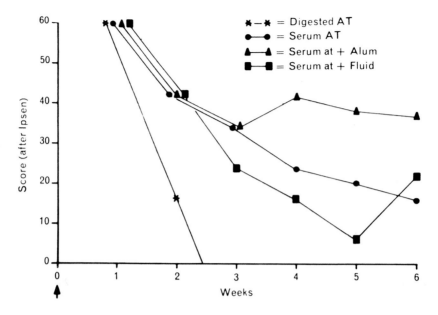

FIGURE 5.   Combined tetanus immunization in mice: 200 units horse antitoxin, 1 Lf toxoid, 20 minimum lethal dose challenge. (From McComb, J. A., *Principles on Tetanus*, Hans Huber, Bern, 1967, 360. With permission.)

elaborated, the battle could be won before any symptoms were ever recognized. MacLennan and co-workers[27] proved this with maternal antibodies in tetanus neonatorum in New Guinea. Obviously, no one can ever be sure of this when the globulin must be given intramuscularly in any size of dose. Neither can one be sure even after extensive testing that the heterologous antitoxin will not cause reactions, although small doses are less likely to cause reactions than larger ones.[28]

A revision of the 1966 recommendations of the Second International Conference on Tetanus was recently published in the *W.H.O. Chronicle*. This was undertaken following the Fourth International Conference in 1975, held in Dakar, Senegal. After reaffirming the value of active immunization and the fact that prevention of tetanus in the unimmunized at the time of injury cannot be guaranteed to provide protection, they recommended that a prophylactic dose of 500 to 1000 units of TIG(H) be administered when available.[29]

The fact that this recommendation comes 10 years after the 250-unit dose was officially adopted decisively indicates the great value of the earlier recommendation both in the matter of protection from tetanus and from the dangers of heterologous antitoxin. Prophylactic "failures" may be due to a previously disregarded, untreated injury rather than to the injury for which treatment was received. These cases of tetanus are most often found in individuals in high-risk, manual occupations. While there can be little risk from a larger dose of human globulin because of reactions, it is well worth repeating that any reduction in the world supply that would limit its use in disasters would penalize underdeveloped countries the most.

REFERENCES

1. **Adams, F., Ed.,** *The Extant Works,* Vol. 1, B. Wertheimer, London, 1856, 246 and 400.
2. **Carle, A. and Rattone, G.,** Studio experimentale sull' eziologia del tetano, *G. Accad. Med. Torino,* 32, 174, 1884.
3. **Nicolaier, A.,** Über Infectiosen tetanus, *Dtsch. Med. Wochenschr.,* 10, 842, 1884.
4. **Kitasato, S.,** Über den tetanus Bacillus, *Z. Hyg.,* 7, 225, 1889.
5. **von Behring, E. and Kitasato, S.,** Über das Zustandelkommen der Diphtherie-Immunität und der Tetanus-Immunität bei Thieren, *Dtsch. Med. Wochenschr.,* 16, 1113, 1890.
6. **Ramon, G. and Zöeller, C.,** L'anatoxin tétanique et l'immunisation active de l'homme vis-a-vis du tétanos, *Ann. Inst. Pasteur Paris,* 41, 803, 1927.
7. **Ramon, G. and Zoeller, C.,** Sur la valeur et la durée de l'immunité conferée par l'anatoxine tétanique dans la vaccination de l'homme contre tétanus, *C. R. Seances Soc. Biol. Paris,* 112, 347, 1933.
8. **Cohn, E., Strong, L., Hughes, W., Jr., Mulford, D., Ashworth, J., Melin, M., and Taylor, H.,** Preparation and properties of serum and plasma proteins. IV. A system for the separation into fractions of the protein and lipoprotein components of biological tissues and fluids, *J. Am. Chem. Soc.,* 68, 459, 1946.
9. **McComb, J. and Dwyer, R.,** Passive-active immunization with tetanus immune globulin (human), *N. Engl. J. Med.,* 268, 857, 1962.
10. **Levine, L., McComb, J., Dwyer, R., and Latham, W.,** Active-passive tetanus immunization, choice of toxoid, dose of tetanus immune globulin and timing of injections, *N. Engl. J. Med.,* 274, 186, 1966.
11. **Mellanby, J. and van Heyningen, W. E.,** Pathogenesis, in *Principles on Tetanus,* Eckmann, L., Ed., Hans Huber, Bern, 1967, 177.
12. **Bytchenko, B.,** Epidemiology, in *Principles on Tetanus,* Eckmann, L., Ed., Hans Huber, Bern, 1967, 21.
13. **Masawe, A.,** Tetanus in Kampala, Uganda. The experience in Mulago Hospital from 1963-1965, *East Afr. Med. J.,* 51, 255, 1974.
14. **Sakurai, N.,** Epidemiology, in *Principles on Tetanus,* Eckmann, L., Ed., Hans Huber, Bern, 1967, 91.
15. **Sergeeva, T. I. and Matveev, K. I.,** Epidemiology, in *Principles on Tetanus,* Eckmann, L., Ed., Hans Huber, Bern, 1967, 77.
16. **van Heyningen, W.,** Pathogenicity and virulence of microorganisms. IV. Bacterial toxins, in *General Pathology,* Florey, L., Ed., 4th ed., Lloyd-Luke, London, 1970, 879.
17. **Struppler, A., Struppler, E., and Adams, R.,** Local tetanus in man, *Arch. Neurol.,* 8, 162, 1963.
18. **Cole, L., Youngman, H., and Gandy, A.,** An attack of tetanus, *Lancet,* 2, 567, 1968.
19. **McComb, J.,** Tetanus in previously immunized persons, *N. Engl. J. Med.,* 273, 452, 1965.
19a. **Berger, S. A., Cherubin, C. E., Nelson, S., and Levine, L.,** Tetanus despite preexisting antitetanus antibody, *JAMA,* 240(8), 769, 1978.
20. **Bonney, V., Box, C., and MacLennan, J.,** Tetanus bacillus recovered from scar ten years after an attack of past operative tetanus, *Br. Med. J.,* 2, 10, 1938.
21. **Creech, O., Glover, A., and Ochsner, A.,** Tetanus: evaluation of treatment at Charity Hospital, New Orleans, Louisiana, *Ann. Surg.,* 146, 369, 1957.
22. **Patel, J., Mehta, B. C., and Modi, K. N.,** Prognosis in tetanus, in *Proc. Int. Conf. on Tetanus,* Patel, J., Ed., Bombay Associated Advertisers and Printers, Bombay, 1965, 181.
23. **Furste, W. and Wheeler, W.,** Tetanus: a team disease, *Curr. Probl. Surg.,* October 1972.
24. **Levine, L., Ipsen, J., Jr., and McComb, J.,** Adult immunization: preparation and evaluation of combined fluid tetanus and diphtheria toxoids for adult use, *Am. J. Hyg.,* 73, 20, 1961.
25. **McComb, J. and Levine, L.,** Adult immunization. II. Dosage reduction as a solution to increasing reactions to tetanus toxoid, *N. Engl. J. Med.,* 265, 1152, 1961.
26. **Hartley, P.,** The effect of peptic digestion on the properties of diphtheria antitoxin, *Proc. R. Soc. London Ser. B,* 138, 499, 1951.
27. **MacLennan, R., Schofield, F., Pittman, M., Hardegree, M., and Barile, M.,** Immunization against neonatal tetanus in New Guinea, *Bull. W.H.O.,* 32, 683, 1965.
28. **Anon.,** Antitoxin in treatment of tetanus, *Lancet* (editorial), 944, May 1, 1976.
29. **Cvjetanovic, B., Bytchenko, B., and Edsall, G.,** Guidelines for the prevention of tetanus, *W.H.O. Chron.,* 30, 201, 1976.

EDITORIAL COMMENT

The World Health Organization reported that there were 400,000 deaths from tetanus world-wide in 1970. Tetanus is a completely preventable disease yet almost one person dies weekly in the U.S. The incidence of disease has declined dramatically in countries where tetanus toxoid is used, but the case fatality rate has remained greater than 50%. One reason for this is that physicians often have not realized that tetanus is not necessarily the result of a deep wound. It may be associated with relatively minor lesions or indolent conditions. Furthermore, about 20% of cases occur without any identifiable site of injury or break in the skin.

Tetanus was formerly associated with accidents on the farm, in automobiles, or hunting. Today, however, in the U.S., 75% of tetanus-associated wounds occur in the home. Injuries involving lawn mowers are the second most frequent type of injury associated with tetanus. These latter, as well as accidents in the home, can be attributed to animal contamination of the premises and in some cases, human contamination. Minor injuries, such as small abrasions or minor puncture wounds, that arouse little concern on the part of the injured may result in fatal tetanus in persons not immunized. Such a case occured in a pharmacist some years ago who had a minor injury caused by a palm frond.

While physicians treat traumatic wounds with prompt immunoprophylaxis, they all too often ignore decubitus ulcers, diabetic skin ulcers, or minor wounds including dental procedures and even ear-piercing. Occasionally tetanus follows routine surgery in man and animals (Figure 1).

The prognosis is related to a variety of factors such as age, wound location, and the rapidity of onset of symptoms. If the incubation period is less than 10 days, the fatality rate is over 60%; if greater than 10 days, the fatality rate is about 35% and even less than 20% in persons with mild spasms. Patients with severe convulsions have a fatality rate of almost 75%.

Adequate immunization is the only way to prevent tetanus, inasmuch as the spores occur in the excreta of all animals including humans and are commonly found in soil and dust. Only a few spores in a wound can result in enough toxin production to cause fatal disease.

The production of this toxin may take place with little or no sign of inflammation to alert the physician or injured person to the threat of tetanus. Hence, the importance of immunization to insure adequate levels of circulating antibodies.

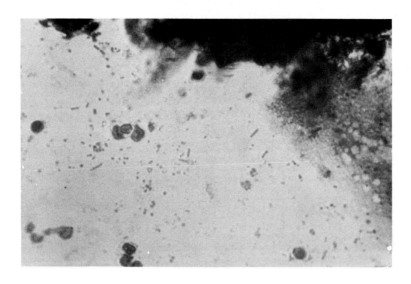

FIGURE 1.   Gram stain of purulent exudate from a small wound on the thumb of a patient with severe tetanus. Note tennis-racket-like Gram-positive rod *(Clostridium tetani)* in the center of the photograph (arrow). (Reprinted from McGee, Z. A. and Melly, M. A., *Consultant,* Vol. 18, No. 6, 1978. With permission, Cliggott Publishing Co., Greenwich, Conn.)

BOVINE TUBERCULOSIS

L. D. Konyha, E. M. Himes, and C. O. Thoen

INTRODUCTION

Bovine tuberculosis is an infectious disease caused by *Mycobacterium bovis* and is usually characterized by formation of nodular granulomas known as tubercles. Although commonly defined as a chronic debilitating disease, bovine tuberculosis can occasionally assume an acute, rapidly progressive course. Any body tissue can be affected, but lesions are most frequently observed in the lymph nodes, lungs, intestines, liver, spleen, pleura, and peritoneum.

Hippocrates (470 to 376 B.C.), a Greek physician who acquired the title "Father of Medicine," apparently was the first to write elaborate descriptions of persons suffering from tuberculosis. He called the disease "Phthisis," meaning to waste away. It was later known as consumption, which has the same meaning. Through the centuries it was given various names such as "Captain of the Men of Death" and "Great White Plague." The word "tuberculosis" was introduced in 1839.[1]

ETIOLOGIC AGENT

Mycobacterium bovis is a slow growing, nonchromogenic, acid-fast bacillus. A confirmative diagnosis of *M. bovis* requires isolation and identification of the mycobacterium. Simplified methods that use 2% sodium hydroxide for treating tissues and body exudates minimize contamination.[2] Colonies usually appear on egg media at 3 to 8 weeks incubation at 37°C. *M. bovis* is inhibited by glycerol; therefore, media without glycerol should be used. Growth of this fastidious microorganism can be enhanced by addition of pyruvate to the culture media.[3]

Smears of colonies should be stained with Ziehl-Neelsen and examined for acid-fast rods. Biochemical and drug susceptibility tests are useful for identification.[2] *M. bovis* does not produce niacin or nitrate reductase and is inhibited by thiophen-2-carboxylic acid hydrazide.

TRUE AND ALTERNATE HOSTS

Cattle are considered to be the true hosts of *M. bovis*; however, the disease has been reported in several other species. In the U.S., the organism has been isolated from swine, cats, horses, dogs, and man.[4] Moreover, isolations have been made fro certain wild nondomestic animals including deer, mink, antelope, and bison. Consequently, when epidemiologic investigations are conducted on premises where *M. bovis*-infected cattle are maintained, it is necessary to consider other domestic and wild animals as potential reservoirs of infection.

Tuberculosis in exotic animals — including nonhuman primates — is reported to be widespread in the U.S. and some other countries.[5-7] *M. bovis* was isolated from exotic animals in 18 states during the 5-year period from 1971 to 1976.[7] Isolations were made from monkeys, baboons, deer, antelope, llamas, kudus, and sitatungas and from one eland, tapir, and elk. These animals came from seven zoos, seven animal parks, and four animal colonies. The source of these infections is unknown; however, it is suspected that the animals were infected during transport from their native habitat to their destination. These infections are of concern to regulatory officials since the offspring of imported animals may be moved interstate without restriction and thereby provide a foci of infection for cattle and other domestic animals.

DISTRIBUTION

Bovine

The world-wide distribution of *M. bovis* infection in cattle (by geographic grouping of countries) is shown in Table 1. Of the 155 countries reporting, 21 indicated bovine tuberculosis to be exceptionally low in occurrence, 68 indicated a low sporadic incidence, 21 indicated moderate incidence, and 3 indicated high incidence.

Man

In most countries where strains of mycobacteria from human patients have been typed, the bovine-type bacillus has been identified. The incidence of pulmonary tuberculosis caused by the bovine bacillus is higher, as might be expected, in farm workers than urban inhabitants.[8] Studies in some Latin American countries (Argentina, Brazil, Chile, Venezuela, and Mexico) indicate that human infection due to the bovine bacillus is not uncommon despite the apparently widespread habit in those countries of boiling milk.[8] Apparently this is because milk products are frequently prepared from raw or inadequately pasteurized milk, and because disease can be transmitted to man in other ways, especially by inhalation. In a more recent study in Sao Paulo, 7 of 200 (3.5%) mycobacterial isolations from tuberculous patients were *M. bovis.*[9]

Workers at the Institute Pasteur de Lille did an epidemiologic study of human tuberculosis cases (extrapulmonary vs. pulmonary) due to *M. bovis* in 25 countries for the period from 1954 to 1970.[10] More than 2% of the cases were pulmonary and 9.4% were extrapulmonary (Table 2). The combined incidence of both forms of *M. bovis* infection ranged from a high of 25.9% to a low of 0.01% with an average of 3.1%.

In the U.S., infection with the bovine tubercle bacillus in man is rare. According to Feldman,[11] humans now infected with *M. bovis* are probably elderly persons 50 to 80 years of age who were infected before the tuberculin testing of cattle and the pasteurization of milk were generally practiced. Exceptions are possible, of course. In rural areas where a family obtains its milk from the "family cow," an occasional such animal that has not been tuberculin tested may harbor tubercle bacilli and could be a source of tuberculosis in man. In 1976, three family members of a family were found to have positive skin tests when checked by U.S. Public Health Service personnel. Since they had been drinking raw milk from a tuberculous cattle herd, they were immediately placed on isoniazid (INH) chemoprophylaxis.

Evidence of rural vs. nonrural incidence is contained in a report from the U.S.S.R. that shows that the incidence of *M. bovis* infection in humans varied from 5% in Moscow to 61% in Kasakh S.S.R. (Siberia).[12] Blagodarny et al.[13] studied the epidemiologic hazards presented by tuberculosis-affected farm animals in Kazakhstan (U.S.S.R.). *M. bovis* was isolated in 9.5 to 15% of the newly identified patients, and the authors concluded that tuberculosis in stock breeders and milkmaids is an occupational disease; they recommended that chemoprophylaxis be carried out.

Other studies were made in Sweden and Germany to investigate whether the risk of tuberculous infection in persons from different areas is related to varying prevalences of tuberculous infection in cattle.[14,15] It was found that the risk of infection in man is related to the prevalence of tuberculous infection in cattle.

Table 1

WORLD-WIDE DISTRIBUTION OF *MYCOBACTERIUM BOVIS* INFECTION IN CATTLE BY GEOGRAPHIC GROUP

	Disease incidence	Disease control
Group 1		
Mauritania	Low, sporadic	
Morocco	Moderate	Systematic testing under official control scheme; quarantine, movement control, and other precautions at frontier and inside of country; slaughter policy; notifiable disease
Algeria	Moderate	Slaughter policy; notifiable disease
Tunisia	Mainly in imported animals	Systematic testing under official control scheme; notifiable disease
Libyan Arab Republic	Low, sporadic	Systematic testing under official control scheme; slaughter policy
Egypt	Low, sporadic	Slaughter policy; notifiable disease; compulsory testing and slaughter of reactors on governmental farms
Sudan	Low, sporadic	Systematic testing under official control scheme; slaughter policy; notifiable disease; compulsory testing and slaughter of reactors on governmental farms
Ethiopia	Low, sporadic	Slaughter policy
French territory of Afars, Issas	Low, sporadic	
Somalia	Disease only recently recognized in country[a]	
Kenya	Not recorded, obviously not present	Quarantine and other precautions at frontier; slaughter policy; notifiable disease
Uganda	Low, sporadic; highest incidence in Ankole Longhorn cattle; small incidence in wild buffalo	Notifiable disease
Tanzania	Exceptional occurrence	
Malawi	Moderate	Systematic testing under official control scheme; vaccination; notifiable disease; BCG vaccination of calves
Zambia	Moderate	Quarantine, movement control, and other precautions at frontier and inside of country; slaughter policy; notifiable disease

Table 1 (continued)
WORLD-WIDE DISTRIBUTION OF *MYCOBACTERIUM BOVIS* INFECTION IN CATTLE BY GEOGRAPHIC GROUP

	Disease incidence	Disease control
Rwanda	Low, sporadic	
Zaire	Low, sporadic	
Congo, P.R.	High	Systematic testing under official control scheme; slaughter policy; notifiable disease
Group 2		
Chad	No information available	
Niger	Low, sporadic	Slaughter policy; notifiable disease
Upper Volta	Low, sporadic	Slaughter policy
Mali	Moderate	
Senegal	Exceptional occurrence	
Gambia	No information available	
Cape Verde	Confined to certain regions	Slaughter policy
Guinea (Bissau)	Mainly in imported animals	
Guinea	Not recorded, probably not present	
Sierra Leone	No information available	Notifiable disease
Liberia	Mainly in imported animals; confirmed only at slaughterhouse in cattle imported for slaughter	
Ivory Coast	Low, sporadic	Slaughter policy; notifiable disease
Ghana	Low, sporadic	Slaughter policy
Togo	Low, sporadic	Systematic testing under official control scheme; notifiable disease
Benin	Low, sporadic	
Nigeria	Low, sporadic	Systematic testing under official control scheme; quarantine, movement control, and other precautions at frontier and inside of country; slaughter policy; notifiable disease
Cameroon	Low, sporadic	Systematic testing under official control scheme; slaughter policy; notifiable disease

Equatorial Guinea	Low, sporadic	Slaughter policy; notifiable disease
Gabon	Not recorded, probably not present	
Central African Republic	Moderate; confined to certain regions	Quarantine, movement control, and other precautions at frontier and inside of country; notifiable disease
Group 3		
Mozambique	Moderate	Systematic testing under official control scheme
Rhodesia	Disease much reduced but still in existence	Systematic testing under official control scheme; slaughter policy; notifiable disease
Botswana	Exceptional occurrence	
Lesotho	Suspected but not confirmed	
Swaziland	Low, sporadic	Quarantine, movement control, and other precautions at frontier and inside of country; slaughter policy; notifiable disease
South Africa	Moderate	Systematic testing under official control scheme; quarantine, movement control, and other precautions at frontier and inside of country; notifiable disease; eradication scheme launched in 1969
Angola	Moderate	Slaughter policy; notifiable disease
Brazil	Confined to certain regions; moderate	
Argentina	Low, sporadic	Systematic testing under official control scheme; quarantine and other precautions at frontier
Uraguay	Low, sporadic	Systematic testing under official control scheme; slaughter policy; notifiable disease[b]
Paraguay	Moderate	Notifiable disease
Chile	High	Systematic testing under official control scheme; notifiable disease
Bolivia	Moderate	
Peru	Low, sporadic; disease in regression, virtually limited to dairy herds	Systematic testing under official control scheme; quarantine, movement control, and other precautions at frontier and inside of country; notifiable disease
Ecuador	Exceptional occurrence	
Columbia	Not recorded, obviously not present	Prohibition of imports from infected countries

Table 1 (continued)
WORLD-WIDE DISTRIBUTION OF *MYCOBACTERIUM BOVIS* INFECTION IN CATTLE BY GEOGRAPHIC GROUP

	Disease incidence	Disease control
Venezuela	Low, sporadic	Systematic testing under official control scheme; quarantine, movement control, and other precautions at frontier and inside of country; slaughter policy; notifiable disease; eradication scheme operating in central and western part of country
Guyana	Low, sporadic	
Surinam	Not recorded, obviously not present	Systematic testing under official control scheme
Group 4		
Iceland	Not recorded, obviously not present; case last recorded in 1959	
Canada	Exceptional occurrence	Systematic testing under official control scheme; slaughter policy; notifiable disease; compulsory official national eradication scheme
U.S.	Exceptional occurrence	Systematic testing under official control scheme; quarantine, movement control, and other precautions at frontier and inside of country; slaughter policy; notifiable disease
Mexico	Moderate	Notifiable disease
Belize	Suspected but not confirmed; no reactors found in the 1938 cattle tested	Notifiable disease
Guatemala	High	Systematic testing under official control scheme; quarantine, movement control, and other precautions at frontier and inside of country; slaughter policy; notifiable disease
El Salvador	Low, sporadic	Systematic testing under official control scheme
Honduras	Low, sporadic	Notifiable disease
Nicaragua	Exceptional occurrence	

Costa Rica	Low, sporadic	Systematic testing under official control scheme; quarantine and other precautions at frontier; slaughter policy
Panama	Exceptional occurrence	Systematic testing under official control scheme; quarantine measures and movement control inside of the country; slaughter policy; notifiable disease
Bermuda	Not recorded, probably not present	Systematic testing under official control scheme; slaughter policy
Bahamas	Not recorded, probably not present	
Cuba	Disease much reduced but still exists[c]	Notfiable disease
Jamaica	Low, sporadic	Notifiable disease
Haiti	Suspected but not confirmed	
Dominican Republic	Moderate	Systematic testing under official control scheme
British Antilles	Disease only recently recognized[d]	
Trinidad and Tobago	Exceptional occurrence	Systematic testing under official control scheme; slaughter policy; notifiable disease
American Virgin Islands	Not recorded, obviously not present; eradicated more than 10 years ago	Systematic testing under official control scheme; quarantine and other precautions at frontier; slaughter policy
Group 5		
Great Britain	Low, sporadic[e]	Systematic testing under official control scheme; control of wildlife resevoirs; slaughter policy; notifiable disease
Isle of Man	Not recorded, obviously not present; case last recorded in 1970	Systematic testing under official control scheme; slaughter policy; notifiable disease
Channel Islands	Not recorded, obviously not present; case last recorded in 1951	Slaughter policy; notifiable disease
Northern Ireland	Exceptional occurrence[e]	Systematic testing under official control scheme; quarantine, movement control, and other precautions at frontier and inside of country; slaughter policy; notifiable disease

Table 1 (continued)
WORLD-WIDE DISTRIBUTION OF *MYCOBACTERIUM BOVIS* INFECTION IN CATTLE BY GEOGRAPHIC GROUP

	Disease incidence	Disease control
Ireland	Disease much reduced but still in existence[f]	Slaughter policy; notifiable disease
Denmark	Not recorded, probably not present; case last recorded in 1974[g]	Systematic testing under official control scheme; prohibition of imports from infected countries; quarantine, movement control, and other precautions at frontier and inside of country; slaughter policy; notifiable disease
Norway	Not recorded, obviously not present	Quarantine and other precautions at frontier; slaughter policy; notifiable disease
Sweden	Not recorded, obviously not present; case last recorded in 1973 (one)	Notifiable disease
Finland	Exceptional occurrence (one case in 1975)	Slaughter policy; notifiable disease
Netherlands	Exceptional occurrence	Systematic testing under official control scheme; slaughter policy
Belgium	Exceptional occurrence	Systematic testing under official control scheme; slaughter policy; notifiable disease
Luxembourg	Not recorded, obviously not present	Slaughter policy; notifiable disease
France	Low, sporadic	Slaughter policy; notifiable disease
Federal Republic of Germany	Exceptional occurrence	Quarantine, movement control, and other precautions at frontier and inside of country; slaughter policy; notifiable disease
Switzerland	Not recorded, obviously not present; case last recorded in 1959	Notifiable disease
Austria	Exceptional occurrence	Systematic testing under official control scheme; slaughter policy; notifiable disease
Italy	Low, sporadic; compulsory notification limited to clinically apparent disease	Systematic testing under official control scheme; slaughter policy; notifiable disease

Country		
Malta	Low, sporadic	Systematic testing under official control scheme
Spain	Disease much reduced but still in existence; compulsory official national eradication scheme	Systematic testing under official control scheme; quarantine and other precautions at frontier; slaughter policy; notifiable disease
Portugal	Disease much reduced but still in existence; dairy cattle are free of the disease	Systematic testing under official control scheme; slaughter policy; notifiable disease
Group 6 U.S.S.R.	Confined to certain regions	Systematic testing under official control scheme; quarantine measures and movement control inside of country; slaughter policy
Poland	Exceptional occurrence	Systematic testing under official control scheme; slaughter policy; notifiable disease
German Democratic Republic	Disease much reduced but still in existence	Systematic testing under official control scheme; slaughter policy; notifiable disease
Czechoslovakia	Exceptional occurrence	Systematic testing under official control scheme; slaughter policy; notifiable disease
Hungary	Low, sporadic	Systematic testing under official control scheme; slaughter policy; notifiable disease
Romania	Moderate	Systematic testing under official control scheme; quarantine, movement control, and other precautions at frontier and inside of country; slaughter policy; notifiable disease
Bulgaria	Low, sporadic	Systematic testing under official control scheme; control of nonvertebrate vectors; quarantine, movement control, and other precautions at frontier and inside of country; slaughter policy
Yugoslavia	Low, sporadic; eradication scheme successfully terminated in 1952	Slaughter policy; notifiable disease
Albania	Disease much reduced but still in existence	Slaughter policy; notifiable disease
Greece	Confined to certain regions	Systematic testing under official control scheme; prohibition of imports from infected countries; notifiable disease

Cyprus	Not recorded, obviously not present	Systematic testing under official control scheme; quarantine and other precautions at frontier; notifiable disease
Turkey	Low, sporadic	Systematic testing under official control scheme; quarantine, movement control, and other precautions at frontier and inside of country; slaughter policy
Syrian Arab Republic	Exceptional occurrence	
Lebanon	Suspected but not confirmed	Notifiable disease
Israel	Not recorded, obviously not present; last case recorded in 1972; for the first year, not a single case was confirmed in 1973	Systematic testing under official control scheme; quarantine and other precautions at frontier; slaughter policy; notifiable disease
Jordan	Low, sporadic	Systematic testing under official control scheme; notifiable disease
Iraq	Low, sporadic	Notifiable disease
Iran	Low, sporadic	Systematic testing under official control scheme; slaughter policy; notifiable disease
Afghanistan	Disease exists; distribution and incidence entirely unknown	
Pakistan	Moderate	
Group 7		
Saudi Arabia	Moderate	Slaughter policy
Yemen Arab Republic	Low, sporadic	
Yemen, Democratic	Low, sporadic	
United Arab Emirates	Suspected but not confirmed	
Qatar	Not recorded, probably not present	Slaughter policy

Country	Occurrence	Control measures
Bahrain	Suspected but not confirmed	Prohibition of imports from infected countries
Kuwait	Low, sporadic	Slaughter policy
Sri Lanka	Exceptional occurrence	
India	Moderate	
Nepal	Moderate	
Bangladesh	No information available	
Burma	Low, sporadic	Systematic testing under official control scheme; slaughter policy; notifiable disease
Thailand	Exceptional occurrence	Slaughter policy
Cambodia	Low, sporadic	
Lao P.D.R.	Disease exists; distribution and incidence entirely unknown	
South Vietnam	Low, sporadic	Slaughter policy
Macao	Exceptional occurrence	
Hong Kong	Low, sporadic	Notifiable disease
Group 8		
Korea	Low, sporadic	Systematic testing under official control scheme; quarantine, movement control, and other precautions at frontier and inside of country; slaughter policy
Japan	Low, sporadic (136 animals in 29 prefectures)	Systematic testing under official control scheme; quarantine, movement control, and other precautions at frontier and inside of country; slaughter policy; notifiable disease
Philippines	Low, sporadic	Systematic testing under official control scheme; slaughter policy; notifiable disease
Indonesia	Low, sporadic; confined to certain regions	Systematic testing under official control scheme; slaughter policy; notifiable disease
Portuguese Timor	Not recorded, obviously not present	
Singapore	Exceptional occurrence	
Malaysia (western)	Exceptional occurrence; mainly in imported animals	Systematic testing under official control scheme
Malaysia (Sabah)	Disease only recently recognized	Systematic testing under official control scheme; prohibition of imports from infected countries; slaughter policy; notifiable disease

Table 1 (continued)
WORLD-WIDE DISTRIBUTION OF *MYCOBACTERIUM BOVIS* INFECTION IN CATTLE BY GEOGRAPHIC GROUP

	Disease incidence	Disease control
New Zealand	Low, sporadic	Systematic testing under official control scheme; slaughter policy; notifiable disease
Australia	Low, sporadic; confined to certain regions	Systematic testing under official control scheme; quarantine, movement control, and other precautions at frontier and inside of country; slaughter policy
Papua (New Guinea)	Not recorded, probably not present; last case recorded in 1963	Quarantine, movement control, and other precautions at frontier and inside of country; slaughter policy; notifiable disease
Fiji	Disease much reduced but still in existence	Quarantine, movement control, and other precautions at frontier and inside of country; imported animal must be negative to test in country of origin
New Hebrides	Low, sporadic	Systematic testing under official control scheme; quarantine, movement control, and other precautions at frontier and inside of country; slaughter policy
New Caledonia	Not recorded, obviously not present	Systematic testing under official control scheme; quarantine and other precautions at frontier; test given to milking cows; negative test required for importation
French Polynesia	Not recorded, probably not present	Quarantine, movement control, and other precautions at frontier and inside of country
Western Samoa	Moderate	
Mauritius	Low, sporadic	Systematic testing under official control scheme; slaughter policy
Madagascar	Moderate	
Reunion	Low, sporadic	Quarantine, movement control, and other precautions at frontier and inside of country

[a] After examining several suspected organs from slaughterhouses, only one specimen proved positive for TB by cultural and biological tests during the year. All other specimens were negative even though some of them showed acid-fast rods under microscopic examination, identified as *Nocardia*.

[b] In dairy farms supplying milk to the National Cooperative of Milk Producers (Conaprole): annual tuberculin testing, slaughter of positive reactors, and milk price incentive. In other commercial dairy cattle and beef cattle: voluntary testing and disposal of reactors.

c   In 1975, more than 3,700,000 tests were carried out with an incidence of positive reactors below 0.04%. About 1,700,000 cattle were officially certified to be free of the disease.

d   Recorded in Antigua since 1974 on post-mortem 1974: 4 bovine cases; 1975: 12 bovine cases. Not recorded on other islands. Sample testings in previous years negative.

e   Virtually eradicated. Country declared an "attested" (i.e., free) area in October 1960.

f   Virtually eradicated. Country declared an "attested" (i.e., free) area in October 1965.

g   Two herds found to be infected in 1974. Before this, the disease had not been recorded since 1971.

From *FAO/WHO/OIE Animal Health Yearbook, 1975*, Food and Agriculture Organization, Animal Health Service, Animal Production and Health Division, Rome, 1976. With permission.

Table 2
FREQUENCY OF *MYCOBACTERIUM BOVIS* IN HUMAN TUBERCULOSIS — GEOGRAGRAPHIC DISTRIBUTION, 1954 to 1970

	Tuberculosis, pleuro-pulmonary (primary thoracic infection)			Tuberculosis, extra pleuro-pulmonary			All forms of tuberculosis		
	T[a]	B[b]	%B[c]	T	B	%B	T	B	%B
South Africa							180	13	7.2
Germany	4,593	193	4.2	2,409	479	19.9	7,300 (298[e])	769	10.5
England	2,000	4	0.2	4,739	64	4.2	12,676	305	2.4
Australia	26[d]	6[d]	23.1				26[d]	6[d]	23.1
Austria							898	5	0.6
Brazil	664	0	0				664	0	0
Congo							408	9	2.2
Denmark	1,967	70	3.5	107	13	12.2	2,074	83	4.0
Egypt	110	4	3.6	37	14	37.8	147	18	12.2
France	18,088	191	1.1	1,859	144	7.7	24,262	388	1.6
Greece	583	11	1.9	16	3	18.7	599	14	2.3
Hungary							2,763	341	12.6
Iraq	2,500	1	0.04				2,500	1	0.04
Italy	165	5		22	3	13.6	2,794	79	2.1
Kenya				57	0	0	57	0	0
Mexico							487	36	7.4
Nigeria				65	0	0	65	0	0
Poland	385 (68[e])	6	1.5	59	34	57.6	603 (187[e])	48 (1[e])	8.0
Romania				27	7	25.9	27	7	25.9
Switzerland	1[e]	1[e]		149	38	25.5	1,216 (1[e])	69 (1[e])	5.7
Czechoslovakia	1,149	44	3.8	275	101	36.7	1,424	145	10.2
Turkey	3,416	204	5.9	271	53	19.5	3,687	257	6.9
U.S.							2,000	2	0.1
Venezuela	1	1					165	9	5.4
Yugoslavia							16,000	3	0.01
Total	35,648	741	2.1	10,092	953	9.4	83,022	2,607	3.1

[a]   Total number of cases studied.
[b]   Number of cases of tuberculosis of bovine origin.
[c]   Proportion of cases of tuberculosis of bovine origin per 100 cases for which species of bacillus was determined.
[d]   Cases of tuberculosis observed in dairy workers.
[e]   Cases of tuberculosis observed in persons living in contact with cattle.

From Gervois, M., Vaillant, J. M., Fontaine, J. F., Laroche, G., and Dubois, G., *Arch. Monaldi Tisiol. Mal. Appar. Respir.*, 27(3), 298, 1972. With permission.

Several pertinent facts on the infectivity of *M. bovis* for humans, as reported by Feldman,[11] are still applicable today:

1. *M. bovis* is an important pathogen for human beings.
2. The marked decrease in the incidence of tuberculosis in cattle has been paralleled by a striking reduction in the incidence of *M. bovis* infections in humans. (The incidence of *M. bovis* in cattle [Table 1] suggests where the greatest likelihood is of finding *M. bovis* infections in persons.)

3. *M. bovis* is capable of producing many forms of tuberculosis.
4. Although the extrapulmonary forms of tuberculosis predominate in the statistics, several hundred cases of human pulmonary tuberculosis caused by *M. bovis* have been recorded.
5. The tuberculous dairy cow is a serious menace to human health and should not be tolerated by an informed society.

DISEASE IN ANIMALS

Symptomatology — Bovine

Clinical evidence of tuberculosis in cattle is seldom encountered in the U.S. today because the intradermal tuberculin test enables presumptive diagnosis and elimination of infected animals before signs appear.[16] Prior to the national tuberculosis eradication campaign, however, the signs associated with this disease were commonly observed.

These signs vary with the distribution of tubercles in the body, but with few exceptions the course of the disease is chronic. In many instances, characteristic signs are lacking even in advanced stages of the disease when many organs may be involved. Lung involvement may be manifested by a cough, that can be induced by changes in temperature or manual pressure on the trachea.

Dyspnea and other signs of low-grade pneumonia are also evidence of lung involvement. In advanced cases, lymph nodes are often greatly enlarged and may obstruct air passages, the alimentary tract, or blood vessels. Lymph nodes of the head and neck may become visibly affected and sometimes rupture and drain. Involvement of the digestive tract is manifested by intermittent diarrhea and constipation in some instances. Extreme emaciation and acute respiratory distress may occur during the terminal stages of tuberculosis. Lesions involving the female genitalia may occur.[16a]

Primary uterine infection may occur following service by an infected bull or even by artificial insemination with contaminated semen.[17] Male genitalia are seldom involved; however, when penile lesions are present, they appear to be limited to the submucosa of the glands, sheath, and adjacent lymphatics.[18]

Pathology — Bovine

Infection may be established by inhalation of *M. bovis* organisms on dust particles or water droplets.[5] Bronchioles cannot stop small particles and microorganisms that air turbulence during inspiration does not force against the mucociliary layer of the terminal bronchioles.[19] Foreign substances that enter alveoli are removed by alveolar macrophages.[20] Alveolar macrophages have been shown to originate from blood monocytes.[21] Ultrastructurally, macrophages in progressively expanding granulomas have enlarged and show enormous increases in lysosomes, Golgi complexes, and vesicles.[20]

Macrophages that are transported via afferent lymphatic vessels into the subcapsular and medullary sinuses of a lymph node may become trapped in the loose reticular cell network that lines the sinuses. Phagocytosis of mycobacteria is followed by "digestive failure," degeneration, and death of the macrophage.[20] Blood monocytes emigrate to the location, transform to macrophages, and rephagocytize the agent and its associated cell debris. New macrophages collect in progressively enlarging foci called granulomas.

It has been reported that tuberculous lesions are dynamic and that macrophages constantly enter and constantly die. The speed with which they become activated and increase their microbicidal ability seems to be of crucial importance.[22] Regional lymph nodes that filter lung lymph are relatively few when the large lung area is considered. Nodes with lesions indicate the portion of lung involved.

Tubercles of cattle are most frequently seen during necropsy in bronchial, mediastinal, and portal lymph nodes, that may be the only tissues affected. Other commonly affected tissues are lung, liver, spleen, and surfaces of body cavities. Bacilli spread throughout the tissues by extension onto surfaces in contact with a lesion, or they may be transported in body cavity fluids and disseminated into the vascular system subsequent to vessel erosion at a lesion site. Other anatomical sites must be considered as having the potential to become infected.

On necropsy, a tuberculous granuloma usually has a yellowish appearance and is caseous, caseocalcareous, or calcified in consistency.[23] Occasionally, its appearance may be purulent. Some nontuberculous granulomas occur in which purulent content with a greenish luster is replaced by granulation tissue that may have a resemblance to tuberculous granulomas. The caseous center is usually dry, firm, and covered by a fibrous connective capsule of varying thickness. Fixed tissues in a tubercle are not easily removed intact, as is the case with some nontuberculous granulomas. A lesion may be small enough to be missed by the unaided eye or so large that it involves the greater part of an organ.

The tuberculous granuloma is an attempt by the host to localize the process and allow inflammatory and immune mechanisms to act for longer periods in an effort to destroy the bacilli. Microscopically, a granuloma may consist of epithelioid cells that contain bacilli, granulocytic cells that respond to inflammation (chiefly neutrophils), lymphocytes, monocytes, and necrotic debris.[24] As a result of fusion, monocytes and macrophages have been shown to give rise to giant cells, and often the nuclei become arranged in a horseshoe or ringed shape around the periphery of the cytoplasm.[25] These are referred to as Langhans' giant cells. Necrosis of cellular elements occurs with lesion progression, and acid-fast bacilli are continually being transported from the granulomatous site to infect other cells.

Fibrous connective tissue usually attempts to encapsulate the lesion and form an outer boundary, but often some bacilli have escaped to new sites and formed daughter tubercles. Occasionally the lesion appears diffuse rather than discreet, and fibrous tissue is not observed. Granulocytic cells are usually replaced by other inflammatory reactive cells during progression of a lesion. However, some lesions that appear well past the developmental stage can contain large numbers of neutrophils.

A fibrous encapsulated tuberculous lesion is usually supplied with a poor vascular system. Cells at the center of the lesion appear to die, and they undergo a change to caseous necrosis. The necrosis may extend to or near a zone of fibroblastic connective tissue. The caseous portion stains a homogeneous pink with eosin and occasionally may have what appears to be epithelioid cell nuclei and giant cells after other cells in the area have become necrotic and indistinguishable. Acid-fast bacilli may be demonstrated throughout a lesion in epithelioid and giant cells and in necrotic debris.

Enlargement of tubercles may occur by additional phagocytes appearing peripherally at a primary site or by coalescence of smaller foci. Irregularly shaped collections of calcium salts may be seen in areas of necrosis, and usually take a characteristic purplish color from the basic hematoxylin, although occasionally the effect of eosin may predominate.

A bronchopneumonia may be seen by macroscopic examination in instances of lung lesions although there may be little evidence of fluid accumulations visible by microscopic examination. Some fluids are removed when processing the tissue for slide preparation. Lesions, which may be situated in any one of the lung lobes (Figure 1), consist of a productive bronchopneumonia, and in turn give rise to lesions in the bronchotracheal tree and regional lymph nodes. The retropharyngeal lymph nodes drain both respiratory and alimentary areas and occasionally become infected.[25a] Tubercle bacilli

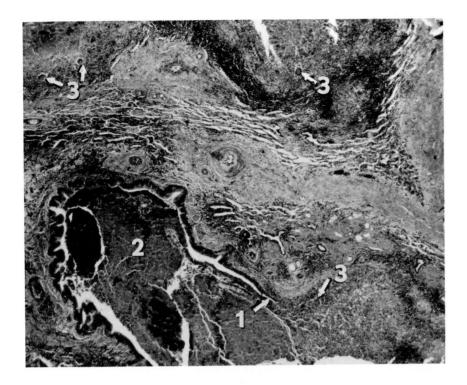

FIGURE 1.   Tuberculous bovine lung. Note erosion of bronchiolar lining (1) with necrotic mass of granuloma filling lumen of bronchiole (2) and Langhans' giant cells (3). (Magnification × 80.)

that become ingested may be absorbed into the intestine and move into the intercellular space that extends along the basement membrane of the absorptive cells and the lamina propria. This could provide access to the lymph system and infect mesenteric lymph nodes as sometimes occurs. The liver and portal lymph nodes may both become infected.

M. bovis lesions in nonhuman primates, when examined microscopically, can exhibit mononuclear cells imbricated along the periphery.[26] In some lesions, the cells appear to adhere to each other and to lack connective tissue encapsulation. Necrotic centers of lesions are usually surrounded by a wide band of mononuclear cells, and inflammatory cells are usually present as observed in the bovine species. Giant cells are often absent or relatively scarce, with some resembling Langhans' type and others having nuclei aggregated in the cytoplasmic centers. These criteria are not a sufficient basis for histologic differentiation between lesions caused by other mycobacteria and those of *M. bovis* and *M. tuberculosis*.[27]

Examined microscopically, it has been observed that exotic animal tissues from another member of the Bovidae family (kudu) and certain nonhuman primates can have tuberculous lesions in the lymph nodes, lung, spleen, and liver that are similar to *M. bovis* infected granulomas in cattle.[26,28] *M. bovis*-infected tissues from other exotic animals (elephant, rhinoceros, vicuna) have been observed microscopically to have incomplete tubercles. Epithelioid cells were scattered loosely in a microscopic field with little or no apparent cohesiveness. Giant cells were difficult to find or absent in tissue sections, and apparent nuclei of epithelioid cells were observed in areas of necrosis. Lymphocytes and other inflammatory cells appeared to be scarce.

DISEASE IN MAN

Symptomatology

M. bovis can produce progressive lung disease in man, that cannot be distinguished clinically from disease caused by *M. tuberculosis*.[8,29] Symptoms observed in man depend upon those tissues involved. Extensive lesions in the pulmonary parenchyma are usually accompanied by dyspnea and coughing with associated fever, anorexia, and nausea. Extrapulmonary lesions involving the meninges, bone, lymph nodes, or genitourinary tract may occur. These are usually characterized by swelling and tenderness, and they may vary from an acute exudative type to chronic proliferative granulomas. Discovery of acid-fast bacilli in an appropriately stained smear is useful in making a presumptive diagnosis; however, bacteriologic tests are necessary to obtain a definitive diagnosis of *M. bovis* infection.

Pathology

Variations from the information provided concerning the pathology in animals may be found in human pathology textbooks.[30,31]

GENERAL MODE OF SPREAD

Cattle

The tuberculous cow is the greatest source of danger to healthy cattle. An infected animal that is not promptly removed from the herd is a source of potential reinfection.

In damp areas such as watering troughs, stagnant ponds, and accumulations of manure, bovine tubercle bacilli may survive for many months under favorable conditions. They will not multiply outside a host's body, however, except on specially prepared media. Active lesions can contain myriads of bacilli and, when they become connected with natural body openings, the organisms can be widely disseminated. This occurs most frequently by way of the respiratory tract in diseased cattle. Bronchial exudates teeming with organisms may be expelled into the manger or watering trough by coughing, or exudates may be swallowed and expelled in the feces.

Animals that ingest contaminated feed or water may contract the disease. Inhalation of contaminated aerosols is also an important way in which the disease is disseminated in closed barns with poor ventilation. Contaminated dust, droplets, or dried secretions can enter the respiratory tract to cause infection in susceptible animals.[5]

Viable organisms can also be eliminated in milk even though there are no lesions in the udder.[16] Calves sometimes are infected during the first few hours or days of life when nursing an infected dam. In the past, many calves were infected by ingestion of unpasteurized skimmed milk from diseased cows, and infrequently, they may be infected as a result of intrauterine exposure.[17]

In one study, 4 of 9 dogs and 24 of 52 cats exposed to cattle infected with bovine tuberculosis were affected with either *M. bovis* or atypical mycobacteria.[32] The study indicated that dogs and cats exposed to *M. bovis*-infected cattle must be considered potential reservoirs for the bovine population and therefore must be appropriately controlled. Dogs and cats exposed to *M. bovis*-infected cattle should also be destroyed if the cow herd is depopulated.

Investigations of cattle reacting to tuberculin testing between 1968 and 1972 were conducted in Hessen, West Germany.[33] It was found that a total of 197 animals had been infected by transmission of tubercle bacilli from man. It should be noted that with *M. tuberculosis*, 26 animals became infected by 6 persons, whereas with *M. bovis*, 114 animals (16 herds) became infected by 12 tuberculous persons. These 114 infected animals amount to nearly 50% of the total number of tuberculous cattle (238 cases) found during this period of time. One farmer infected 16 animals in two herds, and another farmer infected 48 animals in four herds.

In another instance, three herds of cattle became infected by the same owner before he died of pulmonary tuberculosis.[34] Joubert et al.[35] have also reported on the connection between a tuberculous cowhand and enzootic reinfections on six farms.

Man

The ability of the pathogenic *Mycobacterium* sp. to infect one or more heterologous hosts makes tuberculosis in any species of animal a potential threat to other species including man.[4] In fact, the transmissability of tuberculous infections to other than natural hosts constitutes one of the most important problems in the control of this disease.

Human infection by bovine tubercle bacilli is most frequently caused by ingestion of unpasteurized milk or milk products such as cream, cheese, and butter. The first infection most often occurs in childhood. A child's reaction to infection with the tubercle bacillus differs from that of an adult in that in childhood, dissemination of tubercle bacilli outside of the lungs is more likely to occur, whereas in adults, pulmonary tuberculosis is the most common manifestation.[36] Therefore, as tuberculosis is eradicated from the bovine population, this reservoir is eliminated as a future potential source of infection for man. Isolation of *M. bovis* from milk products of nomadic tribes of northern Nigeria has been reported.[37] Unless measures are taken to eradicate the source of this infection in cattle, it will be impossible to eliminate it from the human population.

The public health risk from ingesting tubercle bacillus in the meat of tuberculous cattle is relatively small.[38] It is interesting to note that in those areas of Egypt where buffalo are an important source of meat for humans, 450 carcasses out of a total of 4050 examined (11.1%) were found to be affected with tuberculosis.[39] Moreover, muscle extract was proved to harbor the tubercle bacilli in a virulent form and caused infection in inoculated guinea pigs.

Reference has been made to isolation of *M. bovis* from dogs and cats exposed to cattle affected with bovine tuberculosis.[32] Clinical tests on 64 human contacts revealed that tuberculin reactor rates in this group were significantly greater than reactor rates in the general population. Other reservoirs of the bovine tubercle bacillus are zoo and exotic animals, a large number of which were found to be infected with *M. bovis.* Isolation of this agent has been reported from many different species of zoological animals in the U.S. and Europe.[6,7] Furthermore, the U.S. Public Health Service has reported that the rate of tuberculin conversion from negative to positive is 27 times higher for laboratory workers exposed to monkeys than for the general population.[40]

DIAGNOSIS

Bovine

Clinical evidence of tuberculosis is usually lacking. For that reason, its diagnosis in individual animals and an eradication program were not possible prior to the development of tuberculin by Koch in 1890.[16] Tuberculin, a concentrated sterile culture filtrate of tubercle bacilli grown on glycerinated beef broth and more recently on synthetic media, provides a means of detecting the disease in animals.

Demonstration of the intradermal tuberculin test by Moussu[41] and Mantoux[42] in 1908 provided a convenient and efficient method of identifying infected cattle. In the U.S., the caudal fold is the preferred injection site for the intradermal tuberculin test.

The texture of the skin and relative sensitivity of this area to tuberculin make it particularly suitable.[16] Alhaji[43] has also determined this to be the most suitable site under management conditions existing in Nigeria. The skin of the neck is more sensitive to tuberculin than the caudal fold, and this site is used in many countries for intradermal injections.

Much has been written about the type of tuberculin best suited for conducting the tuberculin test in cattle. It has been reported that a purified protein derivative (PPD) tuberculin is more specific than heat-concentrated synthetic media (HCSM) tuberculin.[44,45] It has also been shown that bovine PPDs are more specific than human PPDs for detecting tuberculous cattle.[46-50]

Heterospecific reactions (i.e., those produced in animals having no gross lesions [NGL] of tuberculosis) to tuberculin tests are a major problem both in areas where tuberculosis has been virtually eliminated and where infection with *M. bovis* is relatively low.[51,52] Heterospecific reactions to tuberculin vary according to ecologic factors in a given situation. These factors include (1) infection with *M. paratuberculosis* (Johne's disease), (2) infection with *M. tuberculosis* and *M. avium*, and (3) various transient sensitizing infections with other mycobacteria. Post-mortem examination of slaughtered NGL reactors and appropriate laboratory studies of tissues are essential to obtain information on the causative agent. In the U.S., animals responding to the caudal fold test in herds not known to be infected with *M. bovis* are retested with the comparative-cervical test either within 10 days of the previous caudal fold injection or after 60 days.[53] PPD tuberculins of equal biologic potency, as determined in sensitized guinea pigs (*M. avium*, D_4 and *M. bovis*, AN_5), are used in conducting the test.

To establish the presence of *M. bovis*, histopathologic and mycobacteriologic examinations should be conducted on reactors from herds of unknown status and on all animals found to have suspicious lesions on routine post-mortem examination. A variety of serologic procedures (gel diffusion, complement-fixation, hemagglutination, hemagglutination inhibition) have been evaluated for the diagnosis of bovine tuberculosis, but none have proven to be successful. Recent studies utilizing the lymphocyte immunostimulation procedure indicate that this test may have some potential as a diagnostic aid.[54,55]

Man

The differential diagnosis of pulmonary infiltration in man is not easy. It must be kept in mind that even if tuberculosis in man has changed its pattern, it has not changed its contagious nature, and definitive diagnosis is very important.[56]

Examination of sputum is an effective case-finding tool of favorable cost effectiveness in many developing countries.[57] Therefore, it is important to always carry out a cultural examination of sputum whenever tuberculosis is suspected.

In public health work as in veterinary medicine, the tuberculin test is accepted as a reliable and specific diagnostic aid.[52] Long[58] has written that "few procedures employed in the campaign to eradicate tuberculosis have been of greater value than the tuberculin test. It has been useful in the diagnosis of tuberculosis in individual patients and valuable in studying the epidemilogy of the disease and laying foundations for public health practices in tuberculosis control."

In the U.S., tuberculin testing of humans is receiving increased emphasis both as a routine screening test and as an epidemiologic tool.[59] Its value as a screening test increases as the prevalence of tuberculosis in a population decreases. In many communities, a positive reaction in a young child may lead to a source of infection either within the household or in someone closely associated with him. The tuberculin test has special value when repeated periodically during surveillance of tuberculin-negative persons likely to be exposed to tuberculosis. All patients who are tuberculin-positive should have a chest X-ray taken. In older populations or in special groups in which at least 50% of the persons are expected to react to tuberculin, simultaneous use of the tuberculin test and chest X-ray may be more practical and economical than use of the tuberculin test followed by a chest X-ray for positive reactors.

Heterospecific sensitivity is also a problem in human tuberculin testing.[59] In the absence of a clear-cut exposure to a case of active tuberculosis, persons with a doubtful or a small positive reaction to human PPD tuberculin who disclose a greater response to simultaneously injected PPD-B can be presumed not to be infected with *M. tuberculosis*.[59] Such an observation must be based on a very careful testing technique and the simultaneous use of two matched antigens. Kantor et al.[60] have shown that bovine PPD in equal protein concentration gives a more specific response than human PPD when applied to persons infected with *M. bovis*.

Since there are no recognizable clinical, roentgenographic, or pathologic features that provide a reliable means to definitely distinguish human from bovine forms of tuberculous infection in man, laboratory procedures are necessary for precise diagnosis.

PREVENTION AND CONTROL

Bovine

Eradication of bovine tuberculosis is a major objective that has nearly been achieved in North America, Australia, Japan, and many countries of Europe. The basis of these eradication programs has been systemic application of the tuberculin test and the slaughter of reactors. Krishnoswamy[61] has reported that the "test and slaughter" method cannot be used in India due to the high incidence of reactors. This procedure would result in the loss of highly productive cows and working animals. The author concluded that in self-contained herds located where there are facilities to segregate reactors, dispose of infected material, and conduct regular tuberculin tests, the policy of "test and segregation" can be adopted. However, this procedure will delay the eradication of bovine tuberculosis if, in fact, it can ever be achieved.

Since 1890, various types of vaccines have been advocated for cattle, but none has produced effective immunity to bovine tuberculosis. Vaccines have been produced from various strains of virulent and avirulent human-type bacillus, metabolic products of bacilli, various portions of disrupted bacilli,[62] the vole bacillus *M. microti*, and bacilli attenuated by growth on bile-containing media. Vaccination experiments with BCG, the vaccine prepared by the Calmette and Guerin method, have been reported.[63] Recent investigations in Malawi[64,65] confirm that BCG vaccine does not eradicate bovine tuberculosis, but it does produce greater resistance to the disease. Therefore, its use may check the spread of infection among herds in this environment. In the latest FAO-WHO-OIE report, Malawi is the only country that reported using BCG vaccine (Table 1).

Besides affording no practical protection to cattle, vaccination induces hypersensitivity to tuberculin and, thus, interferes with the diagnostic test. Countries attempted to use vaccination as the basis of a control program ultimately abandoned the procedure in favor of the "test and slaughter" method.

Experiments in several countries during the past decade have indicated that chemotherapeutic agents found to be effective against human tuberculosis may also be of value against bovine tuberculosis. An extensive and carefully controlled series of trials conducted in the Republic of South Africa showed that excellent prophylactic and therapeutic results were achieved by the administration of INH.[66,67] Basic requirements for its use are the careful administration of INH for long periods, accurate measurement of daily doses, proper identification of cattle, and maintenance of accurate records. Such programs are particularly suitable for large government-operated dairy farms where careful supervision can be maintained. INH therapy may have potential value in countries where the incidence of bovine tuberculosis is high and "test and slaughter" methods are not yet feasible. Use of INH is not recommended for countries like the U.S. where *M. bovis* infection in cattle has nearly been eradicated.[16]

The best preventive measure against bovine tuberculosis is to require a negative tuberculin test before exchange of ownership whether movements are international or local in nature. An epidemiologic investigation, with testing where indicated, should be conducted each time *M. bovis* is reported in persons working or residing on premises where cattle are located as well as each time *M. bovis* is isolated from any other species of animal having contact with cattle.

Man

Elimination of tuberculosis among dairy cattle by the testing and slaughter of reactors and pasteurization of milk has gone a long way in many countries to reduce or eliminate the infection in man. All human exposures on any farm where *M. bovis* is diagnosed should immediately be tuberculin tested and handled accordingly.

Where risk of infection is low, as already reported in many countries of western Europe, North America, Australia, and Japan, mass vaccination with BCG is of limited value. A detailed approach for the determination of when and where to use BCG in man has been reported and should be consulted for details.[68]

At present, there are at least 12 antituberculosis drugs in use throughout the world. Effectiveness of these drugs depends on their antibacterial activity, safety, and acceptability. The recommended dosage for each drug, both for daily and for intermittent treatment, is contained in a report by the Committee on Treatment of the International Union Against Tuberculosis.[69]

EDITORIAL COMMENT

In recent years, it has been demonstrated that *M. bovis* purified protein derivative tuberculin (PPD-B) is more specific for bovine tuberculosis than *M. tuberculosis* PPD. PPD-B is the only tuberculin now being used in the European Economic Community (EEC). Additionally, these countries require that all animals entering the EEC be tested by PPD-B.

There is a slight difference in the processing of PPD-B used in Europe and that used in the U.S. In Europe, the proteins are precipitated by trichloracetic acid, while in the U.S. they are precipitated by ammonium sulfate. Both products appear to be equally effective in detecting tuberculous cattle.

APPENDIX *

Uniform Methods and Rules for the Establishment and Maintenance of Tuberculosis-Free Accredited Herds of Cattle, Modified Accredited Areas, and Areas Accredited Free of Bovine Tuberculosis in the Domestic Bovine

Adopted by the U.S. Animal Health Association on Oct. 17, 1974, and approved by the Animal and Plant Health Inspection Service, Veterinary Services, U.S. Department of Agriculture. Effective Jan. 6, 1975

*   Uniform Methods and Rules — Bovine tuberculosis eradication, U.S. Department of Agriculture, Animal and Plant Health Inspection Service, Veterinary Services, Federal Building No. 1, Hyattsville, Md.

PART I: DEFINITIONS

1. **Bovine tuberculosis** — A disease in cattle caused by *Mycobacterium bovis*.
2. **Bovine tuberculosis eradication** — Eradication is the complete elimination of bovine tuberculosis from cattle in a state of the U.S. so that it does not appear unless introduced from another species or from outside of the state.
3. **Cattle** — Cattle refers to domestic bovine animals of all ages.
4. **Natural additions** — Animals born and raised in the herd.
5. **Herd** — A herd is a group of cattle maintained on common ground for any purpose, or two or more groups of cattle under common ownership or supervision, geographically separated, but with an interchange or movement of cattle without regard to health status (a group is construed to mean one or more animals.)
6. **Tuberculin** — A product that is approved by and produced under license of the U.S. Department of Agriculture for injection into cattle for the purpose of detecting bovine tuberculosis.
7. **Official tuberculin test** — A test for tuberculosis applied and reported by approved personnel in accordance with these Uniform Methods and Rules.
8. **Comparative-cervical tuberculin test** — The injection of standardized mammalian and avian tuberculin at separate sites in the cervical area and a determination as to the probable presence of mammalian tuberculosis by comparing the responses of the two tuberculins.
9. **Passed herd** — Herd in which no animals were classified as reactors or suspects on the herd test.
10. **Annual test** — Tests conducted at intervals of not less than 10 months nor more than 14 months.
11. **No gross lesion (NGL) animal** — An animal in which a lesion(s) of tuberculosis is not found during slaughter inspection. (An animal with skin lesions only will be considered in the same category as an NGL).
12. **Surveillance** — Surveillance refers to all measures used to detect the presence of tuberculosis in a cattle population.
13. **Accredited herd** — An accredited herd is one that has passed at least two consecutive annual tuberculin tests, with no other evidence of bovine tuberculosis disclosed, and that meets the standards of these Uniform Methods and Rules.
14. **Modified accredited area** — A state of the U.S. or portion thereof that is actively participating in the eradication of tuberculosis and that maintains its status in accordance with these Uniform Methods and Rules.
15. **Accredited free state** — A state of the U.S. that maintains full compliance with these Uniform Methods and Rules and where no evidence of bovine tuberculosis has been disclosed for 5 or more years.
16. **Herd depopulation** — Removal of all cattle in the herd direct to slaughter prior to any restocking of the premises with cattle.
17. **Direct to slaughter** — The shipment of cattle from the premises of origin directly to a slaughter establishment without diversion to assembly points such as auctions, public stockyards, and feedlots.
18. **Quarantined feedlot** — A confined area under the direct supervision and control of the state livestock official, who shall establish accounting procedures for all animals entering or leaving such quarantined feedlot. The quarantined feedlot shall be maintained for finish feeding of animals in drylot, with no provision for pasturing and grazing. All animals leaving such feedlot must move only direct to slaughter, in accordance with established procedures for handling quarantined animals.

PART II: OFFICIAL TEST PROCEDURES

A. **Authority to test** — State laws and/or regulations shall provide authority to apply a tuberculin test to any animal or herd at such times as may be deemed necessary by the cooperating state and federal officials. These officials reserve the right to supervise any test conducted by an accredited veterinarian.

B. **Restriction of personnel who may apply tuberculin tests** — Tuberculin tests shall be applied by a veterinarian employed in a full-time capacity by the state, U.S. Department of Agriculture, or by an accredited veterinarian.

C. **Caudal fold test** — The official tuberculin test for routine use shall be the intradermic injection of 0.1 cc of tuberculin in the caudal fold.

D. **Cervical test** — This test is limited to use in herds where bovine tuberculosis has been disclosed except:

1. When the comparative cervical test is used.
2. When special tests such as those applied to animals for export.

For retesting known *M. bovis* herds, 0.2 cc of tuberculin shall be used and applied only by full-time employed state or federal regulatory veterinarians. The comparative and other cervical tests are to be used only as specifically approved by the state-federal cooperating officials.

E. **Requirements for special procedures in infected herds** — All cattle in herds from which tuberculous cattle originate and all cattle that are known to have associated with infected cattle shall be tested promptly. Cattle in feedlots known to be exposed to tuberculous cattle shall be quarantined and shipped under permit directly to slaughter. Disclosure of tuberculosis in any herd shall be followed by a complete epidemiological investigation. Every effort must be made to assure the immediate elimination of the disease from all species of domestic livestock and poultry on the premises.

F. **Tuberculin test interpretation** — Decisions will be based upon the professional judgment of the testing veterinarian, in accordance with the policy established by the cooperating state and federal officials. The injection site on each animal shall be palpated. Observation without palpation is not acceptable. The following are guidelines for classification of cattle tested with the caudal fold test:

1. **Reactor (R)** — Animals showing a circumscribed swelling 5 mm in diameter (3/16 in.) (P_1) or a diffuse swelling twice as thick as the normal caudal fold (X_2) or greater response to tuberculin on routine test should be classified as reactors unless, in the professional judgment of the testing veterinarian, a suspect classification is justified.
2. **Suspect (S)** — Animals showing a response to tuberculin not classified as reactors, with the exception noted below.
3. **Passed**
   a. **Deviator (D)** — Animals showing a minimal response to tuberculin. This is usually designated as a pinpoint (PP) response.
   b. **Negative (N)** — Animals showing no response to tuberculin or those animals with responses which have been classified negative for *M. bovis* by the comparative-cervical tuberculin test.

G. **Report of tuberculin tests** — A report of all tuberculin tests, including the individual identification of each animal by eartag number or tattoo, age, sex, and breed, and a record of the size of the responses shall be submitted in accordance with the requirements of the cooperating state and federal officials.

Part III: DISPOSITION OF TUBERCULIN RESPONSE ANIMALS

A. Disposition of Reactors

1. Reactors must remain on the premises where disclosed until a state or federal permit for movement has been obtaied. Movement for immediate slaughter must be direct to a slaughter establishment where approved state or federal inspection is maintained within 15 days of classification or otherwise the animals must be destroyed under the direct supervision of a regulatory veterinarian to assure that the carcass is either cooked or condemned.
2. No animal classified as a reactor shall be retested.

B. Disposition of Suspects

1. Suspects to the caudal fold tuberculin test shall be quarantined to the premises where found until:
    a. Retested by the comparative-cervical tuberculin test within 10 days of the caudal fold injection, or
    b. Retested by the comparative-cervical tuberculin test after 60 days, or
    c. Shipped under permit direct to slaughter in accordance with state and federal laws and regulations.

C. Deviators

1. Record response for complete animal health history.
2. Movement of deviators classified negative for *M. bovis* by the comparative-cervical tuberculin test should not be restricted.

PART IV: QUARANTINE PROCEDURES

1. All herds in which reactor animals are disclosed shall be quarantined. Exposed animals must remain on the premises where disclosed unless a state or federal permit has been obtained. Movement for immediate slaughter must be direct to a slaughtering establishment where approved state or federal inspection is maintained.
2. Sales of feeder calves from quarantined herds will be restricted. Feeder calves less than 12 months of age that have passed a tuberculin test within 60 days may be permitted to move intrastate to a quarantined feedlot.
3. Herds in which *M. bovis* infection has been disclosed shall remain under quarantine and must pass two tuberculin tests at intervals of at least 60 days and one additional test after 6 months. Minimum quarantine period shall be 10 months from slaughter of lesion reactors. A case will be considered to be ''*M. bovis* infection'' when a pathologic

(granulomatous) lesion suspected of being tuberculosis is found in an animal, unless a satisfactory examination at an accredited laboratory justifies a diagnosis other than bovine-type tuberculosis. Exception — lesions that occur only in the mesenteric lymph nodes.

4. Herds in which only NGL reactor(s) appear and no evidence of *M. bovis* infection has been disclosed may be released from quarantine after a 60-day negative retest of the entire herd.

5. Suspects in herds where only suspect animals are disclosed shall be quarantined to the premises until retested and classified negative or shipped direct to slaughter under permit.

PART V: SPECIAL RETESTS OF HIGH-RISK HERDS

1. In herds in which *M. bovis* infection has been confirmed but the herd has not been depopulated, five annual tests on the entire herd followed by two tests at 3-year intervals shall be applied following the release of quarantine.

2. In herds with history of lesions suspicious of bovine tuberculosis (not confirmed), two complete annual herd tests shall be applied after release of quarantine. The first test is to be applied approximately 1 year after release of quarantine.

3. In a newly assembled herd on a premises where a tuberculous herd has been depopulated, two annual herd tests shall be applied to all cattle. The first test is to be applied approximately 6 months after assembly of the new herd. These tests shall be followed by two complete herd tests at 3-year intervals. If the premises are vacated for one year, these requirements may be waived.

PART VI: CLEANING AND DISINFECTION OF PREMISES

1. Premises where tuberculous cattle have been maintained shall be thoroughly cleaned and disinfected with a disinfectant permitted by the Animal and Plant Health Service, U.S. Department of Agriculture, and in a manner satisfactory to the cooperating state and federal authorities.

PART VII: ORIGIN OF INFECTION

1. Tuberculosis found during slaughter inspection or otherwise in any bovine will be considered to have originated in the state where slaughtered or disclosed, unless successful traceback procedures identify the source to be another state.

PART VIII: IDENTIFICATION OF LIVESTOCK

1. All cattle tested shall be individually identified by official eartag or other satisfactory means. Devices such as neck chains that are easily removed and transferred are not considered to be satisfactory.

2. The state shall* have and enforce dealer control laws and/or regulations that require dealers to maintain the identification of cattle and records of transactions for each animal purchased or sold.

---

* The word "shall" will apply to those states that are to be considered for Accredited Free status. The word "should" may be substituted for states with a Modified Accredited status only.

tions that require dealers to maintain the identification of cattle and records of transactions for each animal purchased or sold.

3. Cattle moved in channels of trade within a state shall be identified and recorded as to origin and destination at the first concentration point (dealer, livestock auction, stockyard, etc.) as follows:

    a. Cattle more than 2 years of age that are returned to farms or ranches, including feeding cattle, shall be identified by official eartag or an official brand. If identified by brand, cattle must be accompanied by an official brand release.

    b. Cattle that are marketed for immediate slaughter shall be identified by eartag, saletag, or official backtag. An official brand release will be acceptable identification for lots of animals of unmixed origin that are shipped directly to slaughter.

    c. Cattle without individual identification may be moved directly to and maintained in a quarantined feedlot under control of the state livestock sanitary official, provided that they are inspected in the feedlot and moved to slaughter under permit at the end of the feeding period.

PART IX: ACCREDITED HERD PLAN

1. Animals to be tested — Testing of herds for accreditation or reaccreditation shall include all cattle more than 24 months of age and any animals other than natural additions less than 24 months of age. All natural additions shall be individually identified and recorded on the test report as members of the herd at the time of the annual test.

2. Additions — Herd additions must originate directly from one of the following:

    a. Accredited herd
    b. Herd in an Accredited Free state
    c. Herd in a Modified Accredited area that has passed a herd test of all animals more than 24 months of age within 12 months, and the individual animals for addition were negative to the tuberculin test conducted within 60 days.
    d. Herd in a Modified Accredited area not meeting the requirements of (a), (b), or (c) — Individual animals for addition must pass a negative test within 60 days prior to entering the premises of the accredited herd and must be kept in isolation from all members of the accredited herd until negative to a test conducted after 60 days of date of entry.
        Animals added under (b), (c), and (d) shall not receive accredited herd status for sale purposes until they have been members of the herd at least 60 days and are included in a herd retest.

3. Accreditation and reaccreditation — To qualify for accredited herd status, the herd must pass at least two consecutive annual tuberculin tests, with no evidence of bovine tuberculosis disclosed. All animals must be bona fide members of the herd. Qualified herds may be issued a certificate by local, state, and federal officials. The accreditation period will be 12 months (365 days) from the anniversary date

and not 12 months from the date of the reaccreditation test. To qualify for reaccreditation, the herd must pass an annual test within a period of 10 to 14 months of the anniversary date.

PART X: MODIFIED ACCREDITED AREA STATUS

1. Testing and Slaughter Surveillance
An annual report shall be submitted for each state or appropriate subdivision at the close of each fiscal year to show the amount of testing and slaughter surveillance that has been conducted.

2. Trace Testing

    a. All cattle in herds of origin or cattle associated with those showing evidence of tuberculosis at time of slaughter must be quarantined and tested.
    b. The testing schedule of all reactor and suspect herds must be current.

3. Revocation or Suspension of Status
Disclosure of tuberculosis in the area and/or failure to take progressive steps to comply with these Uniform Methods and Rules to seek out and eliminate tuberculosis shall be cause for revocation or suspension of the Modified Accredited Status.

PART XI: ACCREDITED FREE STATE

    1. A state may be listed as Accredited Free if the state complies with all of the procedures in these Uniform Methods and Rules and no evidence of tuberculosis has been found for 5 or more years.
    2. Disclosure of tuberculosis in an Accredited Free state will be sufficient justification for revocation or suspension of the Accredited Free status. After all epidemiological studies have been completed and all exposed herds have been tested and it has been established that there has been no spread from the herd, the state may be considered for reinstatement of its Free status.

REFERENCES

1. **Myers, J. A.,** Tuberculosis, in *Tuberculosis and Other Communicable Diseases,* Myers, J. A., Ed., Charles C Thomas, Springfield, Ill., 1959, 3.
2. Laboratory Methods in Veterinary Mycobacteriology, revised ed., U.S. Department of Agriculture, Animal and Plant Health Inspection Service, Veterinary Service Laboratories, Ames, Iowa, 1974.
3. **Lesslie, I. W.,** A comparison of biological and some cultural methods for the primary isolation of *Mycobacterium tuberculosis, J. Comp. Pathol.,* 69, 1, 1959.
4. **Thoen, C. O. and Karlson, A. G.,** The genus *Mycobacterium,* in *Veterinary Microbiology,* Packer, R. A., Mare, C. J., and Merchant, I. A., Eds., Iowa State University Press, Ames, in press.
5. **Francis, J.,** *Tuberculosis in Animals and Man,* Cassell and Company, London, 1958.
6. **Schliesser, T.,** Vorkommen und Bedeutung von Mykobakterien bei Tieren, *Zentralbl. Bakteriol. Parasitenkd. Infektionskr. Hyg. Abt. 1: Orig.,* 271, 184, 1976.

7. **Thoen, C. O., Richards, W. D., and Jarnagin, J. L.**, Mycobacteria isolated from exotic animals, *J. Am. Vet. Med. Assoc.*, in press.

8. **Myers, J. A. and Steele, J. H.**, *Bovine Tuberculosis Control in Man and Animals*, Warren H. Green, St. Louis, 1969.

9. **Correa, C. N. M. and Correa, W. M.**, Human tuberculosis by bovine bacilli in Sao Paulo, Brazil, *Arq. Inst. Biol. Sao Paulo*, 41(3), 131, 1974.

10. **Gervois, M., Vaillant, J. M., Fontaine, J. F., Laroche, G., and Dubois, G.**, Epidemiology of the human infection due to *Mycobacterium bovis*, *Arch. Monaldi Tisiol. Mal. Appar. Respir.*, 27(3), 294, 1972.

11. **Feldman, W. H.**, Tuberculosis, in *Diseases Transmitted from Animals to Man*, Hull, T. G., Ed., Charles C Thomas, Springfield, Ill., 1963.

12. **Kagramanov, A. I.**, Interrelationship of tuberculosis between man and farm animals, *Probl. Tuberk.*, 46, 69, 1968.

13. **Blagodarny, Y. A., Bekmagamberova, Z. Z., Blonskaya, L. I., Sidorkina, E. V., Khivtsova, A. E., Aleeva, A. A., Tulegenov, A. T., and Alimbekova, O. A.**, Tuberculosis in stockbreeders provoked by *Mycobacterium bovis*, *Probl. Tuberk.*, 10, 72, 1975.

14. **Sjogren, I. and Sutherland, I.**, Studies of tuberculosis in man in relation to infection in cattle, *Tubercle*, 56, 113, 1974.

15. **Meissner, G.**, Bovine tuberculosis in man before and after the eradication of tuberculosis in cattle, *Prax. Pneumol.*, 28, 123, 1974.

16. **Konyha, L. D. and Chaloux, P. A.**, Tuberculosis, in *Bovine Medicine and Surgery*, 3rd ed., Amstutz, H. E., Ed., American Veterinary Publications, Santa Barbara, Calif., 1977.

16a. **Seitarides, K.**, Tuberculosis of the reproductive system in cattle, *Ellenike Kteniatr.*, 16(4), 222, 1973.

17. **Roumy, B.**, Une enzootic de tuberculose bovine transmise par insemination artificielle, *Recl. Med. Vet.*, 142(8), 729, 1966.

18. **Thoen, C. O., Himes, E. M., Stumpff, C. D., Parks, T. W., and Sturkie, H. N.**, Isolation of *Mycobacterium bovis* from the prepuce of a herd bull, *Am. J. Vet. Res.*, 38(6), 877, 1977.

19. **Asmundsson, T. and Kilburn, K. H.**, Mucocilliary clearance rates of various levels in dogs' lungs, *Am. Rev. Respir. Dis.*, 102, 388, 1970.

20. **Cheville, N.**, *Cell Pathology*, Iowa State University Press, Ames, 1976.

21. **Godeski, J. J. and Grain, J. D.**, The origin of alveolar macrophages in mouse radiation chimeras, *J. Exp. Med.*, 136, 630, 1972.

22. **Dannenberg, A. M., Masayuki, A., and Kiyoshi, S.**, Macrophage accumulation, division, maturation, and digestive and microbicidal capacities in tuberculous lesions, *J. Immunol.*, 109(5), 1109, 1972.

23. **Davis, C. L.**, Pathology and the differential diagnosis of tuberculosis, in Proc. Tuberculosis Eradication Conf., Publication No. ARS91-20, U.S. Department of Agriculture, Washington, D.C., 1959, 43.

24. **Smith, H. A., Jones, T. C., and Hunt, R. D.**, *Veterinary Pathology*, 4th ed., Lea & Febiger, Philadelphia, 1972.

25. **Davis, J. M. G.**, The ultrastructural changes that occur during transformation of lung macrophages to giant cells and fibroblasts in experimental asbestosis, *Br. J. Exp. Pathol.*, 44, 568, 1963.

25a. **Stamp, J. T.**, A review of the pathogenesis and pathology of bovine tuberculosis with special reference to potential problems, *Vet. Rec.*, 56(47), 443, 1944.

26. **Thoen, C. O., Beluhan, F. Z., Himes, E. M., Capek, V., and Bennett, B. T.**, *Mycobacterium bovis* infection in baboons (*Papio papio*), *Arch. Pathol. Lab. Med.*, 101, 291, 1977.

27. **Lomme, J. R., Thoen, C. O., Himes, E. M., Vinson, T. W., and King, R. E.**, *Mycobacteria tuberculosis* infection in two East African onysex, *J. Am. Vet. Med. Assoc.*, 169(9), 912, 1976.

28. **Himes, E. M., Lyvere, D. B., Thoen, C. O., Essey, M. A., Lebel, J. L., and Freiheit, C. F.**, Tuberculosis in Greater Kudu, *J. Am. Vet. Med. Assoc.*, 169(9), 930, 1976.

29. **Karlson, A. G. and Carr, D. T.**, Tuberculosis caused by *Mycobacterium bovis*: report of six cases, 1954-1958, *Ann. Intern. Med.*, 73, 979, 1970.

30. **Boyd, W.**, *A Textbook of Pathology*, 8th ed., Lea & Febiger, Philadelphia, 1970.

31. **Anderson, W. A. D.**, *Pathology*, 6th ed., C. V. Mosby, St. Louis, 1971.

32. **Snider, W. R., Cohen, D., Reif, J. S., Stein, S. C., and Prier, J. E.**, Tuberculosis in canine and feline populations, *Am. Rev. Respir. Dis.*, 104, 866, 1971.

33. **Schliesser, T.**, Tuberculosis in domestic and wild animals, *Prax. Pneumol.*, 28, 511, 1974.

34. **Tice, F. J.**, Man — a source of bovine tuberculosis in cattle: case report, *Cornell Vet.*, 34, 363, 1944.

35. **Joubert, L., Filleton, R., Steghens, P., Tissot, J., and Viallier, J.**, Tuberculosis caused by bovine bacteria, a reversible zoonosis, *Rev. Med. Vet.*, 36(6), 757, 1973.

36. **Crofton, J.**, Human tuberculosis, in *Tuberculosis in Animals*, Vol. 4, Zoological Society of London, 1961, 57.
37. **Alhaji, I. and Schnurrenberger, P.**, Public health significance of bovine tuberculosis in four northern states of Nigeria: a mycobacteriologic study, *Niger. Med. J.*, in press.
38. **Francis, J.**, Very small public health risk from flesh of tuberculous cattle, *Aust. Vet. J.*, 49, 496, 1973.
39. **El-Mossalami, E., El-Amrousi, S., and Zeidan, M.**, Tuberculosis in buffalo carcasses, *Egypt. J. Vet. Sci.*, 9, 1, 1972.
40. National Archives of the U.S., Code of Federal Regulations, Title 42, Part 71, Oct. 10, 1975.
41. **Moussu, M.**, Sur l'intradermal reaction à la tuberculine, *Bull. Soc. Cent. Med. Vet.*, 26, 649, 1908.
42. **Moussu, M. and Mantorex, C.**, Sur l'intradermal reaction à la tuberculin chez les animaux, *Bull. Soc. Cent. Med. Vet.*, 26, 500, 1908.
43. **Alhaji, I.**, Tuberculin test survey of cattle in four northern states of Nigeria, *Bull. Anim. Health Prod. Afr.*, 24(3), 1976.
44. **Van Wavern, G. M.**, Testing of cattle with PPD tuberculins, in *Proc. 15th Int. Vet. Congr.*, International Veterinary Congress, Stockholm, 1953, 140.
45. **Choi, C. S., Kim, J. H., Lee, H. S., and Jeon, Y. S.**, Studies on the improvement of bovine tuberculin, *Res. Rep. Off. Rural Dev. (Vet.) (Suwon) (Nongsa Shihom Yon'gu Pogo Kach'uk Wisaeng P'yon)*, 17, 101, 1975.
46. **Lesslie, I. W., Herbert, C. N., Burn, K. J., and MacClancy, B. N.**, Comparison of the specificity of human and bovine tuberculin PPD for testing cattle. I. Republic of Ireland, *Vet. Rec.*, 96, 332, 1975.
47. **Lesslie, I. W., Herbert, C. N., and Barnett, D. N.**, Comparison of the specificity of human and bovine tuberculin PPD for testing cattle. II. Southeastern England, *Vet. Rec.*, 96, 335, 1975.
48. **Lesslie, I. W. and Herbert, C. N.**, Comparison of the specificity of human and bovine tuberculin PPD for testing cattle. III. National trial in Great Britain, *Vet. Rec.*, 96, 338, 1975.
49. **O'Reilly, L. M. and MacClancy, B. N.**, A comparison of the accuracy of a human and a bovine tuberculin PPD for testing cattle with a comparative-cervical test, *Ir. Vet. J.*, 29, 63, 1975.
50. **Roswurm, J. D., Kantor, I. N., Spinelli, R., and Spath, E.**, Tuberculin Test Sensitivity in Cattle Naturally Infected with *M. bovis* in Argentina, paper presented to the Committee on Tuberculosis in Animals, International Union Against Tuberculosis, Paris, 1976.
51. **Joint FAO/WHO Expert Committee on Zoonoses**, Third report, FAO Agricultural Study No. 74, *W.H.O. Tech. Rep. Ser.*, 378, 45, 1967.
52. **Karlson, A. G.**, Nonspecific or cross-sensitivity reactions to tuberculin in cattle, in *Advances in Veterinary Science*, Vol. 7, Academic Press, New York, 1962, 147.
53. **Roswurm, J. D. and Konyha, L. D.**, The comparative-cervical tuberculin test as an aid to diagnosing bovine tuberculosis, in *Proc. 77th Annu. Meet. U.S. Animal Health Assoc.*, U.S. Animal Health Association, St. Louis, 1973, 368.
54. **Muscoplat, C. C., Thoen, C. O., Chen, A. W., and Johnson, D. W.**, Development of specific *in vitro* lymphocyte responses in cattle infected with *M. bovis* and *M. avium*, *Am. J. Vet. Res.*, 36, 395, 1975.
55. **Ayivor, M. D., Muscoplat, C. C., Chen, A. W., Rakich, P. M., Thoen, C. O., and Johnson, D. W.**, Whole blood lymphocyte stimulation for the diagnosis of tuberculosis in cattle, in *Proc. 19th Annu. Meet. Am. Assoc. Vet. Lab. Diagnosticians*, American Association of Veterinary Laboratory Diagnosticians, Miami Beach, 1977, 351.
56. **Tala, E. and Kekki, M.**, Tuberculosis — a forgotten disease in differential diagnosis?, *Scand. J. Respir. Dis. Suppl.*, 89, 145, 1974.
57. Technical Guide for Collection, Storage and Transport of Sputum Specimens and for Examinations for Tuberculosis by Direct Microscopy, 2nd ed., International Union Against Tuberculosis, Paris, 1977.
58. **Long, E. R.**, The specificity of the tuberculin reaction (editorial), *Am. Rev. Tuberc.*, 63, 355, 1951.
59. **Anon.**, The tuberculin skin test, *Am. Rev. Respir. Dis.*, 104(5), 769, 1971.
60. **Kantor, I. N., Marchevsky, N., and Lesslie, I. W.**, Response to PPD in tuberculosis patients infected with *M. bovis*, *Medicina* (Buenos Aires), 36, 127, 1976.
61. **Krishnoswamy, S.**, Control of bovine tuberculosis by tuberculin testing and segregation in an organized dairy herd, *Mysore J. Agric. Sci.*, 7, 615, 1973.
62. **Larson, C. L., Baker, M. B., Baker, R., and Rifi, R.**, Studies of delayed reactions using protoplasm from acid-fast bacilli as provoking antigen, *Am. Rev. Respir. Dis.*, 94(2), 257, 1966.
63. **Cotton, E. E. and Crawford, A. B.**, Second report on the Calmette-Guerin method of vaccinating animals against tuberculosis, *J. Am. Vet. Med. Assoc.*, 80, 18, 1932.
64. **Waddington, F. G. and Ellwood, D. C.**, An experiment to challenge the resistance to tuberculosis in B.C.G.-vaccinated cattle in Malawi, *Br. Vet. J.*, 128, 541, 1972.

65. **Ellwood, D. C. and Waddington, F. G.,** A second experiment to challenge the resistance to tuberculosis in B.C.G.-vaccinated cattle in Malawi, *Br. Vet. J.,* 128, 619, 1972.
66. **Kleeberg, H. H.,** Chemotherapy and chemoprophylaxis of tuberculosis in cattle, *Adv. Tuberc. Res.,* 15, 189, 1966.
67. **Kleeberg, H. H.,** Tuberculosis and other mycobacterioses, in *Diseases Transmitted From Animals to Man,* 6th ed., Hubert, W. T., McCulloch, W. F., and Schnurrenberger, P. R., Eds., Charles C Thomas, Springfield, Ill., 1975.
68. **Rouillon, A. and Waaler, H.,** BCG vaccination and epidemiological situation, *Adv. Tuberc. Res.,* 19, 64, 1976.
69. Committee on Treatment, The Chemotherapy of Tuberculosis. Considerations on Antituberculosis Drugs and Recommendations on Chemotherapy Regimens, International Union Against Tuberculosis, Paris, 1975.

HUMAN TUBERCULOSIS IN ANIMALS

J. H. Steele

Human tuberculosis is a world-wide disease that has been well described by Benenson.[1] It is a chronic mycobacterial disease, important as a cause of disability and death in many parts of the world. Primary infection usually goes unnoticed clinically, and tuberculin sensitivity appears within a few weeks. Lesions commonly become inactive, leaving no residual changes except pulmonary or tracheobronchial lymph node calcifications. However, the disease in man may progress to an active pulmonary form, tuberculosis, pleurisy, or lymph-hematogenous dissemination of bacilli to produce miliary, meningeal, or other extrapulmonary involvement. A serious outcome of primary infection is more frequent in infants and adolescents than older persons.

Pulmonary tuberculosis generally arises from a latent primary focus and, if untreated, has a variable and often asymptomatic course with exacerbations and remissions; it may be cured with chemotherapy. Clinical status is established by presence of tubercle bacilli in sputum or by progression or retrogression as detected in serial X-rays following a definitive bacteriologic diagnosis. Abnormal X-ray densities indicative of pulmonary infiltration, cavitation, or fibrosis commonly occur before clinical manifestations. Cough, fatigue, fever, weight loss, hoarseness, chest pain, and hemoptysis may occur, but these symptoms are often absent until the advanced stages.

Presumptive diagnosis is confirmed by demonstration of tubercle bacilli by culture of sputum, tracheobronchial, gastric washings, or other specimens. Smear examination may give a presumptive diagnosis and repeated examinations are often needed to find bacilli. Persons infected with *Mycobacterium tuberculosis* or *M. bovis* react to a low-dose tuberculin test (e.g., with the bioequivalent of 5 IU). The reaction may be suppressed in critically ill tuberculosis patients and during the course of certain acute infectious diseases, especially measles.

Extrapulmonary tuberculosis is much less common than the pulmonary variety. The former includes tuberculosis meningitis, acute hematogenous tuberculosis, and involvement of the bones and joints, eyes, lymph nodes, kidneys, intestines, larynx, skin, or peritoneum. Diagnosis is based upon recovery of tubercle bacilli from lesions or exudates.

Tuberculosis is present in all parts of the world; however, numerous countries have shown downward trends of mortality and morbidity for many years. Mortality rates range from less than 5 to as many as 100 deaths per 100,000 population per year. The mortality and morbidity rate increases with age, is higher in males than females, and is much greater in nonwhites than whites. In 1974, the reported incidence of new cases in the U.S. was 14.2/100,000 population. In developed countries, prevalence of pulmonary tuberculosis is low for persons less than 20 years of age and rises as a person ages, reaching its highest point in males more than 50 years of age. Most postprimary tuberculosis is endogenous, i.e., arises from old latent foci remaining from initial infection, especially in low-incidence areas. Epidemics have been reported among children in crowded classrooms or other groups congregated in enclosed spaces.

Prevalence of infection, as manifested by tuberculin testing, increases with age, and the rate is usually higher in cities than rural areas. There has been a rapid decline in prevalence of the disease in developed countries in recent decades. In the U.S., less than 3% of males aged 17 to 20 years now react positively to 5 tuberculin units (TU) of purified protein derivative (PPD). In areas where human infection with atypical mycobacteria is prevalent, e.g., the southeastern U.S., cross-reactions may complicate the interpretation of the tuberculin reaction.

Table 1
TOTAL NUMBER OF CASES OF
NATURAL TUBERCULOSIS IN
DIFFERENT ANIMALS IN WHICH THE
TYPE OF TUBERCLE BACILLUS HAS
BEEN DETERMINED

Species of animal	Number of cases	Types of tubercle bacilli found		
		Bovine	Human	Avian
Horse	26	24	—	1
Pig	163	118[a]	5	43
Cat	20	20	—	—
Dog	4	1	3	—
Goat	1	1	—	—
Sheep	4	2	—	2
Cattle	52	50	1	1
Fowl	13	—	—	13
Guinea pig	6	5	1	—
Rabbit	8	4	—	4

[a]   Three cases showed mixed types of tubercle bacilli.

From Griffith, A. S., in *Hagan's Infectious Diseases of Domestic Animals,* 6th ed., Bruner, D. W. and Gillespie, J. H., Eds., Comstock, Ithaca, N.Y., 1973, 425. Copyright 1961, 1966, and 1973 by Cornell University. Used by permission of Cornell University Press.

Human infection caused by the bovine tubercle bacillus is rare in the U.S. and many other countries, but it is still a problem in some areas.

M. tuberculosis, the human tubercle bacillus and infectious agent, can affect many species of animals. Some animals, such as chickens, are susceptible to infection with only one type while others, e.g., pigs, are susceptible to all three types: human, bovine, and avian, as shown in Table 1. In general, it can be pointed out that the human-type bacillus is capable of invading a number of species of animals but produces progressive disease only in the dog and rarely in the cat. Cattle are usually sensitized by *M. tuberculosis* and can be infected experimentally by intravenous injection of the organism with a generalized disease resulting. In India, there are reports of generalized disease in cattle that had been stabled in sheds in which the attending dairymen had open cases of tuberculosis.[3] It is thought that the diseased dairymen expectorated in the feed, troughs, or water tanks and that the cows ingested massive numbers of *M. tuberculosis* organisms.

The following summary illustrates the pathogenicity of the human type of *M. tuberculosis* in animals.[4]

Cattle — *M. tuberculosis* causes only minimal lesions in the lymph nodes and is of no importance except for the fact that animals react to tuberculin following exposure. Careless caretakers suffering from pulmonary tuberculosis may cause many animals to become sensitized to tuberculin.

Horses — No cases have been reported, but it is probable that horses would react like cattle.

Swine — Lesions are confined to the lymph nodes of the alimentary tract. These are minimal in nature and unimportant.

Sheep and goats — No cases have been reported in these animals.

Dogs — Progressive tuberculosis is produced. Most respiratory infections are contracted from tuberculous owners.

Cats — Apparently, cats are highly resistant, but a few cases have been recorded.

Birds — All birds except members of the Psittacidae (parrot family) are resistant. Cases have been reported in parrots that were in contact with tuberculous owners.

Studies of *M. tuberculosis* in cattle were first undertaken by Kock in the 1880s, and when he failed to produce disease experimentally, he stated that human tuberculosis was of no threat to cattle. However, he also interpreted his findings to mean that the inverse was also true, i.e., bovine tuberculosis was not infectious to man. This was false reasoning, and in 1898 Theobald Smith presented data that showed *M. bovis* to be a serious public health problem. Some persons even stated that *M. tuberculosis* could be used to immunize cattle. Such a vaccine (the bovovaccine of Von Behring) was used successfully in Europe for several years and did increase resistance until it was demonstrated that *M. tuberculosis* in cattle was being excreted in the milk.

Extensive studies of the effects of *M. tuberculosis* were undertaken by investigators in Europe and the U.S. at the beginning of the century. It was found that cows and calves did not develop the disease when exposed or injected subcutaneously, but they did develop infection and become tuberculin sensitive. Some calves injected intravenously developed generalized disease.

Professor R. Stenius of the pathology department of the Veterinary College, Helsinki, was asked to investigate tuberculin test problems when an increasing number of reactor animals were found to be free of tuberculosis lesions and, consequently, questions were raised regarding the accuracy of the test.

In 1929, within a short time after beginning his study, he reported that human tubercle bacilli, *M. tuberculosis*, caused the inclusive positive tuberculin tests. Isolation of *M. tuberculosis* from reactor cows confirmed Stenius' hypothesis. In 1928, human tuberculosis was not uncommon among farmers, herdsmen, and milkers. Experiments in which healthy calves were placed on farms where tuberculous persons worked demonstrated the importance of human disease in sensitizing or infecting young livestock. Further epidemiological investigation revealed that drain water from tuberculosis sanitariums was the cause of infection and positive tuberculin reactors among cattle.

Beginning in 1933, herds were classified as (1) probably tuberculous or (2) nonspecific positive tuberculin reactors. When reactors appeared in the first group, they were treated as if infected with *M. bovis* until proven otherwise. The second group consisted mainly of herds in which nonspecific tuberculin reactors appeared from time to time. These herds were tested once or twice each year. A concurrent search was made for open cases of human or avian tuberculosis or other possible sources. Usually, after several weeks or even months, the cause of the tuberculin sensitivity would be found and eliminated, the disease would clear up, and the herd would be declared healthy.[5]

In conclusion, bovine disease control programs must be based upon sound epidemiological observations backed by good laboratory support in order to identify the mycobacteria that may be involved. Findings in Europe, North America, and India emphasize the need for investigations in different environmental settings.

Swine are susceptible to all three types of tubercle bacilli.[6] Prevalence of avian, bovine, and human types depends upon the environment surrounding the swine and character of their feed. For example, the human type of infection, where it does appear, almost always occurs in swine that are fed raw garbage. For this reason, it is dangerous to feed swine uncooked garbage from hospitals and sanitariums. Because of their exposure to diseased chickens, the most common type of tuberculosis found in swine is the avian type. However, the bovine form causes the most serious disease in pigs.

Tuberculosis lesions in swine are generally found in the abdominal cavity of hogs. Infections are contracted most commonly by ingestion; hence, the primary lesions are found in the lymph nodes of the throat and abdominal cavity.

Feldman,[7] in a 1939 study of 264 carcasses of garbage-fed hogs, found that 28.4% had tuberculosis. Subsequent studies to determine the types of tubercle bacilli in the diseased carcasses revealed that 74.5% contained the avian type and 25.5% contained the human type. The offal of diseased chickens accounted for the high percentage of avian-type infection. The human-type bacillus was apparently present more frequently in garbage than had been previously assumed.

In another study, Butler and Marsh[8] reported that 30% of hogs that were fed garbage from a tuberculous sanitarium were infected with the human type of disease. It should be remembered that the average life span of most swine is not more than 8 or 9 months, at which time they are sent to slaughter. Because such animals do not live long enough to become active spreaders of the disease, swine-to-swine transmission probably occurs very infrequently. Tuberculosis of swine is a disease contracted from the environment rather than from other hogs, and there has been no report of swine-to-man transmission.

Human tuberculosis in swine is rarely reported today; however, in regions of the world where human tuberculosis is still widespread, it may occur. Regarding human tuberculosis in other animals, animal health officials should consider subhuman primates in zoos and laboratories and other laboratory animals as being susceptible to infection. The disease may spread among subhuman primates when they are held for long periods.[9]

APPENDIX *

The health and welfare of man are closely associated with that of cattle, even more so in a predominantly agrarian state like India where, besides providing a milk supply, cattle are used extensively for agriculture, transport, etc. Contact between man and cattle can be very intimate. In many places, they share the same shelter during the winter and rainstorms, increasing the chances for spread of communicable diseases between each other. The problem of tuberculosis arises in all of these contexts, but milk supply is the main area for concern.

In a number of developed countries like those of the U.K. and others, about 80% of nonpulmonary tuberculosis in children is caused by bovine bacillus. This is due to contamination of milk caused by udder tuberculosis of cattle. Slaughter and segregation of tuberculin-reactor cattle eradicates the danger.

In India, no pulmonary or nonpulmonary case due to infection by bovine bacillus has yet been reported. This may be the result of the Indian habit of drinking boiled milk. In addition, tuberculous mastitis in cattle appears to be very rare here, as compared to its prevalence in developed countries. A total of about 18 cases have been reported to date, mainly from the Indian Council of Agriculture Research Scheme (Annual Report, 1941 to 1942). Obviously, the anatomy of cattle here compared with that of those abroad cannot differ, so the cause of such low a prevalence of tuberculous mastitis in India remains unknown.

Studies on tuberculous infection in cattle have not been sufficiently extensive. Other than a few reports from individual workers, there has been only one planned survey, reported by Lall et al. in a paper presented at the National Seminar on Zoonoses in India (Transactions of the National Institute of Communicable Diseases, 1968). The rates of infection recorded in and around four cities were: Punjab, 20.4%; Bombay, 16.7%; Madras, 2.1%; and Bihar, 2.0%. Additionally, the rates of infection in herds of some organized farms varied from 0 to 55%. Such a wide variation in the infection

* Anon., Tuberculosis in cattle, *Indian J. Tuberc.* (editorial), 16(4), 1969.

rate is unexplainable unless the groups tested were highly selected, especially in relation to the extent of contact with open cases of tuberculosis in the herds. No such information has, however, been made available.

The true rate of infection by *M. tuberculosis* is difficult to determine since the reaction to the test has to be differentiated from false or nonspecific reactions caused by other bacteria, especially anonymous mycobacteria. Attempts should also be made to distinguish infection by bovine bacillus from that caused by human and avian strains. For this purpose, WHO* recommends the use of a standardized test with tuberculin derived from the different types of bacilli mentioned above with a view to draw inferences by comparing qualitative and quantitative reactions. The report endorses the method used in Great Britain** and suggests PPD as the tuberculin of choice for all strains.

Studies on tuberculous disease in cattle in India are not only few, but even the diagnostic criteria used are not entirely reliable. The study by the Madras Veterinary College published in this issue appears to be quite valuable. The investigation includes histological but not bacteriological examinations of 874 consecutive autopsies. The rate of disease detected was about 4.0%. It is, however, difficult to reconcile this rate with the 2.1% infection rate detected in the same area unless the group studied was highly selected in some way.

A positive bacteriological finding is the only absolute evidence of tuberculosis, but information in this regard is quite inadequate. Results of only two studies deserve mention. Of 40 cultures made by the Indian Veterinary Research Institute, 100% showed the causative organism to be bovine bacillus, whereas 27% of 11 cultures studied by the Madras Veterinary College proved to be *M. bovis* while 73% demonstrated the human type. Such a large variation cannot be explained by rural vs. urban habitation of the herds. Findings of the Madras study may be regarded as very important on an least two counts: (1) it challenges the current concept that human bacilli cannot cause progressive disease in cattle and (2) it contradicts the idea that man cannot transmit disease to cattle.

Clearly, more authentic information obtained through epidemiological studies is needed to design a suitable control program for cattle. Because large-scale slaughter or even segregation of positive reactors cannot be undertaken under conditions existing in India, the program should be phased in and initially limited to herds under observation. In this light, it is suggested that infected cattle be segregated and watched carefully without interrupting milk supply from them. Upon manifestation of the disease, they must be slaughtered. The first phase of this program should apply only to large organized farms that supply milk products. Chemoprophylaxis should be considered later, as suggested by WHO.

In a program such as this, the veterinary, agricultural, and medical sciences should be equally interested and jointly plan and execute a proper study in suitably located centers in India. The Indian Council of Medical Research has already conducted some valuable cooperative studies. Possibly, it will take the initiative in this important study also.

---

*   Joint WHO/FAO Expert Committee Report on Zoonoses, *W.H.O. Tech. Rep. Ser.*, 378, 44, 1967.
** Paterson, A. B., Stuart, P., Lesslie, I., and Leach, F. B., *J. Hyg.*, 56, 1, 1958.

REFERENCES

1. **Benenson, A. S., Ed.,** *Control of Communicable Diseases in Man,* 12th ed., American Public Health Association, Washington, D.C,, 1975, 340.
2. **Griffith, A. S.,** cited in Bruner, D. W. and Gillespie, J. H., Eds., The mycobactericeae, in *Hagan's Infectious Diseases of Domestic Animals,* 6th ed., Comstock, Ithaca, N.Y., 1973, 425.
3. **Chandraeskharan, K. P. and Ramakrishan, R.,** Bovine tuberculosis due to the human strain of *Mycobacterium tuberculosis, Indian J. Tuberc.,* 16(4), 103, 1969.
4. **Bruner, D. W. and Gillespie, J. H., Eds.,** The mycobactericeae, in *Hagan's Infectious Diseases of Domestic Animals,* 6th ed., Comstock, Ithaca, N.Y., 1973, 426.
5. **Myers, J. A. and Steele, J. H.,** Tuberculosis — etiology, diagnosis, treatment, and prevention, in *Bovine Tuberculosis Control in Man and Animals,* Warren H. Green, St. Louis, 1969, 41.
6. **Steele, J. H.,** Garbage-borne diseases in swine, *Proc. lst Natl. Conf. Trichinosis,* American Medical Association, Chicago, 1953.
7. **Feldman, W. H.,** Types of tubercle bacillin lesions of garbage-fed swine, *Am. J. Public Health,* 29, 1231, 1939.
8. **Butler, W. J. and Marsh, H.,** Tuberculosis of human type in garbage-fed hogs, *J. Am. Vet. Med. Assoc.,* 70, 786, 1927.
9. **Ganaway, J. R.,** Bacterial zoonoses of laboratory animals — tuberculosis, in *CRC Handbook Series in Laboratory Animal Science,* Vol. 2, Melby, E. C., Jr. and Altman, N. H., Eds., CRC Press, Cleveland, 1974, 245.

APPENDIX 1
INFECTION WITH AVIAN TUBERCLE BACILLI AND THE RELATIVE PATHOGENICITY OF THE MYCOBACTERIA

J. Francis

Both the chapter by Chapman in Section A, Volume I and the excellent account by Kleeberg[1] of tuberculosis and other mycobacterioses recognize the existence of a classical *Mycobacteria avium*, but some medical writers, concerned predominantly with tuberculosis in man, almost fail to recognize such an organism. They speak of the "avium-intracellulare complex" and do not include *M. avium* as one of the "tubercle" bacilli.

In the writer's view this represents an entirely anthropomorphic view that cannot be supported if one looks at the overall evidence in all species of animals — something that is surely necessary to reach sound conclusions. To understand this subject, it is necessary to briefly review the evidence from about 1900 when knowledge of the bacteriology of tuberculosis was still uncertain. At this time tuberculosis was the white plague that threatened the European peoples, and the question of bacteriology and the possibility of transfer of infection from one species to another was a matter of great public importance.

Major investigations were initiated, including those conducted by the British Royal Commission on Tuberculosis, which had to determine:

1. Whether the disease in animals and man is one and the same
2. Whether animals and man can be reciprocally infected with it
3. Under what conditions, if at all, the transmission of the disease from animals to man takes place, and what are the circumstances favorable or unfavorable to such transmission

The book by Francis[2] includes an appendix describing the contents of these reports and the book summarizes the results of the works of the Commission together with other relevant evidence. By about 1910, it was evident that there were three very important types of tubercle bacilli, namely the human, bovine, and avian types. For the next 40 or 50 years, nearly all authoritative texts on tuberculosis accepted and described these three types of tubercle bacilli.

It is realized that the cultural characteristics of the avian type of the tubercle bacillus or *M. avium* are considerably different from those of the two chief mammalian types, but this cannot set aside the great mass of bacteriological, pathological, and epidemiological evidence showing that the avian tubercle bacillus or *M. avium* has produced and can produce a major infectious disease in various types or species of birds associated with typical tuberculous allergy and caseating tubercles with a characteristic histology including Langerhans giant cells. All this evidence on *M. avium* infection of birds and mammals has been presented in a major monograph by Feldman[3] and has been further analyzed on a comparative basis by Francis.[2] The fact that some strains or types of *M. intracellulare* closely resemble *M. avium* cannot alter the fact that classical *M. avium* is one of the three most important types of tubercle bacilli with the capacity to produce tuberculosis in a far wider range of species than the human tubercle bacillis, *M. tuberculosis*.

Francis[2] reviewed evidence on the pathogenicity of the three types of tubercle bacilli for various species of animals following different routes of infection and presented the results in a series of tables the are summarized below.

Route of infection	Number of species infected		Number of species susceptible		
	Mammals	Birds*	Bovine	Avian	Human
Subcutaneous	16	1	12	3	2
Intraperitoneal	6	1	6	4	3
Intravenous**	7	1	6	6	3

*   Domestic fowl.
** At appropriate comparative doses.

It will be seen that the bovine type of tubercle bacilli has much the widest range of pathogenicity. The avian type is accepted as being pathogenic for virtually all species of birds and it will be seen that it also has a considerable range of pathogenicity for mammals. The arithmetic mean of the percentage isolates from the various species gives 63.5% bovine type, 34.2% avian, and 22.3% human type. For a variety of reasons these percentages do not add up to 100. So we see that even from mammalian species (excluding man), the avian type is isolated more frequently than the human type of tubercle bacilli.

The great majority of species of tubercle bacilli isolated from man would obviously be of the human type and from many species of birds of the avian type. The parrot however, is susceptible to the human and bovine as well as the avian types of the tubercle bacilli.

Tuberculosis is characteristically a disease of urban man and his animals and birds. The disease is virtually unknown in wild animals except for voles infected with *M. microtis*. On the other hand, it is probable that *M. avium* produces a naturally perpetuating disease in wild pigeons[2] and possibly in other species of birds. However, if the human tubercle bacillus were eradicated from man, the bovine from cattle, and the avian from domestic fowls, mycobacterial infection of man, animals, and birds would be reduced to an extremely low level and would chiefly be caused by atypical tubercle bacilli or the potential pathogens that exist in the environment.

We thus see that when we look over the various species of animals and birds, the avian tubercle bacillus has much the widest range of pathogenecity although the disease it produces in mammals is less severe than that produced by the bovine bacillus. The latter organism has quite a wide range of pathogenecity for animals but is virtually nonpathogenic to birds except for parrots. Apart from man and other primates, the human tubercle bacillus has a very limited range of pathogenicity.

ATYPICAL TUBERCLE BACILLI

Other parts of this volume deal with bovine tuberculosis, infection of cattle with tubercle bacilli of the human type, and the atypical mycobacteria. It is the last group which causes the most difficulty as is illustrated by the variety of names used to describe it. With the foregoing information in mind, it is possible to consider the name of this group of bacteria. The expressions "anonymous" and "unclassified" mycobacteria are falling into disuse, but the expression "atypical mycobacteria" is widely applied and convenient. However, it is only by usage that it can be understood to describe the group of mycobacteria that sometimes produce lesions indistinguishable from some forms of tuberculosis, but not typical tuberculous disease. When strictly interpreted, this term is incorrect as the organisms concerned are no more "atypical mycobacteria" than is *M. bovis* or *M. phlei*. It has the further disadvantage that it does not specifically exclude the saprophytic mycobacteria.

The term "mycobacteria other than tubercle bacille," or MOTT bacilli, has gained some acceptance. However, it is rather a clumsy acronym and, if strictly interpreted, specifically includes the saprophytic mycobacteria; it is in fact more applicable to the saprophytes than to the "atypicals" so it is obviously an incorrect or inaccurate term.

The term tuberculoid bacilli excludes the saprophytic mycobacteria, but there seems to be some objection to the use of this word. The term "atypical tubercle bacilli" is, therefore, suggested. This term has the great advantage that it says what it means; it includes mycobacteria that produce atypical or tubercle-like lesions but excludes the saprophytic mycobacteria. Use of the expression "atypicals" could still be continued if preferred to "the ATTB."

As indicated above, some medical bacteriologists tend to include *M. avium* or at least the *M. avium* complex, in the atypicals. Facts have been presented to show that *M. avium* must be accepted as one of the classical tubercle bacilli and the one that produces typical tuberculous disease in a far wider range of species than *M. tuberculosis* or even *M. bovis*. However, some people will doubtless continue to include the *M. avium* complex in the "atypical" group and, therefore, make the expression "mycobacteria other than tubercle bacilli" particularly objectionable because classical *M. avium* is obviously a tubercle bacillus. However, there is little objection to including the *M. avium* complex under the term "atypical tubercle bacilli" as *M. avium* has considerable differences in cultural characteristics and pathogenicity from *M. tuberculosis* or *M. bovis*.

THE COMPARATIVE TUBERCULIN TEST

Because avian tubercle bacilli and the atypical tubercle bacilli infect man and animals, there is considerable interest in the comparative tuberculin test that is carried out by making a simultaneous intradermal injection of both avian and mammalian tuberculin in different sites. Each tuberculin has specificity for its own species of organism but those made from the human and bovine types are very similar. That made from the avian type differs considerably from mammalian tuberculin but is similar to that made from many of the atypical tubercle bacilli.

Information on the subject has been presented by Francis et al.[4] The comparative tuberculin test using bovine tuberculin on the one hand, and avian on the other, is the standard test carried out on cattle in Britain and is used as a supplementary test in the U.S. and some European countries. However, as indicated in the chapter on bovine tuberculosis, on the basis of available published evidence, the sensitivity of this test is disappointingly low and the specificity not outstandingly high.

Francis et al.[4] presented evidence indicating that the following results might be expected with different forms of the single intradermal tuberculin test:

	Sensitivity	Specificity
Caudal fold	85%	85%
Cervical	91%	76%
Cervical comparative	72%	88%

In man, evidence suggests that nonspecific sensitization to tuberculin may be most prevalent in the tropical regions. This sensitization, especially in the coastal areas of northern Queensland, is due mainly to organisms of the *M. avium-intracellulare-*

scrofulaceum complex. It is, of course, well known that *M. avium* and *M. paratuberculosis* cause nonspecific sensitization to tuberculin in cattle, especially in moist temperate areas, but infections by these organisms are virtually unknown in cattle in Queensland.

Comparative tuberculin tests are widely used in man in an attempt to distinguish tuberculous reactors from those with nonspecific reactions to tuberculin. Although this approach is usually successful in children, the comparative test in adults appears to have very poor specificity. It is possible that the concept of "original mycobacterial sin," suggested by Abrahams, is applicable to cattle as well as humans and this may be an explanation of the apparently poor results given by the comparative test in cattle. If calves are sensitized with other mycobacteria before they are exposed to *M. bovis,* then subsequent *M. bovis* infection, while resulting in hypersensitivity to *M. bovis* antigen, may boost their sensitivity to avian tuberculin to an even greater extent. Conversely, in calves exposed early in life to *M. bovis,* the tendency to react to mammalian tuberculin may predominate despite the fact that the early *M. bovis* infection had been overcome. Whether or not such explanations are applicable to cattle, it appears that further evidence is required on the sensitivity and specificity of the comparative test and that the single caudal or cervical test may be more efficient, particularly for initial surveys.

REFERENCES

1. **Kleeberg, H. H.**, Tuberculosis and other mycobacterioses, in *Diseases Transmitted from Animals to Man,* 6th ed., Hubbert, W. T., McCulloch, W. F., and Schnurrenberger, P. R., Eds., Charles C Thomas, Springfield, Ill., 1975, 303.
2. **Francis, J.**, *Tuberculosis in Animals and Man: A Study in Comparative Pathology,* Cassell and Company, London, 1958, 357.
3. **Feldman, W. H.**, *Avian Tuberculosis Infections,* Williams & Wilkins, Baltimore, 1938, 483.
4. **Francis, J., Seiler, R. J., Wilkie, I. W., Boyle, D. A., Lumsden, M. J., and Frost, A. J.**, The sensitivity and specificity of various tuberculin tests using bovine PPD and other tuberculins, *Vet. Rec.,* 103, 420, 1978.

APPENDIX 2*

Tuberculosis has been a serious problem among elderly people for centuries. In 1920, S. Peller[1] reported on vital statistical studies in Vienna that revealed that in 1752 to 1753 of those 50 years of age and older at time of death, mortality from tuberculosis accounted for 20.8%. Freedman and Heiken[2] of Philadelphia reported that among 3000 routine necropsies, unsuspected pulmonary tuberculosis was found in 20%. Those who died at the age of 60 years or older comprised one third of the total necropsy incidence but provided 28% of the total incidence of pulmonary tuberculosis. Under the title *Disregarded Seedbed of the Tubercle Bacillus,* Medlar et al.,[3] of New York City, reported large numbers of post-mortem examinations. They wrote:

> Among patients who died from tuberculosis, the clinical diagnosis was incorrect six times more often for persons over 50 than for persons under 30 years. Among patients who died from other diseases but who harbored tuberculosis that was capable of spreading, there was clinical recognition of tuberculosis in only one fourth. Tuberculosis tends to be less explosive in type in old persons than in young adults. Older persons can have progressive disease with so few manifestations of illness that they may not seek the advice of a physician. In these circumstances, they remain unrecognized spreaders of the infection . . . In a high proportion of new cases of tuberculosis in adults in New York City, the disease is apparently contracted from unrecognized sources of infection . . . The seedbed must be controlled if the continuity of the disease is to be broken . . . The seedbed must be eradicated if tuberculosis is to be eradicated.

Early in this century, many persons had communicable pulmonary tuberculosis, but little effort was made to prevent them from disseminating tubercle bacilli among infants, children, and youths with the result that a high percentage were harboring the organism on attainment of young adulthood. It was also learned that many of those young adults would retain living tubercle bacilli in their bodies for the remainder of their lives, and some would develop chronic clinical pulmonary disease at any time including old age.

Obviously, the problem was to prevent infants, children, and youths from becoming infected with tubercle bacilli so that they could pass through all the years of their lives without becoming infected.

SANATORIUMS FOR TREATMENT AND PREVENTION OF TUBERCULOSIS

In 1859, Dr. Herman Brehmer established the first permanent sanatorium in the world for persons suffering from tuberculosis at Gobersdorf, Germany. In 1882, Dr. E. L. Trudeau[4] read in the *English Practitioner* an account of Brehmer's sanatorium. The methods used there so closely approached those employed in the treatment of his personal tuberculosis problem that he conceived the idea of building a similar institution in America. He opened his institution under the name Adirondack Cottage Sanitarium (later "Sanatorium") at Saranac Lake, N.Y. in 1885. Such institutions soon began to spring up across the country. They were built for treatment of patients who had tuberculosis in the early stage. However, a serious problem was encountered, namely, that 80% or more of the applicants to those institutions had the disease in an advanced communicable stage. Practicing physicians were serverely criticized for not making early diagnoses. Patients were also criticized for not having reported to physicians for examination when symptoms first appeared.

*   Reprinted from Myers, J. A., Tapering off of tuberculosis among the elderly, *Am. J. Public Health,* 66(11), 1101, 1976. With permission.

When groups of recent tuberculin-converter children and university students were followed over long periods of time to determine the natural history of tuberculosis in the human body, those destined to develop clinical disease had very small shadow-casting lesions appear and slowly evolve for 2 or more years before symptoms developed or the lesions could be detected by physical signs. The reasons for absence of symptoms were (1) the lungs have no sensory nerve pain fibers so extensive disease may develop without causing pain, (2) normal lungs have a capacity for approximately eight times more air than is inhaled with each breath so extensive disease may develop without causing shortness of breath, and (3) cough with sputum rarely occurs until lesions begin to break down in an advanced stage. Thus, while the disease was in the early stage, patients had no reason to report to physicians for examination.

In the early decades of sanatoriums, 25% of the patients admitted had hopelessly advanced disease and died there. For the remainder, sanatorium routine, collapse therapy including artificial pneumothorax, and extrapleural thoracoplasty played an important role in successful treatment.

An equally if not more important function of sanatoriums was that they received communicable cases from their home communities; those who did not recover remained isolated until death, and the much larger number who recovered were rendered safe associates for infants, children, and youths in their home communities.

BOVINE SPECIES OF TUBERCLE BACILLUS CONTRIBUTED TO SERIOUSNESS OF PROBLEM

Another source of infection by tubercle bacilli in infants, children, and youths was tuberculous cattle in which the disease was rampant.[5] In 1892, Dr. Leonard Pearson and Charles E. Cotton[6] of the University of Pennsylvania administered the first tuberculin tests to cattle in this country. They demonstrated the presence of tubercle bacilli in many animals in which infection with or without clinical disease had not been suspected. Therefore, a campaign was started in a few places to control the disease among cattle. An ordinance was passed in Minneapolis in 1895 forbidding any person to sell milk in that city without a license that required a certificate showing that the cows had been tested with tuberculin and all reactors were removed from the herd. In a short time, other cities adopted similar ordinances, thus protecting infants, children, and youths against *Mycobacterium bovis* infection.[5]

Between 1896 and 1898, Smith[7] of Harvard University isolated the bovine species of tubercle bacillus (*M. bovis*), and in 1901 Ravenel[8] of Philadelphia announced that *M. bovis* causes illness and death in people. It was later shown to be as destructive in various human tissues and organs as the human species — *Mycobacterium tuberculosis*. Park and Krumwiede[9] of New York City made bacteriological analyses and reviewed similar work of others on 1511 fatal cases of tuberculosis among infants and young children. They found that 66% of fatal generalized tuberculosis cases were due to *M. bovis.*

In England, Griffith[10,11] observed that, in addition to causing as serious a disease as *M. tuberculosis* in human extrathoracic organs, *M. bovis* was also a common cause of disease in human lungs, including those of the aged.

SOME OF THE MANY SPECIAL ATTEMPTS TO SOLVE THE PROBLEM

In order to promote the activities of those persons attempting to protect infants, children, and youths against infection with tubercle bacilli, it was necessary to inform the nation's citizenry about tuberculosis. The National Association for the Study and

Prevention of Tuberculosis (later National Tuberculosis Association and now American Lung Association) was organized in 1904. As that organization developed, it had more than 2500 component state, country, and municipal associations and societies across the country. Their main purpose was to disseminate information concerning tuberculosis among the entire citizenry of the nation. Numerous nationwide campaigns were in operation, including anti-spitting, abolishing the public drinking cup, and emphasizing early diagnosis. The latter was established in cooperation with the National Conference of Tuberculosis Secretaries. State, county, and municipal tuberculosis associations cooperated by devoting the month of April to emphasis on early diagnosis. Each year a slogan for the campaign was adopted. For the first year it was "You may have tuberculosis — let your doctor decide." Another was "From whom did he get it, to whom has he given it." These slogans could be seen in bold type most everywhere throughout the nation. The early diagnosis campaign each April was so effective that it continued, and many tuberculosis associations adopted similar procedures for their year-round programs.[12]

In 1935, the Federation of American Sanatoria — later the American College of Chest Physicians — was organized and thereafter devoted much time to providing physicians throughout the country with information on diagnosis, treatment, and prevention of tuberculosis.

Other national organizations had active committees on tuberculosis including the American Academy of Pediatrics, the American College Health Association, the American School Health Association, American Public Health Association, American Nurses Association, American Academy of General (Family) Practice, and the American Medical Association with a section of Diseases of the Chest. In the 1930s and 1940s, many state medical associations had or appointed committees on tuberculosis, and in some states each county medical society had such a committee.

As sanatoriums increased in number, pasteurization of milk was practiced in cities, and control of tuberculosis among cattle was well under way, tapering off of the disease was first observed in infants and children.

ACCOMPLISHMENTS DEMONSTRATED BY MORTALITY RATES

By 1930, a marked decrease in tuberculosis mortality had occurred. Among infants, the mortality rate dropped from 311.6/100,000 in 1900 to 51.6/100,000 in 1930.* Among children of 1 to 4 years, the rate had decreased from 101.8/100,000 in 1900 to 25.9/100,000 in 1930 (Table 1). There was also marked tapering off of mortality rates in all other ages, but less in those of 45 years and older (Table 1). With such large numbers of old people still carrying infections acquired in early life, why did their mortality rate not remain as high as had occurred among those of and preceding 1900? It appears that educational work had created an awareness of the hazards of the disease which had resulted in greater acceptance of sanatorium treatment. Moreover, in addition to the usual sanatorium routine, collapse therapy including artificial pneumothorax and extrapleural thoracoplasty came into extensive use. In large institutions, collapse therapy was employed on 50 to 65% of the patients including the elderly. Therefore, many persons who previously would have entered the old-age period with chronic active disease had been treated successfully. Also, many elderly tuberculous patients had their disease controlled by collapse therapy.[12]

During the fourth decade of this century, the intensity of the anti-tuberculosis campaign was increased, and the accomplishments were such that, in 1935, Dr. Wade

---

* Vital statistics data cited in the text, unless otherwise referenced, were provided by Anthony M. Lowell, Chief, Statistics and Analysis, Tuberculosis Control Division, Center for Disease Control, Atlanta.

Table 1
U.S. TUBERCULOSIS MORTALITY RATES[a]

Age group (years)	Year						
	1900	1930	1940	1950	1959—1961	1970	1973
0—1	311.6	51.6	24.6	8.5	0.9	0.5	0.4
1—4	101.8	25.9	12.3	6.3	0.7	0.3	0.1
5—14	36.2	11.9	5.5	1.8	0.1	0.0[b]	0.0[b]
15—24	205.7	73.3	38.2	11.3	0.6	0.1	0.1
25—34	294.3	102.8	56.3	19.1	2.3	0.7	0.3
35—44	253.6	92.4	59.4	26.1	5.0	1.8	1.2
45—54	215.6	93.2	66.3	35.9	9.2	3.5	2.5
55—64	223.0	97.0	75.8	47.8	15.4	6.2	4.5
65—74	256.1	111.7	81.5	58.2	23.2	10.1	7.3
75—84	279.3	115.5	80.1	63.2	32.2	16.4	11.6
85+	204.5	76.9	63.9	47.7	38.6	20.9	15.2
All ages	194.4	71.1	45.9	22.5	6.0	2.6	1.8

[a] TB death rates per 100,000 population.
[b] Less than 0.05.

Courtesy of Anthony M. Lowell, Chief, Statistics and Analysis, Tuberculosis Control Division, Center for Disease Control, Atlanta.

Frost,[13] eminent epidemiologist of The Johns Hopkins School of Public Health, wrote: "The eradication of tuberculosis is now an expectation sufficiently well-grounded to justify shaping our tuberculosis control program toward this definite end. We have reached the stage at which biological balance is against the survival of the tubercle bacillus . . . and, as demonstrated by the steadily falling morbidity and mortality rates, each existing case has for some time been giving rise to less than one new case of the disease. If this balance can be maintained and the sources of infection further reduced, the control of tuberculosis is within our grasp." There had been numerous opinions expressed concerning prevalence of tuberculosis among old people. The most frequently repeated one pertained to lowered resistance to tuberculosis in that period of life. However, in 1939, Dr. Frost[14] offered the correct explanation. He pointed out that those persons who were in the age group of 50 to 60 years in the 1930s, if followed back to birth, actually experienced their highest mortality at the age of 20 to 30 years. Therefore, he wrote: "The present day 'peak' of mortality in late life does not represent postponement of maximum risk to a later period, but would rather seem to indicate that the present high rates in old age are the residuals of higher rates in earlier life." By 1946, the tuberculosis mortality rate for all ages had decreased from 194.4/100,000 in 1900 to 33.5/100,000 (82.8%).

CASE RATE BETTER THAN MORTALITY RATE AS CRITERION OF MAGNITUDE OF TUBERCULOSIS PROBLEM

Armstrong's[15] report of 1923 on the Framingham, Mass. demonstration that showed that for each death from tuberculosis nine active cases exist in the same community was soon found to obtain in other places. Therefore, it was obvious that mortality rates were not as good a criterion of the tuberculosis problem as case rates. In 1930, the reported case rate for people of all ages in the registration area of the U.S. was 101.5 (124,940 cases), and in 1940 it had dropped to 78.0 (102,984 cases).

By 1940, the number of sanatorium beds had increased to 90,000 (later to 130,433).

Also, 40,000 patients were isolated in general hospitals. The use of general hospitals for tuberculous patients had long been strongly recommended.[16]

The veterinarians' tuberculosis eradication program among cattle was so effective that by 1940 each of the 48 states had been rated as modified accredited areas, which meant that tuberculin reactors among cattle had been reduced to one half of 1% or less.[16] Therefore, infection of infants, children, and youths with *M. bovis* had become almost nil.

When Dr. Herman E. Hilleboe became the first chief of the newly created Tuberculosis Control Division of the U.S. Public Health Service, he devised a plan for control that embraced four principal phases for attacking tuberculosis on a national basis:[12] (1) case finding, (2) medical care and isolation, (3) after-care and rehabilitation, and (4) protection of tuberculous families from economic distress. This was the first nationwide attempt by an official agency to control tuberculosis among people. Over the years, these phases were conducted with remarkable success. For example, under the case-finding phase, he made available photoflurographic units and operating personnel to local workers for examining adults in cities across the country. Those surveys resulted in examination of nearly 9,000,000 persons, and 60,000 individuals were found to have clinical tuberculosis. Dr. Hilleboe strongly promoted and succeeded in having a full-time tuberculosis officer appointed to most state health departments — as well as those of large cities — to carry out all phases of his program.

ANTI-TUBERCULOSIS DRUGS INTRODUCED

In 1946, Hinshaw, Feldman, and Pfuetze[17] of the Mayo Clinic announced that streptomycin had been proved to have a supppressive effect on tuberculosis in man. That same year, Lehmann[18] of Sweden introduced paraaminosalicylic acid; thereafter, these and other drugs were administered by physicians across the country and resulted in postponement of death of many persons including the elderly who would have died from tuberculosis. Thus, the drugs served as an adjunct to the methods that had been employed so effectively, and they continued to result in an ever-increasing number of uninfected persons attaining old age.

The Veterans Administration inaugurated a large tuberculosis case-finding project in 1950.[12] By 1955, more than four million examinations for tuberculosis had been made, including routine chest X-ray inspection of all new patient admissions to Veterans Administration hospitals, in outpatient departments, regional offices, etc. Among those veterans, 15,479 active cases of tuberculosis were found. The program continued for several years with approximately one million chest examinations and about 2000 new cases being found annually.

In 1953, the case rate (both active and inactive) had decreased to 67.5 (106,925 cases). Seven years later, the rate was down to 39.2 (70,124 cases). In 1952, the Public Health Service adopted the policy of reporting previously unknown cases *separately* as a better way of measuring incidence of the disease.

In 1953 among infants and children under 5 years of age, the case rate was 15.4 (2719 cases) (Table 2). The highest rates were among persons of 45 to 64 years with 79.9 (25,838 cases), and those of 65 years and over with a rate of 82.9 (11,322 cases). During the next 10 years, the number of uninfected persons continued to replace those who had moved on in years, and many of the oldest died. That was reflected in the case rates among persons from 45 to 64 years of age and those 65 and over, which had been reduced to 46.2 and 58.2, respectively. In 1974, the case rate for persons of all ages was 12.4, but for those of 45 to 64 years, it was 23.6, and for those of 65 and over, 32.5 (Table 2).

Table 2
U.S. NEW ACTIVE
TUBERCULOSIS CASE RATES[a]

Age group (years)	Year			
	1953	1963	1973	1974
Under 5	15.4	14.9	7.4	7.5
5—14	9.1	9.0	2.8	2.6
15—24	49.5	17.1	6.4	6.3
25—44	67.7	32.4	15.9	15.4
45—64	79.9	46.2	25.3	23.6
65 and over	82.9	58.2	33.4	32.5
All ages	53.0	28.7	14.8	14.2

[a]   TB case rates per 100,000 population.

Courtesy of Anthony M. Lowell, Chief, Statistics and Analysis, Tuberculosis Control Division, Center for Disease Control, Atlanta.

TUBERCLE BACILLUS ATTACK RATE BEST CRITERION OF EXTENT OF TUBERCULOSIS PROBLEM

Veterinarians used the tuberculin test to determine the magnitude of the tuberculosis problem among cattle. Beginning in 1917, the eradication campaign consisted of testing all cattle periodically across the country and removing reactors from the herds. From that year through 1967, they administered the test 470,395,546 times and removed 4,167,200 reactors from the herds.[19] Roswurm and Ranney[20] pointed out that among the carcasses inspected in slaughterhouses, of the 9.3 million tuberculin reactors found that year, 50,000 were "condemned" or "passed for cooking only" because of tuberculosis. Moreover, 1 cow in every 20 was infected. However, in 1971, only 1 in 20,000 cattle reacted to tuberculin, and of the 35 million slaughtered that year, less than 300 carcasses were "condemned" or "passed for cooking only" because of this disease. Thus, over the years and decades there was a constant decrease of infection with *M. bovis* among infants, children, and youths until now it is a rarity.

First infection with tubercle bacilli is the beginning of all forms of tuberculosis that develop in the human body. The infection is identifiable by the tuberculin test a few weeks after the initial invasion of tubercle bacilli occurs. Inasmuch as each recent tuberculin reactor is a potential case of chronic pulmonary tuberculosis, the test provides the best criterion of the magnitude of the tuberculosis problem in a family, community, state, or nation. In the early years of this century, this test was used infrequently because many physicians believed that nearly universal infection occurred by the age of 15 years. That belief was based on von Pirquet's[21] 1908 report showing that 92% of 14-year-old Vienna children reacted to the test. In 1916, Sedgewick[22] tested many Minneapolis infants and children and concluded that the test was practical only among children up to the sixth or seventh year. He believed that there was a 70% prevalence among youths.

However, with the efforts already in vogue to protect infants, children, and youths against exposure to *M. tuberculosis* and *M. bovis*, tuberculin testing in those age groups would be expected to determine whether the first infection attack rate was changing. In 1915,[23] 48% of youths of 13 and 14 years in St. Louis reacted to tuberculin. In the early 1920s, testing in other areas revealed even smaller numbers of reactors.[24] Among many thousands of school children[25] in Massachusetts in 1929, only 22.7% of white and 27.34% of black children reacted to tuberculin. Thus, only approximately one fourth of the children were potential cases of chronic clinical disease later in their lives. The 75% uninfected were replacing older, heavily infected individuals as they moved on to the older age brackets. Soon thereafter, tuberculin testing in schools, colleges, and universities was adopted across the nation. The more than 2500 tuberculosis associations and societies in states, counties, and cities adopted tuberculin testing of school children as their major project. Colleges and universities did likewise, and later extensive tuberculin testing was extended to adults.

In 1934, the newly appointed committee on Tuberculosis of the American School Health Association recommended that all school personnel, both professional and nonprofessional, be tested with tuberculin with appropriate further examination of reactors.[26] That program later resulted in legislation in most states making such examinations of all school personnel mandatory. Among school personnel, cases of clinical pulmonary tuberculosis were discovered in teachers, cooks, janitors, bus drivers, and others. Some of these individuals had communicable disease but were working regularly. For example, bus drivers were found who had infected a considerable percentage of children whom they transported to and from school. Cases were discovered similar to the one reported by Dr. Alfred Hess and related by Dr. George Rosen[27] in his recent centennial tribute to Dr. Hess.

Tuberculin reactor children were referred to family physicians with the suggestion that they examine the children's adult associates in an effort to locate persons responsible for their infections.

To stimulate cooperation and participation, a program was devised for official certification of schools on the basis of tuberculosis work in progress. To obtain a first-class certificate, 100% of personnel members and at least 95% of children had to have been tested. Thousands of certificates were won by schools.

Thus, a method for accurately determining the effectiveness of the tuberculosis program from time to time was in general use. For example, a 28-year study begun by Harrington[28] of Minneapolis revealed that tuberculin reactors among grade school children decreased from 47.3% in 1926 to 7.7% in 1944 and to 3.9% in 1954. Now it has become almost a rarity to find a tuberculin-reactor school child in that city.

From 1956 to 1965, Dr. Carroll Palmer and Dr. Lydia Edwards[29] of the U.S. Public Health Service tuberculin tested 58,000 school children and nearly 15,000 college students in six states. Among the children on entrance to school, 0.5% of those from 6 to 14 years, 1% reacted, while among those from 14 to 18 years old, 2.5% reacted. From 1949 to 1951, they tested 55,706 U.S. Navy recruits from 17 to 21 years old from 31 states, finding only 6.6 reactors. Testing 539,138 recruits from across the country from 1958 to 1964, they found 3.9% reactors.

By that time, the great masses of uninfected people had continued to replace extensively infected groups who had moved on in years. Each year brought death from various causes including tuberculosis among the eldest, who were replaced by the oncoming, mostly uninfected old people. Those newcomers in old age resulted in lower percentages of infection from year to year.

In one state in 1954, 47.7% of the men and 44.1% of the women of 50 to 59 years reacted to tuberculin; whereas in 1964, 24.52% of men and 11.73% of women reacted; and in 1967, 8.5% of men and 4.5% of women reacted.[30] In 1964, among persons of 60 years and older, 35.58% of men and 19.33% of women reacted to tuberculin. By 1967, those percentages had decreased to 15.2 and 7.72, respectively.[30]

On the basis of tuberculin testing, it has been estimated that among the 214 million persons of this country, 16 million are infected with tubercle bacilli with a preponderance among those of 45 years or older. The prevalence of tuberculin reactors is now estimated to be about 0.2% among children of 6 years and 0.7% among youths. With the prevalence of 0.2% of children of 6 years, the current infection rate is estimated to be 0.03%.

At no time, including today, has 100% protection against infection with tubercle bacilli been provided for all infants, children, youths, or other age groups. This is largely due to lack of examination or failure to have the disease diagnosed before it has become communicable. For example, in 1974, 1143 new active cases were first reported at death. Moreover, of the 22,518 new active cases of clinical pulmonary tuberculosis with extent of disease specified, 17,319 were in an advanced stage when first reported. Usually, when the disease is in that stage, it is communicable. Therefore, it is likely that microoutbreaks (epidemics) were caused by many of those persons before their disease was discovered.

If the methods of control that have been so responsible for tapering off of tuberculosis are revived or continued, apparently mortality, case, and infection rates will disappear last among the aged. To insure this accomplishment, it must be remembered that (1) tuberculin reactors are potential cases of chronic clinical tuberculosis caused by endogenous reinfection — a term coined by Dr. Leon Bernard[31] of Paris in the 1920s, and (2) that 80% or more of such clinical cases have no symptom to cause them to report for examination until the disease is in an advanced and usually communicable stage.

SUMMARY

Tuberculosis has long been prevalent among elderly people. When tubercle bacilli first enter human bodies, they usually remain through the rest of their hosts' lives and are capable of causing clinical disease at any time, even in old age. In 1900, a large percentage of people of all ages were harboring tubercle bacilli, and high mortality and case rates obtained among elderly people. The only way to solve the problem among future old people was to protect infants, children, and youths from becoming infected and to enable them to remain so throughout life. As far as possible, that was accomplished by isolating and treating tuberculous patients in sanatoriums and hospitals, with anti-tuberculosis drugs after 1946, and by controlling the disease among cattle. In due time large numbers of children entered adulthood uninfected. From year to year, they replaced those who were heavily infected as they advanced in years. By 1973, the mortality rate was only a fraction of 1.0/100,000 among persons under 34 years of age, but of those 65 to 84 years, it was 9.7; the case rate was 28.1 for those older than 45 years. Although tuberculosis among the elderly has tapered off phenomenally, much time and work are necessary to accomplish eradication.

REFERENCES

1. **Peller, S.,** Zur Kenntnis der stadtischen Mortalitat im 18: Jahrundert mit besonderer Berucksichtigung der Sauglings und Tuberkulose-Sterblichkeit (Wien zur Zeit der ersten Volkszahlung), *Z. Hyg. Infectionskr.,* 90, 227, 1920.
2. **Freeman, J. T. and Heiken, C. A.,** Geriatric aspect of pulmonary tuberculosis, *Am. J. Med. Sci.,* 202, 29, 1941.
3. **Medlar, E. M., Spain, D. M., and Halliday, R. W.,** Disregarded seedbed of the tubercle bacillus, *Arch. Intern. Med.,* 81, 501, 1948.
4. **Trudeau, E. L.,** *An Autobiography,* Doubleday-Page, Garden City, N.Y., 1916.
5. **Myers, J. A.,** *Man's Greatest Victory Over Tuberculosis,* Charles C Thomas, Springfield, Ill., 1940.
6. **Pearson, L.,** Report of first testing of cattle in the United States, *Med. News,* 60, 358, 1892.

7. **Smith, T.,** A culture test for distinguishing the human from the bovine type of bacilli, *J. Med. Res.,* 13, 253, 1905.
8. **Ravenel, M. P.,** The intercommunicability of human and bovine tuberculosis, *Proc. Pathol. Soc. Philadelphia,* 23, 181, 1901.
9. **Park, W. H. and Krumwiede, C.,** The relative importance of the bovine and human types of tubercle bacilli in the different forms of human tuberculosis, *J. Med. Res.,* 23, 205, 1910.
10. **Griffith, A. S.,** Observations on the bovine tubercle bacillus in human tuberculosis, *Br. Med. J.,* 10, 501, 1932.
11. **Griffith, A. S.,** Bovine tuberculosis in man, *Tubercle,* 18, 529, 1937.
12. **Myers, J. A.,** *Captain of All These Men of Death — Tuberculosis Historical Highlights,* Warren H. Green, St. Louis, 1977.
13. **Frost, W. H.,** Outlook for eradication of tuberculosis, *Am. Rev. Tuberc.,* 32, 644, 1935.
14. **Frost, W. H.,** Age selection of mortality from tuberculosis in successive decades, *Am. J. Hyg.* (Section A), 30, 91, 1939.
15. **Armstrong, D. B.,** Framingham Monograph No. 10, Final Summary Report 1917-1923, National Tuberculosis Association, Framingham, Mass., 1924.
16. **Myers, J. A. and Wahlquist, H. F.,** Fifteen reasons why general hospitals should serve tuberculous patients, *Hosp. Manage.,* 23, 34, 1927.
17. **Hinshaw, H. C., Feldman, W. H., and Pfuetze, K.,** Streptomycin in treatment of clinical tuberculosis, *Am. Rev. Tuberc.,* 54, 191, 1946.
18. **Lehmann, J.,** The treatment of tuberculosis in Sweden with para-aminosalicylic acid (PAS): a review, *Dis. Chest,* 16, 684, 1949.
19. **Myers, J. A. and Steele, J. H.,** *Bovine Tuberculosis Control in Man and Animals,* Warren H. Green, St. Louis, 1969.
20. **Roswurm, J. D. and Ranney, A. F.,** Sharpening the attack on bovine tuberculosis, *Am. J. Public Health,* 63, 884, 1973.
21. **von Pirquet, C.,** Frequency of tuberculosis in childhood, *JAMA,* 52, 675, 1909.
22. **Sedgewick, J. P.,** The diagnosis of early tuberculosis in children, *St. Paul Med. J.,* 18, 213, 1916.
23. **Veeder, B. S. and Johnston, M. B.,** The frequency of infection with the tubercle bacillus in childhood, *Am. J. Dis. Child.,* 9, 478, 1915.
24. **Slater, S. A.,** The results of Pirquet tuberculin tests on 1,654 children in a rural community in Minnesota, *Am. Rev. Tuberc.,* 10, 229, 1924.
25. **Chadwick, H. D. and Zacks, D.,** The incidence of tuberculous infection in school children, *N. Engl. J. Med.,* 200, 332, 1929.
26. **Anon.,** Eradication of tuberculosis from the schools of america. Thirty-two years report of the committee on Tuberculosis of the American School Health Association, *J. Sch. Health,* 36, 323, 1966.
27. **Rosen, G.,** The case of the consumptive conductor, or public health on a streetcar. A centennial tribute to Alfred F. Hess, M.D., *Am. J. Public Health,* 65, 977, 1975.
28. **Myers, J. A., Gunlaugson, F. G., Meyerding, E. A., and Roberts, J.,** Importance of tuberculin testing of school children — a twenty-eight year study, *JAMA,* 159, 185, 1955.
29. **Lowell, A. M., Edwards, L. B., and Palmer, C. E.,** *Tuberculosis,* Harvard University Press, Cambridge, Mass., 1969.
30. **Flemming, D. S.,** Minnesota State Department of Health Official Reports for 1964 and 1967.
31. **Bernard, L.,** The onset of tuberculosis in man, *Am. Rev. Tuberc.,* 15, 169, 1927.

TULAREMIA

J. F. Bell

INTRODUCTION

Tularemia is an infectious disease caused by *Francisella tularensis*. The species is now generally conceded to be comprised of two subspecies: *F. tularensis tularensis* (sometimes called type A) and *F. tularensis palearctica* (type B). There is a current effort to designate other subspecies as well as to change the present subspecific names. The type A organism occurs only in nearctic areas and is typically a disease of lagomorphs vectored by ticks. The type B, of holarctic distribution, is typically associated with rodents, especially microtines, and is often transmitted by carnivorism. Both types are often transmitted by other overlapping mechanisms. The nearctic form is more virulent, and that characteristic plus the ability to ferment glycerol and possession of the enzyme citrullineureidase distinguish it from type B. Bacteria of both kinds are notoriously infectious and are considered to penetrate the unbroken skin of man; paradoxically, however, the disease in man is not contagious. The spectrum of syndromes produced in man is extremely wide and depends to a large extent upon the route of infection as well as upon the kind and dose of organism and other less well-defined factors. Serological and skin tests are used for diagnosis. The disease is cured efficiently with antibiotics, especially streptomycin, but not with penicillin. An effective live vaccine is available.

History

Tularemia was recognized and described as a distinct entity by several astute observers in North America and in other areas of the Northern Hemisphere before the etiologic agent was isolated. In Japan, Soken Homma[108] described "hare meat poisoning" in 1837 and the disease came to be known as Yato-byo (hare disease) in Japan. In 1911, Pearse[134] described deer fly fever — later recognized as a form of tularemia — prevalent near Brigham City, Utah between 1908 and 1910. In 1911, McCoy[95] described a plague-like disease of rodents in Tulare County, Calif. McCoy and Chapin[96,97] published further observations on this plague-like disease and in two reports described the etiologic agent and its isolation. They named the organism *Bacterium tularense*. A syndrome that, in retrospect, must have been tularemia was defined by several Russian workers. The first etiologically defined infection in man, the occuloglandular form, was reported in 1914 by Wherry and Lamb[177] in Ohio.

The subsequent early history of tularemia to a large extent revolved around the efforts of one man, Dr. Edward Francis,[67] who entered into extensive surveys, experiments, correspondence, and collaboration with other investigators. In 1925 and 1926, Ohara,[105,106] who had been studying Yato-byo in Japan, recognized the similarity of that disease and its etiologic agent to tularemia, and he sent patients' sera and lymph nodes to Francis in Washington. Thus, the identity of the two diseases was established. In the U.S.S.R., several investigations of diverse syndromes known as Siberian ulcer, polyadenitis, and, especially, the prevalent water-rat-trappers' illness culminated in the isolation, by Suvarov and associates,[169] of a nonmotile coccobacillus that they recognized as similar to the tularemia agent. Zarkhi[188] sent his own postinfection serum and organs of infected cavies to Washington where the inferences of the Russian workers were confirmed.

More recent history of tularemia in the U.S.S.R. has been especially notable for extensive studies of epizoology, including differentiation of various biocoenoses, detection of the presence of the organism in water, and development of an effective vaccine.

EUBACTERIALES

The Organism: Classification

Two organisms, accorded subspecific rank, are now recognized as the etiologic agents of tularemia. The species is now assigned to a new genus, *Francisella,* established for it and for the species *F. novicida*[122] in the order Eubacteriales, as suggested by Dorofe'ev.[34] In *Bergey's Manual of Determinative Bacteriology,*[122] this genus and several others are grouped as "Genera of Uncertain Affiliation" in the Gram-negative aerobic rods and cocci. *Francisella* is separated from the others on the rather tenuous and ambiguous basis that "no growth (occurs) on ordinary media without enrichment." The two subspecies, (1) *F. tularensis tularensis* (type A) of the nearctic and (2) the holarctic subspecies, *F. tularensis palearctica* (type B), seem to be antigenically identical and more closely related, antigenically, to *Brucella* spp. than to *Francisella novicida.* Unfortunately, DNA hybridization studies to determine genomic homology with *Brucella* spp. have not yet been done, although the technique has established that the genomes of *Francisella* and *Pasteurella* are distinct and that close homology exists between *F. tularensis* and *F. novicida.* Genetic relatedness according to the criteria of Sanderson[153] would seem to be the most stable and logical basis for taxonomy.

Differences between the now-established subspecies were not recognized until Kadull et al.[72] noted the significantly higher mortality in American as compared to Eurasian tularemia. Those differences were confirmed by other observers,[118] and subsequent biochemical studies revealed that some American isolates utilized glycerol[117] and possessed the enzyme citrullineureidase (type A),[93] whereas other American and Eurasian isolates were alike in lacking those characteristics (type B). Inoculation of mice, cavies, and domestic rabbits with measured doses of fresh isolates revealed that one viable cell of both kinds of organism would kill the first two species but that several dex[59] bacteria of type B were required to kill rabbits, whereas only one dex bacteria of type A isolates would do so.[13] Epidemiologic data showed an association of the more virulent kind of bacteria with sheep, cottontail rabbits (*Sylvilagus* spp.), hares (*Lepus* spp.), and ticks of the genera *Dermacentor* and *Amblyomma,* whereas the less virulent kind is most often associated with rodent infections and contaminated water.[70] However, those associations are not rigid; epidemiology is of presumptive (but not usually definitive) value in identification of the subspecies involved in a particular human infection or group of cases.

In addition to original inclusion in the taxon *Bacterium* and current assignment to the new genus *Francisella,* the organism has been included at times in the genera *Brucella* and *Pasteurella;*[140] it is not improbable that it will be reassigned. Currently there is an effort to change the subspecific name *F. tularensis palearctica* to *F. tularensis holarctica,* which is a more logical appellation in view of its distribution. There is also some effort to further subdivide that subspecies, based on minor differences such as the rate of glycerol fermentation (recently it has been found that some type B strains slowly ferment glycerol) and on specific antibiotic susceptibilities.

The Organism: Description

F. tularensis of both types is very pleomorphic; the range of shapes and sizes includes some organisms that pass filters impermeable to most other bacteria.[43] McCoy and Chapin[97] noted that large globular forms may commonly occur, an observation that

tion of colony types was said to be favored in liquid media. Correlation of virulence and immunogenicity with colony type is not yet on a secure basis. The completely avirulent strain No. 38 produces both smooth and nonsmooth colonies.

The organism is easily killed by chemical and physical agents that kill other common nonspore-forming bacteria; nevertheless, viability is maintained for weeks or longer in mud, soil, water, and fomites, especially at low temperatures.

Virulence

The stable differences in virulence between types A and B, first seen by Kadull et al.[72] and later confirmed by others, are quantifiable by parenteral inoculation of mice, cavies, and domestic rabbits with graded doses of the bacteria.[13] Animals of the three species succumb to 1 dex 59 organisms of type A, whereas only mice and cavies succumb to 1 dex bacteria of type B. Rabbits ordinarily survive the inoculation of 4 dex or more viable bacteria of the latter type. White rats (*Rattus norvegicus*) are even more resistant than rabbits, but irregularly so; therefore, they are not well suited to quantification of virulence. Loss and recovery of virulence can also be traced with the system, which is expensive if used *in toto*. However, clues derived from the origin of the isolate from the epidemiologic association or other sources usually reduce the number of animals required for evaluation. Green[56] noted a correlation of virulence with the host species even within a biocenose. He used the time from inoculation (of cavies) to death as a criterion of virulence, and his conclusions have been substantiated by evaluation with the three-species titration.

Virulence is lost by frequent subculture, especially on egg medium. According to some authors, virulence can be restored by animal passage, but the conditions of loss and restoration are not well defined. The characteristic is retained when cultures are lyophilized. At least one strain (No. 38, commonly used for serologic antigen production) has entirely lost virulence for animals even when inoculated intraperitoneally in very large doses.

The toxicity of *F. tularensis* is questionable in spite of repeated assertions of its occurrence. Foshay[42] noted that the heat-killed bacteria were excessively toxic, precluding their use in skin tests. He subjected the bacteria to elaborate detoxification to prepare them for use. However, heat-killed organisms of types A and B have been used successfully in Japan.[109] Investigators who claimed demonstrations of toxicity have emphasized evanescence of the characteristic on storage and the need to inject large quantities of the bacteria intravenously or intraperitoneally.[79,101] Toxicity was considered to be related to virulence by Moody and Downs,[101] but not unequivocally so. Landay et al.[79] found that the toxin was not destroyed by γ radiation, and, in fact, they described two toxins, one of which was said to be related to the immunizing capacity of the bacteria. Some doubt may be cast upon the above conclusions in view of the demonstrable efficacy of the relatively avirulent and atoxic live vaccine strain (LVS).

Lability

The bacteria are killed when exposed to 56°C for 10 min. Under natural and simulated natural ambiences, viability may be retained for long periods even under conditions that would seem to be inimical to the minute organism, e.g., in soil, water, and dry litter. Viable bacteria have been demonstrated in water and mud samples stored at 7°C for as long as 14 weeks,[132] in tap water for as long as 3 months,[76] and in dry straw litter for at least 6 months.[143] *F. tularensis* remains viable in salted meat for up to 31 days; rare-cooked meat has been held responsible for many infections.[48] Viability persists longer than infectivity when the bacteria are aerosolyzed. Bacteria thus exposed are more fastidious in substrate requirements; virulence is lost before loss of viability.[63]

Chlorine in the usual concentrations (1.5 mg/ℓ) employed for water treatment kills *F. tularensis* and has been employed for that purpose in the purification of reservoir water in the U.S.S.R.[143] and on beaver farms in North America.[180] The bacteria are also labile to copper and zinc ions and to diethyl ether as used in the virus lability test, and butyl rubber is inimical to cultures.

F. tularensis is preserved very satisfactorily by lyophilization and by freezing. Slow cooling and rapid warming are most favorable for optimum recovery in the latter method, and both the freezing and the rehydrating menstrua affect survival and recovery. A solution containing peptone, ammonium chloride, and thiourea has been found to be best for preserving dried cells.[31] Under field conditions, infectivity of tissues can be preserved conveniently by putting them preferably (spleen or muscle) in pure glycerine. Recovery of *F. tularensis* from contaminating materials, e.g., soil, is favored by the extreme infectivity of the bacteria to mice that serve as selective media for isolation.

The Disease: Clinical — Human

Infection in man is as protean as the morphology of the agent. Severity is related to route of infection, infecting dose, and especially to the subspecies of *F. tularensis* involved. Mortality prior to the advent of antibiotics was 1% or less in Eurasia and about 5% overall in North America where both subspecies occur. It has been estimated that 90% of American cases are caused by type A bacteria, but these cases are most severe, most likely to come to attention, and, therefore, most likely to be reported. Skin test and serologic surveys have detected many reactors without compatible history of illness. Exposure of human volunteers and of animals of one species and of uniform age and history reveals marked differences in individual susceptibility not attributable to known parameters. Observations of natural epizootics in range sheep, voles, and hares strongly suggest that stress plays a significant role in susceptibility.[8,10]

Various authors distinguish different categories of clinical appearance that correlate to a significant degree with route of infection. The common routes of infection and the consequent usual syndromes are listed in Table 1.

Location of the ulcer is often helpful in determining the source of infection, e.g., when on the hand, handling of infected meat is suggested; when on the neck or arms, flying insects are suspect; and in the inguinal region, ticks are a likely source. Pulmonary involvement is especially frequent when infection occurs by inhalation, but pneumonia and pleuritis are common in severe tularemia, regardless of source or associated signs.

In addition to the listed syndromes, others with unique or bizarre signs have been described. Hemorrhagic sinusitis, pseudomembranous ulcerative colitis, and perigastritis are some of the unusual forms.

The course of infection, including prolonged convalescence, typically occurs over a period of 2 or 3 months. The incubation period is usually about 3 days but may be less than 2 days or as long as 3 weeks. Headaches, chills, vomiting, fever, prostration, and aching occur commonly and suddenly. The ulcer at the site of entry becomes punched-out in appearance. Regional lymph nodes enlarge and become tender or painful. The appearance of signs of pneumonia is unfavorable to prognosis. In the absence of specific therapy, symptoms of acute illness persist for 2 or 3 weeks.

Exanthem, reported frequently in some series, usually appears during the first or second week of illness and persists for 2 or 3 weeks. The eruption varies from erythematous to urticarial or to acneform and usually occurs on the upper body, face, neck, and limbs.

Table 1

CLINICAL FORMS OF TULAREMIA AND COMMON ROUTES OF INFECTION

Route	Syndrome
Integumental invasions, by arthropod bite, contaminated knife, or bone splinter, etc.; the ulcer may escape detection when it occurs in obscure sites such as the scalp (sometimes no ulcer can be found)	Ulceroglandular; adenopathy occurs, especially in those nodes proximal to the point of entry
Conjunctival contamination; probably most frequently from contaminated hands or from splash while dressing game	Oculoglandular; cephalic and cervical nodes involved.
Ingestion or other contamination of oral, nasal, and G.I. mucosa	Anginal and typhoidal forms; ulcerative tonsillitis or pharyngitis are characteristic of the former type; the typhoidal form may, presumably, result from non-G.I. route of infection also; abdominal or mesenteric forms are sometimes distinguished

Exceptionally, the course of illness is peracute or fulminant. Inhalation of a large amount of type A organisms, with resultant primary pneumonia, and ingestion of insufficiently cooked wild rabbit meat may cause rapidly fatal infection.

Chronic tularemia is more common and usually consists essentially of purulent adenitis that may persist for months or even years. This form of the disease was common before antibiotics became available and occurs even now in cases treated with tetracyclines but not in those adequately treated with streptomycin. In some cases, an apparent cure is followed several months later by the reawakening of symptoms and signs, notably adenitis. Excision of purulent nodes effects the cure.

Serological and skin test surveys[25,139] have revealed numerous reactors among native peoples in the Arctic and Subarctic regions and among personnel engaged in sheep husbandry. Many of the reacting persons had no recollection of infection that could account for the illness. In Japan, the number of reactors was correlated with frequency of clinical tularemia in the several prefectures surveyed.[109] Subclinical tularemia has also been detected in laboratory workers.[173]

The Disease: Clinical — Animals

The clinical appearance of tularemia in common host-animal species is not diagnostic. The usual admonition to hunters to avoid the taking of hares or rabbits that appear sluggish or apathetic is good advice, but it is only in advanced illness that lethargy becomes obvious, as in experimentally infected laboratory animals. The absence of signs of illness in rodents until the terminal stage, e.g., in beavers during epizootics on beaver farms, has been a handicap to effective therapy. Large animals such as the bovidae are often found to have agglutinins to *F. tularensis* in high titer without a known antecedent history of febrile illness. There are published records of extensive mortality in range sheep. The described signs of illness are not distinctive, but the usual presence of large numbers of ticks (*Dermacentor* spp.) affords a high index of suspicion; it is possible that tick paralysis contributes to the signs, prostration, and mortality. Removal of ticks contributes to rapid recovery,[127] but there has been no reported test of adequate antibiotic treatment without their removal. Experimentally infected sheep do not exhibit the congeries of signs reported in the complicated natural infection.[69]

Pavlovsky[133] states that wild and domestic canidae and felidae show no evident signs of tularemia, but Ditchfield et al.[32] recorded isolation of type B organisms from cats that died after eating muskrat viscera; Girard[52] and Stagg et al.[167] observed patent illness in two of three coyotes (*Canis latran*) exposed to aerosol infection; and Schlotthauer et al.[160] studied an epizootic with mortality in gray foxes (*Urocyon cinereoargenteus*). With few exceptions, no specific signs of illness have been detected, but Johnson[71] isolated *F. tularensis* for long periods from experimentally infected dogs that showed signs characteristic of canine distemper. Apparently, no effort was made to demonstrate concurrent infection with distemper virus. Distemper virus is known to render canines more susceptible to several kinds of bacterial infections.[163]

Diagnosis

Diagnosis of the typical ulceroglandular case of tularemia in man poses no challenge to the physician, especially if a history of intimate contact with a wild animal or of an arthropod bite is elicited. Diagnosis of less typical cases is facilitated when the illnesses are associated with other known cases in time or place. Nevertheless, recorded cases of tularemia have been conspicuously associated with the relatively few physicians who have taken particular interest in the disease. A large but variable proportion of patients presents with signs and symptoms other than the classic ones. It is likely that the ready availability and free use of antibiotics have made definitive diagnoses less frequent.

When a laboratory confirmation of a clinical impression is desired, several specific tests are available. Isolation of the bacteria is accomplished most readily by a subcutaneous inoculation of sputum, ulcer scrapings, scrapings of the walls of abscessed nodes, or, irregularly, of blood into mice, hamsters, or cavies. It is remarkable that sputum is frequently infectious even in the absence of signs of pneumonia.[83] Sometimes the bacteria may be cultured directly from test materials, but the procedure is unreliable. It is obvious that appropriate antibiotic treatment of the patient has an adverse effect on isolation success. *F. tularensis* may often be isolated from contaminants by rubbing the contaminated tissue or fluid onto the freshly scarified skin of laboratory animals. In addition to the confirmation afforded by development of typical lesions, best seen in cavies, pure cultures can usually be obtained from blood, spleen, or liver rubbed on the CGBA medium. The rather typical gray colonies over medium that becomes greenish can be emulsified easily and agglutinated by known specific antiserum. A principal disadvantage of isolation is the great infectivity of the organism that has caused many infections in laboratory personnel. It is noteworthy that the bacteria are sometimes difficult to isolate even on CGBA medium, whereas subcultures grow very well on the same medium. Also, primary isolates or early subcultures may not be agglutinated by laboratory-prepared antiserum[78] possibly because somatic antigens are covered.

The organism may be demonstrated by direct examination of appropriately stained infected materials, such as scrapings from lesions or sputum.[83] The very minute and pleomorphic bacteria are sufficiently distinctive to enable tentative identification, but confirmation, as by use of a direct or indirect FA technique,[24,178] is necessary for unequivocal diagnosis. The technique has also been successfully applied on smears made from the tissues of animals killed, even before the onset of patent illness and after inoculation of suspect materials from patients.

The agglutination test was used by McCoy and Chapin[97] in their earliest studies of tularemia, and it continues to be a reliable and common test. However, the test does not become positive until illness is well advanced: the second week at the earliest and, as in other tests that depend upon antibody formation, a rise in titer is much more reliable than a single test. Antibiotic treatment of a febrile patient does not inhibit development of agglutinins.[17] Contrary to what would be expected of an anamnestic reaction, in repeated infection the rise in titer is delayed and thus may cause confusion. Another cause of confusion in the agglutination test with serum from a tularemia patient is the cross-reaction with *Brucella* sp. antigens.[49] Ordinarily, the agglutination titer drops rather rapidly within a few months after recovery, but residual titers as high as 80 or 160 may remain for many years. A zone phenomenon may cause erroneous results if only low dilutions of higher-titer serum are tested.

Alexander et al.[1] adapted the hemagglutination (HA) test to the diagnosis of tularemia. Saslaw and Carhart[155] found the HA test to be positive earlier and at greater dilutions than the bacterial agglutination reaction in experimental infections of human volunteers. Cells not treated with glutaraldehyde or tannic acid were found to be least likely to give false-positive reactions. The prozone phenomenon was not encountered with the HA test.

A microagglutination technique using stained antigens was devised by Massey and Mangiafico.[94] According to the authors, the advantages are rapidity and ease of performance, economy of reagents, and ease of interpreting specific reactivity.

The complement fixation (CF) test is adaptable to the diagnosis of tularemia and has been used with success by Francis[46] and by Marchette et al.,[92] but it appears to offer no advantage over the simpler tests.

The indirect FA technique is applicable in tularemia as in other infectious diseases.[51]

Antigens for the test may be cultured bacteria or infected tissues although the latter give a better reaction.[51]

The skin test (ST) has been utilized, in particular, for surveys of incidence of tularemia, but it is also useful as an adjunct to serology for diagnosis in certain circumstances. It was first used for that purpose by Foshay.[42] Many different antigens have been prepared and used in the technique in Japan,[109] in the U.S.S.R.,[40] and in North America.[25] A very satisfactory antigen, easy to prepare, is the ether-extracted killed vaccine developed by Larson et al.[85] The standard vaccine is diluted 1:1000 with physiologic saline for use in the ST. The ST technique is similar in application and interpretation to the intradermal tuberculin test: the reaction of erythema and edema is read at 48 hr. It persists for several days and leaves a brown-pigmented area for weeks. Reactivity is sometimes demonstrable in the first week and for years after infection.

The serologic techniques may be used for the diagnosis of disease in animals, but most diagnoses of tularemia in animals, especially wild animals, are done on carcasses. Isolation procedures and direct culture or demonstration of the bacteria in infected tissues by FA techniqueare commonly practiced, and Karlsson[73] employed histopathology in comparison with isolation and FA techniques on animals in various stages of decomposition. Astonishingly, pathology as well as FA techniques were more reliable than isolation. The Ascoli test, in which high-titer serum is reacted with an eluate of heated tissue to form a precipitate, was first used for tularemia by Sarchi[154] and more recently by Larson[84] and by Bell et al.[11] It has the advantages that the dangers of isolation are obviated, decomposed tissues are suitable, and formalin-fixed tissues can be used. Formalin-fixed tissues can also be tested successfully with the FA technique.[178] The Ascoli test depends upon presence of sufficient antigen in the test tissue and, therefore, may not be reliable when applied to an animal killed in an early stage of infection or to a tissue not especially involved in infection.

Pathogenesis and Pathology

F. tularensis is notoriously invasive and infectious; there is evidence that it will penetrate unbroken skin.[147] Numerous experiments[14,148] as well as epidemiologic studies have implicated the enteric route as common for entry of the agent into man[48] and rodents.[75,174] The respiratory tract[144] and the conjunctiva[17] are well-documented avenues for experimental and natural infection of man and animals. However, parenteral inoculation by arthropod vectors and by bone splinters, knife wounds, or through preexisting lesions when skinning or dressing wild animals are probably the most common causes of human infection. The greater efficiency of that mode of infection is strongly indicated by the usual presence of a single ulcer, no doubt at the site of entry, whereas large surfaces are commonly exposed when dressing animals. However, multiple cutaneous ulcerations — in muskrat trappers — have been reported.[187]

The lesion at the portal of entry becomes necrotic and forms a crater sometimes covered by a scab. There is rather sharp demarcation between viable and necrotic tissue, the former consisting of epithelioid and plasma cells and lymphocytes in early stages. The stage of repair is characterized by granulation tissue containing the above cells plus macrophages and mast cells. Integumental penetration is followed by regional adenopathy; the same is probably true of entry by other routes, but node involvement is not always demonstrable in mesenteric or hilar locations.

Infection by *F. tularensis* results in development of an allergy that has marked effects upon histologic reactions.[52] Lillie and Francis,[88] in their extensive study of the pathology of tularemia in various species, described both early coagulation necrosis and swelling and proliferation of reticuloendothelium of the sinuses, the latter a probable manifestation of the hypersensitivity. The nodes more remote from the portal of entry have that reaction more markedly. In advanced lesions, necrotic centers are sur-rounded by proliferation of macrophages and epithelioid cells. Giant cells are found at the periphery of palisaded epithelioid cells. In the stage of repair, an outer fibrous capsule is formed and a collagenous layer separates the amorphous center from epithe-lioid cells. Lymphocytes are found commonly in the periglandular tissue.

There is no consensus on the occurrence and chronology of bacteremia. The bacteria are occasionally demonstrable in blood quite early and commonly in the agonal stage or at necropsy, but isolation from blood during acute or chronic illness is not always feasible.

Whether by the lymphogenous or hematogenous route, or both, infection spreads to other tissues and organs. The spleen, liver, lung, and pleura are most commonly and prominently involved in progressive infection, but others may have extensive le-sions. The extent of involvement depends upon virulence of the agent, dose, route of entry, species infected, physiologic status of the animal, and other factors that can only be referred to (vaguely) as intrinsic factors, i.e., in an apparently uniform group of animals uniformly exposed, a wide spectrum of reactions and tissue involvement may be found.

The most common lesion, focal necrosis, is best seen in the spleen and liver but is also seen at times in bone marrow, kidneys, and the wall of the intestine. Histology of the lesions depends to a large extent upon the acuteness of the infection; necrosis may occur alone in very acute cases while a marginal proliferative reaction is seen in those of longer duration. Both kinds of lesions may occur in the same organ; the former type presumably represents more recent foci. The healing process is similar to that described for the lymph nodes. The pulp is often congested and frequently con-tains lymphocytes and plasma cells, rarely neotrophils, during active infection; multi-plication and swelling of reticuloendothelial cells occur. Follicles are usually small.

In addition to foci of necrosis, the liver may show congestion, cloudy swelling, and fatty changes. Coagulation necrosis in the foci may result in the formation of necrotic cellular thrombi in capillaries. Kidney involvement is irregular.

In man, the most common abnormality is cloudy swelling, but occasionally cortical focal necrosis, proliferative lesions in the glomeruli, and degenerative lesions of the tubules have been reported. Prominent kidney lesions are also unusual in animals, but in recent studies[14] the common occurrence of chronic pyelonephritis in voles (*Microtus pennsylvanicus*) that survive enteric route infection with fully virulent *F. tularensis* type B has been noted. The lesions strongly resemble those of tuberculosis of the kid-ney. Focal lesions are commonly seen in the marrow of rodents and lagomorphs, but not in man.[88]

The respiratory tract is involved to varying degrees in a large proportion of human and animal infections. The appearance of pneumonic signs and symptoms is unfavor-able to prognosis in untreated cases, and the reactions encountered do not depend upon route of infection.[168] In rhesus monkeys exposed to infectious aerosols, the bac-teria impinge on the respiratory bronchiole resulting in focal lesions. Infected bron-chioles and adjacent alveoli become atelectatic and filled with neutrophils and necrotic debris. When extensive, these processes result in confluent bronchopneumonia and pleuritis. The resolution process is accomplished by epithelialization, vascularization, and fibrosis of exudates.

Inflammation of the peritoneum, pleura, and pericardium is recognizable by the extensive serous or serosanguineous exudate often observed at necropsy in man and animals and is often a cause of distress during illness in man. The fluid is sometimes fibrinopurulent. Focal nodular lesions of the pleura have been reported, and fibrosis during recovery may cause extensive thickening of the pleura. Serous membrane nod-

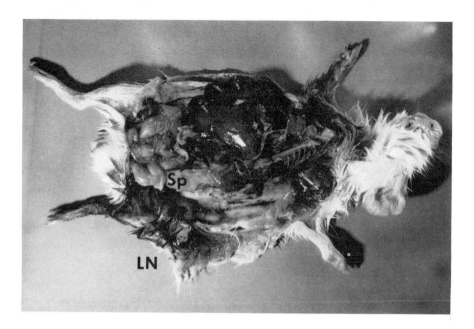

FIGURE 2.   Enlarged necrotic spleen (Sp) and enlarged caseous lymph node (LN) at site of inoculation by scarification of *F. tularensis* type B.

ules can be reproduced rather consistently by intravenous inoculation of large doses of virulent bacteria into partially immunized animals.

Tonsillar ulceration and necrosis of Peyer's patches are frequent results of infection by ingestion. Nonpathognomonic lesions are observed occasionally or rarely in other organs and tissues. Zenker's degeneration and minute focal hemorrhages in skeletal muscle — myelin degeneration, cellular nodules, and hemorrhagic foci in the brain — are among the rare lesions.

The characteristic lesions of tularemia as seen in rodents are plague-like, as noted by McCoy,[95,96] but differ in degree, e.g., the buboes are neither as large nor so extensively inflamed. Lillie and Francis[88] noted the similarity of the lesions in rabbits to those of tuberculosis in man and conjectured that tularemia in man may sometimes be misdiagnosed as tuberculosis. We have seen the reverse mistake made at necropsy. A characteristic picture is best reproduced when mature cavies are inoculated by scarification in the inguinal region (Figure 2). Upon reflection of the skin at necropsy, a plastic condition of that tissue is noted. Homolateral inguinal nodes are enlarged and appear inflamed. The spleen is usually enlarged and thickly studded with foci that vary in size but are usually less than 1 mm in diameter. There may be diffuse areas of necrosis in an enlarged spleen. The liver is also swollen and studded with small foci of necrosis.

Baskerville and Hambleton[6] studied the pathogenesis and pathology of experimental respiratory tularemia in the rabbit (*Oryctolagus cuniculi*) because "the rabbit is a natural host for *F. tularensis* . . . " Although lagomorphs, especially *Sylvilagus* spp. in North America and *Lepus* spp. holarctically, are often naturally infected, the domestic rabbit (*O. cuniculi*) of European origin is relatively resistant to indigenous *F. tularensis palearctica* (type B), rarely found infected, and plays no significant role in the epidemiology of tularemia in palearctic regions. Virulent *F. tularensis* A (strain Schu S-4) was administered by aerosol with 90% of the droplets 1 to 2 μm in diameter. Groups of organisms were found at the alveolar duct level 5 and 10 hr after exposure. Areas of necrosis and infiltration by polymorphonuclear leukocytes (PMN) developed in peripheral alveoli at least 24 hr earlier than changes in the walls of airways and then disseminated and spread to involve much of the lung with bronchopneumonia. The disease caused by virulent *F. tularensis* A in rabbits is acutely fatal and, therefore, the processes of healing has not been described. Pulmonary arteritis reported previously in human infection[88] was a prominent feature of the infection in these rabbits. Lesions were present in the nasal mucosa and trachea of the rabbits from the second day, and the infection extended to cervical lymph nodes that became necrotized.

Studies have been done on the biochemical changes in tularemia,[18,135,158,179] with some indication that the affinity of *F. tularensis* for cystine may result in the depletion of essential amino acids. In man, serum iron concentration and iron-binding capacity fall very early in infection and again during the onset of severe illness.[135] Free amino acids, nonprotein nitrogen (NPN), and total serum proteins are decreased in infected rats.

Therapy

The discovery of therapeutic efficacy of streptomycin by Heilman[61] has made the discussion of other therapeutic measures academic. No other antibiotic has proved superior. Tetracyclines have been tested extensively and have ameliorative effects, but often they do not eradicate infection. Penicillin, as well as the sulfonamides, has no therapeutic effect. The singular effectiveness of streptomycin, as compared to some of the other bactericidal but less effective antibiotics, may be partially attributable to the stimulation of phagocytosis by macrophages.

Historically, treatment of ulcers and buboes with mercurial ointment was considered beneficial in the U.S.S.R. Foshay used serotherapy in 1931 and claimed it reduced mortality and shortened the illness. Some experimental tests afforded limited support to the claim, but a preponderance of data fails to demonstrate the benefit. Foshay also treated patients by desensitization, i.e., repeated injections of antigen, but the regimen was difficult and of doubtful value.

Untreated tularemia and tularemia treated by antibiotics other than streptomycin often have protracted courses characterized, in particular, by persistent adenopathy. Surgical removal of affected nodes is curative.

Immunology

The desirability of an effective vaccine to prevent tularemia in man became obvious early in the history of the disease because its exceptional infectivity resulted in disease in laboratory personnel at a time when effective specific therapy was not yet available. The need became urgent when it was recognized that thousands of cases occurred each year in the U.S.S.R. No serious effort was made to develop an attenuated live vaccine in North America, possibly because no reliable measure of virulence was available. Instead, killed vaccines of several kinds were tested. Foshay et al.[44] tested a heat-killed, formalinized bacterial suspension, but because of severe systemic reations in apparently normal (nonsensitized) recipients, they prepared another antigen "detoxified" with nitrous acid. No significant protection against experimental infection was conferred on laboratory animals by the product, but results of tests in man were viewed as favorable. An ether-extracted vaccine prepared by Larson,[81] by a method successful with rickettsiae, was tested in mice. Rapid development of resistance to challenge by the attenuated strain 425 — but not to fully virulent challenge — was obtained,[85] and the vaccine was employed in experimental studies on volunteers.[38] High titers of antibody and some degree of reduction in the severity of illness were achieved, but parallel studies of live vaccine developed in the U.S.S.R. at about that time clearly demonstrated the superiority of the latter type of vaccine. Gotschlich et al.[55] used living attenuated cultures of North American strains of *F. tularensis* as live vaccines. Their success spurred further efforts, and an indigenous strain (type B) was selected for further study. It was lost during World War II, but after the war El'bert, Gaiskiy, and others renewed their efforts to find and evaluate a live vaccine. Gaiskiy finally chose "strain 15" ("bul'onnyi"), isolated from *Arvicola terrestris* in 1936, as most suitable, and descendants of that culture provide the live vaccine used in North America and Japan as well as in the U.S.S.R. The organism was brought to the U.S. by R. E. Shope and K. F. Meyer in 1956. Gaiskiy attenuated virulence of the organism by repeated subculture. The culture was taken to Japan in 1962[112] and is commonly referred to as the live vaccine strain (LVS).

LVS has been administered to man and animals by several routes including oral and respiratory. The usual route for animals, e.g., beavers on fur farms, is by subcutaneous inoculation of 4 to 5 "dex"[59] viable organisms.[12] When applied to man, the multiple puncture mode is used in common practice. The area to be vaccinated, usually the deltoid, is cleaned with acetone, alcohol, or ether, and care must be taken to insure that all antiseptic is gone before a drop of bacterial suspension is deposited on the site. Fifty superficial punctures are made with a slanted needle through the drop, and the liquid is allowed to dry without dressing. The local reaction is ordinarily mild with papule formation, a slight vesiculation, and a small crust. The reaction is not significantly greater in previously sensitized persons and does not preclude LVS revaccination for exceptional exposure. Precautions include assurance that the recipient is not receiving antibiotics inimical to *F. tularensis* and, theoretically, assurance that normal immunologic capability is not compromised, e.g., by corticosteroids, X-ray, or intrinsically. Transfer of the LVS liquid to the conjunctiva should be avoided. Followup inspection of the vaccination site obviates many difficulties.

The rate of development of immunity is not known exactly and is probably variable. Maximum agglutinin titers are present at 21 to 28 days, 1 week or more later than comparable titers after those of the less effective ether-extract vaccine.[180]

Although LVS has proven very effective in widespread use in the U.S.S.R. and in experimental exposures,[121,171] absolute protection should not be expected in view of the known occurrence of reinfections from natural exposure of man[47] and experimental reinfection in rats.[36] Second and postvaccination infections are generally mild but may be locally distressing. Appropriate antibiotic therapy has made the subject of academic interest only. Killed vaccine and LVS have been combined with other vaccines, including those for brucellosis, anthrax, plague, pertussis, and Venezuelan equine encephalomyelitis,[104,125,142,157] with satisfactory antibody elicitation to the component antigens.

Epidemiology

The epidemiology of tularemia is as diversified as the morphology of *F. tularensis,* including water-borne, air-borne, arthropod-vectored, and contact infections. Epizootic forms are intimately related to susceptibility of the common hosts and to their ectoparasites, especially the *Ixodidae.*

Microtine rodents are generally considered to play the most important role in epidemiology of *F. tularensis* B in Eurasia, where *Arvicola terrestris,* the water rat, has been the most common animal source of infection, partly because it comes in direct contact with man. In eastern Siberia and in North America, rodents of the genus *Microtus* are the predominant hosts. However, in Japan and frequently in Europe, hares of the genus *Lepus* are the principal source of human infection, probably because of frequent contact with humans. A common impression that "rabbits" (*Oryctolagus cuniculi*) are hosts and a reservoir of tularemia in Europe is a result of confusion caused by the colloquial misuse of the terms rabbit and hare.

In North America, where both recognized subspecies of *F. tularensis* occur, the epidemiologic characteristics have been of generally different but not always clearly distinct modes. Examples of type A epizootics are those in which *F. tularensis* is transmitted to sheep by *Dermacentor andersoni* ticks, those occurrences in which *F. tularensis* A is transmitted among cottontail rabbits (*Sylvilagus* spp.) by *Haemaphysalis, Amblyomma,* and *D. variabilis* ticks, and to man by contact with the rabbits or by tick bites. The subspecies, *F. tularensis* B, is typically an infection of rodents — especially microtine animals (*Microtus, Ondatra*) — and also of beavers (*Castor*). No type A organisms have been isolated from water that is frequently contaminated with type B bacteria, and no type B agent has been isolated from sheep during epizootics. However, there are records of occurrence of strains of relatively low virulence (type B) in the same biocoenose where others of maximum virulence (type A) are found.[30,56,170] At present, the environment and circumstances in which disease occurs are helpful — but not usually definitive — in identifying the subspecies of *F. tularensis* involved.

Although tularemia of each kind is typically associated with relatively few species of reservoir animals and vectors, the total spectrum of species infected is much larger. Mammals of the listed families have been found infected, some of them rarely and under unusual circumstances (see Table 2). The list is in accordance with taxonomy as it appears in *Mammals of the World*,[176] but it differs from the taxonomic assignments in the lists by Olsuf'jev,[133] Burroughs et al.,[21] and Reilly,[149] from which much of the data were taken.

There is some disagreement in the literature as to the susceptibility of canids, felids, mustelids, and carnivores that frequently must come into close contact with infected prey. Serologic surveys have convincingly demonstrated that many animals of those families survive that contact,[98,170] and experimental infections, even with type A bacteria, confirm the usual mildness of tularemia in them.[92] Olsuf'jev[133] states that "even on receipt of massive doses of the pathogen (type B), the disease may proceed without clinical manifestations." Parker and Francis[128] produced lethal infection in coyote pups (*Canis latrans*) by oral exposure. Marchette et al.[92] caused mortality in very young pups by subcutaneous inoculation, but Stagg et al.[167] found them resistant to aerosol exposure. Lundgren et al.[89] were unable to kill full-grown adults by oral or subcutaneous routes. Foxes and minks exposed to large quantities of infected jackrabbit (*Lepus* spp.) meat in their feed have suffered severe mortality,[54,161] and wild gray foxes (*Urocyon* sp.) in Minnesota died with tularemia infection.[160] Johnson[71] described a tularemia syndrome similar to that of canine distemper in experimentally infected dogs, but no attempt was made to ascertain that the virus was not present concurrently. Distemper virus is notorious for causing depression of resistance to bacterial infection.[102] Hopla[66] recorded failure of normal ticks to become infected by feeding on dogs inoculated with virulent *F. tularensis*, and it seems unlikely that the canids are of direct importance in exchange of infection. However, as pointed out by Calhoun,[22] they serve to disseminate the vectors, and Brown[19] noted the importance of large mammals as essential hosts for adult stages and, therefore, for population maintenance of *Dermacentor* spp. and some other ticks.

Domestic cats (*Felis catus*) have been found infected in nature,[32,162] killed by inoculation of virulent bacteria, and have transmitted infection by bite.[19] Mortality from the disease seems to be the exception,[92] although the natural infection may be severe and chronic.[58]

Ungulates, with the exception of sheep, rarely suffer mortality from uncomplicated tularemia, although serology indicates frequent infection.[170] Foals (*Equus* sp.) heavily infested with ticks have died of tularemia,[27] and cattle (*Bos* sp.) and deer (*Odocoileus*

Table 2
MAMMALS KNOWN TO BE INFECTED WITH *FRANCISELLA TULARENSIS*

Family	Common names	Comments
Soricidae	Shrews	Several species naturally infected in Old and New World
Talpidae	Moles	Occasionally found infected
Callithricidae	Marmosets	One record in a domiciled squirrel monkey
Hominidae	Humans	About 1% mortality in Old World (*Francisella tularensis* B) and about 5% in New World (*Francisella tularensis* A and B) before antibiotics
Leporidae	Rabbits, hares	*Lepus* spp. commonly infected in Old and New World and *Sylvilagus* spp. in New World; susceptibility variable among genera; *Oryctolagus cuniculi* native of Europe, not important in epidemiology in Old World; domestic form rather resistant to *Francisella tularensis* B
Erethizontidae	New World porcupines	Isolation of *Francisella tularensis* reported
Didelphidae	Opossums	Seropositive and a rare source of human infection
Canidae	Dogs, wolves, coyotes, foxes	Occasional evidence of infection; some with mortality (*Urocyon* sp.), but adult animals in good condition usually suffer little from experimental infection
Mustelidae	Weasels, polecats, mink, martens, badgers	Sparse evidence of infection in wild, but epizootics have occurred on fur farms (mink)
Felidae	Cats, lynx	Irregularly susceptible; fatal infection recorded after large oral doses
Suidae	Pigs	Not fatally susceptible in limited trials but a source of human infection
Procyonidae	Raccoons	Seropositive and a rare source of human infection
Sciuridae	Squirrels, ground squirrels, prairie dogs, chipmunks, marmots, susliks	Ground squirrels (*Citellus [Otospermophilus] beecheyi*) were the first source of cultures by McCoy and Chapin; not prominently reported since the studies of McCoy and Chapin[96]
Heteromyidae	Pocket mice, kangaroo rats	Occasional infection
Castoridae	Beavers	Epizootics in wild and on fur farms
Cricetidae	New World rats and mice, hamsters, voles, lemmings, gerbils	Various species probably the most commonly infected of all animals in Old and New World, especially *Microtus* spp. and *Arvicola* sp.
Dipodidae	Jerboas	Old World
Muridae	Old World rats and mice	*Mus musculus* very susceptible; suffers epizootics; *Rattus norvegicus* and *R. rattus* relatively resistant
Zapoidae	Jumping mouse	Isolation
Cervidae	Deer	White tail and mule deer (*Odocoileus* spp.) occasionally source of human infection when animals are dressed
Antilocapridae	Pronghorn antelope	Serologic evidence of infection
Bovidae	Cattle, buffalo, goats, sheep	Evidence (serology) of nonlethal infection is common in all species, especially in sheep; high mortality has been documented in sheep on range, but folded, well-fed sheep are resistant
Equidae	Horses	Foals heavily infested with ticks have succumbed to tularemia
Camelidae	Camels	Culture isolated

spp.) have been found infected in nature[170] and have been killed with massive parenteral inoculations.[137] Ewes (*Ovis* sp.) on the range have suffered high mortality when heavily infested with ticks during the lambing and shearing season, but folded sheep on good rations resist infection by large inoculations of fully virulent type A bacteria.[10]

It is inferred that stress of lambing, and probably tick infestation per se,[103] contribute to the apparent greater susceptibility of range sheep.[10] Buffaloes (*Bubalus* sp.) may become chronically infected when inoculated and can shed *F. tularensis* in the urine for as long as 37 days.

Lagomorphs constitute a reservoir of tularemia and a source of infection for man. Generalizations about susceptibility in the various genera and species cannot be made, but the most commonly infected species are well known. Infection in *Lepus brachyurus* is the common source of human infection in Japan. In Europe, *L. timidus* (the varying hare), *L. capensis tolai*, and *L. europaeus* are the species involved, both directly as infected game animals and as sources of vector-transmitted infection. *Oryctolagus cuniculi*, the European wild (and domestic) rabbit, is relatively resistant to infection by the indigenous type B bacteria and is not a common source of human disease. As mentioned previously, the common terms "hare" and "rabbit" are often used loosely and interchangeably, which has led to much confusion. In the New World, *L. americanus*, the snowshoe hare, and *L. californicus*, a species of "jackrabbit" (actually, a hare), are often infected, but cottontail rabbits (*Sylvilagus* spp.) are more frequent sources of human tularemia. "Rabbit fever" is one of the colloquial names for tularemia. The relatively high mortality (about 5%) in patients thus infected probably implies that type A infection is the usual kind.

Epidemiologic studies[57] indicate that susceptibility of *L. americanus* to tularemia is dependent to some extent upon the physiologic status of the animals, as determined by lactation, age, crowding, and other less well-defined parameters. Marchette et al.[92] found differences in susceptibility to experimental infection between two subspecies of *L. californicus*.

Rodents of the family Cricetidae are probably the species most often infected in nature and the most common sources of human infection in Eurasia. The water rat (*Arvicola terrestris*) is a species trapped for its fur, and the infection is thus transmitted directly to man; this is also true of muskrats (*Ondatra zibethica*), native to North America and introduced into the Old World. Various species of voles (*Microtus*) are more widely distributed and often infected, but infection is usually indirectly transmitted to man by contamination of the environment. Occasionally, large numbers of agriculturists contract tularemia when processing grain or stacked hay contaminated by voles and other rodents.[143] It seems probable that widespread contamination of water is attributable to bacteriuria in infected voles.[14] However, Pavlovsky[133] believes that water contamination is derived from infected carcasses. Contaminated vegetables were the probable source of infection in an epizootic of tularemia in a closed hamster (*Mesocricetus auratus*) breeding colony.

Many other rodents including those from other families (Sciuridae, Castoridae, and Muridae, in particular) are sometimes infected, occasionally in large numbers. Beavers (*Castor canadensis*) suffer high mortality on fur farms and in the wild, and house mouse (*Mus musculus*) infection may be extensive at times.

Birds of several families, even including anserine and passerine representatives, have been found infected or serologically positive and serve as hosts of infected ticks. Mortality from natural infection has occurred in galliforms: grouse of several species (*Bonasa*, *Pediocetes*, *Centrocercus*, *Lagopus*, and *Dendragapus*) have been found to be susceptible to laboratory infection or infected in nature, but *F. tularensis* isolated from sage grouse (*Centrocercus* sp.) during the epizootic in that species may not have been essentially responsible for the mortality observed.[129] The same seems to be true of infections reported in bob white "quail" (*Colinus virginianus*),[129] ruffed grouse (*B. umbellus*), Japanese pheasants, the domestic hen (*Gallus domesticus*), pheasants (*Phasianus colchicus*), and other species from which isolates of *F. tularensis* have been obtained or that have been apparent sources of human infection.[133,170] However, fatal infections have been induced in blue grouse (*D. obscurus*) and bob white "quail" in the laboratory.[129]

The low virulence of isolates obtained from grouse (*B. umbellus*) has been noteworthy and especially remarkable because of occurrence in the biocoenose of highly virulent *F. tularensis* in snowshoe hares (*L. americanus*) that share the common tick vector, *H. leporispalustris*.[57] Divergence of virulence in the two hosts is enigmatic.

Infection, demonstrated by isolation or serology, is common among raptors and opportunistic avian predators. We have observed very extensive predation on small rodents by gulls (*Laridae* sp.) during an epizootic of tularemia in the mammals[68] and have taken infected voles from the gullets of the gulls.[28] Predation or scavenging on carcasses probably accounts for the antibodies to *F. tularensis* and for isolates obtained from flesh-eating birds including passerine shrikes (*Lanius* sp.).[66,133,170]

Serologic evidence of infection among anserine species is puzzling because they resist large doses of orally administered virulent *F. tularensis*, a presumed natural mode of infection. However, several species of ducks, geese, and terns are fatally susceptible to parenterally induced tularemia. Chronic shedding tularemia involving the liver, gall bladder, kidneys, and cloaca has been produced in terns (*Laridae*) by parenteral inoculation.[66] The direct relevance of tularemia in birds to human infection or to maintenance of *F. tularensis* in nature appears to be slight, but serologic studies of predators afford useful indices to currency of the disease in prey species.[170]

Transmission of tularemia is extremely diversified; much of the cycle of exchange between vectors and hosts is unknown or known only superficially. It is understandable, therefore, that unanimity of concept does not exist. In a major attempt to bring order to the multitudinous elements that affect maintenance and spread of tularemia, several Russan workers have developed the theory of "nidality" (essentially the biocoenosis or ecosystem of each epidemiologic type) of the epidemiology of zoonoses. The epidemiologic nidi vary in different geographic areas and become important at different times. To a large degree, they are brought to human awareness only during epizootics and when man becomes involved directly, by infection, or indirectly, by mortality in valuable wild or domestic animals. The nidi, based on human infections, as outlined by Olsuf'jev and Dunaeva,[116] are listed as follows: (1) arthropod-borne, (2) trapping (direct contact), (3) hunting-eating, (4) water, (5) agriculture, (6) domestic, (7) "productory," (8) productive, and (9) trench or foxhole (wartime).

There is much overlap, theoretically and actually, between the various categories, e.g., an infected hare could infect arthropod vectors, infect a hunter who killed and dressed it, and contaminate others when marketed (productive). Infected carcasses of hares found around a haystack could cause "productory" infection in man.

Maksimov[91] and Olsuf'jev and Dunaeva[116] used ecologic criteria in differentiating nidi. The latter categorized the following epidemiologic modes: (1) floodplain — swamp, (2) meadow and field, (3) forest, (4) steppe (ravine), (5) piedmont — river, and (6) tugaian (desert — floodland).

In Japan, epidemiology is much simpler; insofar as man is concerned, tularemia is essentially a disease of hares transmitted by direct contact to hunters and their families. Arthropod- and water-borne tularemia and infection of man from agricultural activities are absent or rare although infection is occasionally contracted from other infected animals. Ticks on hares are known to be infected. In North America, the widespread, susceptible cottontail rabbits, frequent tick-borne infection, and infections contracted from sheep are prominently related to clinical tularemia.

Arthropod-borne tularemia was discovered soon after the disease was recognized as an entity. In retrospect, it seems clear that an infectious syndrome, attributed by R.

A. Pearse[134] to bites by horseflies, was tularemia. Diptera have been incriminated in many localized epidemics since then. There is a consensus that transmission by mosquitoes and biting flies is mechanical although experimental infection of several species has established that infection can be retained for weeks or months.

The source of dipteran infection is commonly thought to be sick mammals, especially hares, but Olsuf'jev[115] presents evidence that infection could be obtained from contaminated water. Tabanids have been observed to feed on carcasses of animals even 48 hr after death and have experimentally transmitted infection from carcasses to normal animals. Pavlovsky[133] emphasizes that agonistic behavior of animals attacked by irritating diptera probably increases the frequency of multiple feedings, and transmission is probably accomplished by bite in most cases; however, crushing an infected insect adjacent to a bite and ingestion by a host are possible mechanisms of transfer. Deer flies have been efficient vectors in circumscribed areas, especially in Utah, whereas mosquitoes are notorious in Scandinavia,[16,113] and tabanids are significant vectors in the U.S.S.R. Pavlovsky[133] lists *Chrysops relictus, Tabanus autumnalis, T. flavoguttatus, T. bromius,* and *Chrysozona pluvialis* as known vectors. A deer fly, *Chrysops discalis,* has caused numerous infections in Utah. Mosquitoes of the genera *Aedes, Mansonia, Theobaldia,* and *Anopheles* have been shown to be capable of transmission or retention of *F. tularensis,*[41,114,120,138] Presumably, since transmission is mechanical, any mosquito that feeds on susceptible hosts is a potential vector. That mode of transmission would be most effective when donor and recipient hosts are in close proximity. Krinsky's[77] recent review of tabanid-carried infections should be consulted for comprehensive references to the pertinent literature.

The terms "gnat" and "midge" are often used interchangeably; this has led to some confusion as to their role as vectors. However, there is circumstantial evidence that *Culicoides* spp. sometimes convey infection from hares to man and, presumably, between hares.[2] *Culicoides pulicaris, Eusimulium* spp., and *Simulium* spp. have been found infected in western Siberia.[133]

It is characteristic of dipteran-transmitted infection that the site of inoculation is usually on parts of the body not covered by clothing, but the Ceratopogonidae (gnats) have a predilection for hairy parts of the head and neck. Characteristically, tularemia from those sources occurs in the warmest months.

There is no doubt that fleas can be infected experimentally, are infected in nature, and can retain the infection for long periods of time. However, evidence that fleas transmit infection by bite is weak[66] and mostly circumstantial.[170,175] McCoy[95] thought that transfer of infection by fleas was accomplished by ingestion of the infected insect.

Lice of the genera *Hoplopleura,*[53] *Pediculus, Neohematopinus, Hemodipsus,* and *Polyplax* have been investigated with conflicting results as regards their ability to transmit infection among their native hosts. Because lice are markedly host-specific, any lice that are potential vectors would be of greatest significance for spread of infection among individuals of one species. Price[145] found that experimentally infected *Pediculus humanus* could shed infectious feces for as long as 20 days, but there is no evidence that the species is an important source of human infection. Francis and Lake[50] found that bedbugs (*Cimex lectularius*) were capable vectors. It appears that infection is transmitted to the host who ingests contaminated feces.[29]

Despite a wide spectrum of modes of transmission, it would not be an exaggeration to state that tularemia, particularly the type A form, is essentially a tick-borne disease. In 1924, Parker et al.[131] reported the presence of infection in *Dermacentor andersoni* in Montana. Since then a large number of species of the family Ixodidae have been found to be infected or have been infected experimentally.[8,66] Ixodids of the genera *Amblyomma* and *Dermacentor* are those usually responsible for transmission to man in North America. Nearctic *Ixodes* and *Haemaphysalis* spp. attack man infrequently but are often found infected on normal as well as infected hosts. *H. leporispalustris* on varying hares (*Lepus americanus*) and on ruffed grouse (*Bonasa umbellus*) sometimes achieves populations of several thousand,[57] and the potential for exchange of infection is tremendous.

Tick-borne infection is of minimal direct importance to man in Japan, but infected *Ixodes* and *Haemaphysalis* spp. are found on hares. Tularemia infection from tick bites is unusual in the U.S.S.R. The vectors among rodents and lagomorphs are ticks of these genera important in North America, plus *Rhipicephalus* and *Hyalomma*.

Experimentally, ticks become infected by ingestion of bacteremic blood; infection is most successful when satiation of the ticks coincides with the terminal stage of illness. Animals that are relatively resistant to tularemia, e.g., dogs, do not serve as effective hosts for infection of ticks.[66,136] There is general agreement that transstadial infection occurs. Petrov[66] concluded that small infections could be lost during molting, and Bell's studies[7] led to the conclusion that infection could be lost by feeding on immune hosts.

Infection occurs in both the gut and in body tissues and hemolymph fluid, and Hopla[65] observed propagation of the bacteria in ticks. Infection is known to persist for many months and even years in some species.[5,114]

Parker and Spencer[130] asserted that gravid *Dermacentor andersoni* transmit infection to the progeny, and several other investigators confirmed this phenomenon in that species and others.[66] However, transovarial infection could not be demonstrated in later tests of *D. andersoni, D. variabilis,* and *R. sanguineus*.[66] Calhoun and Alford[22] found infected, wild, unfed larvae of *A. americanus*, excellent proof of maternal origin of infection.

There is also disagreement regarding the effects of infection upon the tick. In some experiments, no mortality could be attributed to presence of *F. tularensis,* whereas selective mortality was evident in others. It would seem that intensity of primary infection and perhaps the instar infected, conditions of tick maintenance, virulence of the bacterium, and other less well-defined factors could cause variations in experimental results.

Argasid ticks can be infected in the laboratory; *Ornithodoros parkeri* can remain infected for at least 701 days. Burgdorfer and Owen[20] demonstrated the vectoral ability of four species of *Ornithodoros*, but it is generally held that argasid ticks are of minimal or no importance in the maintenance of tularemia in nature or as a cause of infection in man.

Coxal fluid and feces of infected ticks contain viable *F. tularensis* and are deposited during feeding. Transmission by contamination of the bite wound can no doubt be accomplished in this way. Petrov[66] established that saliva, injected during feeding, is infectious to the host.

The various nidal cycles are inadequately known because, with certain exceptions, they have not been studied adequately. Green and associates[57] conducted an investigation of the cycle involving snowshoe hares (*Lepus americanus*) and *H. leporispalustris*, in particular, but also *D. variabilis, Sylvilagus* sp., and *Bonasa umbellus* in Minnesota. The complex cycle in a Utah desert area has been studied continuously for many years,[2,3] and a discrete habitat in mountainous Montana has been subjected to intensive scrutiny:[166] however, only small fragments of the total diversified picture are known. Better information and unifying concepts have been developed in the U.S.S.R., notably by scientists at the Gamaleya Institute, but much more needs to be done.

Several species of mites have been found to be infected when removed from infected animals, and Hopla[64] found the tropical rat mite, *Ornithonyssus bacoti,* capable of

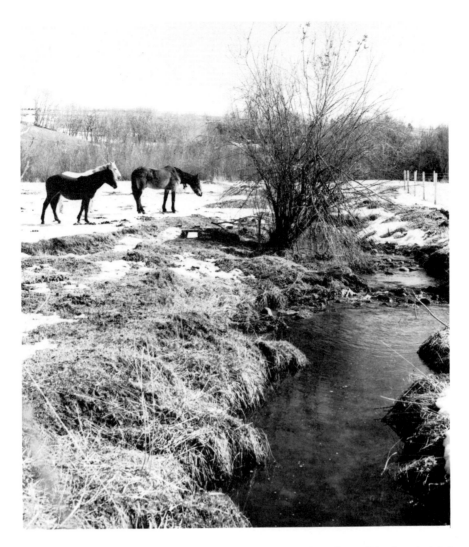

FIGURE 3.   A brook in the foothills of Western Montana. *F. tularensis* type B has been isolated from this stream annually during the cold seasons for 15 years. The stream arises in excellent vole habitat.

retaining and transmitting the infection. The current and rather general belief that mites are unimportant in the ecology of *F. tularensis* may be based on inadequate evidence. Maksimov[91] considers the gamasid mites to be principal vectors in some associations.

The anomalous discovery that tularemia can be contracted from water, as well as from arthropod vectors and infected carcasses, was made by P. V. Somov[99] and by Karpoff and Antonoff[74] at about the same time. This source of human infection has been of great significance in Eurasia where many thousands of cases have been attributed to it: tularemia thus contracted was a major cause of troop disability in World War II; wells and drinking water reservoirs have required chlorination to eliminate *F. tularensis* contamination. The problem does not exist in Japan. In North America, certain streams have been known to be contaminated for long periods, one of them annually for 15 years (Figure 3), but human infection from that source is rare. The seasonal occurrence of *F. tularensis* over a period of 3 years is shown in Figure 4.[15]

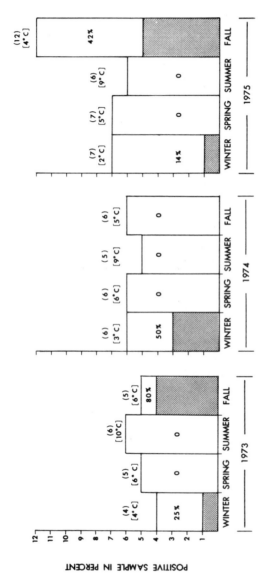

FIGURE 4.   Seasonal prevalence of *F. tularensis* type B in a brook during a 3-year period of sampling. Number of samples in parentheses. Average water temperature in brackets.

Contaminated water causes human infection when consumed, as attested by stomatitis, pharyngitis, and tonsillitis in patients who contract the disease not only by drinking from streams[143] but also when the water is used as a spray to clean beets in a sugar factory.[146] Other routes of infection from water are the conjunctiva and breaches of the integument, either preexisting or coinciding with exposure to water, e.g., injury by fishhook or fin prick. Theoretically, infection could enter through unbroken skin, but it has been observed repeatedly that colonies of muskrats or beavers may thrive for long periods in contaminated waters. However, epizootics do occur in those animals at times, and it appears that fortuitous infection of one animal, perhaps through a wound, may result in sequential amplification of the contamination of water to more infectious levels.

Infection by ingestion is frequent and serious in man. This mode of infection is, presumably, responsible for many *F. tularensis* antibody titers found in various carnivores although they are also hosts to infectious ticks. Incorporation of the meat of rabbits infected with *F. tularensis* into the rations fed to mink and foxes on fur farms has caused high mortality.[54] Carnivorism, and especially cannibalism, appear to be the most frequent cause of spread of infection among various species of rodents during epizootics. We have noted the relative rarity of vector parasites on rodents but there is significant evidence indicating cannibalism of infected vole carcasses in nature and among captive voles.[68] Carnivorism has also been held responsible for transmission in other species.[164,174] Quan and Von Fintel[148] conducted experiments on the susceptibility of rodents by the oral route and found that the doses required for infection were several dex larger than the minimal infectious parenteral dose.

The source of contamination of water is conjectural. Russian workers have favored the concept that carcasses of animals dead of tularemia contaminate streams; they present evidence that one small rodent can thus contaminate 5 dex liters of water.[133] Most studies indicate that poikilothermic aquatic vertebrates and invertebrates become contaminated in water containing *F. tularensis* but that proliferative infection does not occur. Parker et al.[132] believed that *F. tularensis* multiplied in water-mud medium and thus maintained the bacterial population. Our own[14] studies led us to conclude that chronic nephritis and bacteriuria in voles that results from ingestion of *F. tularensis* is a likely source of water contamination. This form of infection was detected in a naturally infected vole and was reproduced in the laboratory. Adjuvant evidence for bacteriuria, rather than the other mechanisms, as the source is based on (1) the absence of detectable carcasses in the stream so frequently contaminated, (2) rapid (overnight) disappearance of rodent carcasses placed in the stream, (3) long duration of bacteria in the stream, (4) presence of bacteria in earth of the watershed, (5) failure of *F. tularensis* to grow in the laboratory on excellent media at the low temperature of the streams, and (6) occurrence of contamination in streams only in vole habitats. Bacteriuria has also been detected in man,[110] water buffaloes (*Bubalus* sp.),[43] and other species.

Airborne infection has resulted from aerosolized water in beet factories and from dust in haystacks infested with rodents.[144] The syndrome produced in one such event was characterized by conjunctivitis, ulcers in the mouth, sore throat, and pneumonia. Studies on monkeys and volunteers confirm infectivity by the respiratory route[155,156] that has led to infection in laboratory workers.[72] The feasibility of airborne spread of tularemia among rodents was demonstrated by Owen and Buker.[123]

Tularemia has been notorious as a laboratory infection and, in spite of relative rarity among routine laboratory cultures, it has ranked first as a cause of laboratory-acquired bacterial infections.[141]

In spite of great invasiveness and infectivity by a number of routes and the fact that a high proportion of patients, even those without overt signs of pneumonia, have infectious sputum,[83] nosocomial infection is rare.[43]

Geographic Distribution

One of the peculiarities of tularemia is its strict holarctic distribution. In the New World, there is authentic evidence from above the Arctic Circle to Mexico; purported occurrence in Venezuela cannot be substantiated.[9] Latitudinal palearctic distribution is generally similar to the nearctic, ranging from northern Siberia to Mediterranean Africa, but no further south. In view of the known infection of migratory birds and of their ectoparasites, absence of the disease in South America, Australia, and the great mass of Africa is puzzling. We have not been able to confirm quoted reports of tularemia in Thailand, but recent investigations[4] have extended the known range to Iran. In North America, all continental states and provinces are known to be within the range of tularemia; in Europe, Iberia is singularly free of infection. The British Isles are also free, in spite of the proximity to infection on the continent.

Economic Significance

The direct economic importance of tularemia to man has diminished greatly since the discovery of an effective antibiotic therapy and development of an effective vaccine. Prior to these discoveries, very extensive epidemics had occurred in the U.S.S.R., and there were serious focal outbreaks in Scandinavia. In North America, the disease was at one time common among purveyors of game animals, in trappers, and in sheep-husbandry workers. Tularemia not treated with antibiotics is, ordinarily, quite enervating for long periods. Its occurrence as an occupational disease among trappers and husbandmen was serious because it resulted in work incapacity during periods of greatest activity. In a large proportion of clinical disease, prostration required hospitalization and protracted medical care. In Japan, surgery was often needed to terminate persistent adenitis. Economically, the disease is still indirectly significant. On the negative side is the epizootic occurrence among fur bearers in nature and on fur farms, lesser utilization of game animals — with loss of recreation and of meat as a result of fear — "broken" fleeces, and loss of animals in focal outbreaks among range sheep.

The positive economic impact of tularemia is more difficult to measure and is, very likely, underestimated. Because it is, primarily, a disease of rodents and lagomorphs (animals that are destructive to forests, meadows, and cultivated crops, sometimes in very spectacular ways), anything that contributes to decimation of those populations is an economic benefit (Figure 5). In an extreme example of destruction by high rodent populations, those population foci that were not poisoned still experienced near eradication by several infectious diseases and especially by tularemia.[68] The presence of plague (*Yersinia pestis*) infection in the same population[75] suggests that it might have assumed greater proportion with more serious effects if tularemia had not been so effective in population control.

Control

Control of tularemia is no longer as urgent as it was before effective therapy and prophylaxis were available. Incidence of reported cases of tularemia has declined dramatically from a peak of nearly 20/100,000 in 1939 to less than 1 in the past decade. Nevertheless, human cases do occur, and sometimes protracted illness or disability develops before a correct diagnosis is made and appropriate therapy is applied. Vaccination with LVS has resulted in nearly complete cessation of epidemic tularemia in man in the U.S.S.R.[143] Similar extensive and severe outbreaks have not occurred in North America. Use of LVS has removed the threat of infection among laboratory workers and could be used more widely by trappers, hunters, sheep husbandmen, and

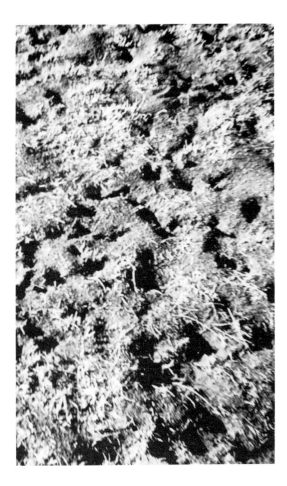

FIGURE 5.   A clover field riddled by tunnels of voles.

residents or sojourners in remote areas. General education regarding the dangers of
tick bite and game meat and measures to avert infection from those sources are appropriate and useful, but instructions regarding the use of rubber gloves in dressing game
are inadequate if the precautions entailed in the proper use of the gloves are not given
in detail. Also, advice to avoid sick animals or animals with "spots on the liver" may
give a false sense of security. Insect and tick repellents are undoubtedly helpful, but
the latter should be supplemented by careful examination of the body to remove ticks;
clothing that excludes ectoparasites is also useful. Freezing or hanging game animal
meat does not rid it of *F. tularensis*. When such meat is handled, mouth, nares, and
eyes should not be touched before thorough hand washing. Possibly dangerous meat
should not be eaten rare. Avoidance of epizootic areas is implicit but depends upon
adequate epidemic intelligence. Occurrence of unexplained die-off of wild animals
should be reported to health authorities. There is little or no practical justification for
isolation of patients with tularemia, but the potential for contagion, from a theoretical
standpoint, suggests a cautionary attitude.

   Epizootic tularemia is severe in proportion to the total population and concentration
of susceptible animals. It follows that agricultural practices and policies in regard to
predators have significant effects upon the occurrence and spread of disease. Severe
outbreaks of tularemia in rodents have been the conspicuous result of concentration
of rodents around unprotected piles of grain or stacks of unthreshed grain.[91] Where

grain monoculture is practiced, leaving bales of straw in the fields furnishes the necessary cover that, together with abundant food grain, is conducive to rodent population increase. Modern agricultural policies that destroy habitat for predators or that favor killing of predators also favor the increase of rodents and epizootic disease among them. It is noteworthy that disease was much more efficient than was widespread use of poison in eradicating a severe plague of rodents in a wide area of the northwestern U.S. in 1958.[68] Moreover, application of poison was very expensive and caused severe mortality of game and songbirds.

FRANCISELLA NOVICIDA

This organism shares with *F. tularensis* type A the distinction of strict nearctic occurrence. Unlike *F. tularensis* type B, it is known to occur in only one site, the Ogden Bay Bird Refuge, north of the Great Salt Lake in Utah. In fact, the organism has been isolated only once from a water sample inoculated into cavies and white mice.[86] The two cavies and three of eight mice became ill; at necropsy, foci of necrosis similar to those of tularemia were seen on the liver and spleen. Similar pure cultures were obtained from one cavy and two mice. Suspensions of the cultures were obtained from one cavy and two mice. Suspensions of the cultures failed to agglutinate with *F. tularensis*-specific antiserum, and tissues of the animals gave nil reactions in the Ascoli test.

The organism in culture is Gram-negative and pleomorphic, principally rod-shaped, and nonmotile. No spores or flagellae are formed. As is true of *F. tularensis*, clear areas are observed around cells in smears from infected tissues, but capsule stains do not demonstrate a capsule. In tissue smears, bacteria are ovoid to coccoid, 0.28 μm in length, 0.20 to 0.28 μm in width, and arranged singly or in small clusters. In liquid media they are larger — 0.7 × 1.7 μm, predominantly short, thick rods with slightly bulging sides — and occur singly or in pairs. On solid media the rods are 0.47 to 0.84 0.47 μm.

On primary isolation, growth is good on CGBA but not on "nutrient" agar. Fresh liver or spleen from an infected animal supports growth on horse meat infusion agar; cystine, yeast extract, and whole blood are also effective supplements for growth. Colonies on CGBA resemble those of *F. tularensis*, i.e., gray with a blue cast, smooth, slightly elevated, glistening, amorphous, and with entire edges. They are butyrous or viscid and are easily emulsified in water. Appreciable growth occurs aerobically in 24 hr at 37°C. There is no hemolysis.

Fermentation of sucrose by *F. novicida* serves to differentiate it from *F. tularensis*. Dextrose, levulose, and mannose are fermented; glycerol, maltose, lactose, dextrin, and mannitol are not. Nitrates are not reduced, the indole test is negative, H_2S is formed, ammonia is not produced, methylene blue is reduced, the catalase test is positive, unenriched gelatin supports growth but is not liquified, and litmus milk is unchanged; methyl red and Voges-Proskauer tests are negative. Olsuf'jev et al.[119] showed citrullineureidase activity.

Growth occurs on suitable media at 25 to 41°C. Suspensions of bacteria are killed by exposure to 60°C for 10 min and to 1% phenol for 20 min. There is no evidence of toxin formation. Mice, cavies, and hamsters succumb to inoculation of 1 or 2 dex bacteria. Rabbits, white rats, and pigeons die only when inoculated with much larger doses. At necropsy, mice inoculated subcutaneously have congestion of subcutaneous tissues, hemorrhages at the site of entry, enlargement and congestion of local lymph nodes, hemorrhages and congestion of lungs, and enlargement of the spleen with multiple small foci of necrosis. There are no gross lesions in the liver. Lesions in other animals are generally similar, but the cavy liver is usually spotted.

Immunologic studies show slight antigenic relationship to *F. tularensis* and even less of a relationship to members of the *Yersinia* group. High-titer anti-*novicida* sera react only slightly or not at all with *F. tularensis* and *Y. pestis* antigens in agglutination and precipitin tests. The reverse is also true. Acetone-precipitated preparations of *F. tularensis* and *F. novicida* show common antigens in agar-gel diffusion tests.[111] CF tests with antisera prepared in rabbits show some cross-reaction, but sera of cavies give only specific reactions.[124] PCA tests are highly specific. Hemagglutination and hemagglutination-inhibition tests are specific.

Close genomic similarity between *F. tularensis* and *F. novicida* has been demonstrated by DNA hybridization[150] and by transformation.[172]

REFERENCES

1. **Alexander, M. M., Wright, G. G., and Baldwin, A. C.**, Observations on the agglutination of polysaccharide treated erythrocytes by tularemia antisera, *J. Exp. Med.*, 91, 561, 1950.
2. **Anon.**, Ecology Studies in Western Utah, Annu. Rep., Ecodynamics Series No. 72-1, 1972.
3. **Anon.**, Reports to the Department of the Army, Ecology and Epizoology Series, Department of the Army, Dugway, Utah, 1972.
4. **Arata, A., Chamsa, M., Farhang-Azad, A., Mischeryakova, I., Neronov, V., and Saidi, S.**, First detection of tularemia in domestic and wild mammals in Iran, *Bull. W.H.O.*, 49, 597, 1973.
5. **Balashov, Y. S.**, Bloodsucking ticks (Ixodoidea), in *Vectors of Diseases of Man and Animals*, Nauka Publishers, Leningrad Department, Leningrad, 1968; Translation 500, Medical Zoology Department, U.S. Navy Medical Research Unit No. 3, Cairo, 1972.
6. **Baskerville, A. and Hambleton, P.**, Pathogenesis and pathology of respiratory tularemia in the rabbit, *Br. J. Exp. Pathol.*, 57, 339, 1976.
7. **Bell, J. F.**, The infection of ticks (*Dermacentor variabilis*) with *Pasteurella tularensis*, *J. Infect. Dis.*, 76, 83, 1945.
8. **Bell, J. F.**, Ecology of tularemia in North America, *J. Jinsen Med.*, 11, 33, 1965.
9. **Bell, J. F.**, personal communication, 1976.
10. **Bell, J. F., Wikel, S. K., Hawkins, W. W., and Owen, C. R.**, Enigmatic resistance of sheep to infection by virulent *Francisella tularensis*, *Can. J. Comp. Med.*, 1977, 42, 310, 1977.
11. **Bell, J. F., Jellison, W. L., Owen, C. R., and Larson, C. L.**, Applicability of the Ascoli test to epizootic tularemia in wild rodents, *J. Wildl. Manage.*, 23, 238, 1959.
12. **Bell, J. F., Owen, C. R., Jellison, W. L., Moore, G. J., and Buker, E. O.**, Epizootic tularemia in pen-raised beavers, and field trials of vaccines, *Am. J. Vet. Res.*, 23, 884, 1962.
13. **Bell, J. F., Owen, C. R., and Larson, C. L.**, Virulence of *Bacterium tularense:* a study of *Bacterium tularense* in mice, guinea pigs, and rabbits, *J. Infect. Dis.*, 97, 162, 1955.
14. **Bell, J. F. and Stewart, S. J.**, Chronic shedding tularemia nephritis in rodents: possible relation to occurrence of *Francisella tularensis* in lotic waters, *J. Wildl. Dis.*, 11, 421, 1975.
15. **Bell, J. F. and Stewart, S. J.**, unpublished data.
16. **Berglund, A.**, Tularemia near the Arctic Circle, in *Contributions to Microbiology and Immunology*, Vol..2, S. Karger, Basel, 1973, 232.
17. **Bost, R. B., Percefull, S. C., and Leming, H. E.**, Tularemia in the Ozarks region, *JAMA*, 137, 352, 1948.
18. **Bowden, J. P.**, Biochemical studies of host-parasite interaction in tularemia, *J. Infect. Dis.*, 110, 23, 1962.
19. **Brown, J. H.**, The susceptibility of fur bearing animals and game birds to tularemia, *Can. Field Nat.*, 58, 55, 1944.
20. **Burgdorfer, W. and Owen, C. R.**, Experimental studies of Argasid ticks as possible vectors of tularemia, *J. Infect. Dis.*, 98, 67, 1956.
21. **Burroughs, A. L., Holdenried, R., Longnecker, D. S., and Meyer, K. F.**, A field study of latent tularemia in rodents with a list of all known naturally infected vertebrates, *J. Infect. Dis.*, 76, 115, 1945.
22. **Calhoun, E. L. and Alford, H. J.**, Incidence of tularemia and Rocky Mountain spotted fever among common ticks of Arkansas, *Am. J. Trop. Med. Hyg.*, 4, 310, 1955.

23. **Calhoun, E. L., Mohr, C. O., and Alford, H. J.,** Dogs and other mammals as hosts of tularemia and of vector ticks in Arkansas, *Am. J. Hyg.,* 63, 127, 1956.

24. **Carter, C. H. and Leise, J. M.,** Specific staining of various bacteria with a single fluorescent antiglobulin, *J. Bacteriol.,* 76, 152, 1958.

25. **Casper, E. and Philip, R. N.,** A skin test survey of tularemia in a Montana sheep-raising country, *Public Health Rep.,* 84, 611, 1969.

26. **Chamberlain, R. E.,** Evaluation of live tularemia vaccine prepared in a chemically defined medium, *Appl. Microbiol.,* 13, 232, 1965.

27. **Claus, K. D., Newhall, J. H., and Mee, D.,** Isolation of *Pasteurella tularensis* from foals, *J. Bacteriol.,* 78, 294, 1959.

28. **Craighead, J. J.,** Predation by hawks, owls, and gulls, in *The Oregon Meadow Mouse Irruption of 1957—1958,* Publication of the Oregon State College, Corvallis, 1958, 25.

29. **Davis, G. E.,** Further attempts to transmit *Pasteurella tularensis* by the bedbug (*Cimex lectularius*), *J. Parasitol.,* 29, 395, 1943.

30. **Davis, G. E., Philip, C. B., and Parker, R. R.,** The isolation from the Rocky Mountain wood tick (*Dermacentor andersoni*) of strains of *Bacterium tularense* of low virulence for guinea pigs and domestic rabbits, *Am. J. Hyg.,* 19, 449, 1934.

31. **Dearmon, I. A., Orlando, M. D., Rosenwald, A. J., Klein, F., Fernelius, A. L., Lincon, R. E., and Middaugh, P. R.,** Viability and estimation of shelf-life of bacterial populations, *Appl. Microbiol.,* 10, 422, 1962.

32. **Ditchfield, I., Meads, E., and Julian, R.,** Tularemia of muskrats in eastern Ontario, *Can. J. Public Health,* 51, 474, 1960.

33. **Dominowska, C.,** Properties and typing of *Francisella tularensis* colonies. I. Development of dynamism and morphology of colonies of various *F. tularensis* strains, *Bull. Inst. Mar. Trop. Med. Med. Acad. Gdansk,* 18, 131, 1967.

34. **Dorofeev, K. A.,** On classification of the microbe of tularemia, *Symp. Res. Works,* Vol. 1, Institute of Epidemiology and Microbiology, Chita, U.S.S.R., 1947, 170.

35. **Downs, C. M. and Bond, G. C.,** Studies on the cultural characteristics of *Pasteurella tularensis, J. Bacteriol.,* 30, 485, 1935.

36. **Downs, C. M., Coriell, L. L., Pinchot, G. B., Maumenee, E., Klauber, A., Chapman, S. S., and Owen, B. J.,** Studies on tularemia. I. The comparative susceptibility of various laboratory animals, *J. Immunol.,* 56, 217, 1947.

37. **Drozhevkina, M. S.,** Liquid yolk medium for cultivation of *B. tularense, Gov. Anti Plague Inst. Bull.,* Rostov-on-Don, U.S.S.R., 4, 51, 1945.

38. **Eigelsbach, H. T.,** Tularemia prophylaxis — alpha to omega, in *Essays in Microbiology in Honor of Morris Scherago,* University of Kentucky Press, Lexington, 1968, 81.

39. **Eigelsbach, H. T., Braun, W., and Herring, R. D.,** Studies on the immunogenic properties of *Bacterium tularense* variants, *J. Infect. Dis.,* 91, 86, 1952.

40. **Federow, V. N. and Gol'dshtern, G.,** Spezifische Hantreaktion bei Tularmie, *Klin. Wochenschr.,* 48, 1723, 1934.

41. **Federow, V. and Siwolobow, V.,** The role of mosquitoes in the epidemiology of tularemia, *Vestn. Mikrobiol. Epidemiol. Parazitol.,* 14, 65, 1935.

42. **Foshay, L.,** Tularemia: accurate and earlier diagnosis by means of the intradermal reaction, *J. Infect. Dis.,* 51, 286, 1932; *Am. J. Sci.,* 187, 235, 1932.

43. **Foshay, L.,** Tularemia, *Annu. Rev. Microbiol.,* 4, 313, 1950.

44. **Foshay, L., Hesselbrock, W. H., Wittenberg, H. J., and Rodenberg, A. H.,** Vaccine prophylaxis against tularemia in man, *Am. J. Public Health,* 32, 1131, 1942.

45. **Francis, E.,** Cultivation of *Bacterium tularense* on mediums new to this organism, *Public Health Rep.,* 37, 102, 1922.

46. **Francis, E.,** Tularemia: a new disease of man, *Int. Clinics,* 2, 73, 1923.

47. **Francis, E.,** Immunity in tularemia, *Trans. Assoc. Am. Physicians,* 51, 394, 1936.

48. **Francis, E.,** Sources of infection and seasonal incidence of tularemia in man, *Public Health Rep.,* 52, 103, 1937.

49. **Francis, E. and Evans, A. C.,** Agglutination, cross-agglutination, and agglutinin absorption in tularemia, *Public Health Rep.,* 41, 1273, 1926.

50. **Francis, E. and Lake, G. C.,** Transmission of tularemia by the bedbug, *Cimex lecturlarius, Public Health Rep.,* 37, 83, 1922.

51. **Franek, J. and Prochazka, O.,** Fluorescent antibody demonstration of *Pasteurella tularensis, Folia Microbiol.,* 10, 77, 1965.

52. **Girard, G.,** Comportement *in vivo* and *in vitro* de *Pasteurella tularensis* Isolee au cours de l'evolution de la tularemie chez des hotes diversement receptifs, *Ann. Inst. Pasteur Paris,* 89, 137, 1955.

53. **Golov, D. A.,** Contribution to the question of the role of the water rat in the epidemiology of tularemia, *Med. Zh. Kazakstana,* Alma Ata, No. 1—2, 1935; *Rev. Appl. Entomol., Series B,* (Abstr.), 25, 276, 1937.

54. **Gorham, J.,** Mink, fox susceptible to tularemia, *Am. Nat. Fur Mktg. J.,* 28, 21, 1949.

55. **Gotschlich, E., Golem, S. B., and Berkin, T.,** Immunization experiments on laboratory animals with living attenuated strains of *Bacterium tularense, Turk. Z. Hyg. Exp. Biol.* (Ankara), 2, 145, 1940; *Bull. Hyg.,* 16, 97, 1951.

56. **Green, R. G.,** Virulence of tularemia as related to animal and arthropod hosts, *Am. J. Hyg.,* 38, 282, 1943.

57. **Green, R. G., Evans, C. A., Bell, J. F., and Larson, C. L.,** Minnesota Wildlife Disease Investigation, Monthly Reports, March, 1933—1938, 17.

58. **Gutman, L.,** personal communication, 1976.

59. **Haldane, J. B. S.,** "Dex" or order of magnitude, *Nature,* 187, 879, 1966.

60. **Halmann, M. and Mager, J.,** An endogenously produced substance essention for growth initiation of *Pasteurella tularensis, J. Gen. Microbiol.,* 49, 461, 1967.

61. **Heilman, F. R.,** Streptomycin in the treatment of experimental tularemia, *Proc. Staff Meet. Mayo Clin.,* 19, 553, 1944.

62. **Hesselbrock, W. and Foshay, L.,** The morphology of *Bacterium tularense, J. Bacteriol.,* 49, 209, 1945.

63. **Hood, A. M.,** Infectivity of *Pasteurella tularensis* clouds, *J. Hyg.,* 59, 497, 1961.

64. **Hopla, C. E.,** Experimental transmission of tularemia by the tropical rat mite, *Am. J. Trop. Med.,* 31, 768, 1951.

65. **Hopla, C. E.,** Experimental studies on tick transmission of tularemia organisms, *Am. J. Hyg.,* 58, 101, 1953.

66. **Hopla, C. E.,** The ecology of tularemia, *Adv. Vet. Sci. Comp. Med.,* 13, 25, 1974.

67. **Jellison, W. L.,** Tularemia: Dr. Edward Francis and his first 23 isolates of *Francisella tularensis, Bull. Hist. Med.,* 46, 477, 1972.

68. **Jellison, W. L., Bell, J. F., and Owen, C. R.,** Mouse disease studies, in *The Oregon Meadow Mouse Irruption of 1957—1958,* Publication of the Oregon State College, Corvallis, 1958, 71.

69. **Jellison, W. L. and Kohls, G.,** Tularemia in sheep and in sheep industry workers in Western United States, *Public Health Monogr.,* 28, 1, 1955.

70. **Jellison, W. L., Owen, C., Bell, J. F., and Kohls, G. M.,** Tularemia and animal populations, *Wildl. Dis.,* 17, 1, 1961. (Microcard)

71. **Johnson, H. N.,** Natural occurrence of tularemia in dogs used as a source of canine distemper virus, *J. Lab. Clin. Med.,* 29, 906, 1944.

72. **Kadull, P. J., Reames, H., Coriell, L. L., and Foshay, L.,** Studies on tularemia. V. Immunization of man, *J. Immunol.,* 65, 425, 1950.

73. **Karlsson, K.-A.,** Studies on the Immunofluorescent Technique as a Diagnostic Tool in Bacteriology, monograph (collected papers), National Veterinary Institute, Stockholm, 1975.

74. **Karpoff, S. P. and Antonoff, N. J.,** The spread of tularemia through water, as a new factor in its epidemiology, *J. Bacteriol.,* 32, 243, 1936.

75. **Kartman, L., Prince, F. M., and Quan, S. F.,** Epizootiologic aspect, in *The Oregon Meadow Mouse Irruption of 1957—1958,* Publication of the Oregon State College, Corvallis, 1958, 43.

76. **Khatenever, L. and Levchenko, L.,** Experiments on study of vital capacity of *B. tularense, Zh. Mikrobiol. Epidemiol. Immunobiol.,* 20, 3, 1938.

77. **Krinsky, W. L.,** Disease agents transmitted by horse flies and deer flies (Diptera: Tabanidae), *J. Med. Entomol.,* 13, 225, 1977.

78. **Labzoffsky, N. A. and Sprent, J. A. F.,** Tularemia among beaver and muskrat in Ontario, *Can. J. Med. Sci.,* 30, 250, 1952.

79. **Landay, M. E., Wright, G. G., Pulliam, J. D., and Finegold, M. J.,** Toxicity of *Pasteurella tularensis* killed by ionizing radiation, *J. Bacteriol.,* 96, 804, 1968.

80. **Larson, C. L.,** The growth of *Pasteurella tularensis* in the yolk sac of developing chick embryo, *Public Health Rep.,* 60, 587, 1945.

81. **Larson, C. L.,** Immunization of white rats against infection with *Pasteurella tularensis, Public Health Rep.,* 60, 725, 1945.

82. **Larson, C. L.,** The relative value of liquid media, glucose-cystine blood agar and mouse inoculation in the titration of *Pasteurella tularensis, Public Health Rep.,* 60, 863, 1945.

83. **Larson, C. L.,** Isolation of *Pasteurella tularensis* from sputum; a report of successful isolation from three cases without respiratory symptoms, *Public Health Rep.,* 60, 1049, 1945.

84. **Larson, C. L.,** Studies on thermostable antigens extracted from *Bacterium tularense* and from tissues of animals dead of tularemia, *J. Immunol.,* 66, 249, 1951.

85. **Larson, C. L., Bell, J. F., and Owen, C. R.,** The development of resistance in mice immunized with soluble antigen derived from *Bacterium tularense, J. Immunol.,* 73, 221, 1954.

86. **Larson, C. L., Wicht, W., and Jellison, W. L.,** A new organism resembling *P. tularensis* isolated from water, *Public Health Rep.,* 70, 253, 1955.

87. **Levin, M. A., Trupin, J. S., and Cabelli, V. J.,** A Clear Medium for the Cultivation of *Pasteurella tularensis,* Tick Report, DPGR 273, U.S. Army Chemical Corps., Dugway, Utah, 1960, 1.

88. **Lillie, R. D. and Francis, E.,** The pathology of Tularaemia, National Institute of Health Bulletin No. 167, U.S. Treasury Department, Public Health Service, Washington, D.C., 1936, 1.

89. **Lundgren, D. L., Marchette, W. J., and Smart, K. L.,** Tularemia in the coyote, *Canis latrans lestes,* Merriam, *J. Infect. Dis.,* 101, 154, 1957.

90. **Makismov, A. A.,** The Main Types of Tularemia. Foci, Characterization of Them and Geographic Distribution of Them in the RSFSR Dan SSSR, Reports of the Academy of Sciences, U.S.S.R. (new series), 56, 501, 1947.

91. **Maksimov, A. A.,** Role of agriculture in the formation of the meadow-field type of natural foci of tularemia, in *Proceedings of a Symposium,* Rosicky, B. and Heyberger, K., Eds., Czechoslovak Academy of Sciences, Prague, 1965, 337.

92. **Marchette, N. J., Lundgren, D. L., Nicholes, P. S., and Vest, E. D.,** Studies on infectious diseases in wild animals in Utah. I. Susceptibility of wild animals to experimental tularemia, *Zoonoses Res.,* 1, 49, 1961.

93. **Marchette, N. J. and Nicholes, P. S.,** Virulence and citrulline ureidase activity of *Pasteurella tularensis, J. Bacteriol.,* 82, 26, 1961.

94. **Massey, E. D. and Mangiafico, J. A.,** Microagglutination test for detecting and measuring agglutinins of *Francisella tularensis, Appl. Microbiol.,* 27, 25, 1974.

95. **McCoy, G. W.,** A plague-like disease of rodents, *Public Health Bull.,* 43, 53, 1911.

96. **McCoy, G. W. and Chapin, C. W.,** Studies of plague, a plague-like disease and tuberculosis among rodents in California. V. *Bacterium tularense —* the cause of a plague-like disease of rodents, *Public Health Bull.,* 53, 17, 1912.

97. **McCoy, G. W. and Chapin, C. W.,** Further observations on a plague-like disease of rodents with a preliminary note on the causitive agent, *Bacterium tularense, J. Infect. Dis.,* 10, 61, 1912.

98. **McKeever, S., Schubert, J. A., Moody, M. D., Gorman, G. W., and Chapman, J. F.,** Natural occurrence of tularemia in marsupids, carnivores, lagomorphs, and large rodents in southwestern Georgia and northwestern Florida, *J. Infect. Dis.,* 103, 120, 1958.

99. **Miller, A. A.,** Tularemia and its new epidemiology, *Sovetskaiaa Urachebusia Gazeta,* 39, 187, 1935.

100. **Mizuhara, M.,** Relationship between terminal oxidation system and virulence of *Pasteurella tularensis, Jinsen Igaku,* 10, 323, 1961.

101. **Moody, M. D. and Downs, C. M.,** Studies on tularemia, I. The relation between certain pathogenic and immunogenic variants of *Pasteurella tularensis, J. Bacteriol.,* 70, 297, 1955.

102. **Munyer, T., Dolan, T., Mangi, R., and Kantor, F. S.,** Suppression of delayed hypersensitivity in MMR-vaccinated children and canine distemper virus infected dogs, *Clin. Res.,* 22(Abstr.), 425A, 1974.

103. **Neitz, W. O.,** The Different Forms of Tick Toxicosis: A Review, Rep. 2nd Meet. FAO/OIE Panel Tick-Borne Diseases, Cairo, 1962, 24.

104. **Nutter, J. E.,** Agglutinin responses of rabbits to combined *Pasteurella tularensis — Brucella abortus* vaccination, *Appl. Microbiol.,* 19, 250, 1970.

105. **Ohara, H.,** Concerning an acute febrile disease transmitted by wild rabbits: a preliminary report, *Jikken Iho V,* 11, 508, 1925.

106. **Ohara, H.,** Human inoculation experiment with a disease of wild rabbits, with a bacteriologic study, *Kinsei Igaku,* 12, 401, 1925.

107. **Ohara, H., Kobayashi, T., and Kudo, J.,** A study on pleomorphism of *Bacterium tularense, Tohoku J. Exp. Med.,* 25, 520, 1935.

108. **Ohara, S.,** "Yato-Byo" Ohara's disease, tularemia in Japan, *Annu. Rep. Ohara Hosp.,* 40, 1, 1965.

109. **Ohara, S. and Hoshishima, K.,** Diagnosis of Yato-Byo (Ohara's disease, tularemia in Japan), *Fukishima J. Med. Sci.,* 4, 51, 1957.

110. **Ohara, S. and Sato, T.,** Isolation of *Pasteurella tularensis* from man, animals and ticks, in Japan, Symp., 11th Kanto Branch Meet, Jpn. Bacteriol. Assoc., Yamamoto Shoten, Tokyo, 1959, 1.

111. **Ohara, S., Sato, T., and Homma, M.,** Serological studies on *Francisella tularensis, Francisella novicida, Yersinia philomiragia* and *Brucella abortus, Int. J. Syst. Bacteriol.,* 24, 191, 1974.

112. **Ohara, S., Suzuki, T., Akutsu, H., Ichikowa, K., Sato, T., Hoshishima, K., and Bell, J. F.,** Study of tularemia live vaccine, *Annu. Rep. Ohara Hosp.,* 14, 3, 1965.

113. **Olin, G.,** Studies on the origin and mode of propagation of tularemia in Sweden, *Bull. Mens. Off. Int. Hyg. Publique,* 30, 2804, 1938.

114. Olsuf'jev, N. G., Parasitology of tularemia, in *Tularemia Infections*, Khatenever, L. H., Ed., State Publisher of Medical Literature, Moscow, 1943, 74.

115. Olsuf'jev, N. G., Tularemia, in *Human Diseases with Natural Foci*, Pavlovsky, Y. N., Ed., Foreign Languages Publishing House, Moscow, 1966, 219.

116. Olsuf'jev, N. G. and Dunaeva, T. N., Epizootiology (natural nidi) of tularemia, in *Tularemia*, Olsuf'jev, N. G. and Rudnev, G. P., Eds., State Publisher of Medical Literature, Moscow, 1960, 136.

117. Olsuf'jev, N. G. and Emelyanova, O. S., Further studies of strains of tularemic bacteria of the Old and New World, *J. Hyg. Epidemiol. Microbiol. Immunol.*, 6, 193, 1962.

118. Olsuf'jev, N. G., Emelyanova, O. S., and Dunayeva, T. N., Comparative study of strains of *B. tularense*. II. Evaluation of criteria of virulence of *Bacterium tularense* in the Old and New World, *J. Hyg. Epidemiol. Microbiol. Immunol.*, 3, 138, 1959.

119. Olsufiev, N. G., Emelyanova, O. S., Mescheryakova, T. S., and Rodionova, I. V., A study on the tularemia-similar *F. novicida* Larson et al. micro-organism, *J. Microbiol. Epidemiol. Immunobiol.*, (U.S.S.R.), 8, 92, 1968.

120. Olsuf'jev, N. G. and Golov, D. A., The role of mosquitoes in the transmission and preservation of tularemia, in *Problems of Regional Parasitology*, Vol. 3, Department of the VIEM, Moscow, 1938, 213.

121. Olsuf'jev, N. G. and Rudnev, G. P., Eds., *Tularemia*, State Publisher of Medical Literature, Moscow, 1960, 1.

122. Owen, C. R., Genus Francisella Dorofe'ev 1947, 176, in *Bergey's Manual of Determinative Bacteriology*, 8th ed., Buchanan, R. E. and Gibbons, N. E., Eds., Williams & Wilkins, Baltimore, 1974, 283.

123. Owen, C. R. and Buker, E. O., Factors involved in the transmission of *Pasteurella tularensis* from inoculated animals to healthy cage mates, *J. Infect. Dis.*, 99, 227, 1956.

124. Owen, C. R., Buker, E. O., Jellison, W. L., Lackman, D. B., and Bell, J. F., Comparative studies of *Francisella tularensis* and *Francisella novicida*, *J. Bacteriol.*, 87, 676, 1964.

125. Pannell, L., Studies on protection against experimental tularemia in mice. I and II, *J. Infect. Dis.*, 102, 162, 1958.

126. Parker, R. R., Quail as a possible source of tularemia infection in man, *Public Health Rep.*, 44, 999, 1929.

127. Parker, R. R., Brooks, C. S., and Marsh, H., The occurrence of *Bacterium tularense* in the wood tick (*Dermacentor occidentalis*) in California, *Public Health Rep.*, 44, 1299, 1929.

128. Parker, R. R. and Francis, E., The susceptibility of the coyote (*Canis lestes*) to tularemia, *Public Health Rep.*, 41, 1407, 1926.

129. Parker, R. R., Philip, C. B., and Davis, G. E., Tularemia: occurrence in the sage hen, *Centrocercus urophasianus*, also reports of additional cases following contacts with quail, *Colinus virginianus*, *Public Health Rep.*, 47, 479, 1932.

130. Parker, R. R. and Spencer, R. R., Hereditary transmission of tularemia infection by the wood tick, *Dermacentor andersoni* Stiles, *Public Health Rep.*, 41, 1403, 1926.

131. Parker, R. R., Spencer, R. R., and Francis, E., XI. Tularemia infections in ticks of the species *Dermacentor andersoni* Stiles in the Bitterroot Valley, Montana, *Public Health Rep.*, 39, 1057, 1924.

132. Parker, R. R., Steinhaus, E. A., Kohls, G. M., and Jellison, W. L., Contamination of natural waters and mud with *Pasteurella tularensis*, and tularemia in beavers and muskrats in the Northwestern United States, *Natl. Inst. Health Bull.*, 193, 1951.

133. Pavlovksy, E. N., V. Some natural nidal diseases, in *Natural Nidality of Transmissible Diseases*, Levine, N. D., Ed., University of Illinois Press, Urbana, 1966, 93.

134. Pearse, R. A., Insect bites (with discussion by Dr. E. C. Rich), *Northwest Med.*, 3, 81, 1911.

135. Pekarek, R. S., Bostian, K. A., Bartelloni, P. J., Calia, F. M., and Beisel, W. R., The effects of *Francisella tularensis* on iron metabolism in man, *Am. J. Med. Sci.*, 258, 14, 1969.

136. Petrov, V. G. and Dunaeva, T. N., The relationship between infection of ixodid ticks and characteristics of the course of tularemia in animal donors, in *Problems of Regional, General and Experimental Parasitology and Medical Zoology*, Moscow, 1955, 153.

137. Philip, C. B., unpublished.

138. Philip, C. B., Davis, G. E., and Parker, R. R., Experimental transmission of tularemia by mosquitoes, *Public Health Rep.*, 47, 2077, 1932.

139. Philip, R. N., Huntley, B., Lackman, D. B., and Comstock, G. W., Serologic and skin test evidence of tularemia infection among Alaskan Eskimos, Indians and Aleuts, *J. Infect. Dis.*, 110, 220, 1962.

140. Philip, C. B. and Owen, C. R., Comments on the nomenclature of the causative agent of tularemia, *Int. Bull. Bacteriol. Nomencl. Taxon.*, 11, 67, 1961.

141. Pike, R. M., Sulkin, S. E., and Schulze, M. L., Continuing importance of laboratory-acquired infections, *Am. J. Public Health*, 55, 190, 1965.

142. **Pilipenko, V. G.,** The effect of pre-existing immunity against tularemia and brucellosis on the efficacy of vaccination with plague E B vaccine in a combination of plague, tularemia and brucellosis vaccine, *Zh. Mikrobiol. Epidemiol. Immunobiol.,* 45, 101, 1968.

143. **Pollitzer, R.,** General prophylaxis, in *History and Incidence of Tularemia in the Soviet Union: A Review,* The Institute of Contemporary Russian Studies, Fordham University, Bronx, 1967, 280.

144. **Prag, S.,** Clinical observations during an airborne epidemic of tularemia in Sweden from 1966—1967, in *Contributions to Microbiology and Immunology,* Vol. 2, S. Karger, Basel, 1973, 239.

145. **Price, R. D.,** The multiplication of *Pasteurella tularensis* in human body lice, *Am. J. Hyg.,* 63, 186, 1956.

146. **Puntigam, F.,** Erkrankugen an Thorakalen Formen der Tularemie bei Arbeitnehmern in Zuckerfabriken, *Z. Hyg.,* 147, 162, 1960.

147. **Quan, S. F., McManus, A. G., and Von Fintel, H.,** Infectivity of tularemia applied to intact skin and ingested in drinking water, *Science,* 123, 942, 1956.

148. **Quan, S. F. and Von Fintel, H.,** Quantitative oral infectivity of tularemia for laboratory animals, *Am. J. Hyg.,* 59, 282, 1954.

149. **Reilly, J. R.,** Tularemia, in *Infectious Diseases of Wild Mammals,* Davis, J. W., Karstad, L. H., and Trainer, D. V., Eds., Iowa State University Press, Ames, 1970, 175.

150. **Ritter, D. B. and Gerloff, R. K.,** Deoxyribonucleic acid hybridization among some species of the genus *Pasteurella, J. Bacteriol.,* 92, 1838, 1966.

151. **Saito, T., Kojima, M., Yamagata, Y., Kusonoki, N., Ohara, S., Ueno, T., Shiba, H., and Takagi, Z.,** Pathology of kidney lesions in experimental shedding tularemia, *Annual Report of Ohara Hospital,* Fukushima, in press.

152. **Sakurai, N. and Tanami, Y.,** The effects of the supernatant from grown cultures on the growth of *Bacterium tularense.* An attempt to analyze these effects by absorption phenomena, *Naturwissenschaften,* 43, 87, 1956.

153. **Sanderson, K. E.,** Genetic relatedness in the family Enterobacteriaceae, *Annu. Rev. Microbiol.,* 30, 327, 1976.

154. **Sarchi, G. I.,** Die Epizootie der Tularemie unter den Wasserratten und die Methodik ihrer Untersuchung, *Zentralbl. Bakteriol. Parasitenkd. Infektionskr. Hyg. Abt. Orig.,* 117, 367, 1930.

155. **Saslaw, S. and Carhart, S.,** Studies with tularemia vaccines in volunteers. III. Serologic aspects following intracutaneous or respiratory challenge in both vaccinated and nonvaccinated volunteers, *Am. J. Med. Sci.,* 241, 689, 1961.

156. **Saslaw, S., Eigelsbach, J. T., Prior, J. A., Wilson, H. E., and Carhart, S.,** Tularemia vaccine study. II. Respiratory challenge, *Arch. Int. Med. Exp.,* 107, 702, 1961.

157. **Sawyer, W. D., Kuehne, R. W., and Gochenour, W. S.,** Simultaneous aerosol immunization of monkeys with live tularemia and live Venezuelan equine encephalomyelitis vaccines, *Mil. Med.,* 129, 1040, 1964.

158. **Sbarra, A. J. and Woodward, J. M.,** The host-parasite relationship in tularemia, *J. Bacteriol.,* 69, 363, 1955.

159. **Scharer, J. M., Klein, F., and Lincoln, R. E.,** Growth and metabolism of live vaccine strain of *Pasteurella tularensis, Appl. Microbiol.,* 16, 855, 1968.

160. **Schlotthauer, C. F., Thompson, L., and Olson, C.,** Tularemia in wild grey foxes: report of an epizootic, *J. Infect Dis.,* 56, 28, 1935.

161. **Schmuter, M. V. and Abramova, C. G.,** Case of isolation of a culture of *B. tularense* from the American mink, *Collect. Pap. Anti Plague Inst.,* Rostov-on-Don, U.S.S.R., 10, 229, 1956.

162. **Schuller, A. and Erdmann, B.,** Beobachtungen bei einer Tularemie-Epidemie, *Zh. Hyg. Infektkr.,* 124, 624, 1943.

163. **Schultz, R. D.,** Immunosuppression Induced by Canine Distemper Virus, Paper E136, 75th Annu. Meet., Am. Soc. Microbiology, New York, April 27 to May 2, 1975.

164. **Smith, T. C. and House, E. W.,** The care and breeding of wild rodents under laboratory conditions, *Lab. Anim.,* 4, 32, 1975.

165. **Snyder, P. L., Penfield, R. A., Engley, F. B., and Creasy, J. C.,** Cultivation of *Bacterium tularense* in peptone media, *Proc. Soc. Exp. Biol. Med.,* 63, 26, 1946.

166. **Sonenshine, D. E., Yunker, C. E., Clifford, C. M., Clark, G. M., and Rudbach, J. A.,** Contributions to the ecology of Colorado tick fever virus, *J. Med. Entomol.,* 12, 651, 1976.

167. **Stagg, G., Tanner, W. S., and Lavender, J.,** Experimental infections of native animals with *P. tularensis, J. Infect., Dis.,* 99, 34, 1956.

168. **Stuart, B. M. and Pullen, R. L.,** Tularemic pneumonia: review of American literature and report of 15 additional cases, *Am. J. Med. Sci.,* 210, 223, 1945.

169. **Suvarov, S. V., Volfertz, A. A., and Voronkova, M. M.,** Plague-like lymphadenitis of the Astrikhansky Region Vestnik Mikrobiol., *Epidemiol. Parazitol.,* 7, 293, 1928.

170. Thorpe, B. D., Sidwell, R. W., Johnson, D. E., Smart, K. L., and Parker, D. D., Tularemia in the wildlife and livestock of the Great Salt Lake Desert region 1951—1964. *Am. J. Trop. Med.*, 14, 622, 1965.

171. Tigertt, W. D., Soviet viable *Pasteurella tularensis* vaccines, *Bacteriol. Rev.*, 26, 354, 1962.

172. Tyeryar, F. J., Jr. and Lawton, W. D., Transformation of *Pasteurella novicida, J. Bacteriol.*, 100, 1112, 1969.

173. Van Metre, T. E. and Kadull, P. J., Laboratory-acquired tularemia in vaccinated individuals: a report of 62 cases, *Ann. Intern. Med.*, 50, 621, 1959.

174. Vest, E. D. and Marchette, N. J., Transmission of *Pasteurella tularensis* among desert rodents through infective carcasses, *Science*, 128, 363, 1958.

175. Volfrz, A. A., Kolpakova, S. A., and Flegontoff, A. A., On epizootiology of tularemia. The role of ectoparasites in the tularemic epizootic of ground squirrels, *Rev. Mikrobiol. Epidemiol. Parasitol.*, 13, 103, 1934.

176. Walker, E. P., in *Mammals of the World*, Vol. 1, 2, and 3, Johns Hopkins Press, Baltimore, 1964.

177. Wherry, W. B. and Lamb, B. H., Infection of man with *Bacterium tularense, J. Infect. Dis.*, 15, 331, 1914.

178. White, J. D. and Blundell, G. P., The use of fluorescent antibody technic for demonstration of *Pasteurella tularensis* in formalin-fixed tissues, *Bacteriol. Proc.*, 136, 1958.

179. Woodward, J. M., Sbarra, A. J., and Holtman, D. F., The host-parasite relationship in tularemia I A. Study of the influence of *Bacterium tularense* in the amino acid metabolism of white rats, *J. Bacteriol.*, 67, 58, 1954.

180. Woodward, T. E., Randall, R., McCrumb, F. B., and Snyder, M. J., Studies on tularemia vaccines, Annual Report to the Commission on Epidemiological Survey of the Armed Forces Epidemiological Board, February 1, 1958 to January 15, 1959.

181. Yamanaka, M., Mikami, H., Aoshima, S., and Ohara, S., Electron microscopic observation of *Bacterium tularensis* with a special reference to the morphology of the flagellum, *Bull. Osaka Med. Sch.*, 1, 24, 1954.

187. Young, L. S., Bicknell, D. S., Archer, B. G., Clinton, J. M., Leavens, L. J., Feeley, J. C., and Brachman, P. S., Tularemia epidemic: Vermont 1968. Forty-seven cases linked to contact with muskrats, *N. Engl. J. Med.*, 280, 1253, 1969.

188. Zarkhai, G. I., Tularemia among water rats; methods of studying them, *Bull. Hyg.*, 5, 875, 1930.

VIBRIO INFECTIONS

B. D. Firehammer

DISEASE

The members of the genus *Vibrio* known to cause disease in human beings are *V. cholerae* and *V. parahaemolyticus*. Both organisms cause enteritis in man and have been isolated from certain species of animals.

ETIOLOGIC AGENTS

V. cholerae Biotypes *cholerae* and *eltor*

The species contains four biotypes that can be identified by their physiologic and serologic characteristics.[1] Two of the biotypes, *cholerae* and *eltor*, are called "cholera vibrios." The other two biotypes, *proteus* and *albensis*, are commonly referred to as "noncholera vibrios" although they can cause gastroenteritis in man.

The organisms are short, slightly curved to straight Gram-positive rods of 1.5 to 2 μm in length with a polar flagellum that may be several times the length of the cell. The cells occur singly or in short chains. Spheroplasts with a flagellum are sometimes present after a period of incubation.[2] The colonies are smooth, low, entire, and transparent. When viewed by obliquely transmitted light, they have a characteristic internal structure and chromatic refraction that is helpful when picking colonies from plates of mixed cultures.[3]

The organisms are sensitive to the vibriostatic compound 0/129 and novobiocin. Gelatin is liquefied, hydrogen sulfide and indole are produced, and lactose is slowly fermented. Nutritional requirements are not exacting.

The organisms of biotype *cholerae* do not hemolyze blood in the tube hemolysis test, and the serogroup is 0:1 that by combinations of the antigen factors A, B, and C give three serotypes: ogawa, inaba, and hikojima. Most of the biotype *eltor* isolates are hemolytic and also of serogroup 0:1, and they have the same range of serotypes as biotype *cholerae*.

Noncholera Vibrios (NCV)

Vibrios not belonging to serogroup 0:1 have been isolated from individual cases of gastroenteritis and during outbreaks of diarrheal disease. For years they have been informally designated as nonagglutinable in 0 group 1 antisera (NAG).[4] This term is misleading because they are agglutinable by homologous antisera although as a group they are serologically quite heterogenous. In recent years, these organisms have been commonly referred to as NCV because human enteric disease caused by members of the group is less severe than classical cholera. In the eighth edition of *Bergey's Manual of Determinative Bacteriology*, two NCV organisms were designated as biotypes of *V. cholerae* (*V. cholerae* biotypes *proteus* and *albensis*).[1] The term NCV is used in this chapter as a general term to designate isolates of *V. cholerae* biotypes *proteus* and *albensis* as well as any other closely related *Vibrio* organisms that do not cause classical cholera and have not been given species rank in the *Vibrio* genus. The NCV organisms are similar to biotypes *cholerae* and *eltor* in morphology and physiology, but they are not in serogroup 0:1 and produce a negative cholera red reaction.

Vibrio parahaemolyticus

These organisms are Gram-negative rods with little or no curving of the long axis of the cell and resemble *V. cholerae* in morphology. Bipolar staining of the organisms is sometimes evident, and when the first isolations were made in 1951 by Fuijino et al.,[5] they were classified as *Pasteurella*. The colonies are entire, convex, as large as 3 mm in diameter, and range from translucent to opaque.[6] Rough colonies are sometimes present. When grown in liquid media, the cells have a single, polar, sheathed flagellum, but on solid media, unsheathed peritrichous flagella are also present.[7] These organisms are halophilic, and most tolerate 8% NaCl in growth media. Starch is hydrolyzed, and catalase, oxidase, and lysine decarboxylase are produced.

Most isolates of *V. parahaemolyticus* from patients are hemolytic on specially prepared media (Kanagawa phenomenon-positive) although isolates from seawater or seafood, even when associated with outbreaks of enteritis, are usually nonhemolytic (Kanagawa phenomenon-negative).[8,10] This apparent contradiction has not been satisfactorily resolved although it has been the subject of considerable comment and experimentation. The hemolysis is influenced by the type of blood used, concentration of NaCl, and presence of calcium ions, so the problem might be due in part to procedures for performance of the Kanagawa test.[8,11]

Evaluation of a large number of isolates led to the conclusion that *V. parahaemolyticus* consists of two subgroups and that subgroup 1 is pathogenic but subgroup 2 is not.[6,12] Subgroup 2 was later given the species designation *V. alginolyticus*.[13]

TRUE AND ALTERNATE HOSTS

These organisms are most commonly isolated from the feces and G.I. tracts of persons suffering from cholera. Isolations of *V. cholera* biotype *eltor* have been made from the feces of cattle, dogs, and chickens,[14] but there is no specific evidence to indicate that animal carriers suffer from the infection. Cholera can be reproduced experimentally in dogs by oral inoculation,[15] but a heavy inoculum is required, and the length of the illness is usually shorter than it is in man.[16] Although isolations of cholera vibrios have been made from dogs, the incidence of infection appeared low,[14] and one fairly extensive study failed to result in any isolations other than NCV from dogs.[16]

Noncholera Vibrios (NCV)

NCV organisms have been isolated from human beings, dogs, crows, chickens, and goats.[14,16]

V. parahaemolyticus

The first isolation of *V. parahaemolyticus* was made in Japan from partially dried sardines called *shirasu*.[5] Many of the isolations since that time have been made from seafoods including crabs, shrimp, clams, oysters, mussels, squid, and various saltwater fish. Although evidence indicates that shellfish may harbor *V. parahaemolyticus* under natural conditions, the situation is less clear with ocean fish, and the possibility exists that some, if not most, of the isolations have resulted from contamination of fish after they were caught and handled. Cultures of market fish cannot be expected to yield information concerning the relationship between *V. parahaemolyticus* and populations of fish in nature. Bockemuhl and Triemer[17] found that, although 47.5% of fish and shellfish from lagoons were positive for *V. parahaemolyticus* on culture, only 0.5% of freshly caught Atlantic Ocean fish were positive. These findings are in agreement with the known association of *V. parahaemolyticus* with coastal waters and sediments.

DISTRIBUTION

V. cholerae Biotypes cholerae and eltor

Cholera has been endemic in the deltas of the Ganges and Brahmaputra Rivers in eastern India and East Pakistan since the beginnings of recorded history.[18] An endemic focus of infection due to *V. cholerae* biotype *eltor* on the island of Sulawesi (Celebes) in Indonesia was the origin of the seventh pandemic of cholera that commenced in 1961 and had reached Korea, Taiwan, and the Philippines by 1963.[18] By 1966, it had reached West Pakistan, Afghanistan, Iran, Iraq, and portions of the U.S.S.R. In 1970, Lebanon, Israel, Syria, Jordan, Saudi Arabia, Libya, Tunisia, Guinea, Sierra Leone, Liberia, the Ivory Coast, Mali, Toga, Dahomey, Nigeria, Niger, Turkey, and Czechoslovakia had all reported cases.[19] In 1974, cholera appeared in Portugal, South Africa, Tanzania, and the Cape Verde Islands.

Noncholera Vibrios (NCV)

Most isolations of NCV organisms have been made during the course of outbreaks of cholera. This is probably because NCV organisms, like the true cholera vibrios, are spread by the fecal-oral chain, carried by water, and isolated from feces on media commonly used for the diagnosis of cholera. In general, countries with cholera also have NCV organisms.

V. parahaemolyticus

Isolations of *V. parahaemolyticus* have been made from seafoods, coastal waters, and coastal sediments in many parts of the world.[6,17,20-28] It is probable that *V. parahaemolyticus* is ubiquitous in coastal waters throughout the world, but compared to prevalence rates in warmer regions, the population of organisms in regions of lower water temperatures is low.[29] Isolation of *V. parahaemolyticus* from seafood and coastal sediments or water does not necessarily infer that enteric disease is present in the region. Differences in food-handling procedures, as well as the eating habits and customs of a population, probably determine to a significant degree the incidence of the disease in specific regions.

The annual incidence of food poisoning outbreaks in Japan due to *V. parahaemolyticus* ranged from 266 to 558 in the period from 1963 to 1972.[30] The significance of the problem can be appreciated by the fact that this country has had as many as 14,000 cases in 1 year.[30] The first confirmed outbreak of gastroenteritis due to *V. parahaemolyticus* in the U.S. occurred in 1971, and through 1972 a total of 13 outbreaks were reported.[23,31] Outbreaks have also been reported from India, Malaysia, the Philippines, South Vietnam, Australia, Togo, and Thailand.

DISEASE IN ANIMALS

V. cholerae Biotypes cholerae and eltor

Although the *eltor* vibrios have been isolated from cattle, dogs, and chickens,[14] there is no proof that the infection causes overt disease in these animals. It is possible that some evidence of disease might be found if the infections were studied more thoroughly. Dogs inoculated orally with adequate numbers of cholera vibrios develop clinical cholera with vomiting, massive diarrhea, and consequent depletion of fluids that sometimes results in death. Experimental canine cholera has been used as a model for study of the disease.[15] The inoculum necessary to produce cholera in dogs is very large, and the experimentally produced disease has a somewhat shorter duration than that in human beings.[15] The incidence of natural infection with cholera vibrios in dogs is probably quite low.[16]

Noncholera Vibrios (NCV)

Isolations of NCV have been made from cows, dogs, goats, crows, and chickens.[14,16] Presently, there is no specific evidence available to indicate that NCV cause disease in these animals under natural conditions. Positive ileal loops in rabbits have been obtained with NCV.

V. parahaemolyticus

There are numerous reports concerning the isolation of *V. parahaemolyticus* from oysters, clams, shrimp, crabs, and other marine species used as food, but there is very little information concerning the possibility of pathogenic potential for the host animals. There are two reports of disease in crabs and shrimp in holding tanks. Isolations of *V. parahaemolyticus* were made from necrotic claws and hemolymph of lethargic and moribund crabs retained in commercial tanks during the "shedding" period of soft crabs.[32] Mortality in some of the tanks was in excess of 50%.

The second incidence of disease due to *V. parahaemolyticus* occurred in brown shrimp (*Penaeus aztecus*) held in laboratory aquariums for use on nutrition experiments. The source of the infection was traced to bits of white shrimp (*Penaeus setiferus*) used to feed the brown shrimp.[33] Addition of *V. parahaemolyticus* cultures to the holding tanks resulted in uneasy behavior by the brown shrimp in less than 1 hr and death occurred within 3 hr. Cultures from the cephalothorax region of the shrimp yielded nearly pure cultures of *V. parahaemolyticus*.

Both of these outbreaks involved marine species held under unnatural conditions and do not prove that *V. parahaemolyticus* causes disease in nature. However, until more information becomes available, *V. parahaemolyticus* should be considered as a possible pathogen of marine animals.

DISEASE IN MAN

V. cholerae Biotypes *cholerae* and *eltor*

Ingestion of cholera vibrios is followed by multiplication in the small intestine and liberation of enterotoxin. It is thought that the enterotoxin increases adenyl cyclase activity resulting in excessive production of adenosine 3',5'-cyclic-monophosphate (cAMP) followed by hypersecretion of water and salts.[34-40] The secretion exceeds the absorptive ability of the large intestine and a watery diarrhea results. The incubation period from ingestion of organisms to development of symptoms may vary from 1 to 5 days. In some instances the diarrhea is relatively mild, but in the more typical cases, its swift onset (sometimes with vomiting) results in rapid dehydration, diminished skin turgor, cold extremities, high pulse rate, and low blood pressure. Fluid loss may exceed 1 ℓ/hr and lead to hypovolemic shock and metabolic acidosis resulting in death.[41]

Due to poor renal perfusion, many patients died from uremia prior to 1960, but since that time, death due to this cause has declined remarkably, probably due to the use of massive fluid and electrolyte-replacement therapy.[42]

Studies on the pathology of cholera have revealed that intestinal water and electolyte transport are altered without structural damage to the gut mucosa. Acute inflammation is not involved in the production of fluid by the gut, and there is no apparent damage to the epithelial junction sites or basement membranes. However, there may be distention of capillaries at the tips of the villi.[43]

Cholera vibrios are quite sensitive to low pH, and there is evidence that the acidity of the stomach may function as a first line of defense.[16] It may be that the pH of the gastric fluids, when vibrios are ingested with food or water, determines the outcome of exposure.

Noncholera Vibrios (NCV)

Although disease due to NCV in human beings was recognized some time ago,[44,45] the causative organisms have seldomly been adequately described and identified in literature. For this reason, it is impossible to accurately differentiate between *V. cholera* biotypes *proteus* and *albensis*, or possibly undescribed NCV, on a retrospective basis. It is therefore necessary for the sake of convenience to view the NCV as a group although it might eventually prove to be a rather heterogeneous one.

NCV organisms have been isolated from the stools of persons with diarrheal disease during epidemics of cholera, as well as during limited outbreaks of diseases that were obviously not cholera. In 1965, an explosive outbreak of "gastroenteritis" that involved 56 young men at a training center in Czechoslovakia resulted in isolation of NCV organisms.[46] All of these cases developed within 1 day, and although six severe cases required hospitalization, there was no acidosis, dehydration, or indication for the administration of intravenous fluids. Most of the patients were free of symptoms by the second day. Although there is no doubt that NCV can cause severe diarrheal disease, there is some evidence that these organisms are usually not quite as pathogenic as classical cholera vibrios.[47-49]

Although NCV are not related to *V. cholerae* biotypes *cholerae* or *eltor* by common O antigens, they are related to the cholera vibrios by virtue of possession of common enzymes,[50] DNA base compositions, polynucleotide sequence relationships, and biochemical characteristics.[51-53] Because of these relationships, NCV have been given the status of biotypes of *V. cholerae*.

V. parahaemolyticus

Since 1950 when *shirasu* food poisoning was first recognized in Japan, *V. parahaemolyticus* has been incriminated as an important cause of food-borne enteritis in that country and to a lesser extent in other countries as well. The incubation period can range from 1 to 2 hr through several days, but it is usually less than 24 hr. Diarrhea, abdominal pain, and nausea are the most common symptoms. The diarrhea is usually watery, but in some cases, mucus and even blood may be present. Headache and fever are not uncommon. The illness usually lasts for 2 or 3 days, but in exceptional cases it may persist for 10 days or longer. Dehydration is usually mild to moderate in severity. Although a few deaths occurred in the initial outbreak,[5] fatalities are rare.

Isolations of *V. parahaemolyticus* have been made from lesions of the extremities and discharges of the eyes and ears of individuals who apparently acquired infection as a result of recreational contact with a marine environment.[54] Following bathing in a bay, gangrene of the leg and endotoxin shock due to *V. parahaemolyticus* were reported.[55]

Ligated rabbit ileal loop techniques have been used in attempts to determine the relative pathogenicities of Kanagawa-positive and -negative cultures and to detect enterotoxic activity in various culture-derived preparations, with rather confusing results. This is probably due in part to the fact that broth filtrates concentrated by lyophilization prior to evaluation in ileal loops may contain concentrations of NaCl capable of causing loop distention.[56,57] Enterotoxin activity was not found in unconcentrated broth filtrates.[56] However, the hemolytic ability of a strain appears to be related to its capability to produce dilation of ligated ileal loops in rabbits,[57] and a thermolabile direct hemolysin has been isolated from filtrates of Kanagawa-positive isolates.[58-60] Cell-free filtrates from Kanagawa-positive cultures fail to produce distention of ileal loops but crude lysates cause dilation and produce hemolysis, indicating that a toxic factor is associated with cell particles and resembles the Kanagawa hemolysin.[57] The purified hemolysin is cardiotoxic and can cause death in animals.[61]

GENERAL MODE OF SPREAD

V. cholerae Biotypes *cholerae* and *eltor*

Cholera has been considered a water-borne disease since Snow[62] mapped the incidence of cases in London in 1854 and concluded that fecal contamination of water supplies was probably associated with the contagion. In an attempt to stop the epidemic, he recommended that the handle of the Broad Street pump be removed.

Water contaminated with fecal material, seafood from areas contaminated by sewage, and food prepared with contaminated water are the major sources of infection. Fomites are not a significant source of infection, and the vibrios do not survive long in water containing large numbers of other bacteria. They can survive for as long as 17 days in clean water at room temperature, however.[63] It appears that improperly processed bottled water might spread the infection. Direct person-to-person spread of cholera is probably extremely rare.

NCV

The mode by which infection with NCV organisms is spread has not been investigated as thoroughly as has the mode of classical cholera, but it is generally assumed that it also involves ingestion of water or food contaminated by feces.

V. parahaemolyticus

Gastroenteritis results from the ingestion of seafood containing a pathogenic (Kanagawa-positive) strain of *V. parahaemolyticus*. Although *V. parahaemolyticus* is virtually ubiquitous in coastal seafoods and waters, it is thought that infection with approximately 10^5 organisms is required to produce clinical illness, indicating the likelihood that multiplication during processing and storage of food precedes outbreaks. The Japanese custom of eating certain seafoods raw probably contributes to the relatively high incidence of enteritis due to *V. parahaemolyticus* there.

EPIDEMIOLOGY

V. cholerae Biotypes *cholerae* and *eltor*

India was the source of six pandemics of cholera between 1817 and 1923, but the seventh started in Indonesia in 1960 and had reached Portugal, Tanzania, and the Cape Verde Islands by 1974. This pandemic was caused by the biotype *eltor*. India was invaded by the pandemic in 1964, and the entire country was covered within 1 year.[19] The main route of spread was by land travel; El Tor cholera invaded areas where the disease had never occurred before and regions that had been free of it for some time.[19] Although Bangladesh, West Pakistan, and India were endemic for classical cholera for quite a long time, they responded differently to the El Tor pandemic. The classical *V. cholera* predominated in Bangladesh, both biotypes survived in West Pakistan, and classical cholera was replaced with the *eltor* biotype in India.[19] In both in vitro and in vivo experiments, Basu and co-workers[64] found that in mixed culture, *eltor* vibrios from cholera cases overgrew and eliminated classical cholera vibrios. Gallut and Quiniou[65] confirmed the inhibition of classical cholera vibrios by *eltor* and found that NCV are even more effective at inhibition than *eltor*. They also found that NCV inhibit the *eltor* biotype.[65] The mechanism of inhibition is not understood, but the possibility that it might alter the course of epidemics has been suggested.[4]

Cholera caused by biotype *eltor* is generally of a milder nature than the classical cholera caused by *V. cholerae* biotype *cholerae*. The high frequency of unrecognized El Tor ogawa infections and the more prolonged survival of El Tor vibrios in the environment have been suggested as possible reasons for the dissemination of El Tor cholera throughout Southeast Asia and the Middle East.[14,66]

Although the significance of human carriers in the transmission of cholera is a subject of controversy, the carrier does constitute a reservoir of infection and chronic carriers may contribute to the endemicity of the infection.[16] Carriers or individuals with mild or subclinical cases of El Tor cholera could be transported by air transportation to distant regions within a few hours. However, the establishment of a new epidemic would be dependent upon a rather exacting set of circumstances. In many countries of the world, the fecal-oral cycle could not take place to any appreciable extent because of effective handling of sewage and water supplies. In less advanced countries, the lack of appropriate sanitation facilities and practices could lead to the establishment of a cholera epidemic.

Isolations of *V. cholerae* biotype *eltor* have been made from household cows, dogs, and chickens so there is a possibililty that these animals might serve as sources of human infection.[14] However, only 8 isolations of biotype *eltor* and 46 of NCV organisms were made from 1287 examined specimens, so the sampled animal population did not contain a high proportion of carriers.[14]

NCV

The epidemiology of disease caused by NCV vibrios has not been investigated nearly as thoroughly as classical cholera. NCV vibrios have sometimes been called "water vibrios" because of their prevalence in surface waters in some areas.[45] These organisms have been isolated at a considerably higher rate from cows, goats, dogs, chickens, and crows than have vibrios of the *eltor* biotype.[14,15] The nonhuman sources of infection with NCV probably exceed those of classical cholera. There is little information available concerning the incidence of human NCV carriers, but inasmuch as diarrheal disease due to NCV is usually less severe than in classical cholera, infected individuals may be somewhat more mobile than cholera patients. Consequently, they facilitate the spread of the infection.

NCV appeared to replace cholera vibrios during the decline of a cholera epidemic in Iran in 1966, and these organisms are capable of eliminating *V. cholera* biotypes *cholerae* and *eltor* in mixed culture.[4,65] Their ability to compete effectively with classical cholera vibrios, establish carrier status in animals, and possibly survive in surface waters present ample opportunities to establish infection in man.

V. parahaemolyticus

Available evidence indicates that *V. parahaemolyticum* is commonly present in coastal marine sediments and shellfish but is far less common in the open ocean. Organisms surviving in coastal sediments during the cold months of the year are released into the water column as the water warms and become associated with the copepod populations.[67] The ability of *V. parahaemolyticus* to adsorb onto chitin is considered to be a factor in determining the annual cycle of distribution.[68] Populations of *V. parahaemolyticus* in oysters and sediments are related to water temperature,[25,28] and *shirasu* food poisoning in Japan is most prevalent during the warm months of the year. Multiplication in raw or poorly cooked seafood is also more likely during the warmer seasons. Even 3 hr at a temperature of 20°C can result in infective levels if the initial population is 10^2 to 10^3 organisms per gram.[69] Chilling and freezing reduce populations of *V. parahaemolyticus* on fish and shellfish, with chilling being the more lethal of the two.[69]

Serological typing of isolates has revealed a tendency for new K serotypes to appear each year, or every other year, and to become the major cause of disease in humans the same year.[70,71] Different serotypes may also be isolated during the course of a single outbreak or even from an individual patient.[31,70] The reasons for the change in predominant K serotypes and for the frequent appearance of new serotypes are unknown. Baross et al.[72] found that oysters can accumulate both *V. parahaemolyticus*. and specific bacteriophages. Through their ability to filter large volumes of water, oysters and clams actually facilitate the contact between bacteria, bacteriophages, and different types of bacteria. This contact presents opportunities for both transduction and conjugation with subsequent increased potentiality for adaptation to changing environmental conditions.[72] One can speculate that similiar mechanisms might lead to the appearance of "new" serotypes of *V. parahaemolyticus.*

DIAGNOSIS

V. cholerae Biotypes *cholerae* and *eltor*

Immediate diagnosis is not essential prior to initiation of supportive therapy, but it is of value when cholera has not been diagnosed in the region. About 80% of the cases can be diagnosed correctly by dark-field examination of fecal material if the sample is collected early in the course of the disease; even more cases can be diagnosed following 6 to 18 hr enrichment.[73] Fecal smears can also be used for a slide agglutination test with O-group serum.[73]

Although cholera vibrios can be grown on nutrient agar, their growth is inhibited on media such as MacConkey, SS, and EMB, that are commonly used for culturing fecal matter.[74] In regions where cholera is uncommon, bacteriologists might not only be using inappropriate media but, because they may not be anticipating the possibility of cholera, may discard *V. cholerae* cultures under the assumption that they are nonpathogenic organisms.

Stool samples or rectal swabs should be cultured in enrichment broth and on both selective and nonselective agar media.[73,75] Alkaline peptone water can be used as an enrichment and also a transport medium, but several other media are satisfactory for transportation.[73,75] Nutrient and gelatin agars are satisfactory nonselective media. Selective media such as thiosulfate-citrate-bile-salt sucrose (TCBS) agar or taurocholate-gelatin agar (TGA) have proven to be of value. Agar plates containing gelatin are useful in detecting cholera vibrios because of the cloudy zones caused by gelatinase activity. Oblique-light microscopy may be useful in recognizing colonies for picking.[3,74] Consideration of the numerous isolation procedures available is beyond the scope of this chapter, but such information has been published in detail.[48,73-76] In general, the methods and media satisfactory for isolation of classical cholera vibrios can also be used for isolation of NCV.

V. parahaemolyticus

V. parahaemolyticus can be isolated from stools and marine specimens on TCBS and bromthymol blue (BTB) Teepol agars, but enrichment in a salt-Teepol buffer (STB) may be useful for isolation from sparsely-infected materials.[77] Hydrolysis of starch is a characteristic of *V. parahaemolyticus* that has been considered in the formulation of a salt-starch-agar medium that can be used, with the addition of penicillin, for isolation from sea water, marine sediments, and seafood.[28,78]

Isolation of heat- or cold-stressed cells of *V. parahaemolyticus* is more effective on a salt-starch medium (without penicillin) than on TCBS medium.[79] The use of salt-starch medium for culturing fresh commercial seafood may result in large numbers of false-positive isolations, but this can be avoided by enrichment in trypticase soy broth containing 7% NaCl followed by streaking on TCBS plates.[79]

Isolates of Gram-negative pleomorphic rods that are oxidase-positive, hydrolyze starch, liquefy gelatin, produce lysine decarboxylase, ferment glucose, and tolerate 7% NaCl can tentatively be considered to be *V. parahaemolyticus.* Several authors have presented the characteristics of *V. parahaemolyticus* and the procedures useful for identification.[5,12,28,51,54,80]   It is not surprising that there are several discrepancies in the characteristics attributed to *V. parahaemolyticus, V. alginolyticus,* and *V. anguillarum.*[25,28,51]   The Center for Disease Control (CDC), Atlanta, has received cultures of an unnamed halophilic bacterium isolated from the blood of persons in the U.S.[81] This organism can be differentiated from *V. parahaemolyticus* by a lower tolerance for NaCl and by fermentation of lactose.

PREVENTION AND CONTROL

Cholera

Cholera carriers or individuals with milder forms of the disease can be quickly transported to distant sites by air travel and release large numbers of viable organisms into the environment. Modern sewage disposal and water-treatment practices prevalent in many parts of the world prevent the establishment of epidemics even though carriers or obviously ill persons may be present at times. In other regions, poor sanitation facilities and practices permit spread of the disease. Under these conditions, health authorities should (1) make laboratory personnel aware of the possible occurrence of cholera and (2) provide training in appropriate diagnostic procedures. Plans should be made for the isolation and treatment of cholera patients. Treatment is effective and deaths are preventable by prompt replacement of fluids and electrolytes if trained personnel and the necessary equipment are available at the site of the outbreak. Cholera cots can be useful for measuring the loss of G.I. fluid, but if cots and calibrated buckets are unavailable, intravenous fluids should be given at a rate sufficient to maintain a normal radial pulse volume and normal skin turgor.[82] In rural areas where intravenous fluids are not readily available, administration of glucose-electrolyte fluid by mouth or nasogastric tube can be used effectively for replacement therapy.[83-85]

Tetracycline therapy can result in a significant reduction in fluid loss and elimination of *V. cholerae* from the stools of most patients.[86-88] Although antibiotic therapy reduces fluid needs, these needs are still large, and availability is sometimes the limiting factor in management of patients during outbreaks.[82]

Outbreaks of cholera can be controlled by breaking the fecal-oral chain. The use of portable field toilets and water purification apparatus can do much to halt the spread of infection. These measures, although effective, are difficult to initiate under conditions existing during an outbreak; tenacity on the part of the responsible authorities is required. Because *V. cholerae* may survive for several weeks in milk, milk products, seafood, or certain frozen foods, it is important that proper sanitation measures be observed during production and handling. A common hazard is the use of contaminated water for the production and washing of foods. Adequate cooking of foods is recommended.

Controlled field trials with vaccines have indicated that a degree of protection can be obtained by vaccination, but the immunity is of relatively short duration. Although cholera is probably best controlled by initiation of appropriate sanitation, in some instances vaccination may be of value in management of outbreaks. Long-term prevention can probably be best approached by (1) education of the population in the principles of basic sanitation and (2) gradual development of safe facilities for production of drinking water and sewage disposal.

NCV

Prevention of disease due to NCV is dependent upon effective facilities for disposal of sewage and production of drinking water. Emphasis should also be placed upon the role of animals as carriers and as potential sources of human infection. As with cholera, application of the principles of basic sanitation within the household is a useful preventive measure. Some of the factors involved in contamination of surface water with NCV and the survival time of the organisms in water are not well understood.

V. parahaemolyticus

Gastroenteritis due to *V. parahaemolyticus* can be prevented by sanitary food-handling procedures, refrigeration, and adequate cooking of seafood. The generation time of *V. parahaemolyticus* is relatively short and growth at temperatures of 20 to 30°C can be rapid.[23,66] Poorly cooked seafood or seafood that has been contaminated after cooking can become infective within a few hours if not properly refrigerated.

Superficial wounds and abrasions acquired in a marine environment should not be taken lightly since entry of *V. parahaemolyticus* can result in a serious wound infection and even endotoxin shock.

APPENDIX*

A 61-year-old truck driver was admitted to a Montgomery, Ala. hospital on April 19, 1977, with a 6-day history of fever, chills, and right upper quadrant pain. A clinical diagnosis of cholecystitis was made, and on April 25 the gall bladder was removed and bile cultured. On May 2, a Gram-negative rod isolated from the culture was identified as *Vibrio cholerae*. This identification was confirmed by both the state laboratory in Alabama and by the Bureau of Laboratories, Center for Disease Control (CDC).

The patient denied any recent history of severe diarrhea, but he had experienced episodes of recurrent diarrhea approximately once a month for at least 14 years. The patient made many transcontinental trips each year but denied any travel outside of the U.S. except for brief trips into Mexico more than 30 years ago. Although he was in the armed forces during World War II, he did not serve overseas. However, he did have contact with persons in prisoner-of-war camps who came from countries where cholera was endemic. The patient also had eaten large quantities of raw oysters for many years.

An investigation conducted by the Alabama State Department of Health and the CDC did not demonstrate vibrios in stool cultures from the patient or his family. Cultures of sewage from the patient's home and neighborhood sewage system were negative for *V. cholerae*.

CDC Editorial Note

This is the second case of nonlaboratory-acquired infection with *V. cholerae* in the U.S. since 1911; the first occurred in Port Lavaca, Tex. in 1973. Although the source of infection of the Alabama case has not yet been identified, the patient, as with the Port Lavaca case, gave a history of eating large quantities of raw oysters. Shellfish have previously caused cholera epidemics in Italy and Portugal.[89,90]

---

* Center for Disease Control, *Vibrio cholerae*—Alabama, in Morbidity and Mortality Weekly Report, Publication No. (CDC) 77-8017, U.S. Department of Health, Education, and Welfare, Public Health Service, Atlanta, 1977, 159.

Chronic carriage of *V. cholerae* is rare, but studies suggest that carriage can occur in the gall bladder, with or without evidence of excretion of the bacteria in the stool.[91,92] The occurrence of a carrier in the U.S. poses little risk because of generally adequate water sanitation and sewage treatment practices.

REFERENCES

1. **Shewan, J. M. and Veron, M.**, Genus I, Vibrio Pacini 1854, in *Bergey's Manual of Determinative Bacteriology*, 8th ed., Buchanan, R. E. and Gibbons, N. E., Eds., Williams & Wilkins, Baltimore, 1974, 340.

2. **Gallut, J. and Giuntini, J.**, Etude de *V. cholerae* au microscope electronique et relation entre l'aspect morphologique et l'agglutinabilite O, *Bull. W.H.O.*, 29, 767, 1963.

3. **Lankford, C. E.**, The Henry oblique light technique as an aid in bacteriological diagnosis of cholera, *J. Microbiol. Soc. Thailand*, 3, 10, 1959.

4. **Gallut, J.**, The cholera vibrios, in *Cholera*, Baru, D. and Burrows, W., Eds., W. B. Saunders, Philadelphia, 1974, 17.

5. **Fujino, T., Okuno, Y., Nakada, D., Aoyama, A., Fukai, K., Mukai, T., and Ueho, T.**, On the bacteriological examination of shirasu food poisoning, *Med. J. Osaka Univ.*, 4, 299, 1953.

6. **Sakazaki, R., Iwanami, S., and Fukumi, H.**, Studies on the enteropathogenic, facultatively halophilic bacteria, *Vibrio parahaemolyticus*. I. Morphological, cultural and biochemical properties and its taxonomical position, *Jpn. J. Med. Sci. Biol.*, 16, 161, 1963.

7. **Allen, R. D. and Baumann, P.**, Structure and arrangement of flagella in species of the genus *Beneckea* and *Photobacterium fischeri*, *J. Bacteriol.*, 107, 295, 1971.

8. **Mizamoto, Y., Kato, T., Obara, Y., Okiyama, S., Takizawa, K., and Yamai, S.**, *In vitro* hemolytic characteristic of *Vibrio parahaemolyticus*: its close correlation with human pathogenicity, *J. Bacteriol.*, 100, 1147, 1969.

9. **Sakazaki, R., Tamura, K., Kato, T., Abara, S., Yamai, S., and Hobo, K.**, Studies on the enteropathogenic facultatively halophilic bacteria, *Vibrio parahaemolyticus*. III. Enteropathogenicity, *Jpn. J. Med. Sci. Biol.*, 21, 325, 1968.

10. **Barrow, G. I. and Miller, D. C.**, Growth studies on *Vibrio parahaemolyticus* in relation to pathogenicity, in *Int. Symp. Vibrio parahaemolyticus*, Fuijino, T., Sakaguchi, G., Sakazaki, R., and Takeda, Y., Eds., Saikon, Tokyo, 1974, 205.

11. **Chun, D., Chung, J. Y., Tak, R., and Seol., S. Y.**, Nature of the Kangawa phenomenon, *Infect. Immun.*, 12, 81, 1975.

12. **Zen-Yoji, H., Sakai, S., Terayama, T., Kudo, Y., Ito, T., Benoki, M., and Nagasaki, M.**, Epidemiology, enteropathogenicity, and classification of *Vibrio parahaemolyticus*, *J. Infect. Dis.*, 115, 436, 1965.

13. **Sakazaki, R.**, Proposal of *Vibrio alginolyticus* for the biotype 2 of *Vibrio parahaemolyticus*, *Jpn. J. Med. Sci. Biol.*, 21, 359, 1968.

14. **Sanyal, S. C., Singh, S. J., Tiwari, I. C., Sen, P. C., Marwah, S. M., Hazarika, U. R., Singh, H., Shimada, T., and Sakazaki, R.**, Role of household animals in maintenance of cholera infection in a community, *J. Infect. Dis.*, 130, 575, 1974.

15. **Sack, R. B. and Carpenter, C. C. J.**, Experimental canine cholera. I. Development of the model, *J. Infect. Dis.*, 119, 138, 1969.

16. **Sack, R. B.**, A search for canine carriers of *Vibrio*, *J. Infect. Dis.*, 127, 709, 1973.

17. **Bockemuhl, J. and Triemer, A.**, Ecology and epidemiology of *Vibrio parahaemolyticus* on the coast of Togo, *Bull. W.H.O.*, 51, 353, 1974.

18. **Mosley, W. H.**, Epidemiology of cholera, in Principles and Practice of Cholera Control, Public Health Paper No. 40, World Health Organization, Geneva, 1970, 23.

19. **Kamal, A. M.**, The seventh pandemic of cholera, in *Cholera*, Baru, D. and Burrows, W., Eds., W. B. Saunders, Philadelphia, 1974, 1.

20. **Atthasampunna, P.**, *Vibrio parahaemolyticus* food poisoning in Thailand, in *Int. Symp. Vibrio parahaemolyticus*, Fuijino, T., Sakaguchi, G., Sakazaki, R., and Takeda, Y., Eds., Saikon, Tokyo, 1974, 21.

21. **Bonang, G., Lintong, M., and Santoso, U. S.,** The isolation and susceptibility of various antimicrobial agents of *Vibrio parahaemolyticus* from acute gastroenteritis cases and from sea food in Jakarta, in *Int. Symp. Vibrio parahaemolyticus,* Fuijino, T., Sakaguchi, G., Sakazaki, R., and Takeda, Y., Eds., Saikon, Tokyo, 1974, 27.

22. **Muic, V. and Zekic, R.,** Isolation of *Vibrio parahaemolyticus* from the northern Adriatic, Croatia, Yugoslavia, in *Int. Symp. Vibrio parahaemolyticus,* Fuijino, T., Sakaguchi, G., Sakazaki, R., and Takeda, Y., Eds., Saikon, Tokyo, 1974, 41.

23. **Barker, W. H., Jr.,** *Vibrio parahaemolyticus,* outbreaks in the United States, in *Int. Symp. Vibrio parahaemolyticus,* Fuijino, T., Sakaguchi, G., Sakazaki, R., and Takeda, Y., Eds., Saikon, Tokyo, 1974, 47.

24. **Fishbein, M., Wentz, B., Landry, W. L., and MacEachern, B.,** *Vibrio parahaemolyticus* isolates in the U.S.: 1969-1972, in *Int. Symp. Vibrio parahaemolyticus,* Fuijino, T., Sakaguchi, G., Sakazaki, R., and Takeda, Y., Eds., Saikon, Tokyo, 1974, 53.

25. **Sutton, R. G. A.,** Some qualitative aspects of *Vibrio parahaemolyticus* in oysters in the Sydney area, in *Int. Symp. Vibrio parahaemolyticus,* Fuijino, T., Sakaguchi, G., Sakazaki, R., and Takeda, Y., Eds., Saikon, Tokyo, 1974, 71.

26. **Leistner, L. and Hechelmann, H.,** Occurrence and significance of *Vibrio parahaemolyticus* in Europe, in *Int. Symp. Vibrio parahaemolyticus,* Fuijino, T., Sakaguchi, G, Sakazaki, R., and Takeda, Y., Eds., Saikon, Tokyo, 1974, 83.

27. **Kristensen, K. K.,** Semiquantitative examinations on the contents of *Vibrio parahaemolyticus* in the sound between Sweden and Denmark, in *Int. Symp. Vibrio parahaemolyticus,* Fuijino, T., Sakaguchi, G., Sakazaki, R., and Takeda, Y., Eds., Saikon, Tokyo, 1974, 105.

28. **Baross, J. and Liston, J.,** Isolation of *Vibrio parahaemolyticus* from the northwest Pacific, *Nature* (London), 217, 1263, 1968.

29. **Vasconcelos, G. J., Stang, W. J., and Laidlaw, R. H.,** Isolation of *Vibrio parahaemolyticus* and *Vibrio alginolyticus* from esturine areas of southeast Alaska, *Appl. Microbiol.,* 29, 557, 1975.

30. **Okabe, S.,** Statistical review of food poisoning in Japan—especially that by *Vibrio parahaemolyticus,* in *Int. Symp. Vibrio parahaemolyticus,* Fuijino, T. Sakaguchi, G., Sakazaki, R., and Takeda, Y., Eds., Saikon, Tokyo, 1974, 5.

31. **Molenda, J. R., Johnson, W. G., Fishbein, M., Wentz, B., Mehlman, I. J., and Dadisman, T. A., Jr.,** *Vibrio parahaemolyticus* gastroenteritis in Maryland: laboratory aspects, *Appl. Microbiol.,* 24, 444, 1972.

32. **Krantz, G. E., Colwell, R., and Lovelace, E.,** *Vibrio parahaemolyticus* from the blue crab *Callinecta sapidus* in Chesapeake Bay, *Science,* 164, 1286, 1969.

33. **Vanderzant, C., Nickelson, R., and Parker, J. C.,** Isolation of *Vibrio parahaemolyticus* from Gulf Coast shrimp, *J. Milk Food Technol.,* 33, 161, 1970.

34. **Finkelstein, R. A.,** The role of choleragen in the pathogenesis and immunology of cholera, *Tex. Rep. Biol. Med.,* 27 (Suppl. 1), 181, 1969.

35. **Pierce, N. F., Greenough, W. B., III, and Carpenter, C. C. J.,** *Vibrio cholerae* enterotoxin and its mode of action, *Bacteriol. Rev.,* 35, 1, 1971.

36. **Schafer, D. E., Lust, W. D., Sincar, B., and Goldberg, N. D.,** Elevation of adenosine 3'5'-cyclic monophosphate concentration in intestinal mucosa after treatment with cholera toxin, *Proc. Natl. Acad. Sci. U.S.A.,* 67, 851, 1970.

37. **Sharp, G. W. G. and Hynie, S.,** Stimulation of intestinal adenyl cyclase by cholera toxin, *Nature* (London), 229, 266, 1971.

38. **Kimberg, D. V., Field, M., Johnson, J., Henderson, A., and Gershon, E.,** Stimulation of intestinal mucosal adenyl cyclase by cholera enterotoxin and prostaglandins, *J. Clin. Invest.,* 50, 1218, 1971.

39. **Chen, L., Rohde, J. E., and Sharp, G. W. G.,** Properties of adenyl cyclase from human jejunal mucosa during naturally acquired cholera and convalescence, *J. Clin. Invest.,* 51, 731, 1972.

40. **Field, M., Fromm, D., Al-Awqati, Q., and Greenough, W. B., III,** Effect of cholera enterotoxin on ion transport across ileal mucosa, *J. Clin. Invest.,* 51, 796, 1972.

41. **Carpenter, C. C. J.,** Cholera and other enterotoxin-related diseases, *J. Infect. Dis.,* 126, 551, 1972.

42. **Norris, H. T.,** Changing patterns of autopsy findings in patients dying of cholera after 1960, *Am. J. Trop. Med. Hyg.,* 22, 215, 1973.

43. **Elliot, H. L., Carpenter, C. C. J., Sack, R. B., and Yardley, J. H.,** Small bowel morphology in experimental canine cholera, *Lab. Invest.,* 22, 112, 1970.

44. **Dutta, N. K., Panse, M. V., and Jhala, H. I.,** Choleragenic property of certain strains of El Tor, non-agglutinable, and water vibrios confirmed experimentally, *Br. Med. J.,* (Suppl. 1), 1200, 1963.

45. **McIntyre, O. R., Feeley, J. C., Greenough, J. C., III, Benenson, A. S., Hassan, S. I., and Saad, A.,** Diarrhea caused by non-cholera vibrios, *Am. J. Trop. Med. Hyg.,* 14, 412, 1965.

46. **Aldova, E., Laznickova, K., Stepanokova, E., and Lietava, J.,** Isolation of nonagglutinable vibrios from an enteritis outbreak in Czechoslovakia, *J. Infect. Dis.,* 118, 25, 1968.

47. Hornick, R. B., Music, S. I., Wenzel, R., Cash, R., Libonati, J. P., Snyder, M. J., and Woodward, T. E., The Broad Street pump revisited: response of volunteers to ingested cholera vibrios, *Bull. N.Y. Acad. Sci.,* 47, 1181, 1971.

48. Smith, H. L., Jr. and Goodner, K., on the classification of vibrios, in *Proc. Cholera Res. Symp.,* Publication No. 1328, U. S. Public Health Service, Washington, D.C., 4.

49. Finkelstein, R. A., Cholera, *Crit. Rev. Microbiol.,* 2, 553, 1973.

50. Hsieh, H. and Liu, P. V., Serological identities of proteases and alkaline prosphatases of the so-called nonagglutinable (NAG) vibrios and those of *Vibrio cholerae, J. Infect. Dis.,* 212, 251, 1970.

51. Colwell, R. R., Polyphasic taxonomy of the genus *Vibrio:* numerical taxonomy of *Vibrio cholerae, Vibrio parahaemolyticus,* and related *Vibrio* species, *J. Bacteriol.,* 104, 410, 1970.

52. Citarella, R. V. and Colwell, R. R., Polyphasic taxonomy of the genus *Vibrio:* polynucleotide sequence relationships among selected *Vibrio* species, *J. Bacteriol.,* 104, 434, 1970.

53. Sakazaki, R. Gomez, C. Z., and Sebald, M., Taxonomical studies of the so-called NAG vibrios, *Jpn. J. Med. Sci. Biol.,* 20, 265, 1967.

54. Twedt, R. M., Spaulding, P. L., and Hall, H. E., Morphological, cultural, biochemical, and serological comparison of Japanese strains of *Vibrio parahaemolyticus* with related cultures isolated in the United States, *J. Bacteriol.,* 98, 511, 1969.

55. Roland, F. P., Leg gangrene and endotoxin shock due to *Vibrio parahaemolyticus* — an infection acquired in New England coastal waters, *N. Engl. J. Med.,* 282, 1306, 1970.

56. Johnson, D. E. and Calia, F. M., False-positive rabbit ileal loop reactions attributed to *Vibrio parahaemolyticus, J. Infect. Dis.,* 133, 436, 1976.

57. Brown, D. F., Spaulding, P. L., and Twedt, R. M., Enteropathogenicity of *Vibrio parahaemolyticus* in the ligated rabbit ileum, *Appl. Environ. Microbiol.,* 33, 10, 1977.

58. Zen-Yoji, H., Hitakoto, S., Morozumi, S., and Le Clair, R. A., Purification and characterization of a hemolysin produced by *Vibrio parahaemolyticus, J. Infect. Dis.,* 123, 665, 1971.

59. Sakurai, J., Matsuzaki, A., and Miwatani, T., Purification and characterization of thermostable direct hemolysin of *Vibrio parahaemolyticus, Infect. Immun.,* 8, 775, 1973.

60. Honda, T., Taga, S., Takeda, T., Hasibuan, M., Takeda, Y., and Miwatani, T., Identification of lethal toxin with the thermostable direct hemolysin produced by *Vibrio parahaemolyticus,* and some physiochemical properties of the purified toxin, *Infect. Immun.,* 13, 133, 1976.

61. Honda, T., Gohsima, K., Takeda, Y., Sugino, Y., and Miwatani, T., Demonstration of the cardiotoxicity of the thermostable direct hemolysin (lethal toxin) produced by *Vibrio parahaemolyticus, Infect. Immun.,* 13, 163, 1976.

62. Snow, J., On the mode of communication of cholera, in *Snow on Cholera. A Reprint of Two Papers by John Snow,* Hafner, New York, 1965, 1.

63. Barua, D., Survival of cholera vibrios in food, water and fomites, in Principles and Practice of Cholera Control, Public Health Paper No. 40, World Health Organization, Geneva, 1970, 29.

64. Basu, S., Bhattachorya, P., and Mukerjee, S., Interaction of *Vibrio cholerae* and *Vibrio El Tor, Bull. W.H.O.,* 34, 371, 1966.

65. Gallut, J. and Quiniou, J., Interactions de *Vibrio cholerae* classique, *V. cholerae* biotype El Tor et vibrions, NAG, *Bull. W.H.O.,* 42, 464, 1970.

66. Bart, K. J., Huq, Z., Khan, M., and Mosley, W. H., Seroepidemiologic studies during a simultaneous epidemic of infection with El Tor Ogawa and classical Inaba *Vibrio cholerae, J. Infect. Dis.,* Suppl. 121, 17, 1970.

67. Kaneko, T. and Colwell, R. R., Incidence of *Vibrio parahaemolyticus* in Chesapeake Bay, *Appl. Microbiol.,* 31, 251, 1975.

68. Kaneko, T. and Colwell, R. A., Adsorption of *Vibrio parahaemolyticus* onto chitin and copepods, *Appl. Microbiol.,* 29, 269, 1975.

69. Liston, J., Influence of U.S. seafood handling procedures on *Vibrio parahaemolyticus,* in *Int. Symp. Vibrio parahaemolyticus,* Fuijino, T., Sakaguchi, G., Sakazaki, R., and Takeda, Y., Eds., Saikon, Tokyo, 1974, 123.

70. Zen-Yoji, H., Sakai, S., Kudoh, Y., Itoh, T., and Terayama, T., Antigenic schema and epidemiology of *Vibrio parahaemolyticus, Health Lab. Sci.,* 7, 100, 1970.

71. Kudoh, Y., Sakai, S., Zen-Yoji, H., and Le Clair, R. A., Epidemiology of food poisoning due to *Vibrio parahaemolyticus* occurring in Tokyo during the last decade, in *Int. Symp. Vibrio parahaemolyticus,* Fuijino, T., Sakaguchi, G., Sakazaki, R., and Takeda, Y., Eds., Saikon, Tokyo, 1974, 9.

72. Baross, J. A., Liston, J., and Morita, R. Y., Some implications of genetic exchange among marine vibrios, including *Vibrio parahaemolyticus,* naturally occurring in the Pacific oyster, in *Int. Symp. Vibrio parahaemolyticus,* Fuijino, T., Sakaguchi, G., Sakazaki, R., and Takeda, Y., Eds., Saikon, Tokyo, 1974, 129.

73. **Barua, D.**, Laboratory diagnosis of cholera cases and carriers, in Principles and Practice of Cholera Control, Public Health Paper No. 40, World Health Organization, Geneva, 1970, 47.
74. **Feeley, J. C.**, Isolation of cholera vibrios by positive-recognition plating procedures, *J. Bacteriol.*, 84, 866, 1962.
75. **Balows, A., Herman, G. J., and De Witt, W. E.**, The isolation and identification of *Vibrio cholerae*—a review, *Health Lab. Sci.*, 8, 167, 1971.
76. **Schrank, G. D., Stager, C. E., and Verwey, W. F.**, Differential medium for *Vibrio cholerae*, *Infect. Immun.*, 7, 827, 1973.
77. **Chun, D., Chung, J. K., and Seol, S. Y.**, Enrichment of *Vibrio parahaemolyticus* in a simple medium, *Appl. Microbiol.*, 27, 1124, 1974.
78. **Twedt, R. M. and Novelli, R.**, Modified selective medium for *Vibrio parahaemolyticus*, *Appl. Microbiol.*, 22, 593, 1971.
79. **Vanderzant, C., Nickelson, R., and Hazelwood, R. W.**, Effect of isolation-enumeration procedures on the recovery of normal and stressed cells of *Vibrio parahaemolyticus*, in *Int. Symp. Vibrio parahaemolyticus*, Fuijino, T., Sakaguchi, G., Sakazaki, R., and Takeda, Y., Eds., Saikon, Tokyo, 1974, 111.
80. **Vanderzant, C. and Nickelson, R.**, Procedure for isolation and enumeration of *Vibrio parahaemolyticus*, *Appl. Microbiol.*, 23, 26, 1972.
81. **Hollis, D. G., Weaver, R. E., Baker, C. N., and Thornsberry, C.**, Halophilic *Vibrio* species isolated from blood cultures, *J. Clin. Microbiol.*, 3, 425, 1976.
82. **Carpenter, C. C. J.**, Cholera: diagnosis and treatment, *Bull. N.Y. Acad. Med.*, 47, 1192, 1971.
83. **Nalin, D. R. and Cash, R. A.**, Oral or nasogastric therapy for cholera, in Principles and Practices of Cholera Control, Public Health Paper No. 40, World Health Organization, Geneva, 1970, 73.
84. **Sack, R. B., Cassells, J., Mitra, R., Merritt, C., Butler, T., Thomas, J., Jacobs, B., Chaudhuri, A., and Mondal, A.**, The use of oral replacement solutions in the treatment of cholera and other severe diarrhoeal disorders, *Bull. W.H.O.*, 43, 351, 1970.
85. **Nalin, D. R., Cash, R. A., and Rahman, M.**, Oral (or nasogastric) maintenance therapy for cholera patients in all age-groups, *Bull. W.H.O.*, 43, 361, 1970.
86. **Greenough, W. B., III, Gordon, R. S., Jr., Rosenberg, I. S., Davies, B. I., and Benenson, A. S.**, Tetracycline in the treatment of cholera, *Lancet*, 1, 355, 1964.
87. **Lindenbaum, J., Greenough, W. B., and Islam, M. R.**, Antibiotic therapy of cholera in children, *Bull. W.H.O.*, 37, 529, 1967.
88. **Wallace, C. K., Anderson, P. N., Brown, T. C., Khanra, S. R., Lewis, G. W., Pierce, N. F., Sanyal, S. N., Segre, G. V., and Waldman, R. H.**, Optimal antibiotic therapy in cholera, *Bull. W.H.O.*, 39, 239, 1968.
89. **Blake, P. A., Rosenberg, M. L., Bandiera Costa, J., et al.**, Cholera in Portugal, 1974. I. Modes of transmission, *Am. J. Epidemiol.*, 105, 337, 1977.
90. **Baine, W. B., Zampieri, A., Mazzotti, M., et al.**, Epidemiology of cholera in Italy in 1973, *Lancet*, 2, 1370, 1974.
91. **Azurin, J. C., Kobari, K., et al.**, A long term carrier of cholera: cholera Delores, *Bull. W.H.O.*, 37, 745, 1967.
92. **Gangarosa, E. J., Saghori, H., et al.**, Detection of *Vibrio cholera* biotype El Tor by purging, *Bull. W.H.O.*, 34, 363, 1966.

PSEUDOTUBERCULAR YERSINIOSIS

P. L. Stovell

THE DISEASE

Definition

This zoonotic bacterial disease is characterized principally by necrotizing, granulomatous abscesses. Typically, the clinical signs indicate a lymphadenopathy of the ileocecal area with pain focalized in the right lower quadrant (RLQ) of the abdomen. Its spread is apparently through direct or indirect contact with a wide range of potential animal hosts. The disease probably arose in Europe where with the exception of the Mediterranean littoral, including the Iberian Peninsula,[1] the prevalence of human pseudotuberculosis remains high.[2] Current awareness of human infection dates from the 1953 diagnosis of *Yersinia pseudotuberculosis* infection in abscess-forming reticulocytic lymphadenitis of the mesentary (ARLM) in Germany.[3,4]

First Discovery

The disease was first discovered almost a century ago in laboratory guinea pigs in France, wherein it undoubtedly represented an exaltation of latent infection, following the inoculation of human tubercular material.[5,6] Yersinial pseudotuberculosis due to *Y. pseudotuberculosis* in guinea pig production herds or laboratory colonies has been frequently reported since that historic event. The triggering of latent infections by inoculation or other stresses imposed on guinea pigs and rabbits is now generally recognized.[2,7] This raises potential problems in the use of latently infected animals for bacterial isolation or virulence-testing purposes.

The first recognized human infection with *Yersinia pseudotuberculosis,* a terminal case of the rare septicemic form, was diagnosed in 1909.[8] About the same time Albrecht[9] observed the first localized form which presented itself as a pseudoappendicitis in a 15-year-old boy. This report with its commendable clinical microbiology and epidemiological deductions concerning possible animal hosts (cats) and reservoirs (synanthropic rodents) evidently did not receive the attention it deserved until 40 years later. In recent years the RLQ syndrome of pseudotuberculosis has been termed pseudoappendicitis by several clinicians.

Relative Importance in Animals and Man

In many species of mammals and birds this disease reachs epizootic proportions, often on a large scale and accompanied by extremely high mortalities.[10-13] In man, with the exception of the rare septicemic form that usually appears in patients predisposed from other causes, the normally sporadic disease usually runs a benign course and epidemics of the clinical infection are rare. Sporadic cases in lower animals including primates are by contrast frequently fatal and usually first diagnosed at post-mortem.

Comparisons with Other Key Yersinioses — Plague and Enterocolitis

Y. pseudotuberculosis lacks the lethal virulence of the plague bacillus for man and synanthropic rodents. It has no known arthropod cycle and no pneumonogenic capability or the associated aerogenic transmission route of *Yersinia pestis*. On the other hand, *Y. pseudotuberculosis* has a considerably greater host range. This extends beyond the rodents and lagomorphs to numerous wild and exotic mammals and birds and a number of species of domestic livestock and pets. In marked contrast to plague, the usual transmission route is apparently oral, principally, it must be assumed, through the fecal connection, whereas the severe primary gastrointestinal lesions with clinical signs are so characteristic of enterocolitis due to *Yersinia enterocolitica;* these are absent in human pseudotuberculosis where symptoms of pseudoappendicitis are typically first to appear.

While both diseases may cause an RLQ syndrome in humans, this is proportionately more frequent in pseudotuberculosis than enterocolitis.[1,2] *Y. pseudotuberculosis* produces characteristic necrogranulomatous lesions in an extremely wide spectrum of hosts, including birds. While in some species such lesions are found to involve *Y. enterocolitia,*[14] in general these features are absent or reduced in enterocolitis.[12] Yersinial enterocolitis has by contrast a wider geographic occurrence[1] but lacks some of the seasonal influences that cause marked annual or biannual fluctuations in the prevalence of pseudotubercular yersiniosis.

Despite the foregoing, recent information seems to indicate that in Northeast Europe the proportionate incidence of *Y. enterocolitica* involvement in the syndrome has increased dramatically. Current observations of human *Y. enterocolitica* infections in North America seem to indicate seasonal fluctuations similar to those accepted in Europe for *Y. pseudotuberculosis* of both man and animals.

THE ETIOLOGIC AGENT

Classification and Terminology

Yersinia pseudotuberculosis is still occasionally referred to as the bacillus of Malassez and Vignal but was actually termed by these discoverers "the organism of tuberculose zoogleique" in 1883.[5] Eberth,[15] 2 years later, first used the term pseudotuberculosis, considered by some to be semantically incorrect,[16] for the lesions in rabbits and guinea pigs. The name pseudotuberculosis is considered inappropriate for the organism as well as for the disease process;[13] however, it later became quite commonly used for both purposes.

After numerous reports under several generic designations,[17] this organism was named for the genus *Pasteurella* in 1929.[18] It thus joined the closely related[19] plague bacillus of Yersin, the isolation of which, in 1894, followed that of the pseudotuberculosis bacillus by 11 years. There was a period of further confusion during which additional generic designations were used. Workers meanwhile became aware of another etiologic entity, now known as *Yersinia enterocolitica,* in association with certain pseudotuberculosis-like cases as well as the more typical gastroenteritis or enterocolitis. Following a taxonomic study of the genus *Pasteurella* with recommendations,[19] the original agent of pseudotuberculosis, *P. X* and *P. pestis* were transferred to form the genus *Yersinia.*[18] This genus was later listed with the Enterobacteriaceae in the eighth edition of *Bergey's Manual.*[24] Meyer[21] indicated that the term pseudotuberculosis must be reserved strictly for infections caused by *Pasteurella* (now *Yersinia*) *pseudotuberculosis,* whereas Wetzler[22] suggested the inclusion of *Y. enterocolitica.* Mair[1] devoted a special footnote to the confusion in the veterinary literature caused by the use of the term pseudotuberculosis for other entities than *Y. pseudotuberculosis* infection. These entities have even included aspergillosis.[23] The alternate designation yersiniosis was recommended for infections due to either the *pseudotuberculosis* or the *enterocoliticum* spp.;[1] however, this also suffers from the disadvantage of nonspecificity that may become compounded should new members be added to the genus. The name pseudotuberculosis remains the species epithet and the term is deeply embedded in both the early and recent literature (of this disease). Clearly, the clinician, laboratorian, epidemiologist, and others should expect to encounter yersiniosis caused by either of the two species just mentioned. In some areas, or in rodents and their arthropods, they should also be prepared to deal with *Y. pestis.* For specific discussions, probably Meyer's suggestion should be followed. This is to reserve use of the term pseudotuberculosis for general reference to the disease and immunogenic processes of *Y. pseudotuberculosis.*

For clinical assessment and diagnostic bacteriology of cases resembling pseudotuberculosis, the suggestion of Wetzler[12,13] may be most practicable. The term pseudotuberculosis should be reserved exclusively for zoonotic disease in man, lower mammals, or birds caused by either of the two *Yersinia* species, *Y. pseudotuberculosis* or *Y. enterocolitica.* The more specific terms yersiniosis due to *Y. enterocolitica* or simply enterocolitis would naturally take precedence when appropriate.

Cell Morphology and Staining

The cells are generally coccobacillary, pleomorphic, round-ended, straight of axis, noncapsulated, and nonspore-forming. They stain Gram negative. Strains vary in the presentation of groups, short chains or filaments with straight or curved axis.[16,24] Long, curved filaments are not uncommon.[25] Cell sizes according to various authors are for some strains 0.8 to 2.0 × 0.8 μm, and for others 1.5 to 5.0 × 0.6 μm,[25] 0.8 to 6.0 × 0.8 μm,[16] or 1.5 to 5.0 × 0.5 μm.[21]

Most cells are coccobacilli or ovoid forms of less than 1.0 μm in length. Cells are motile at 22 to 27°C by means of one to six peritrichate flagella[25] or one to two mostly parapolarly located flagella four to five times longer than the bacterium, with occasional single rods showing peritrichous flagella.[21] A viscous layer or envelope may be visible in india ink preparations of growth at 22°C incubation.[21]

The cells stain with bipolarity of various degrees in Gram's counterstain, whereas with Wayson's plague stain[26,27] the bipolarity is distinct to dramatic;[11] especially notable are the banded, filamentous forms.[11,25] A mild acid-fastness can be discerned with Cook's method[28] and this quality can be further accentuated with the use of Macchiavello's rickettsia stain.[11] *Y. pseudotuberculosis* and in some cases also *Y. enterocolitica* bacilli in tissues may stain satisfactorily for visibility with the following: Hansen's brucella stain,[29] routine H & E,[11,30] Gram's method for sections,[14,30] Ollett's modification of Twort's stain for Gram-negative bacteria,[11] and occasionally the blue counterstain for regular acid-fast smears with suspect mycobacteria.[31]

Y. pseudotuberculosis is thought to be less regular than *Y. pestis,* the plague bacillus, in its uptake of bipolar stain;[21] however, some freshly isolated animal strains (canary and guinea pig) show intense bipolarity.[11,32] Wetzler[22] states that most isolates of *Y. pseudotuberculosis* are markedly bipolar with Wayson's stain, whereas *Y. enterocolitica* rarely demonstrates this phenomenon.

Growth Physiology

This microorganism is aerobic and facultatively anaerobic,[16] growing especially well in the presence of abundant oxygen.[21] The optimal pH range is thought to be as great as 6.0 to 8.0[21] although a somewhat narrower range, 6.3 to 7.3, is also given.[25] Acidification is thought to favor rough dissociation.[21] Optimum growth temperature is 27 to 30°C[17,25] with a growth range of 5 to 43°C[25] or below 42°C.[16] The optimum temperature for abundant growth may be as high as 37°C,[24] but this temperature favors and accelerates dissociation. The optimum temperature for motility is probably 22°C with a range of 18 to 27°C. Wetzler[22] states that the yersiniae may be cultivated in the temperature range 4 to 40°C, with optimal production of structures assured in the narrow range of 20 to 28°C. It can thus be seen that *Y. pseudotuberculosis* is a psychrotroph and isolation should be performed routinely at room temperatures in order to conserve the virulence potential and to preserve the smooth somatic antigenic components.[22] Also of considerable interest is the characteristic in vivo environment of *Y. pseudotuberculosis* that is a facultatively or electively intracellular parasite.[33-37] This fact is related to various characteristics of virulence, latency, and immune response in the disease pathogenesis. *Y. pseudotuberculosis* produces good growth on ordinary media and its nutritional requirements may be less at 28°C than at 37°C.[38] It attacks carbohydrates fermentatively without gas production and is oxidase negative and catalase positive.

Cultivation

Strains of *Y. pseudotuberculosis* grow easily on meat-extract media; in broth the S phase produces a uniform turbidity and after several days a sediment. The R phase strains grow without producing turbidity.[24] Fresh isolants give a uniform turbidity for 1 to 2 days in beef heart-infusion broth incubated at routine temperatures (35 to 37°C). Following this, the broth usually clears leaving a ring at the surface and a heavily flocculent sediment.[11] Growth is diffuse at 22°C; clumped masses and occasionally ring and pellicle formation are seen.[21] On solid medium containing serum or blood, most smooth to slimy, light, transparent colonies reach a diameter of 2 to 3 mm by 48 hr; at 37°C the colonies are thin, dry, irregular with rough edges.[21] Colonies observed from 24 to 72 hr on nutrient and blood agar develop from low convex to umbonate; from smooth shiny to granular (sometimes coarsely so); from being completely translucent to greyish-yellow and opaque; and from having entire edges to showing effusive edges with radial striations stretching back to the umbonate center.[11] No hemolysis is produced on blood agar.

Occasionally, rare chromogenic cultures may develop at temperatures below 24°C and possess unusual biochemical or fermentative characteristics.[39] Normally pigmentation, especially of virulent cultures, occurs only on a special medium containing hemin with incubation at 28°C.[40] Shifts from S to R or intermediate types are largely influenced by high temperatures, composition of the media, and age of the cultures.[21] The factor of acidification was mentioned under discussion of pH.

The pseudotuberculosis agent propagates readily on all the usual enteric selective media at ambient temperatures achieving maximal and characteristic growth in less than 48 hr. Preferred media would include eosin methylene blue (EMB), MacConkey, desoxycholate citrate (DCC), Endo, and tergitol 7 agar.[22]

On MacConkey medium colonies are inclined to show granularity at 24 hr; they are more effusive at the edges and inclined to lyse after 72 hr.[11] Both MacConkey and deoxyribonuclease agar have been used for primary differentiation of *Y. enterocolitica* from other lactose-negative bacterial colonies. Both media may be modified by the addition of Tween-80® and in the case of the latter medium also sorbitol.[41] Meyer considered Endo to be the most satisfactory of the salmonella-diagnostic media; whereas DCC agar, recommended for differentiation of *Y. pestis* from *Y. pseudotuberculosis,* may suppress visible colony formation of the latter.[21]

Biocharacterization

Details and procedures for the generic identification, biodifferentiation, and serotyping of cultural isolants can be found in a number of readily available publications.[16,21,24,25,42]

Serotypes and Antigenic Structure

The optima in temperature and pH for antigen production and the general antigenic

Table 1
ANTIGENIC STRUCTURE OF *YERSINIA PSEUDOTUBERCULOSIS*

O group	O subgroup	R antigen	Thermostable O antigens	Thermolabile H antigens
I	A	(1)	2, 3	a, c
	B	(1)	2, 4	a, c
II	A	(1)	5, 6	a, d
	B	(1)	5, 7	a, d
III	—	(1)	8	a
IV	A	(1)	9, 11	b or a, b
	B	(1)	9, 12	a, b, d
V	A	(1)	10, 14	a; a, e, (b)
	B		10, 15	a
VI	—	(1)	13?	a

Note: By the indirect hemagglutination test a heat-stable somatic antigen common to all types can be demonstrated.[46]

From Thal, E. and Knapp, W., *Symposia Series in Immunological Standardization*, S. Karger, Basel, 1971, 219. With permission.

relationships between members of the yersiniae are adequately discussed in various publications.[25,39,43,44] Table 1 shows the currently accepted antigenic structure of *Y. pseudotuberculosis* as outlined by Thal and Knapp.[45] According to Mollaret and Thal,[24] serological cross-reactions with other organisms and certain of the six serotypes of *Y. pseudotuberculosis* are common. The similarity between antigen (1), present in all types of *Y. pseudotuberculosis,* and a similar (R) antigen complex of *Y. pestis* accounts for the ability of the former to stimulate cross-protection against plague.[24,47]

Relationships exist between *Y. pseudotuberculosis* type II and O-factors 4 and 27 of the *Salmonella* B group and between *Y. pseudotuberculosis* type IV and O-factors 9 and 46 of the *Salmonella* D group and O-factor 14 of the *Salmonella* H group. Cross-reactions have been found between *Y. pseudotuberculosis* type IV A and *Escherichia coli* O groups 17 and 77, and *Enterobacter cloacae.*[48] Recently, an antigenic relationship was reported by Mair[48] between *Y. pseudotuberculosis* type VI (Japanese strains) and *E. coli* O-group 55.[48]

Infectivity and Virulence Including Toxicity

Recently, Mair isolated a number of avirulent, apathogenic, and atoxic type III strains from healthy swine in Britain.[49] Thal has discussed studies of a type III strain isolated from a field mouse by Mair.[47] This strain was avirulent and atoxic but immunogenic, being protective for nontoxic strains. Thus the qualities of infectivity are not necessarily bound to those of virulence, at least insofar as gut infections are concerned.

Among the six properties of virulence in plague strains noted by Jackson and Burrows (1956) and still considered valid[25] are two related characteristics that apply to *Y. pseudotuberculosis*. These are the formation of V and W antigens (i.e., VW+) and resistance to phagocytosis. The former probably applies fully, whereas the latter is somewhat modified in *Y. pseudotuberculosis*. A loss of virulence analagous to that observed with *Y. pestis* takes place with the mutation from VW+ to VW- of *Y. pseudotuberculosis*.[50] Brubaker and Yang's in vitro experiments suggested that these antigens are only produced within phagocytic cells. Accordingly, VW antigens may be necessary to ensure long-term intracellular survival or they may be associated with the ability to multiply within fixed macrophages of the reticuloendothelium system.[34]

When conditions were created in media to resemble the mammalian intracellular environment, the growth of VW⁺ cells was favored. The virulence antigens may evolve in preparation for intracellular residence.[34] The role of toxins in the pathogenesis of yersinial pseudotuberculosis is not clear. This is principally because of inadequate studies of endotoxins.[21] Thal studied the exotoxins of type III strains in bacterial-free filtrates.[51] Meyer felt that some type III strains possessed both endo- and exotoxins, the thermolabile (latter) component being easily converted into toxoid by formaldehyde. This is highly lethal for rabbits, rats, and mice and to a lesser degree for guinea pigs.[21] Wilson and Miles[25] discussed the phage lysates of some strains of *Y. pseudotuberculosis* that were found by Lazarus and Nozawa (1948) to be toxic to mice. The toxin was inactivated by heating to 60°C for 30 min; it was thus more heat labile than the murine toxin of the plague bacillus. The toxicity appears to be associated with the polysaccharide present in each of the five serological types of the pseudotubercle bacillus (Davies 1958). That present in group III seems to be particularly potent. Polysaccharides extracted from rough strains differ from the smooth polysaccharides and are related to the rough polysaccharide of *Y. pestis*.[25]

Wetzler[12] feels there is no reason to believe that *Y. pseudotuberculosis* strains are enhanced in virulence by animal passage. He suspects the reverse to be true if the major parasitic virulence factor is the VW antigen. Either an extremely virulent strain of *Y. pseudotuberculosis* must be disseminated among highly sensitive hosts or a prestressing of the susceptible population must be assured, with or without a strain of extreme virulence, in order for epizootics to occur of disease with high mortality, examples of which are given. The pathogenicity for laboratory animals is discussed below.

HISTORY AND WORLD DISTRIBUTION

Origin of Agent

The apparent origin and one of the heaviest concentrations of the *Yersinia pseudotuberculosis* agent is in Northern and Central Europe. This could well be due to an original (transmutation) source of this bacillus in the agent of medieval plague. The theories of Devignat and others in this regard[52,53] were supported by Mollaret[2] and the work of Burrows and Bacon[50] in the study of virulence factors. The studies of Korobkova[54] and others concerning transmutation of *Y. pestis* to *Y. pseudotuberculosis* embrace this theory that has received recent favorable comment.[1,55] In any case, whether or not correct or provable, this theory is a useful one for its effect in underlining the close similarities between these organisms. It stimulates further research into immunogenic cross-protection and bacterial genetics. The cross-protective capabilities against plague of avirulent but invasive strains of *Y. pseudotuberculosis*[21,47] make the role of reservoir hosts of current and future importance. Dynamics of the sylvatic forms of both plague and pseudotuberculosis may be profoundly influenced by the natural immunization of reservoir populations.

Dynamics of Pseudotuberculosis

Examination of some first or early reports of pseudotuberculosis in various species and areas has yielded more questions than answers on most aspects of the dynamics of this disease. A few examples follow. There seems no cause to doubt the established preexistence of the agent, in European rodents and wild birds at least, at the time of the first discovery in 1883. This occurrence came in the dawn of pathogenic bacteriology, less than 5 years after the works of Kitt[56] and of Pasteur, whose name was given to the former genus of *Y. pseudotuberculosis*. As early as the following year (1884), Zuern was reported to have encountered this disease agent in canaries in Dresden.[57]

In 1885 Eberth,[15] as previously mentioned, reported disease of rabbits and guinea pigs in Germany and Nocard reported infections in birds in the Low Countries.[58] By the end of that decade, an infected horse in Leipzig[59] and another canary epizootic in Dresden[60] were reported. This rapid sequence of reports seems to suggest preexistence also in canaries, rabbits, and guinea pigs, now recognized as susceptible victims of synanthropic carrier hosts. During the next 30 years, infections were reported in a cow in 1897[61] and more guinea pigs in 1900,[7] both in Italy; yellow buntings in Germany[62] in 1903; pigeons in Hanover[63] in 1916, and a cat in France in 1920.[64] Meanwhile, a series of additional reports on canary outbreaks came from Germany and neighboring countries up to the outbreak of World War I in 1914. In this period came the first report of pseudotuberculosis in canaries in North America by Kinyoun in 1906.[65] The reported occurrences of human pseudotuberculosis commencing in 1909 are discussed elsewhere. Up to 1953 they were few in number because only the rare, often-fatal septicemic form was recognized. Only in areas where the localized forms and manifestations of infection are readily recognized and regularly reported can the human prevalence (sentinels) serve as an indication of disease dynamics in the animal population. As will be seen, such indications are currently revealing in Europe.

The disease in turkeys was first reported in 1924, also in Germany,[66] and this was followed by a series of reports during the next decade from Germany, France, and Sweden. Not until 1944 did the disease appear in turkeys in the U.S., when a massive outbreak occurred in Oregon involving 19 flocks.[67] Apart from one additional turkey death in California 10 years later,[68] the disease seems not to have recurred generally in North American turkeys. In Europe meanwhile, in 1925, the importation of live poultry into Denmark was banned because of pasteurellosis including pseudotuberculosis. Sporadic chronic or subacute infections were still occurring in fowl in that country 29 years later.[69] Also in 1925, Wayson revealed the presence of this bacterium in wild rats of the San Francisco Bay area.[70] The disease was reported in a goat in 1927 in Germany,[71] field hares in Croatia, Yugoslavia in 1929,[72] the muskrat in Germany in 1934,[73] and further hare outbreaks in Hungary in 1938[74] and Yugoslavia in various years.[72] Also in 1938, the first isolation was made from a synanthropic rodent, also a rat, in the U.S.[75] In the following year a single case was reported in a blackbird in New Jersey.[76] This infection was considered so rare in North American birds that the author wrote a full review of avian pseudotuberculosis. At this point, one could be inclined to pause and wonder what, if anything, was taking place just across the English Channel in Britain and across the Baltic in the Scandinavian Peninsula. At the same time it could be wondered if the widespread disease did really exist at that time in North America or was only occasionally introduced in ship-borne rats or infected animal stocks from Europe. Subsequent events provided data that exceeded expectations for the first question, eliminated hopes of answering the second, and raised additional questions. Within the next decade the disease was recorded in swine in Scandinavia[77] and, in response to appropriate research, in rodents in the U.S.S.R.[78] In 1948, a case was reported in a chinchilla in the U.S.[79] and this was followed in quick succession by further reports from Oregon in 1950 and Washington in 1952.[80] Meanwhile in Britain, Blaxland in 1947 reported outbreaks on eight turkey premises in the English midlands and in synanthropic rodents (rats) on two of those premises.[81] In 1953, Clapham[82] studied an avian epizootic among stock doves and other wild birds in England, including a wood pigeon. These findings were extended in 1962 by the report of Paterson and Cook[83] involving losses of 1000 experimental guinea pigs in repeated epizootics. The disease had its source in the dietary field greens that were soiled with droppings of infected wood pigeons (*Columba palambus*). Six years after the localized form of human pseudotuberculosis was reported in Germany in 1953,

Mair recognized the first human cases in England.[84] In the next 6 years (1961 to 1966 inclusive) Mair[85] received 188 isolants of animal origin in addition to 11 from guinea pigs in the home laboratory. Of the total 199 isolants, 58 came from farm animals and domestic pets, 46 from experimental animals, 45 from free-living species, and 50 from wild animals living in captivity. Returning to events in Scandinavia at the beginning of the 1950s, Thal[51,86] worked on 186 strains of which 119 were of Swedish origin. The hares were represented by 75 strains and turkeys by 16. The non-Swedish strains were mostly from Denmark, Germany, Holland, and England. In North America, the disease in chinchillas was widely recognized and acknowledged in breeder-organization bulletins and by one veterinary biologics company that put out a chinchilla mixed killed bacterin containing no less than nine species of bacteria including *Y. pseudotuberculosis*.[87] A number of infections came to light in Canada commencing in 1953 with an isolant in British Columbia from a bovine mesenteric lymph node[31] that had been sent to the laboratory for tuberculosis examination and found negative. From 1955 to 1956, Langford obtained isolants from three chinchillas, a beaver, a muskrat, and a hare in Alberta. The following year he isolated it again from chinchillas in British Columbia.[88] In 1958, Stovell[11] isolated the pseudotuberculosis bacillus from large numbers of canaries in three British Columbia aviaries (the second one diagnosed by Langford)[88] and carried out investigative and experimental work on fecal transmission in canaries. He also diagnosed infection in a herd of guinea pigs on a dairy farm.[32] Imported birds were not involved in the canary epizootics studied; however, on several separate occasions then, and over the next 10 years, additional cases came to light in British Columbia canaries and other cage birds, some of which were imported from Europe,[11] and chinchillas and cattle, some of which were reported by Langford.[88,89] Meanwhile, human cases of ARLM (or acute appendicitis) due to pseudotuberculosis came to light in British Columbia and Alberta.[39,90,91] Also during this time (1959 to 1960) a massive epizootic of pseudotuberculosis took place in grackles occupying a large icterid roost in Maryland.[10] By 1967, Wetzler[39] had accumulated data on nine human strains isolated in North America (including one from Alberta), 10 from birds, and 19 from wild and domestic animals. Meanwhile, it was the common impression among Scandinavian workers that chinchillas imported to Denmark and Sweden from the North American Pacific Northwest subseqeuently proved infected with the bacilli of both pseudotuberculosis and enterocolitis (both types of yersiniosis infection).[92] Some additional and more recent episodes of pseudotuberculosis are listed or discussed in special groupings under species distribution.

Conclusions and Questions

The prevalence of the disease in humans apparently reflects the level of infection in the animal hosts in areas of clinical and microbiological awareness. The closeness of this reflection may be related in some cases to rural location and community agriculture, rather than to purely ethnic or economic factors. However, sanitation levels for both farms and communities must have a major influence. A number of questions arise from even this miniscule attempt to examine the dynamics of the disease in animals.

1. Is pseudotuberculosis an ancient or a relatively new disease?
2. Was pseudotuberculosis in animals actually on the move of its own volition during the last 75 years, or was the diagnostic increase merely a reflection of disruptive wars and scientific, technological, economic, and sociologic changes? Is the disease in fact quite slow moving or virtually static?
3. Was the disease prevalence in North America less than in Europe at the time of first discovery? If so, is it still less or likely to remain less?

4. Can the relatively late appearance of the disease in England and its high current incidence or prevalence in humans and many animals all be attributed to recently acquired awareness? If so, can the former hypothetical lack of awareness of the disease in animals in Britain be attributed merely to island insularity and language communication difficulties? If so, to what extent can this be blamed on the two world wars?

5. Are most or all of these questions pointless until the basics of predisposition, stress, and pathogenesis of clinical infections, especially epizootics, become better understood?

6. Is it possible that transmission takes place in lower animals at subclinical levels so that exhaustive surveys of trapped animals, road-kills, and animals dead of other causes is required to assess incidence?

7. If such surveys for pseudotubercular and enterocolitic yersiniosis become more general, will this pay dividends also in a better assessment of residual sylvatic or synanthropic plague?

Disease Distribution

A partial list of the animal hosts that are known to suffer epizootics, sporadic, or latent infections is presented in arbitrary groupings. These allocations for both wild and managed populations are based primarily on considerations of habitat and epidemiological potential. They relate to probable roles in the interspecies spread of infection and possibilities of human contact.

Sylvatic Reservoir Hosts

Beaver and muskrat — Beaver and muskrat infections were reported in Finland[93] and Sweden.[51] Beaver alone in Canada; Alberta,[88] British Columbia,[11] and Ontario.[94]

Field mice — Field mice infections were detected in Czechoslovakia[95] and Russia (meadow vole),[78] and in Germany fecal isolations were made.[96]

Wild rats — The available information on rats is slight and most of that appears to represent synanthropic rats. Only Wayson discovered infection in wild rats (San Francisco).[70] Haas reported infection in a domestic rat in the U.S.[75]

Squirrels — One mention only came to attention. This appeared in Wetzler's table;[13] however, no reference is given.

Lagomorphs (other than when taken as game) — Occurrences in hares have been reported from Denmark,[97] Germany,[98] Poland,[99] Italy,[7] Scotland,[100] and Yugoslavia.[72]

Wild rabbit — Infections have occurred in France,[2] Poland,[99] and Italy.[7]

Other mammals — Marten and hedgehog infections were reported from Switzerland.[101]

Birds (wild) — Pigeons and doves appear to be the most common hosts with outbreaks being reported in England,[82] Denmark,[69] Germany,[63] France,[102] and the U.S.[30] Infections in buntings were reported in England,[103] Denmark,[69] and Germany.[62] The organism has been detected in various galliformes in England,[104] Denmark,[69] France,[105] and Sweden.[106] Miscellaneous species such as waxwings in Denmark,[69] swans in France,[107] an owl in Sweden,[92] crows and martens in Canada,[94] jackdaws and rooks in England,[82] and grackles in the U.S.[10] have also been been reported to harbor the organism.

Hosts Involved in Sylvatic Epizootics

Rodents — It may be some time before the question of natural epizootics in rodents can be resolved. It appears that apart from the U.S.S.R. and some countries wholly in Eastern Europe, the role of rodents, even as reservoir hosts, has been very little explored although most writers emphasize their importance in this role. On a number of occasions, rodent epizootics have been suspected on the basis of appearance of the disease in associated hosts coupled with recorded drops from peak population densities. Two examples from the Canadian Pacific Northwest are drops in muskrat population associated with diagnosis in a beaver and a field mouse population drop associated with epizootics in canaries.[11] On other occasions laboratory populations of species normally sylvatic have suffered severe losses, as in the case of *Microtus aggrestis*.[108] There seems little doubt that *Yersinia pseudotuberculosis* requires the presence of stressor factors to reach epizootic proportions.[11,12] To what extent this may be due to the prior presence of low-virulence or avirulent immunogenic strains[47,109] in the natural milieu or population is conjectural at present.

Lagomorphs — Most of the available information is on hares; epizootics have been recorded in Scandinavian countries,[97] Yugoslavia,[72] Italy,[7] possibly in Hungary[74] that was the source of infected hares imported to the game reserves in Italy, and in many other countries.

Birds — Epizootics in wild birds undoubtedly far outnumber the cases that have come to attention. The latter include grackles in Maryland,[10] stock doves in Hampshire, England; probably also wood pigeons[82] and martins in Ontario, Canada.[94] It is important to note the presence of wild birds of other species that did not suffer mortalities in the icterid roosts[10] and of species not far removed from the wild in canary aviaries where mortalities of that principal species approached 100%.[11] There is probably little point in distinguishing among the frequency of epizootics in sylvatic, farm, and zoological environments or aviaries exposed to the exterior because of the greater mobility of birds and the degree of mingling that takes place between wild and domestic or zoo species.

Game Animals

The significance of sylvatic species that are reservoir hosts and/or suffer sporadic or epizootic losses is increased considerably when such birds or mammals are taken as game and the carcasses and viscera are disposed of in human and domestic animal-food use.[110] Hares, rabbits, deer, wild and park animals,[39,98,101,110,111] mufflons, pheasants and other galliformes,[12] and pigeons and doves[11,12] are some examples of animals taken in considerable numbers for primarily sporting or subsistence purposes.

Livestock Production Enterprises

From the point of view of distribution and epidemiological significance, the farmed animals (excluding supply colonies for laboratory use) should be considered in four general groups.

1. Production enterprises with food species that supply meat and milk (dairy products), including rabbitries
2. Fancy species that are sold as breeding stock or pets, including commercial aviaries for cage birds
3. Fur animals that are killed on location for the recovery and preservation of pelts only
4. Recreational, demonstration, or institutional farms that are visited by varying numbers of people and may be staffed in part by unskilled, voluntary, or juvenile helpers

Food Production (Farms)

Cattle infections have been encountered on a few occasions in widely separated areas such as British Columbia,[31,89,112] Britain,[113] and Germany.[114,115] In addition, there have been several recent reports of atypical isolants from cattle.[116,117] The two reports from Germany were both concerned with udder lesions or mastitis; however, this is probably rare. Swine are frequently found to be infected with *Y. pseudotuberculosis*. Most recent reports are concerned with the isolation from healthy swine of both virulent and avirulent strains.[39,49,91,118-120] There have been reports of losses also.[77,121] Other farm food mammals involved are sheep[2,99,112,122-125] and goats.[119] There is one recent report of pseudotuberculosis in a foal in England.[126] At least two older reports of infection in horses are available.[11]

Farm epizootics or sporadic infections in domestic rabbits raised for meat production have been reported principally from Japan;[119,127] however, the writer is aware of at least one such epizootic that took place in the Canadian Maritime Provinces within the last decade.[128] Among the domestic fowl, infections of sporadic and epizootic nature have been reported on numerous situations involving chickens, turkeys, and ducks. The disease in chickens is usually slow moving or sporadic and for this reason the dozen or so reports that have come to hand are fragmentary and may not indicate the true prevalence.

Chickens may be quite refractory to experimental infection with virulent turkey or canary strains.[11,81] Among the more recent encounters is a flock infection in Alberta, Canada in 1960.[11] More recently still, there were two mentions of chicken infections in Poland,[99,129] in the latter case associated with human infections.

In turkeys the infection has been more extensive than in other domestic poultry in North America;[39,130] one epizootic involved ten flocks in Oregon[67] and a sporadic case occurred in California.[68] In 1947, Blaxland reported outbreaks involving eight flocks in England.[81] However, as one would expect, there have been many more reports from Continental Europe commencing a little over 50 years ago (perhaps when turkey raising first developed into an industry). Most cases were in Germany, France, and Sweden.

Ducks are considered to be an important host of pseudotuberculosis in France.[131] Infections have also been reported in Yugoslavia, Poland, and Germany[132] where it is encountered in enzootic form.

Fancier Breeding Establishments

The best examples of infections in establishments selling breeding stock or pets are epizootics in canaries and occasionally other cage species including (rarely) budgerigars.[11,88,99] Undoubtedly, many sporadic infections in this class of establishment go unreported because of the critical matter of reputation in selling of breeding stock assumed to be free from disease. In the case of epizootics in canaries and finches, the mortality is often so high[11] as to make a cover-up pointless.

Fur-Farm Animals

There are numerous references in the literature to sporadic and occasionally epizootic infections in mink and nutria (coypu) and at least one involving incidents in silver foxes.[11] Chinchillas have been most frequently involved in fur-farm epizootics, particularly in the North American Pacific Northwest.[11,88] In Europe *Y. enterocoliticum* infection is encountered with even greater frequency than classical pseudotuberculosis in this species.

Recreational, Demonstration, or Institutional Farms

It is difficult to ascertain from the literature to what extent this type of livestock enterprise has been the source of infections reported; however, the possibilities of stress could be similar to those in zoological gardens or game farms and the actual human exposure probably higher.

Synanthropic Animals
Rodents

Most of the studies on synanthropic rodents were carried out in the U.S.S.R. or Eastern Europe. Norway rats *(R. norvegicus)*[133,134] and black rats *(R. rattus)*[134] were found to be reservoirs or main sources of infection in other species. In Poland, *Y. pseudotuberculosis* was isolated from Norway rats only; no isolants were obtained from culturing black rats. House mice *(Mus musculus)* were incriminated as carriers or reservoir hosts in the U.S.S.R.[78,133,134] and in Germany[96] (isolated from 10 of 30 mixed house and field mice). Somov and Martinevsky[133] noted that of 182 strains of *Y. pseudotuberculosis* received in 8 years, 123 came from synanthropic animals and 27 from their parasites.

In England in 1947, Blaxland[81] isolated *Y. pseudotuberculosis* from rats trapped at the only two premises (out of eight) where this was done following outbreaks of the disease in turkeys. Recently, Baskin[30] isolated *Y. pseudotuberculosis* from all of six Norway rats trapped from the area of an outbreak of pseudotuberculosis in exotic mammals at the National Zoological Park, Washington, D.C. These animals had mild or chronic lesions in four naturally occuring cases. Synanthropic species should be studied as part of any investigation of this disease in animals.

Others

The isolation of *Y. pseudotuberculosis* from two pigeons, also by Baskin at the National Zoological Park, points up the fact that in some cases birds also are synanthropic. In this case the rats were more suspect as the source of infection because of their milder lesions; however, in all cases where synanthropic animals are studied in association with outbreaks under way, the issue arises as to whether they initiated the outbreak or merely served as incidental indicators. The cultural data of terminal bowel content or shed-feces samples would be most useful in this regard.

Laboratory Animals — Study Colonies and Supply Herds

Guinea pigs — In laboratory or supply herds, guinea pigs may harbor latent infection or suffer a sporadic or epizootic disease incidence, a fact well known since the original discovery by Malassez and Vignal in France. As in virtually all other hosts, this is especially common in Europe. Reports at hand include England,[83,135] Japan,[119,136] Yugoslavia,[72] Poland,[99] Italy,[7] and British Columbia.[11] Rigby[135] commented on a survey conducted by Seamer and Chesterman in 1967. Of 33 responding laboratories only 20 routinely autopsied dead or culled animals. This could suggest a more widely prevalent disease than is commonly believed. This is especially true in cases of chronic cervical lymphadenitis when animals remain grossly asymptomatic and may even produce exterior-draining cervical abscesses in the manner of plague buboes. The main external source of infection in a guinea pig colony is food and water contaminated with feces of wild birds and rodents.

Rabbits — It is suspected that some of the reports of pseudotuberculosis in Europe, Japan, and elsewhere took place in domestic rabbit stocks that may at times provide replacements or foundation stock for laboratory holding or breeding operations. It is not known, however, whether sporadic or epizootic infections have actually arisen or persisted in rabbits held under laboratory conditions. The disease in wild rabbits has been reported from Poland.[99] Other reports of disease in rabbits emanating from Europe are probably in reference to wild rabbits.[137]

Gerbils — Wetzler[13] reported high susceptibility of mongolian gerbils (*Meriones unguiculatus*) to experimental infection with *Y. pseudotuberculosis;* however, no reports of spontaneous infection have come to attention.

Hamsters — One author[99] has claimed to encounter infection in one or more breeding colonies of hamsters in Poland. This is surprising as hamsters are generally considered to be refractory to artificial infection.[16]

Mice — Only from Poland[99] was a report available indicating infection in breeding colonies of white mice. An epizootic in a managed colony of field mice (*Microtus aggrestis*)[108] is mentioned earlier in this section.

Primates — Wetzler[13] cites two reports dated 1963 of epizootic infection and widespread serological titers, respectively, in primate colonies that took place in Europe; one involved baboons and the other cyanomologous monkeys. The baboon epizootic was repeated a year later among newly arrived animals in the same colony. Hirai[138] reported the loss of 41 patas monkeys over an 8-year period in a Japanese primate center. During 1977 an outbreak of pseudotuberculosis occurred in squirrel monkeys of a primate center in southern California. This has been confirmed as type III *Y. pseudotuberculosis*.[139] Most other reports on primates are thought to represent zoological gardens or other nonexperimental or breeding facilities.

Zoological Gardens

Zoological gardens or parks represent a unique situation where a number of indiginous and exotic species are in close proximity, where frequent additions take place with varying application of quarantine measures, and where control of general sanitation and wild or synanthropic birds and rodents is most difficult to enforce. In addition, the aspects of extremely diverse dietary sources and (prohibited) public feeding pose great problems in feed hygiene. On top of all this there are continuous stresses due to proximity of predator or competitive species, including man, with the boredom and relative claustrophobia of exhibition quarters. For all these reasons coupled with the wide host spectrum of *Y. pseudotuberculosis,* it is not surprising to note that in zoos in England, for example, pseudotuberculosis is consistently reported as most frequent cause of bacterial deaths in mammals and second only to *Mycobacterium tuberculosis* in birds.[140-143] Some of the key zoological species to be infected with *Y. pseudotuberculosis* are toucans,[104,141,144] canaries,[142,143] various primate species such as colobus monkey,[143] patas monkeys,[142,143] wooly monkeys,[141,142] a lemur,[142] marmosets,[143] bush baby[142] and a douricouli,[142] and rodent species sporadically. Deaths in the London Zoo have occurred in a bush-tailed porcupine, an Indian gerbil, an Erxleben's guinea pig, European hares, and in larger numbers in chinchillas.[143]

Pet Animals

Pet animals are of particular importance as potential hosts of zoonotic disease in that they share some or all of the human living areas and to a greater or lesser extent the board. Excretions are frequently voided on the property, on soil surface, or in containers that are handled for disposal. Some pets, such as cats, are predatory hunters and may be free roaming in the area and taking, if not eating, reservoir hosts, such as rodents or birds. Others, such as dogs, may be garbage scavengers and/or eaters of carrion. Dogs and cats, possibly, and others such as rabbits eat feed compounded from cereals of lower grade in terms of, for example, rodent feces or stored subsequent to formulation in conditions below those required for human food standards in terms of protection from rodent and bird feces. Rabbits and others, such as guinea pigs, may be fed raw, green feed of reject material from human food vegetables, such as outside leaves of lettuce or cabbage that are more likely to be fecally soiled in the field, especially from avian sources. On the credit side, pets may be subjected to fewer general physical and reproductive stresses and may benefit from better nutrition, observation, and veterinary care than many other managed animals.

Cats — As noted previously, cats were suspected as a source for the first localized human infection in 1910. A brief review by Mair[145] one decade ago noted the first authenticated case in a cat in Amsterdam in 1902 and subsequent reporting of some 70 additional clinical cases mostly in France and Germany. Further cases have been reported more recently, including three in Britain,[36,146] that with Mair's two, bring the total to five, and one in Australia.[147] One might conservatively estimate, therefore, that the confirmed cases for the Western World could total less than 100. This low figure, in light of a presumably high exposure level, may be partly explained by the observations of Goret[148] that cats are refractory to artificial infection. On the other hand, Mollaret[149] pointed out that cats can become subclinical carriers of pseudotuberculosis, thus extending chronologically the potential spread of infection. Mair felt that the absence of reports may be due to the low percentage of post-mortems conducted on cats dying of chronic illness. Obviously, there is a need for exhaustive fecal-culture surveys of cats and other pets known to be susceptible to natural pseudotuberculosis. Pets that are predatory on rodents and birds may suffer intestinal contusions that would serve as a portal of entry for the infection.[148]

Canaries — Both epizootic and sporadic cases of canary pseudotuberculosis have been widely reported especially in Europe, but also in North America,[11,12,88] especially Canada. Both endemic and import (European) sources have been reported in the Pacific Northwest area (British Columbia). Canaries have a particularly close relationship to living, dining, and in some cases, food preparation areas of domestic dwellings.

Guinea pigs — The incidence of classical yersinial pseudotuberculosis in guinea pigs maintained as pets is strictly conjectural. Probably only a small proportion of guinea pigs culled or dead due to various infections are ever submitted for examination. There is no reason to suppose that pet guinea pigs collectively are better protected or cared for than those in laboratory supply, holding, or experimental colonies. Many pet guinea pigs may come from laboratory supply sources. On the other hand, the degree of exposure of susceptible-age humans to these potential sources of infection is much higher in pet maintenance and breeding situations.

Conclusion

The foregoing list of animal hosts should be sufficient to illustrate the enormous potential for spread of infection in endemic areas. Obviously, the production of overt disease depends on additional elements in the equation such as stress and poor sanitation in the immediate environment of those at risk.

From the sporadic or latent infections alone, one could predict the occurrence of occasional significant or even dramatic outbreaks of clinical yersiniosis in certain conditions. These include entry of the agent to a new area, a major increase in exposure of population to an animal environment, and a specific critical breakdown in hygiene.

HUMAN DISEASE

Susceptibility

Probably most previously unexposed individuals can develop transitory subclinical or latent infections. Children and the aged or debilitated are most susceptible to clinical disease. The establishment of expanding focal lesions and occasional generalized infections must depend somewhat on strain virulence and degree of exposure. General or specific stress factors undoubtedly play a major role in deciding the outcome of preliminary infections.

Prevalence

The higher prevalence among male adolescents[1] may equally reflect cultural sex-bias in type and degree of exposure as much as the level of innate susceptibility in boys. In an outbreak of pseudotubercular yersiniosis involving patients 6 to 15 years of age in three Hungarian villages, 13 of 30 cases (43%) were girls.[74]

The geographic variations of occurrence are tremendous. In the Soviet Far East, 5000 human cases were thought to have appeared up to 1972.[133] In the U.S. up to 1975, both localized and generalized cases reported totaled 14 or 15.[1,150] While prevalence in Europe is generally high, the human disease is almost unknown in the Iberian Peninsula, Italy, and Greece. The African Continent, India, and Southeast Asia are almost free of human infection.[1] A genesis of *Yersinia pseudotuberculosis* related to the dying thrusts of the medieval plague may well explain the high but uneven prevalence in Europe.[1,2] Even there, the full awareness of human involvement dates back only 25 years. Lack of clinical familiarity elsewhere may give a false impression, and such may be the case in parts of Canada and the U.S. It is doubtful if this lack will continue, however, in light of the publicity recently brought to the yersinioses, especially enterocolitis.

Surveys of the incidence of *Y. pseudotuberculosis* infections in sylvatic and domestic animals, human serological surveys, and development of improved stool-culture techniques could provide the necessary perspective. Increased knowledge of the distribution and role of avirulent strains should be one of the objectives.

Incubation Period and Pathogenesis

The incubation period remains largely conjectural in natural human cases due to the usual uncertainty on source of infection. In some cases, the circumstantial evidence may be strong but the times or duration of exposure and (assumed) ingestion are unknown. The long interval between death of a pet animal and the onset of symptoms, while suggesting a prolonged incubation period, may also eliminate the chance of diagnostic proof.[1] In the case of the gardener and the diarrheic cat cited by Mair,[1] the incubation period could have been as little as 8 days. While high dosage and/or virulence of the infective strain may shorten the period, the fact is that significant antibody titers are usually developed by the time of clinical onset.[1] Such was the case in the recent schoolboy outbreak in England reported by Andrews and Mair.[151] This would suggest an incubation period of at least 10 days.* A latent infection might be followed while still extant by stress factors sufficient to precipitate clinical disease. This would cause a prolonged incubation period, perhaps of several weeks. Generally, the seasonal peaks of animals and human incidence follow each other closely in the colder months (November to April) in Europe.[1,74,131] This suggests that incubation periods are not greatly prolonged, e.g., beyond one month. In consequence, the incubation period is thought to be variable, perhaps 7 to 21 days.

Y. pseudotuberculosis seemingly lacks the invasiveness of the plague bacillus that allows that organism to spread following percutaneous implantation. The pseudotubercle bacillus probably enters the intestinal lymphatic drainage in the manner suggested by Daniels.[1,153] This could allow the development of focal lymphatic abscess with a low infective dosage. It is possible that a primary, rapidly healing intestinal lesion that has been frequently suggested[153,154] but seldom observed is the usual progenitor of lymphatic invasion. Such a beachhead could be preceded in turn by a transient subclinical enteritis. This sequence would form a close parallel to the established pathogenesis for *Y. enterocolitica*.

Intestinal multiplication or transient enteritis would be of key importance in any

---

* This is indirectly supported by Winblad's comparative observations in Sweden[152] on *Y. pseudotuberculosis* and *Y. enterocolitica* titers. In the enterocolitis cases, antibodies are seldom seen at the time of the acute symptoms, but arise 7 to 12 days afterwards.

Table 2
CLINICOPATHOLOGICAL EXPRESSIONS
OF PSEUDOTUBERCULAR YERSINIOSIS

Primary Acute Manifestations

Focalized infection — pseudoappendicitis or RLQ syndrome
    Acute mesenteric lymphadenitis
    Acute terminal ileitis (complication or primary?)
Generalized infections
    Septicemia (rare)
    Scarlatiniform fever (limited to Russian Far-East?)

Secondary Immunological Complexities

Cutaneous manifestations
    Erythema nodosum (EN)
Arthralgic manifestations
    Arthralgia with EN, polyarthritis (scarlatiniform)

human-to-human transmission. Its existence should be provisionally assumed in the interests of sound hygiene and also as motivation for the bacteriological monitoring of persons at risk in outbreaks.

Clinical Pseudotubercular Yersiniosis

Seven clinical entities or groups are listed in Table 2 under two principal classifications, *viz.*, primary acute and secondary immunological. Pseudoappendicitis or RLQ syndrome, a primary acute condition, is comprised of two pathological entities that often occur together.[2]

Acute Mesenteric Lymphadenitis
    ARLM of Masshoff and Dolle.[3]

Acute Terminal Ileitis
The clinical presentation consists of abdominal pain, primarily of the RLQ, vomiting (usually), and a rapid rise in temperature to 38 to 40°C. This syndrome represents approximately 90% of the fully developed clinical infections with *Y. pseudotuberculosis*. In a series of 17 consecutive cases of acute mesenteric lymphadenitis, 3 (18%) were found to be infected with this bacterium.[84] The mesenteric lymphadenitis may simulate an abdominal tumor in up to 10% of cases.[121] Hodgkin's disease, lymphosarcoma, tuberculosis, or Crohn's disease may all be diagnosed initially in up to 15% of cases. In some situations, ileoceal resection precedes the correct diagnosis.[155] Most cases of RLQ syndrome or pseudoappendicitis run a benign course. Many are investigated or treated surgically with the occasional finding of appendiceal involvement. In either case, antibiotics are unnecessary except where there is evidence of continued infection.

Septicemia
This generalized infection is considered to be an extension of a primary acute focus involving the ileocecal area. Until 1953, this was the only generally recognized manifestation of pseudotubercular yersiniosis. Only 30 cases were recorded in the last 60 years.[156,157] Most cases occur in older people, particularly those with liver damage. Probably in normal subjects the integrity of the liver RE system is necessary to prevent dissemination of the microorganisms into the peripheral blood vessels.[158] Patients with

blood diseases, including children, may also contract a septicemic infection. This may be related to iron overload that can enhance pathogenicity of yersinias.[157] The clinical picture is usually dominated by a severe septicemic typhoidal course. An excellent summary of clinical findings was provided by Meyer;[21] however, it is quite possible that some of the earlier cases were due to *Y. enterocolitica*. Up to 50% mortality should be expected in septicemic cases even with use of antibiotics.

Scarlatiniform Fever of the Far East (U.S.S.R.)

Y. pseudotuberculosis has been identified as the cause of an acute generalized infection first recognized in 1959[133] and reported recently by Russian workers. This is a syndrome characterized by fever, scarlatiniform eruptions, and acute polyarthritis with arthralgia. In addition, symptoms may appear consistent with liver and G.I. lesions, especially icterus and abdominal pain. There are a few generalized cases. All cases except for a few of the typical form are accompanied by the scarlet-fever-like rash. There seems to be a close epidemiological association with rodents in the areas involved. The ingestion of cultures of *Y. pseudotuberculosis* from scarlatiniform cases has reproduced the disease symptoms in human volunteers.[159,160]

Erythema Nodosum (EN)

Among the secondary immunological complexities of pseudotubercular yersiniosis, an EN of short duration is the commonest, occurring in perhaps 15 to 20% of cases of acute infection. It follows a prodromal phase that is variable in its duration and manifestations but usually last about a week (range 2 to 21 days). Typically, a case is initially one of mesenteric lymphadenitis in a young male.* Occasionally, however, the eruption may be the first clinical sign, accompanied by high serum agglutinin titers. After a prodromal period, the eruption accompanied by moderate fever and fatigue reaches its maximum in a few days. One to three successive crops occur, finally subsiding along with the systemic illness in 2 to 3 weeks. Relapses have not been recorded.

Arthralgia Accompanying EN — Polyarthritis

Joint involvement is not a commonly reported immunological complexity in pseudotubercular yersiniosis except for an arthralgia often associated with EN. The polyarthritis reported as part of the scarlatiniform fever of the Far East is mentioned again because of its potential importance in different diagnosis. If both types of yersiniosis are geographically dynamic, an overlay might occur with areas where the severe migratory polyarthritis of *Y. enterocolitica* is also prevalent.

Pathological Changes

In pseudoappendicitis there may be a minor degree of peritoneal irritation but little or no abnormality of the appendix. In contrast, the mesenteric nodes, especially those in the ileocecal angle and the mesentery, frequently show redness, either diffuse or limited to the region of the affected nodes.[1] A clear or slightly purulent peritoneal exudate is often present. Affected lymph nodes may be several centimeters in diameter. Cut surfaces show follicular hyperplasia and typical miliary abscessations. These are the characteristic necrotizing abcesses of ARLM.[3,162]

The terminal ileum and cecum may show gross swelling due to hyperemia and edema. The total effect of hyperemic tissues in the right iliac fossa may easily simulate a tumor mass preoperatively. According to Daniels,[153] the swelling and redness of the terminal ileum result from obstruction of the afferent lymph drainage to infected nodes

---

* In Sweden, there is by contrast a high incidence of yersinial EN in middle aged and elderly women caused by *Y. enterocolitica* not *Y. pseudotuberculosis*.[161]

and does not constitute a primary bacterial lesion. In the septicemic cases of pseudo-tubercular yersiniosis, the pathological changes are profound with many organs and regions being affected. At autopsy, the nodular caseous or abscessed necrotic foci, from 1 to 10 mm in diameter, in the enlarged liver and spleen, occasionally also mesenteric lymph nodes and pancreas, are pathognomonic.[21]

According to Mair,[1] the histologic changes, while characteristic, are not specific since similar lesions are also found in cat-scratch disease and lymphogranuloma inguinale. Their presence in a mesenteric lymph node is strongly suggestive of yersinia infection. Nodes distant from the ileocecal angle may yield the organism in the absence of the characteristic necrotic lesions. Only two records were mentioned of extramesenteric lymph node involvement, one being inguinal and the other cervical.[1]

Immunity

Agglutinating antibodies to one or more of the six serologic types of *Y. pseudotuberculosis* usually appear in the serum by the time the clinical manifestations of acute infection reach a peak. The rapid declination of agglutinin levels during the following 3 to 4 months adds to the value of serology in diagnostic confirmation as well as for epidemiological studies. The persistence of agglutinins at high levels probably indicates persistent infection in the lymph nodes. The usual rapid disappearance of circulatory agglutinins does not preclude a retrospective diagnosis since the subject remains sensitized to intradermal antigen for a prolonged period.[1,74] There seems to have been no attention paid to levels of local immunity that would be expected to appear, particularly in the bowel, prior to clinical signs of the *Y. pseudotuberculosis* RLQ syndrome. Possibly some of the difficulties encountered in isolation of this organism from feces may relate to the interaction of coproantibody, such as secretory IgA, in cold enrichment or direct-plating procedures.

Diagnosis and Resolution

Serum-agglutination tests carried out with live smooth strains or formalin- or phenol-killed suspension normally indicate the presence of diagnostic titers at the clinical outset. These titers may vary from 1/160 or lower to 1/10,240 or higher.[21,104]

Isolation of the organism from the blood, mesenteric lymph nodes, effusions from serous cavities, and organ specimens can usually be achieved with little difficulty in the acute stages of illness. This applies also to blood cultures in disseminated or generalized infection.

Fecal-culturing methods require further investigation. This source would probably be fruitful during the prodromal phase when the presence of a short-lived, primary intestinal lesion may be the rule rather than the exception. If a short phase of multiplication occurs in the intestinal lumen, possibly preceding invasion of the intestinal lymph channels, it would make fecal isolation attempts worthwhile in early contacts. If such is the case, this type of cultural approach could be particularly valuable in establishing epidemiological relationships with lower animals. The characteristic histological changes in lymph nodes and occasionally organs require serological and/or cultural support for diagnostic confirmation.[1] Direct smears of lesions stained to successfully demonstrate bacterial bipolarity, however, could allow a provisional diagnosis when area, history, and clinical syndrome all indicate a high probability of *Y. pseudotuberculosis*. Use of the intradermal test with *Y. pseudotuberculosis* allergen provides conclusive evidence of previous infection by demonstrating a persistent skin sensitivity. This does not fix the time of episodes but is useful for indicating areas and situations where families or groups have contracted *Y. pseudotuberculosis* in food or the environment.

Five different serotypes have so far been reported in isolations from human infection. The vast majority (over 75%) of these are serotype I. The proportions of serotype II strains vs. reports of types III, IV, and V combined, are approximately 2:1, respectively. Of these, type III is probably commonest and type V least common. Since most human infections with the exception of the rare septicemic form involve a benign course, the use of surgery and antibiotics treatment are usually unnecesary and, therefore, waived in cases of early clinical diagnosis. It can be seen that in this situation, early diagnosis can alleviate considerable uncertainty and distress; other more serious conditions are eliminated and the specific confirmatory tests indicated can proceed at a stage when the chances of cultural recovery are high.

Current Dispersal and Prevalence in North America

While there is plenty of indication that isolations of the yersinias are being actively pursued in environmental, fecal, and surgical specimens, the available data are quite sparse in the latter two categories. It would be particularly interesting to know whether the infection was geographically concentrated or widely, if somewhat thinly, dispersed in contrast to the situation in Northeast Europe. In the Greater Vancouver area, yersinias are being isolated regularly if infrequently.[163] The preponderance of isolants from surgical or blood cultures of generalized or RLQ syndrome are *Y. enterocolitica*. They exceed the isolants of *Y. pseudotuberculosis.* The ratio is about 4:1. It is understood that a similar preponderance of *Y. enterocolitica* is being encountered elsewhere in Canada. This is believed to reflect the current situation is Northeast Europe with regard to mesenteric lymphadenitis.

DISEASE IN ANIMALS

Epizootics

In the epidemiology of human infections there is little doubt that epizootics in lower animals provide the basic source of ingestive infected material. Directly or indirectly, such epizootics lead to massive contamination levels due to the intensity of fecal shedding.[11] In addition, they may spawn off numerous infected carriers of the species involved and sporadic cases in contact or predator species.

Birds

There is well-substantiated evidence of yersinial pseudotuberculosis epizootics in wild birds. One example, the grackles of New England,[10] illustrates the importance of this type of source. Dead birds were found in large numbers scattered throughout the neighborhood of a large icterid roost, including the vicinity of a hog feeder where swine subsequently died of an unidentified disease. In such a situation there is enormous potential for the infection of other wild birds, rodents, and domestic animals. It must not be supposed, however, that contact with natural infection always leads to disease. In the grackle roost, there were three other species of wild birds that were apparently not suffering mortalities or clinical effect. The high-stress conditions imposed on the grackles in the late winter, just prior to migration, was considered responsible for their susceptibility. Other wild bird epizootics have occurred in Hampshire, England,[82,83] involving stock doves, pigeons, and other birds and in Eastern Canada[94] involving purple martins. Doves have also been involved in high-mortality disease in California.[164] Undoubtedly, many other episodes have gone unnoticed or unreported due to the obvious difficulties involved in detection and jurisdiction of wildlife disease events. Epizootics have been better studied among captive and domestic birds. These include turkeys in Europe, on the Continent, in Britain,[81] and in Oregon;[67] canaries and finches in numerous European reports, Washington, D.C.,[65] and British Columbia;[11,88] and ducks in France.[131] Chickens are probably less susceptible than turkeys; however, several episodes with significant mortalities have been reported in France in the 1930s and one in Alberta, Canada in 1960. Domestic flocks of pigeons also have been afflicted with high mortalities in Germany, Denmark, and France. Toucans appear to be highly susceptible; however, there are seldom sufficient numbers grouped together to classify the losses as epizootics. The same situation applies to many other susceptible avian species in zoological gardens.

Mammals

Epizootics in wild mammals are not as common or as well known as in birds. However, the generally high incidence of infection and occasional heavy mortalities of hares in Europe, from Scandinavia[97] and Britain[1,123] to Italy,[7] well illustrates the potential. The decimation of populations from pseudotuberculosis has also been suspected in other mammals, such as field mice, beaver, and muskrats.[11,88] Many workers have reserved judgment on the possible existence of epizootics in wild mice. Wetzler[13] expresses strong doubt on this issue. He includes managed populations of field mice, also, and comments that it is difficult to explain satisfactorily. One outbreak is known to the writer that involved severe losses in a captive colony of *Microtus aggrestis* in England.[108]

It is quite possible that in rats and mice widespread population infections accompanied by low mortalities are common.[133,134] Captive colonies of exotic species are often vulnerable to outbreaks of pseudotuberculosis. An example of this was the loss of six black-faced kangaroos in California.[164] The disease is a potential threat to primates in zoos, medical-laboratory colonies, and experimental groups. At the time of writing, an outbreak is in progress involving squirrel monkeys in California.[139]

Sporadic Infections

The numbers of animal species involved in occasional and sporadic infections or presenting single cases that might be representative of population involvements is too numerous to list. A partial list in arbitrary groupings is given under World Distribution. These include wild and domestic animals in Europe; North, Central, and South America; North Africa; North and Eastern Asia; and Australia and New Zealand. Probably the combined reports of Mair, Hubbard, Wetzler, and the western European and Russian workers would add up to well over 100 species of birds and mammals that are known to become infected. In reports of zoological gardens alone, 42 affected species of mammals were noted.[141-143] This infection runs first in causes of death due to bacterial disease in mammals and second only to tuberculosis in birds in zoological gardens in the U.K. Particular attention should be directed to the presence of disease in pet and food animals. These include cats, dogs, pet birds, sheep, cattle, pigs, hares, rabbits, and poultry, to name a few only.

Isolation from Healthy Animals

Recently, considerable attention has been paid to isolants of both virulent and avirulent strains of *Y. pseudotuberculosis* from healthy pigs. It is quite possible that these and other animals may pose a potential threat to humans in addition to the epizootic and sporadic cases mentioned.

Serotypes

As in man, the majority of serotypes encountered in animals are type I strains. On a recent compilation from the literature it appears that the percentages of the six serotypes reported are type I—64%, type II—17%, type III—12%, type IV—7%, type V—2%, and type VI—1%. Type I is probably virulent for all species since no single species with the possible exception of *Apodemus agrarius* has infections exclusively with other serotypes. Type I isolants come about 54% from mammals and 46% from birds. Type II is the next most common in birds and mammals outside North America. Type III is almost as common as Type II in mammals but quite rare in birds (only one canary in U.S. has been reported). Type IV is fourth most common in mammals and third commonest in birds. Type V occurs only in rabbits and guinea pigs, no avian. Neither type IV or V has been reported in North America. Type VI occurs only in guinea pigs in Japan, no avian.

Pathogenesis and Clinical Course of Natural Infections
Incubation Period
The incubation periods in naturally infected wild animals of many species are almost completely unknown. In captive or domestic populations, it can probably best be deduced at times of disease outbreaks following the introduction of infected or susceptible stock, as the case may be, to existing colonies. In other situations, the infection is associated with the presence of infected pigeons and rodents without the time of first exposure being established.[30,81] In one canary aviary, deaths commenced about 2 weeks following the finding of two dead field mice in the flight cage.[11] From this, one might estimate an incubation period of 6 to 8 days in this species. A rare situation involving feeding known infected viscera of hares to mink occurred in Denmark.[92] The mink became obviously sick in just a few days and about 75 died in a herd of unknown size. The estimate of 5 to 10 days for incubation period in guinea pigs[165] is probably reasonable for many mammals.

Stress
Undoubtedly, the shorter incubation times and more severe disease are functions of general-host susceptibility, virulence of the strain, and the intervention of stress mechanisms. The latter includes climatic and nutritional factors, reproductive or migratory activity, and competition due to overcrowding, feed shortage, or overpopulation. In guinea pigs, both injection of various inocula and oral dosing with Aureomycin® are known to cause exaltation of latent pseudotuberculosis.[7] Ectoparasitism has been associated with disease in goats and the feeding of G.I. irritants, such as mustard or paprika, with onset of disease in cage birds.

Clinical Disease
Available information on the clinical course of pseudotuberulosis is scanty in both wild and captive or domestic populations. In most cases, animals are not seen by clinicians prior to death. Exceptions to the above are managed colonies of guinea pigs, rabbits, primates, and possibly aviary species. In some cases, outbreaks of disease in domestic fowl are accurately observed and recorded. Some of the cases in zoological gardens are examined and possibly treated. In the more rare focalized infections that sometime occur in farm animals and the cases occurring in pets, some receive clinical assessment. As one might expect from the multiplicity of avian and mammalian species involved, the clinical signs are quite variable. They almost negate attempts to find common features in speed of onset, clinical signs and rapidity, or otherwise, of termination.

Birds
According to Obwolo,[55] birds generally show ruffled feathers, dyspnea, and appar-

ent lameness. Heddleston discussed clinical signs in two main classes.[17] In the very acute cases, diarrhea may suddenly appear followed by manifestations of septicemia. More usually, the course extends over 2 weeks or more with signs appearing only 2 to 4 days before death. Weakness, dull and ruffled feathers, difficult breathing, and diarrhea are seen. In the most protracted cases, emaciation and extreme weakness or possibly paralysis may be evident. Droopiness, somnolence, constipation, and skin discoloration have been seen in such cases. The birds may eat normally until 1 or 2 days before death. In turkeys, according to Blaxland, the disease was sudden in onset with inappetence and a dejected stance. There was also a yellowish diarrhea. Less acute cases showed lameness. This author also described some hyperacute cases that were well in the morning, unable to walk by noon, and dead 3 hr later.[81] Rosenwald and Dickinson described the disease in turkeys as one of anorexia, diarrhea, droopiness, occasional lameness, and sudden death in some cases.[67]

Mammals

Clinical signs were described for guinea pigs by Kunz and Hutton.[165] In the acute septicemic form, the animals were coughing and showed rapid breathing with death occurring in 24 to 48 hr. In the classical form, there was diarrhea and emaciation with death delayed for 3 to 4 weeks. Obwolo[55] described sick guinea pigs as suffering diarrhea, thirst, rapid emaciation, dyspnea, and a staring coat. Baboons were described in sickness by at least two authors. In Mollaret's case[13] the animals remained immobile in the corner of the cage, heads bent on chest, hair erect, and eyelids swollen. The baboons described by Nouvel and Rinjard[13] apparently showed no signs until the day before death. They displayed marked depression, dull fur, slightly distended abdomen, and dysentery. It is interesting that in both of the above episodes, the animals retained their appetite almost to the point of death that in Mollaret's study was described as sudden.

Chinchillas with pseudotuberculosis due to *Y. pseudotuberculosis* were described by Chapman.[79] The animals showed inappetence, a resultant steady drop in fecal output, and lassitude. Chinchillas in British Columbia in the Pacific Northwest were noted to be listless, developing emaciation and occasionally abdominal pain, and dysentery. The associated peritonitis and enteritis may have been partly due to giardia and salmonellas or other enteroopportunitists or pathogens.[166] Some cases of great similarity in terms of gross pathological changes were undoubtedly due to *Y. enterocolitica* infection.[167]

A fatal case of pseudotuberculosis in a dog reported by Collett[168] showed gastroenteritis and anemia. Although pigs have been infrequently associated with clinical disease when infected with *Y. pseudotuberculosis,* a case reported in Japan showed edema of the eyelids.[118]

Pathological Changes

A listing of the gross lesions of pseudotuberculosis due to *Y. pseudotuberculosis* (Table 3), while not exhaustive, is sufficient to indicate the frequency of occurrence in various organs and systems of mammals and birds. Obviously, any attempt to draw comparative conclusions between mammals and birds, between species, and even between individual episodes must begin with the entry of infections.

Portal of Entry

There is one virtually certain and four possible routes of entry that seem to have some support by consideration of the epidemiological picture, species habits, and disposition of the lesions.

Table 3
GROSS LESIONS — VARIOUS ANIMAL SPECIES

System or general location	Family	Species involved (common names)	Ref.
Respiratory tract	Mammals	Anteater (giant)	30
		Baboon	169
		Blesbok	30
		Cat	146
		Chinchilla	164
		Cow	89, 164
		Horse	59
		Mouse (allergic)	170
	Birds	Chicken (trachea)	105
		Crow	94
		Grackle	10
		Pigeon	63
		Turkey	81
Cardiovascular system	Mammals	Pigs (enlarged ventricles)	55
	Birds	Chickens (heart lesions)	105
G.I. tract and mesentery	Mammals	Anteater (giant)	30
		Blesbok	30
		Cat	1, 164
		Chinchilla	79
		Cow	31,164
		Dog	55
		Fallow deer	164
		Hare	1, 92
		Horse	59
		Mink	92
		Monkey	138
		Nutria	171
		Rodents	13
		Sheep	164
	Birds	Canary (cecum)	11
		Chicken	172
		Purple martin	94
		Turkey	81
		Birds (general)	1
Abdominal organs			
Liver and/or spleen	Mammals	Anteater (giant)	30
		Baboon	169
		Beaver	94, 166
		Blesbok	30
		Cat	147, 164
		Chinchilla	79, 80, 164
		Dog	168
		Horse	59
		Kangaroo	164
		Mink	92
		Mouse	170
		Nutria	171
		Sheep	164
	Birds	Blackbird	76
		Chicken	173
		Crow	94
		Dove	164
		Grackle	10
		Pigeon	164
		Purple martin	94
		Turkey	81

Table 3 (continued)

GROSS LEGIONS-VARIOUS ANIMAL SPECIES

System or General Location	Family	Species Involved (common name)	Ref.
Kidney	Mammals	Beaver	166
		Cat	146
		Mink	92
		Mouse	170
		Nutria	171
	Birds	Chicken	105
		Grackle	10
		Purple martin	94
Adrenal	Mammals	Guinea pigs	55
Reproductive tract	Mammals	Cow (aborted fetus)	89, 113
		Cow (mastitis)	4, 115
		Sheep (aborted fetus)	125
		Ram (epididymo-orchitis)	123
Nervous system	Mammals	Sheep (brain)	112

Oral (Enteric) Route

With the main source being excreted feces and the secondary source carrion (see epidemiological chart below), the infective organism can be supplied to the mouth through food or water or indirectly through various grooming activities.

In man, no one doubts the enteric route of infection.[153] The vast majority of animal infections appear to be acquired through the same route, entering the parenchyma through the lower bowel and focalizing in the posterior mesenteric lymph system. Goret[148] suggests that natural infection in the cat is promoted by intestinal lesions induced by bone or toxic (endotoxin?) products.

From the mesenteric, usually ileocecal area, the spread is hematogenous to the liver and the spleen and, when not contained there, to more remote locations including kidney, muscles, adrenals, and possibly lung and reproductive tract.

In canaries studied by Stovell[11] in and following epizootics, both natural and experimental disease states were consistent with an oral-enteric route of fecally contaminated feed.[12] The initial source of contamination was probably mouse feces with the infected canaries themselves fueling the continuing process.

Percutaneous Route

The presence of caseous granulomas in cervical lymph nodes of the guinea pig[165] or both cervical and thoracic nodes[21] (glandular form) is considered by the latter authority to be probably transmitted by bites. The possibility of arthropod-borne *Y. pseudotuberculosis* has been examined experimentally;[174-178] however, at the moment the apparent inability of this agent to establish an arthropod cycle is one of the main differences in its pathogenesis from that of plague. An unusual epididymo-orchitis of rams was conjecturally associated with the tick season in England.[123] Experimentally, the rat flea (*Xenopsylla cheopis*) can remain a carrier for up to 35 days but is incapable of transmitting *Y. pseudotuberculosis*.[179] It was isolated from *Ixodid* ticks collected in the outskirts of Leningrad.[1] One human case was associated with bites from the owner's dog that had a positive serum titer.[1]

Ocular Route

Ocular infection has not been reported in animals with the exception of man. In

Italy, a unique oculoglandular syndrome (Parinaud) has been described that developed 8 days after contact of the conjunctiva with an insect.[7]

Inhalatory Route

The relatively large number of species of both mammals and birds involved with respiratory tract lesions supports conjecture in this area of the pathogenesis.[180] Experimentally, canaries were readily infected in the lung by inadvertent tracheal inspiration due to esophageal regurgitation. The follow-up oral inoculum with smaller dosage in subsequent groups yielded only classical lesions with no gross pulmonary involvement.[11]

Coital Route

The occurrence of bovine and ovine abortions due to *Y. pseudotuberculosis* infection would not of itself lead to conjecture of a potential coital route; however, the report of epididymo-orchitis in ten rams is another matter.[123] Certainly, the infecting organism would be present in semen from an affected case.

Typical Gross Lesions

There is considerable variation in the length of the disease course that can vary all the way from a day or two to many weeks. Mair[1] described the fulminating septicemic form in hares with death in 1 to 3 days with intestinal congestion the only lesion. He also mentioned the subacute and chronic forms with their clinicopathological signs, such as weight loss over a period of days or weeks, severe diarrhea, respiratory distress, etc. Unfortunately he did not describe the chronic lesions in hares. However, Knox[92] noted that yellowish, caseous nodules may be found in the spleen, liver, kidneys, and wall of the intestinal tract. The mink that Knox reported to have contracted pseudotuberculosis from consumption of infected hare viscera suffered a slight enteritis as the first sign. It is not known whether a marked intralumenal multiplication of *Y. pseudotuberculosis,* a specific catarrhal, and/or hemorrhagic enteritis[30,81] or distinctive primary lesions of the Peyers patches[21] or bowel lining is essential in natural infections for extension to the mesenteric lymphatics. However, the development of intestinal nodules in hares and birds, for example,[1] and the cecal abscesses of a low percentage of canaries[11] probably indicate sequelae to such primary foci, especially those that have spawned pyoembolic granulomas in the spleen, liver, and other organs. In the naturally infected (assumed oral route) guinea pig, both septicemias, fatal in 24 to 48 hr, and classic (chronic) forms with emaciation, diarrhea, and death in 3 to 4 weeks were also noted by Meyer.[21] He considered the whitish nodules in liver, spleen, and occasionally lungs to be pathognomonic for the *Y. pseudotuberculosis* form of yersiniosis.

In the canary the pathognomonic lesion noted was the classical pinpoint to millet-sized yellowish tubercles in the spleen. In some cases the liver was similarly affected.[11]

Histopathology

Meyer[21] distinguishes between acute and chronic typical pseudotubercles in guinea pigs. The former represents only areas of focal necrosis, including fragmented polynuclear leukocytes, surrounded by foamy reticulum cells but rarely epithelioid cells. Giant cells are always absent; this observation is in agreement with that of Baskin[30] for the livers and spleens of various naturally infected animals. The chronic lesions, according to Meyer, show extensive fibroblast and epithelioid proliferations that sometimes become granulomatous but never calcify. Bacilli are numerous in such lesions.[21] Baskin also observed numerous colonies of Gram-negative, pleomorphic coccobacilli throughout intestinal lesions.[30] There was a severe necrosis of the mucosa of the small intestine with edema of the lamina propria and submucosa and massive infiltration of neutrophils, lymphocytes, and macrophages. Some bowel segments were hemorrhagic, and in some areas penetration of the muscle layers by the necrotic process led to serosal extension and peritonitis. The lymphatics beneath the serosa were distended with neutrophils, mononuclear cells, and necrotic debris. Many veins contained thrombi.[30]

The structure of typical splenic and liver pseudotubercles in canary infections is provided for epizootics occurring in British Columbia.[11] Of those spleens and livers that were examined from field cases, all showed a marked granulomatous response. Mononucleic macrophages predominated in the cellular mass. Scattered about were numerous, small areas of caseation necrosis, eosinophilic in tone and with areas of blue smudging probably due to degenerating masses of bacteria. The cellular response was more diffuse about the necrotic foci in the spleen than in the liver. In the latter organ, intense cellular cuffing could be noted. Kupffer cells were absent, doubtless due to their cytometamorphosis to form larger macrophages. The liver cords were completely disrupted with marked vacuolar degeneration of the hepatic cells. The appearance of the macrophages suggested intense bacteriophagia although clearly defined microorganisms were not visible in the way noted in the experimental disease. Extensive hemorrhages were noted in the spleen along lines of fracture due to structural weakening of the organ. A cecal abscess and an extremely enlarged spleen were also described histologically.[11] The left cecal lumen of one canary was filled with a mass of macrophages that had infiltrated and replaced the mucosal tissues and extended back into the muscularis mucosa. Centrally located was a necrotic center that stained pink with H & E. At the periphery was a ring of large macrophages showing marked granularity indicative of bacteriophagia. Many giant cells of the Langhans type were noted in the median area. The spleen showing greatest enlargement had a microscopic picture typical of other spleens. The changed organ was seen to be made up of a mass of expanding granulomas with caseating centers. An intense mass of macrophages with lessening degrees of degeneration extended out in concentric rings from the necrotic center. At the periphery, a ring of such cells contained ingested bacteria. The same tissues, when stained with Twort's method using fast green for a counterstain, showed the central necrotic zone staining blue and the peripheral giant cells with their bacterial load showing as an intense red ring on low power. High magnification of the mass of red-staining bacteria showed the typical pattern of bipolarity.[11]

LABORATORY DIAGNOSIS

The laboratory diagnosis of infection due to *Yersinia pseudotuberculosis* has been discussed to a limited extent only. In covering this subject in a general way, little reference is made to any particular species as source of diagnostic material. An attempt has been made to list many of the more commonly used or investigated diagnostic procedures. This is considered to serve only as a general guide for obtaining more specific or detailed information. For this purpose, some references have been supplied in most areas of approach. Table 4 is thus a mixture of common sense and developmental ideas from one person's viewpoint. It may form a basis for development of more precise and succinct schemes for practical use. It will be noted that the diagnostic procedures are listed under four general headings:

1. Bacteriological D.C.I. — a large section dealing with the demonstration, culture, and identification of *Y. pseudotuberculosis*. This is the best substantiation or confirmation for carrier (clinical and/or surgical) or post-mortem diagnosis in man.

Table 4

LABORATORY DIAGNOSTIC PROCEDURES

A. Bacteriological D.C.I.

Step	Objectives	Principle	Specifications	Recommendations, information	Ref.
1.	Demonstration in lesions	a. Aniline stains	Acid fast smear (Cook)		28
			Hansen's brucella stain		29
			Gram's smear		
			Wayson's smear	See Etiologic Agent	26, 27
			Gram's sections	See Cell Morphology and Staining	14, 30
			Ollett/Twort's sections	See Pathological Changes	11
		b. FA stain	Direct FA with anti-*Y. pseudotuberculosis* conjugate.	Satisfactory in plague-free area	129
				No X reaction with *Y. pestis* but high-titer anti-O required	181
				False-positive *Y. pestis* reaction	182
				Not serotype or genus specific	183
		c. Passive HI test	Detection of antigens in infected materials	Discussed by Zaremba	184
2.	Culture of lesions	Heavy and light inoculations, early and chronic lesions, pref. margin to necrotic center; note smears	Incubation plates at:	Pref. blood agar (see Agent cultivation)	
			22°C	Best preservation in vivo characteristics	
			28—30°C	Optimum growth and preservation of structures	
			35—37°C	Comparison of growth only	
			Include culture of human appendix	Two cases recorded as successful	185, 186
3.	Culture of blood	Application mostly in human, especially in absence of available lesions; important for early diagnosis	Routine b/c media	Easily obtained early in cases of septicemia	21
			Ideally carried out in replicate for incubation at room and intermediate temperatures.	Obtained in some generalized cases (Vancouver metropolitan hospitals)	163
				Should attempt early in RLQ syndrome (pseudoappendicitis)	Personal view
4.	Culture of intestinal/fecal samples	a. Selective plate medium	Paterson & Cook's modified Morris medium (mycostatin and crystal violet)	Satisfactory for guinea pig feces	83

Table 4 (continued)
LABORATORY DIAGNOSTIC PROCEDURES

Step	Objectives	Principle	Specifications	Recommendations, information	Ref.
	Clinical cases		Saline dilution fecal sediment to MacConkey agar	Highly satisfactory for fresh canary feces; typical colonies producing acid no gas in maltose broth invariably *Y. pseudotuberculosis*	11
	Symptomless potential carriers of same species	b. Cold enrichment holding	10% fecal suspension in pH 7.6; PB held 7—28 days at 3—4°C (also used trypsinized meat broth); plate on modified Morris	Paterson and Cook also discovered by chance that *Y. pseudotuberculosis* multiplied and other fecal bacteria died during holding time at refrigerator temperature	83
	Synanthropic, domestic, or sylvatic contact animals		Isotonic saline with or without 25 µg/m*l* potassium tellurite hold in refrigerator	For holding and enrichment of any specimens (after Wetzler 1970)	16 187
	Human survey extra determination		10% suspension in M/15 PB 3 weeks at 5°C. (pH 7.6) followed by plating on MacConkey agar.	Best method for guinea pig feces; the MacConkey plate (of particular Japanese formula) performed better than Paterson and Cook's plate medium.	186
				This procedure worked well for isolation from healthy contacts in recent squirrel monkey outbreak southern California	
5.	Primary recognition in culture	a. Colonial morphology	Stereomicroscopic examination both transmitted and reflected light	See Cultivation	139
		b. Cellular morphology	Compound microscopy; aniline staining, darkfield/phase for motility	See Cell Morphology and Staining	

6.	Initial differentiation of cultures	a. Apply preliminary cultural and biochemical criteria to separate out *Yersinia*	Comparison of plates grown at 3 temperatures Motility tests, 22°C in semisolid or broth Lactose Fermentative for, e.g., glucose, mannitol Oxidase test H$_2$S in TSI Urea (Christensen's) Phenylalanine agar (PAA slant)	Any lactose-negative, Gram-negative, oxidase-negative fermentative rod (or cb) which does not produce H$_2$S in TSI, is motile only at room temperature (not 35—37°C), is urease positive in 3—24 hr and PA negative is suspect as *Y. pseudotuberculosis* or *Y. enterocolitica* *Y. pestis* produces colonies which are less granular than *Y. pseudotuberculosis*; it is nonmotile at all temperatures and usually urea-negative. Various rapid diagnostic systems available in kit form might be tried by those already experienced with standard methods, e.g., API 20 Enteric[a] — a rapid semimicro identification kit.	16
		b. Scanning electronmicroscopy	Detect envelope in *Y. pestis* (Fraction 1 antigen) Detect flagella in *Y. pseudotuberculosis* at 22°C.	*Y. pestis* produces most envelope at 37°C whereas this is absent in *Y. pseudotuberculosis* at any temperature May be of use in certain poorly motile strains of *Y. pseudotuberculosis*	188
		c. Preliminary serological differentiation	Widal reaction microslide agglutination	Polyvalent antiserum with antibodies against types I—VI or type-specific O antiserum agglutinates live smooth suspension; is negative to specific antiplague serum	
		d. Preliminary animal inoculation	Inoculation of PC in 1—2 susceptible and 1—2 refractory species of commonly available laboratory animals.	Production of typical lesions with cultural recovery in susceptible species, e.g., gerbils, guinea pigs, and resistance of others, e.g., albino (ab) rats and hamsters, indicates virtually certain diagnosis of *Y. pseudotuberculosis*	21

[a]   Analytab Products Inc., Carle Place, New York.

Table 4 (continued)
LABORATORY DIAGNOSTIC PROCEDURES

Step	Objectives	Principle	Specifications	Recommendations, information	Ref.
7.	Special tests for differentiation	Growth in tissue culture	Use subcutaneous and intraperitoneal routes		
			Entry and survival in cells	Studied uptake and survival in HeLa cells; considered cell systems useful for study of antibiotic or antibody effect and pathogenicity in intracellular state	33
			Multiplication in tissue culture cells	Infection intensity depends on virulence, dose, and sensibility of cells	133
				Multiplied well in dispersed rabbit spleen and kidney cell cultures	35
				Atmospheric control of generation time effected by varying O_2 level (95% vs. 20% O_2 with 5% CO_2)	35
			Determination of degree of virulence	Can be effected with use of cells	133
8.	Identification and typing	a. i. Differentiation between yersinias	Battery of differentiating CHOs for yersinias fermentation	List of 11 carbohydrates (Table 4)	42
				List of 15 carbohydrates (Table 2)	16
	Biochemical profile for biotyping		Additional biochemical differentiation	Decarboxylases, ornithine, and lysine; arginine dihydrolase, hydrolysis of esculin and gelatin; indole, methyl red, VP test at 22°C; catalase; β-galactosidase, nitrate reduction, Simmons citrate, utilization.	16, 42, 189
		ii. Differentiation between Y. pseudotuberculosis and Y. enterocoliticum	Full, growth, biochemical, and fermentative criteria	List of 21 CHOs and 19 other growth and biochemical tests (Table 1); actual differences in only 10 CHOs and 3 biochemical tests of this table.	190
				Limited to 3 key tests, sucrose, rhamnose, and ornithine decarboxylase	14

				Ref.
8. Identification and typing	iii. Differentiation between *Y. pseudotuberculosis* and *Y. pestis*	DNA hybridization test and others	Characterization by DNA hybridization in addition to usual biochemical tests	191
			See details and references	191
		Adenosine deaminase test		192
	b. Antibiotic sensitivity differentials[b]	General sensitivity	In vitro sensitivity to C, S, P, Ne, K, and T; resistant to E and No	193
			All Japanese strains typical Gram-patterns of antibiotic sensitivity and all were urease positive	74, 194
		Specific sensitivity	*Y. enterocolitica* resist to P and Am	195, 196
			Minimum values: *Y. enterolita* > 6.25 μg/ml, *Y. pseudotuberculosis* < 0.78 μg/ml	195
			Resistance developed over several years and some strains now resistant to P, Am, B, and some other synthetic Ps	197
		Sensitivity variations	Strains inhibited for VW production are highly sensitive to P but relatively resistant to S. Cells static for DNA and protein synthesis (but producing VW antigens) resistant to P but acutely sensitive to S	34
		Aureomycin effect	Use of oral Au tends to produce overt disease in latently infected guinea pigs	7, 55, 198
	c. Phage sensitivity and typing	Use of *Y. pestis* phage to differentiate between yersinias incubated at 2 temperatures (25° and 37°C)	One phage 4FLU 1927 will distinguish between the species	24
			Criteria listed in Table 4	42
			Strains of *Y. pestis* bacteriophage lyse all known strains of *Y. pestis* as well as *Y. pseudotuberculosis* at 37°C only	187
		Use of *Y. pseudotuberculosis* phages	Lyses all strains of *Y. pseudotuberculosis* but not *Y. pestis* or *Y. enterocolitica*	16
		Y. enterocolitica phages	Do not act on *Y. pestis* or *Y. pseudotuberculosis*	25

[b] Code: Au-aureomycin; Am-ampicillin; B-benzylpenicillin; C-chloramphenicol; E-erythromycin; K-kanamycin; Ne-neomycin; No-novobiocin; P-penicillin; S-streptomycin; and T-tetracycline.

Table 4 (continued)
LABORATORY DIAGNOSTIC PROCEDURES

Step	Objectives	Principle	Specifications	Recommendations, information	Ref.
		d. Serotyping and differentiation	Antigenic analysis of the organism	Agglutination or hemagglutination can be used Antisera containing antibodies against types I—VI agglutinate *Y. pseudotuberculosis* but not *Y. pestis* or *Y. enterocolitica*	187
		B. Immulological Procedures			
1.	Detection of immune serum titers	a. Agglutination tests	Live smooth strains; phenol- or formalin-killed organisms of the six serotypes	For detection of antibodies in acutely or chronically infected subjects; titers drop quickly with successful resolution of the infection	16
		b. Passive hemagglutination	Erythrocytes coated with supernatant fractions of heat-killed or autoclaved cell suspensions	No antigens or antisera commercially available at present The microhemagglutination test was recommended for detection of serum antibodies	16 199
		c. Indirect FA tests		Use was satisfactory in plague-free area	200
		d. Growth test	Use of strains on *Y. pseudotuberculosis* of different O groups	In guinea pigs the growth test is considerably more sensitive than the agglutination test	47
		e. Gel precipitin reaction	Research test with specific antigens (purified) for diagnostic use.	The three *Yersinias* possess very similar antigenic structure indicated by 12—16 bands in common, whereas only 3—6 are in common with Enterobacteria; this is not a practicable test for diagnostic labs at present	201
		f. Immunoelectrophoresis to solve problems in certain human sera	Absorption agglutination followed by gel precipitin	Common occurrence of (nonspecific) agglutinins in healthy people against live *Y. pseudotuberculosis* type II. Occasional sera simultaneously agglutinates	202

				Ref.
2.	Retrospective determination of immune response in patient.	Testing of patient in clinical facility	many *Yersinia* serotypes; this technique may offer a solution	
			After 24 hr produces an erythematous zone 3.5 cm in diameter with a central red and tender area 1 cm; after 48 hr erythema zone 5 cm, central zone more indurated and tender	104
		Intradermal inoculation with Mollaret's skin-test antigen	Skin sensitivity may persist for at least 5—6 years; this compensates for brevity of persistence of serum agglutinins; intradermal sensitivity may persist 10 years	1, 74

C. Pathology of Classic Pseudotubercular Yersiniosis

				Ref.
1.	Detection or recognition of gross changes	Selection of tissues for histopathology and microbiology	Especially important are any gross lesions which allow discharge of infective organisms into bowel; early initial bowel lesions are of great interest in human cases of RLQ syndrome	11
2.	Histologic, pathognomonic, or indicative of *Y. pseudotuberculosis*	Confirm presence of typical pseudotubercles, intracellular bacteria	H & E stains for bacterial bipolarity, stains for Gram-negative bacteria	See A-1 of this table

D. Assessment of Virulence in Strains

				Ref.
1.	Determine infectivity for laboratory animals	Select fully virulent population of *Y. pseudotuberculosis*, i.e., VW⁺	Calcium dependency procedure of Higuchi and Smith	
		Inoculation intranasal, intraperitoneal, subcutaneous, and intravenous	Virulence testing in mice, gerbils, white rabbits, and guinea pigs will produce characteristic experimental disease states by a variety of routes	22
			White rats and hamsters are refractory to infection	22
			Mini pigs produce only an immune response	203
	Preserve full virulence in newly isolated or recovered	Low-temperature culture on blood or serum supplementary me-	The recovered virulent strain may be titrated in suspectible homologous or other species by oral or parenteral routes, e.g., canaries,	11

Table 4 (continued)
LABORATORY DIAGNOSTIC PROCEDURES

Step	Objectives	Principle	Specifications	Recommendations, information	Ref.
		Y. pseudotuberculosis	dium; one passage only on artifical medium	budgies, chickens, guinea pigs	37
		Introduce experimental virulence factor(s)	Injection of Fe into mice		
		Simulate human oral route	Fed fresh human isolants to mice	Concluded strains enterogenic and assumed a primary intestinal focus	154
2.	Determine toxicogenicity for lab animals	Test for presence of toxins	Inoculate type III into mice	Terminal in 1—10 days depending on dose	204
		Infectivity experiments	Accidental overdose of inoculum	Often kills experimental subjects in 24 hr or less, e.g., mice inoculated with ground-up canary spleens	11
			Toxicosis presumably?	Death in mice after 2—3 days, only slight swelling of liver (yielded pure culture)	76

This approach should also be pursued for evidence or incrimination of suspected epidemiological source. There are also specific and confirmatory diagnostic possibilities in the following approaches

2. Immunological procedures
3. Pathology procedures
4. Assessment of virulence — considered to have its principal application in research

EPIDEMIOLOGICAL RELATIONSHIPS

Disease Investigations

Several cardinal features of *Yersinia pseudotuberculosis* interrelate closely in the epidemiological (and epizootiological) expression of the disease. These include the extremely wide host spectrum of birds and mammals, including primates and man; the undoubted and predominant fecal-enteral route in transmission and pathogenesis; the high incidence of latent, subclinical, or misdiagnosed disease; the stress-plus-virulence mechanism spawning epizootics in animals; and the marked seasonal character to the incidence of clinical disease.[1] The general epidemiological relationships have been dealt with to some degree in the foregoing, particularly in Disease Distribution that is classified on a practical epidemiology basis and Pathological Changes in Animals that is related to the portal(s) of entry of the infection.

Two decades ago, Meyer observed that "the vast animal reservoir with its carriers and shedders is of course suspected as the source of human infections".[21] As stated previously, the seemingly, quite variable incubation time in man and animals and the difficulties of clinical diagnosis have in many cases prevented emergence of a clear picture of epidemiological connections. However, there are a number of episodes on record that are accompanied by sufficient observation or investigative detail to bear some analysis; 15 such reports and situations were selected and assigned to four arbitrary groups. These were based on the confirmed or apparent source and means (vehicle) of transmission. The clinical, pathological, and diagnostic features of both hosts, including laboratory confirmation of infection, were considered and a simple letter code assigned. In some cases, the information being incomplete, certain assumptions were required. The individual episodes are listed in Table 5 under four provisional classes of epidemiological connections according to circumstances and caliber of proof.

All the new information introduced to the table consists of the assumptions, indicated (?), that relate to both vehicle and diagnostic information and a few reciprocal arrows. The latter indicates questions that come to mind as to whether, e.g., synanthropic rodents or wild birds might be specific or common recipients instead of, or in addition to, being the source of infection. The conclusions were as follows:

1. There is very little incontestable proof of the exact vehicle and portal of entry in the epidemiological connections for most episodes.
2. On the other hand, there is no reason to doubt the almost universal assumption of fecal-enteral modus of transmission.
3. The tremendous value of sound and imaginative investigative and experimental work in connection with episodes is well illustrated in a number of those listed.

The complexity of factors assumed to be involved in the epidemiology of human *Y. pseudotuberculosis* and the epizootiology of animal infections are illustrated in the accompanying chart. Some key animal hosts are listed in eight arbitrary groups around

Table 5
EPIDEMIOLOGICAL CONNECTIONS FROM SELECTED PUBLISHED REPORTS[a]

	Source species	Vehicle	Victim species	Country	Ref.
	Reasonably Certain Connections				
1.	Pigeons of source area F-I	Fecally contaminated field greens I	Laboratory guinea pigs D, L, I, F-I	England	83
2.	Sheep D, L, I	Pecked flesh of hides Fecal contamination feed? water?	Magpies D, L, I	Australia	205
3.	Field hares (Assumed L)	Pooled viscera (Assumed L)	75/? Farm mink D, L, I	Denmark	92
4.	Lab culture I	Per orum? Inhalatory? Cutaneous?	Laboratory technician C, S, I (?)	U.S.	206
	Strongly Circumstantial Connections				
1.	Widespread in synanthropic rats, mice K, D, L, I	Contamination food? water?	Thousands of human cases C, SF, L, I	U.S.S.R.	133, 178
2.	Cat C, L, I	Diarrhetic garden soil?	Male gardener Sept., D, L, I	England	1
3.	Rabbit	Dissection handling	8 schoolboys in biology class	England	151

	C? D? K?	L?			
4.	Pigeons Rats L, I	Fecal contamination feed? water?	3 species of exotic animals in zoological park C, L, I, S?	C, RLQ, Surg., L, S, I	Washington, D.C.	30
5.	Dog S (or infection from a common source)	Bite (mouth cult?)	Owner C, Sept, L, I		England	1
6.	Canary F, I	Fecal contamination food?	Owner C, RLQ, F, I		England	207
7.	Rats L, I	Contamination feed? water?	Turkeys C, D, L, I		England	81

Logical Connections

1.	Vast numbers grackles C, D, L, I	Fecal contamination feed trough	Swine D (no diagnosis)		U.S.	10
2.	Field mice D in canary flight (no diagnostic 10 days before first canary case)	Fecal contamination canary feeders	Canaries C, D, L, I		Canada	11
3.	Cats not studied	No sanitation control in home	Boy C, RLQ, I		Germany	9

Table 5 (continued)
EPIDEMIOLOGICAL CONNECTIONC FROM SELECTED PUBLISHED REPORTS[a]

	Source species	Vehicle	Victim species	Country	Ref.
4.	Cow with mastitis S, C	Milk on hands drunk unpasteurized?	Male milker C, RLQ, L, I	Germany	114
Highly Conjectural Connections					
1.	Family pets D (previously)	Contamination general home environment	Number of human cases (confirmed)	England	1
2.	Turkey farm nearby	Access to feed? and water?	Free-flying palm dove[b] C, K, L, I	Israel[b]	208

[a] Code: C—clinical; F—fecal; SF—scarlatiniform fever; Surg—surgical; I—isolation— Y. pseudotuberculosis; L—typical lesions; RLQ—right lower quadrant; D—deaths; K—killed; S—serological; and Sept—septicemia.

[b] This is the first reported infection with Y. pseudotuberculosis in Israel. The health or carrier status of turkeys or possibly of newly introduced birds or livestock of any kind to the area is not known.

the periphery of the chart with arrows showing established or logical connections. The infectivity potentials in the eating of carrion and proximity to flyways of migratory birds[164] are represented by symbols at the top of the outer circle.

Fecal sources and contaminated vehicles for human oral contact are represented within a modified ring structure symbolizing the universal, collective alimentary canal of many species. The human family is represented at table within domicile, the food supplies for which are threatened by many sources of contamination. An accompanying list of symbols explains the relationships of human activities and contacts with animal feces or tissues.

Environmental Monitoring

Available information on the persistence of *Y. pseudotuberculosis* in the external environment has recently been discussed at length by Mair.[1] This agent as a vegetative form is highly resistant to normally adverse environmental conditions such as those encountered in soil and water. This fact, coupled with the established psychrotrophic character of *Y. pseudotuberculosis,* raises important questions as to the dangers of refrigerator conditions for prolonged holding of foodstuffs that are to be consumed without subsequent heating. For this reason, the home-family environment as depicted by symbols on the epidemiology chart includes a domestic refrigerator with accompanying interrogation point. It would be impossible to overemphasize the importance of surveys such as that of Barre, Louzis, and Tuffery that was recently reported from France.[137] Deaths due to *Y. pseudotuberculosis* were studied through laboratory examination of dead and dying animals. Positive diagnoses were made on no less than 31% of over 4400 hares, 17% of 77 rabbits, and 7% of 728 woodpigeons. Red-legged and grey partridges, pheasants, and red squirrels were also found to be infected.

PREVENTION AND CONTROL

According to Mair,[1] no effective preventive measures are known for *Yersinia pseudotuberculosis* infections. The epidemiology chart (Figure 1) and Table 5 fairly well illustrate the almost infinite number of possible connections between reservoir or carrier host and the susceptible animal and human populations. Mair does, however, discuss the value of normal hygiene standards in connection with food-borne infection, education with regard to the hazards of pets, systematic eradication of mice (and rats?), and better protection of food from rodents and birds. The inadvertent importation of disease into hitherto *Yersinia*-free areas may be effected through importation of animals into hunting reserves for breeding purposes and for laboratory experiments. These kinds of situations require surveillance, but latent infections may defeat such an effort.[1]

In the same recent discourse, Mair noted the absence of *Y. pseudotuberculosis* in the Near and Middle East. A case now reported from Israel[190] indicates the continued ability of the disease to extend itself in new geographical areas (Table 5). Several suggestions might be made that would follow up the objectives of Mair. These are in addition to the previously mentioned proposal under Dynamics of Pseudotuberculosis, *viz.,* exhaustive surveys of trapped animals, road-kills, and animals dead of other causes. The purposes of that proposal would include detection of all the yersinias. The concept of spread by carrion is important. The additional suggestions include:

1. Increased education at the clinical and laboratory levels in the fields of human and veterinary health

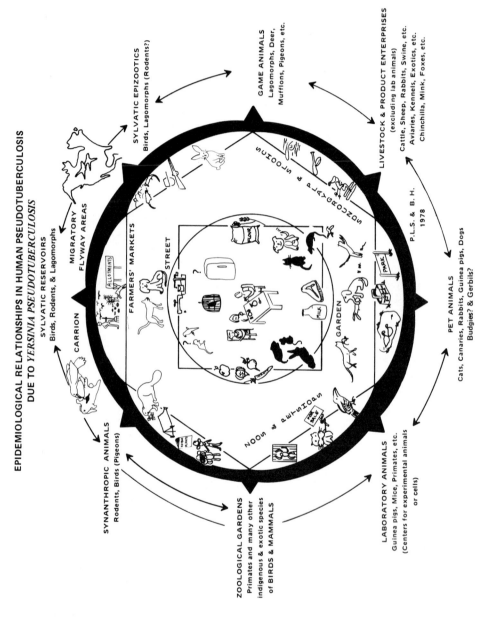

EPIDEMIOLOGICAL RELATIONSHIPS IN HUMAN PSEUDOTUBERCULOSIS DUE TO *YERSINIA PSEUDOTUBERCULOSIS*

Figure 1.   Potential fecal or tissue sources of infection, resultant animal cycles, and potential human contacts.

Boundary of human domicile

Home-grown, procured, or stored food supplies for domicile and direct animal involvement

Area of daily, routine human activities in an urban environment

Extensions of human activities beyond the urban neighborhood that promote animal contact:
1. Allotment or colony gardens
2. Garbage dumps, hunting, trapping of game
3. Outdoor sports activities
4. Parks, picnics, games
5. Zoos, pet stores
6. Riding, hiking, camping

The collective, universally present animal alimentary canal thought to be the predominant delivery system for shed or excreted viable *Y. pseudotuberculosis*

?

Unknown but potential roles of budgerigars, gerbils, and domestic refrigerators in source or multiplication of psychrotrophic *Y. pseudotuberculosis*

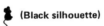 (Black silhouette)

Synanthropics (rats, mice) or pets (canary, cat, guinea pig, rabbit) that are circumstantially or statistically incriminated in human infections

 (Animals in outline)

Susceptible to epizootic or sporadic natural infection with *Y. pseudotuberculosis* but have not yet been directly incriminated in human infections

2. Continuation of the international symposia with publication of complete proceedings in several languages
3. Encouragement by public health and veterinary agencies for more background investigation in tracing back the origin of infections
4. Specialized fecal surveys in animals and man to detect carrier states and delineate areas of possible future outbreaks
5. Development of faster, simpler, and more effective methods for fecal culture
6. Alignment with and inclusion in existing fecal, bacteriological, and serological surveys for, e.g., salmonellosis, enteroparasitism, brucellosis, etc. This includes environmental surveys of surface waters, foodstuffs, and animal feeds
7. Individual testing of import animals to countries with low or nil incidence and/or use of new techniques, such as artificial insemination, embryo transplant, etc., to reduce movement of animals

REFERENCES

1. **Mair, N. S., Hubbert, W. T., McCulloch, W. F., and Schnurrenberger, P. R., Eds.,** *Diseases Transmitted from Animals to Man,* Charles C Thomas, Springfield, Ill., 1975, 174.
2. **Mollaret, H. H.,** L'infection humaine et animal a bacille de Malessez et Vignal en France de 1959 a 1967, in *Int. Symp. Pseudotuberculosis,* Regamey, R. H., Ed., S. Karger, Basel, 1968, 45.
3. **Masshof, W. and Dolle, W.,** Uber eine besondere Form der sogenannte mesenterialen Lymphadenitis: die abscedierende reticulocytare Lymphadenopathie, *Virchows Arch. Pathol. Anat. Physiol.,* 323, 664, 1953.
4. **Knapp, W. and Masshoff, W.,** Zur etiologie der abszedierenden retikulozytare Lymphadenitis eine praktisch wichtigen, vielfach unter dem Bild eine akut Appendezitis verlaufender Erkrankung, *Dtsch. Med. Wochenschr.,* 79, 1266, 1954.
5. **Malassez, L. and Vignal, W.,** Tuberculose zoogléique (forme ou espece de tuberculose sans bacilles), *Arch. Physiol. Norm. Pathol.,* 2, 369, 1883.
6. **Malassez, L.,** Sur le micro-organisme de la tuberculose zoogléique., *Arch. Physiol. Norm. Pathol.,* 81, 1884.
7. **Grancini, L. E.,** La pseudotuberculose en Itale, in *Int. Symp. Pseudotuberculosis,* Regamey, R. H., Ed., S. Karger, Basel, 1968, 75.
8. **Saisawa, K.,** Uber die Pseudotuberkulose beim Menschen, *Z. Hyg. Infektionskr.,* 73, 353, 1913.
9. **Albrecht, H. Z.,** Aetiologie der Enteritis follicularis suppurctiva, *Wein Klin. Wochenschr.,* 23, 991, 1910.
10. **Clark, G. M. and Locke, L. N.,** Case report: observations on pseudotuberculosis in common grackles, *Avian Dis.,* 6, 506, 1962.
11. **Stovell, P. L.,** Epizootiological factors in three outbreaks of pseudotuberculosis in British Columbia canaries *(Serinus canarius),* Masters thesis, University of British Columbia, 1963.
12. **Wetzler, T. F.,** *Infections and Parasitic Diseases of Wild Birds,* Davis, J. W., Anderson, R. C., Karstad, L., and Trainer, D. O., Eds., Iowa State University Press, Ames, 1971, 75.
13. **Wetzler, T. F.,** *Infectious Diseases of Wild Mammals,* Davis, J. W., Anderson, R. C., Karstad, L., and Trainer, D. O., Eds., Iowa State University Press, Ames, 1970, 224.
14. **McLure, H. M., Weaver, R. C., and Kaufman, A. F.,** Pseudotuberculosis in non-human primates: infection with organism of the *Y. enterocoliticum* group, *Lab. Anim. Sci.,* 21, 376, 1971.
15. **Eberth, C. J.,** Zwer mykosen des meerschweinchens, *Virchows Arch. Pathol. Anat. Physiol.,* 100, 15, 1885.
16. **Sonnenwirth, A. C.,** *Manual of Clinical Microbiology,* 2nd ed., Lennett, E. H., Spaulding, E. H., and Truant, J. P., Eds., American Society for Microbiology, Washington, D.C., 1974, 222.
17. **Heddleston, K. L.,** in, *Diseases of Poultry,* 6th ed., Hofstad, M. S., Calnek, B. W., Helmboldt, C. F., Reid, W. M., and Yoder, H. W., Jr., Eds., Iowa State University Press, Ames, 1972, 241.
18. **Buchanan R. E., Holt, J. G., and Lessel, E. F.,** *Index Bergeyana,* Williams & Wilkins, Baltimore, 1966, 791.

19. Smith, J. E. and Thal, E., A taxonomic study of the genus *Pasteurella* using a numerical technique, *Acta Pathol. Microbiol. Scand.*, 64, 213, 1965.

20. Ferber, D. M. and Brubaker, R. R., The effects of pesticin on *Y. enterocolitica* and *Y. pseudotuberculosis* strains, in *Microbiology and Immunology*, Vol. V, S. Karger, Basel, in press.

21. Meyer, K. F., *Bacterial and Mycotic Infection of Man*, 3rd ed., Dubos, R. J., Ed., Lippincott, Philadelphia, 1958, 400.

22. Wetzler, T. F., Rosen, M. N., and Marshall, J. D., *Diagnostic Methods in Medical Microbiology*, Graber, C. D., Ed., Williams & Wilkins, Baltimore, 1970, 67.

23. Baker, E. T., *Sheep Diseases*, Campbell, D. M., Ed., American Veterinary Publishing, Chicago, 1920, 232.

24. Mollaret, H. H. and Thal, E., *Bergey's Manual of Determinative Bacteriology*, 8th ed., Buchanan, R. E. and Gibbons, N. E., Eds., Williams & Wilkins, Baltimore, 1974, 330.

25. Wilson, G. S. and Miles, A., *Topley and Wilson's Principle of Bacteriology, Virology and Immunity*, Vol. 1, 6th ed., Butler and Tanner, Great Britain, 1975, 998.

26. Newman Dorland, W. A., Wayson's staining method, in *The American Illustrated Medical Dictionary*, 21st ed., W. B. Saunders, Philadelphia, 1947, 1387.

27. Paik, G. and Suggs, M. T., *Manual of Clinical Microbiology*, 2nd ed., Lennett, E. H., Spaulding, E. H., and Truant, J. P., Eds., American Society for Microbiology, Washington, D.C., 1974, 940.

28. Cook, R., The naturally occurring diseases of laboratory animals and practical measures for the control of the diseases, *J. Med. Lab. Technol.*, 11, 30, 1953.

29. Van der Schaaf, A., A specific staining method of *Pasteurella pseudotuberculosis*, in *Int. Symp. Pseudotuberculosis*, Regamey, R. H., Ed., S. Karger, Basel, 1968, 193.

30. Baskin, G. B., Montali, R. J., Bush, M., Quan, T. J., and Smith, E., Yersiniosis in captive exotic mammals, *J. Am. Vet. Med. Assoc.*, 171, 908, 1977.

31. Stovell, P. L., Unpublished data concerning an isolant of *Y. pseudotuberculosis* from a bovine mesenteric lymph node, 1953.

32. Stovell, P. L., Unpublished data concerning epizootic of canary pseudotuberculosis and an outbreak in guinea pigs in the Fraser Delta, 1963.

33. Bovallius, A. and Nilsson, G., Ingestion and survival of *Y. pseudotuberculosis* in HeLa cells, *Can. J. Microbiol.*, 21, 1997, 1975.

34. Brubaker, R. R. and Yang, C. H., Expression of the virulence antigens of pasteurellae, in *Symp. Ser. Immunobiological Standardization*, Vol. 15, Regamey, R. H., Stanic, N., and Ungar, J., Eds., S. Karger, Basel, 1971, 223.

35. Richardson, M. and Harkness, T. K., Intracellular *Pasteurella pseudotuberculosis*: multiplication in cultured spleen and kidney cells, *Infect. Immun.*, 21, 631, 1970.

36. Robinson, M., *Pasteurella pseudotuberculosis* infection in the cat, *Vet. Rec.*, 91, 676, 1972.

37. Surgalla, M. J., Andrews, A. W., and Cavanaugh, D. M., Studies on virulence factors of *Pasteurella pestis* and *Past. pseudotuberculosis*, in *Int. Symp. Pseudotuberculosis*, Regamey, R. H., Ed., S. Karger, Basel, 1968, 293.

38. Burrows, T. W. and Gillett, W. A., The nutritional requirements of some *Pasteurella* species, *J. Gen. Microbiol.*, 45, 333, 1966.

39. Wetzler, T. F. and Hubbert, W. T., *Pasteurella pseudotuberculosis* in North America, in *Int. Symp. Pseudotuberculosis*, Regamey, R. H., Ed., S. Karger, Basel, 1968, 33.

40. Burrows, T. W., Observations on the pigmentation of *Yersinia pseudotuberculosis*, *Contrib. Microbiol. Immunol.*, 2, 184, 1973.

41. Lee, W. H., Two plating media modified with Tween 80 for isolating *Y. enterocoliticum*, *Appl. Environ. Microbiol.*, 33, 215, 1977.

42. Frankel, S., Reitman, S., and Sonnenwirth, A. C., *Clinical Laboratory Methods and Diagnosis*, 7th ed., Mosby, St. Louis, 1970, 1275.

43. Chen, T. H. and Meyer, K. F., An evaluation of *Pasteurella pestis* fraction-1-specific antibody for the confirmation of plague infections, *Bull. W.H.O.*, 34, 911, 1966.

44. Wetzler, T. F., Eitzen, H. E., and Currie, T. A., Lipopolysaccharide-like antigens from *Pasteurella pseudotuberculosis* shared by various genera of enterobacteriaceae as demonstrated by hemagglutination tests, in *Int. Symp. Pseudotuberculosis*, Regamey, R. H., Ed., S. Karger, Basel, 1968, 155.

45. Thal, E. and Knapp, W., A revised antigenic scheme of *Yersinia tuberculosis*, in *Symp. Ser. Immunobiological Standardization*, Regamey, R. H., Stanic, N., and Ungar, J., Eds., S. Karger, Basel, 1971, 219.

46. Bader, R. E., A common factor in types I to V of *Pasteurella pseudotuberculosis*, *Abstr. Hyg.*, 47, 1056, 1972.

47. Thal, E., Observations on immunity in *Y. pseudotuberculosis*, *Contrib. Microbiol. Immunobiol.*, 2, 190, 1973.

48. **Mair, N. S. and Fox, E.**, An antigenic relationship between *Y. pseudotuberculosis* type VI and *E. coli* O-group 55, *Contrib. Microbiol. Immunobiol.*, 2, 180, 1973.

49. **Mair, N. S.**, personal communication — isolations of *Y. pseudotuberculosis* from healthy swine, 1977.

50. **Burrows, T. W. and Bacon, G. A.**, V and W antigens in strains of *Pasteurella pseudotuberculosis*, *Br. J. Exp. Pathol.*, 41, 38, 1960.

51. **Thal, E.**, Untersuchungen über *Pasteurella pseudotuberculosis*, Ph.D. thesis, Lund, 1954.

52. **Devignat, R.**, Ancient plague of the Belgian Congo in the framework of history and geography, *Mem. Inst. Royal Col. Belge*, 23, 1953.

53. **Devignat, R. and Boivin, A.**, Comportement biologique et biochemique de *P. pestis* et de *P. pseudotuberculosis*, *Bull. Org. Mond. Sante*, 10, 463, 1954.

54. **Korobkova, E., Lenskaja, G. N., and Sololova, N. M.**, *Int. Symp. Pseudotuberculosis*, Regamey, R. H., Ed., S. Karger, Basel, 1968, 245.

55. **Obwolo, M. J.**, A review of yersiniosis *(Y. pseudotuberculosis* infection), *Vet. Bull.*, 46, 167, 1976.

56. **Kitt, T.**, Septikamie der vogel (Huhnercholera), in *Handbuch der Pathogenen Mikroorganismen*, Vol. 2, Kolle and Wasserman, Eds., 1903, 543.

57. **Beck, A.**, Die Pseudotuberkulose der Nagetiere und ihre Beziehungen zur Paracholera der Puten, Tauben und Kanarie vogel, *Z. Infekt.-Kr. Haustiere*, 33, 103, 1925.

58. **Nocard, E.**, Sur une tuberculose zoogleique des oiseaux de bsse-cour, *Bull. Soc. Centr. Med. Vet.*, 39, 207, 1885.

59. **Pfeiffer, A.**, *Über die bacillare Pseudotuberkulose bei den Nagetieren*, Leipzig, 1889.

60. **Rieck, M.**, Eine infektiöse Erkrankung der Kanarienvögel, *Dtsch. Z. Tiermed. Vergleich. Pathol.*, 15, 68, 1889.

61. **Mazzini, G.**, Pseudotuberkulose beim Rind, *Gior. R. Soc. Acad. Vet. Ital.*, 758, 1897.

62. **Wasielewski, T. von, and Hoffman, W.**, Über eine seuchenhafte Erkrankung bei Singvögeln, *Arch. Hyg.*, 47, 44, 1903.

63. **Dolfen, H.**, Über eine Pseudotuberkulose, seichenhafte Erkrankung bei Tauben, inaugural dissertation, Hannover, 1916, 5.

64. **Leblois, C.**, La pseudo-tuberculose zoogleique chez le chat, *Rec. Med. Vet.*, 96, 307, 1920.

65. **Kinyoun, J. J.**, Bird plague (a preliminary note), *Science*, 23, 217, 1906.

66. **Krage, P. and Weisgerber, F.**, Eine Putenseuche mit Diplo-Streptobazillenbefund, *Tieraerztl. Rundsch.*, 20, 1924.

67. **Rosenwald, A. S. and Dickinson, E. M.**, A report of *Pasteurella pseudotuberculosis* infection in turkeys, *Am. J. Vet. Res.*, 5, 246, 1944.

68. **Mathey, W. I. and Siddle, P. I.**, Isolation of *Pasteurella pseudotuberculosis* from a California turkey, *J. Am. Vet. Med. Assoc.*, 125, 482, 1954.

69. **Marthedal, H. E. and Velling, G.**, Pasteurellose og pseudotuberkulose i husfjerkrae in Danmark (Pasteurella infection in domestic fowls in Denmark), *Nord. Vet. Med.*, 6, 651, 1954.

70. **Wetzler, T. F. and Hubbert, W. I.**, *Int. Symp. Pseudotuberculosis*, Regamey, R. H., Ed., S. Karger, Basel, 1968, 343.

71. **Baumann, R.**, Ein Fall von Pseudotuberkulose bei einer jungen Ziege, *Z. Infektionskr.-Kr. Hyg. Haustiere*, 31, 141, 1927.

72. **Stropnik, Z.**, *Int. Symp. Pseudotuberculosis*, Regamey, R. H., Ed., S. Karger, Basel, 1968, 103.

73. **Claussen, S.**, Über Bakteriaemie durch das *Bact. pseudotuberculosis rodentium* bei der Biberratte, *Dtsch. Tieraerztl. Wochenschr.*, 42, 243, 1934.

74. **Zoltai, N., Rudnai, O., Szita, J., and Svidro, A.**, *Int. Symp. Pseudotuberculosis*, Regamey, R. H., Ed., S. Karger, Basel, 1968, 85.

75. **Haas, V. H.**, A study of *Pseudotuberculosis rodentium* recovered from a rat, *Public Health Rep.*, 53, 1033, 1938.

76. **Beaudette, F. R.**, A case of pseudotuberculosis in a blackbird, *J. Am. Vet. Med. Assoc.*, 97, 151, 1940.

77. **Wramby, G. and Fredricson, M.**, Ett fall av pseudotuberculos hos svin, *Skand. Vet. Tidskr.*, 31, 590, 1941.

78. **Juscenko, G. V.**, *Int. Symp. Pseudotuberculosis*, Regamey, R. H., Ed., S. Karger, Basel, 1968, 107.

79. **Chapman, M.**, *Pseudotuberculosis rodentium* in chinchilla, *N. Am. Vet.*, 29, 493, 1948.

80. **Leader, R. W. and Baker, G. A.**, A report of two cases of *Pasteurella pseudotuberculosis* infection in the chinchilla, *Cornell Vet.*, 44, 262, 1954.

81. **Blaxland, J. D.**, *Pasteurella pseudotuberculosis* infection in turkeys, *Vet. Rec.*, 59, 317, 1947.

82. **Clapham, P. A.**, Pseudotuberculosis among stock doves in Hampshire, *Nature (London)*, 172, 353, 1953.

83. **Paterson, J. S. and Cook, R.**, A method for the recovery of *Pasteurella pseudotuberculosis* from faeces, *J. Pathol. Bacteriol.*, 85, 241, 1963.

84. **Mair, N. S., Mair, H. J., Stirk, E. M., and Gorson, J. G.**, Three cases of acute mesenteric lymphadenitis due to *Pasteurella pseudotuberculosis, J. Clin. Pathol.*, 13, 432, 1960.

85. **Mair, N. S.**, Pseudotuberculosis in free-living wild animals, *Symp. Zool. Soc. London*, 24, 107, 1968.

86. **Thal, E.**, Untersuchungen über *Pasteurella pseudotuberculosis, Proc. 15th Int. Vet. Congr.*, Part 1, Vol. 1, 67, 1955.

87. **Langford, E. V.**, personal communication, 1966.

88. **Langford, E. V.**, *Pasteurella pseudotuberculosis* infections in western Canada, *Can. Vet. J.*, 13, 85, 1972.

89. **Langford, E. V.**, *Pasteurella pseudotuberculosis* associated with abortion and pneumonia in the bovine, *Can. Vet. J.*, 10, 208, 1969.

90. **Hnatko, S. I. and Rodin, A. E.**, *Pasteurella pseudotuberculosis* antibody titres in man, *Can. Med. Assoc. J.*, 86, 725, 1962.

91. **Toma, S. and Diedrick, V. R.**, Incidence of *Y. enterocolitica* and *Y. pseudotuberculosis* infections in Canada, *Can. Med. Assoc. J.*, 114, 16, 1976.

92. **Knox, B.**, personal communication, 1963.

93. **Rislakki, V.**, Pseudotuberculosis in rodents and foxes, *Suom. Elanlaakarile*, 48, 182, 1942.

94. **Hacking, M. A. and Sileo, L.**, *Y. enterocolitica* and *Y. pseudotuberculosis* from wildlife in Ontario, *J. Wildl. Dis.*, 10, 453, 1974.

95. **Karen-Heyberger, E.**, *Int. Symp. Pseudotuberculosis*, Regamey, R. H., Ed., S. Karger, Basel, 1968, 81.

96. **Weidenmuller, H.**, *Pasteurella pseudotuberculosis* infection in animals and man, *Tieraerztl. Umsch.*, 14, 256, 1959.

97. **Borg, K.**, Silvatic psuedotuberculosis in Scandinavia, in *Int. Symp. on Pseudotuberculosis*, Regamey, R. H., Ed., Paris, 129, 1968.

98. **Weidenmuller, H.**, Pseudotuberkulose bei Wildtieren, *Tieraerztl. Umsch.*, 9, 447, 1966.

99. **Fertig, S.**, *Int. Symp. Pseudotuberculosis*, Regamey, R. H., Ed., S. Karger, Basel, 1968, 91.

100. **Flux, J. E. C.**, Life history of the mountain hare (*Lepus timidus scoticus*) in northeast Scotland, *J. Zool.*, 161, 75, 1970.

101. **Schneider, P. A.**, *Int. Symp. Pseudotuberculosis*, Regamey, R. H., Ed., S. Karger, Basel, 1968, 59.

102. **Lesbouyries, G.**, Pseudotuberculosis du pigeon, *Bull. Acad. Vet.*, 7, 103, 1934.

103. **Keymer, I. F.**, Specific diseases of the canary and other passerine birds, *Mod. Vet. Pract.*, 40, 33, 1959.

104. **Mair, N. S.**, *Int. Symp. Pseudotuberculosis*, Regamey, R. H., Ed., S. Karger, Basel, 1968, 121.

105. **Truche, C. and Bauche, J.**, Le bacille pseudotuberculeux chez la poule et faisan, *Bull. Acad. Vet. Fr.*, 6, 43, 1933.

106. **Karlsson, K. F.**, Pseudotuberculosis in gallinaceous birds, *Skand. Vet. Tidskr.*, 36, 673, 1947.

107. **Truche, C.**, Pseudotuberculose du cygne, *Bull. Acad. Vet. Fr.*, 8, 278, 1935.

108. **Chitty, D.**, personal communication, University of British Columbia, Department of Zoology, Vancouver, 1962.

109. **Marshall, J. D., Currie, J. A., and Quy, D. V.**, *Int. Symp. Pseudotuberculosis*, Regamey, R. H., Ed., S. Karger, Basel, 1968, 309.

110. **Van Haaften, J., Poelma, F. G., and Zwart, P.**, *Int. Symp. Pseudotuberculosis*, Regamey, R. H., Ed., S. Karger, Basel, 1968, 117.

111. **Szita, J. and Svidro, A.**, A 5-year survey of human *Y. enterocolitica* infections in Hungary, *Acta Microbiol. Hung.*, 23, 191, 1976.

112. **Avery, R. J. A.**, personal communication, 1970.

113. **Mair, N. S. and Harbourne, J. F.**, The isolation of *Pasteurella pseudotuberculosis* from a bovine fetus, *Vet. Rec.*, 75, 559, 1963.

114. **Graber, H. and Knapp, W.**, Die abscedierende retikulocytare Lymphadenitis mesenterialis (Masshoff) als Bestandteil eines enteralen Primarkomplexes und Folge einer Infektion mit *Pasteurella pseudotuberculosis, Frankf. Z. Pathol.*, 66, 399, 1955.

115. **Messerli, J.**, *Y. pseudotuberculosis*, Erreger einer Mastitis beim Rind, *Zentralbl. Bakteriol. Parasitenkd. Infektionskr. Hyg. Abt. 1: Orig. Reihe A*, 222, 280, 1972.

116. **Gelev, I.**, Bacterial infection in cows associated with abortion, endometritis and infertility, *Vet. Bull.*, 46, 1975, 1976.

117. **Jayaraman, M. S. and Sethumadavan, V.**, The B. L. organism — the casual agent of bovine lymphangitis in Tamil Nadar, *Indian Vet. J.*, 51, 347, 1974.

118. **Morita, M., Nakamatsu, M., and Goto, M.**, Pathological studies on *Pseudotuberculosis rodentium*. Three spontaneous swine cases, *Jpn. J. Vet. Sci.*, 30, 233, 1968.

119. **Tsubokura, M., Itagaki, K., and Kawamura, K.,** Studies on *Yersinia* (*Pasteurella*) *pseudotuberculosis*. Sources and serological classification of the organism isolated in Japan, *Jpn. J. Vet. Sci.,* 32, 227, 1970.

120. **Tsubokura, M., Otsuki, K., Fukuda, T., Kubota, M., Imamura, M., Itagaki, K., Yamaoka, K., and Wakatsuki, M.,** Studies on *Yersinia pseudotuberculosis.* IV. Isolation of *Y. pseudotuberculosis* from healthy swine, *Jpn. J. Vet. Sci.,* 38, 549, 1976.

121. **Mollaret, H. H. and le Pennec, J.,** A propos d'un cas s'infection a bacille de Malassez et Vignal chez le porc, *Rec. Med. Vet.,* 144, 429, 1968.

122. **Dennis, S. M.,** Recovery of *Pasteurella pseudotuberculosis* from a premature Merino lamb, *Vet. Rec.,* 79, 273, 1966.

123. **Jamieson, S. and Soltys, M. A.,** Infectious epididymo-orchitis of rams associated with *Pasteurella pseudotuberculosis, Vet. Rec.,* 59, 351, 1947.

124. **Watson, W. A. and Hunter, D.,** Isolation of *Pasteurella pseudotuberculosis* from an ovine fetus, *Vet. Rec.,* 72, 769, 1960.

125. **Watson, W. A.,** Ovine abortion, *Vet. Rec.,* 74, 1403, 1962.

126. **Mair, N. S. and Ziffo, G. S.,** Isolation of *Y. pseudotuberculosis* from a foal, *Vet. Rec.,* 94, 152, 1974.

127. **Itagaki, K., Tsubokura, M., Sasaki, T., and Nagai, T.,** *Int. Symp. Pseudotuberculosis,* Regamey, R. H., Ed., S. Karger, Basel, 1968, 27.

128. **Butterwick, D.,** personal communication, 1972.

129. **Zaremba, M. and Borowski, J.,** *Y. pseudotuberculosis* in man in Poland, *Contrib. Microbiol. Immunol.,* 2, 217, 1973.

130. **Wise, D. R. and Uppal, P. K.,** Osteomyelitis in turkeys caused by *Y. pseudotuberculosis, J. Med. Microbiol.,* 5, 128, 1972.

131. **Joubert, L.,** Bird-transmitted pseudo-TB held frequent, *Mod. Vet. Pract.,* 48, 32, 1967.

132. **Winkenwerder, W.,** *Int. Symp. Pseudotuberculosis,* Regamey, R. H., Ed., S. Karger, Basel, 1968, 69.

133. **Somov, G. P. and Martinevsky, I. L.,** *Contributions to Microbiology and Immunology,* Winblad, S., Ed., Vol. 2, S. Karger, Basel, 1973, 214.

134. **Timofeeva, L., Mironova, L., and Golovaceva, V.,** *Int. Symp. Pseudotuberculosis,* Regamey, R. H., Ed., S. Karger, Basel, 1968, 219.

135. **Rigby, C.,** Natural infections of guinea pigs, *Lab. Anim.,* 10, 119, 1976.

136. **Sasaki, J., Nagai, T., Itakaki, K., and Tsubokura, M.,** *Int. Symp. Pseudotuberculosis,* Regamey, R. H., Ed., S. Karger, Basel, 1968, 167.

137. **Barre, N., Louzis, C., and Tuffery, G.,** Epidemiological study of *Y. pseudotuberculosis* infection of wild animals in France, *Rev. Med. Vet. Mycol.,* 128, 1545, 1977.

138. **Hirai, K., Suzuki, Y., Kato, N., Yagami, K., Miyoshi, A., Mabuchi, Y., Nigi, H., Inagaki, H., Otsuki, K., and Tsubokura, M.,** *Y. pseudotuberculosis* infection occurred spontaneously in a group of patas monkeys (*Erythrocebus patas*), *Jpn. J. Vet. Sci.,* 36, 351, 1974.

139. **Buhles, W. C.,** in preparation, 1978.

140. **Jones, D. M. and Manton, V. J. A.,** Whipsnade Park, 1973 and 1974, *J. Zool.,* 178, 494, 1976.

141. **Keymer, I. F.,** Report of the pathologist 1969 and 1970, *J. Zool.,* 166, 515, 1972.

142. **Keymer, I. F.,** Report of the pathologist 1971 and 1972, *J. Zool.,* 173, 51, 1974.

143. **Keymer, I. F., Jones, D. M., and Manton, V. J. A.,** Report of the pathologist 1973 and 1974, *J. Zool.,* 178, 456, 1977.

144. **Borst, G. H. A., Buitelaar, M., Poelma, F. G., Zwart, P., and Dorrestein, G. M.,** *Yersinia pseudotuberculosis* in birds, *Vet. Bull.,* 47, 507, 1977.

145. **Mair, N. S., Harbourne, J. F., Greenwood, M. T., and White, G.,** *Pasteurella pseudotuberculosis* infection in the cat: two cases, *Vet. Rec.,* 81, 461, 1967.

146. **Obwolo, M. J. and Gruffydd-Jones, T. J.,** *Yersinia pseudotuberculosis* in the cat, *Vet. Rec.,* 100, 424, 1977.

147. **O'Sullivan, B. M., Rosenfield, L. E., and Green, P. E.,** Concurrent infection with *Y. pseudotuberculosis* and *Platynosomum fastosum* in a cat, *Aust. Vet. J.,* 52, 232, 1976.

148. **Goret, P., Collet, P., Joubert, L., and Pilet, C.,** Diagnostic experimental et pathologenique de la pseudotuberculose du chat, *Bull. Soc. Sci. Vet. Lyon,* 57, 205, 1955.

149. **Mollaret, H. H.,** Infection of cats with the bacillus of Malassez and Vignal (*Pasteurella pseudotuberculosis*). I. Natural infection. II. Experimental, *Rec. Med. Vet.,* 141, 1079 and 1187, 1965.

150. **Triplett, D. A. and Paff, J. R.,** Clinical and laboratory aspects of *Y. pseudotuberculosis* infections, *Annu. Meet. Abstr. Lab. Invest.,* 32, 458, 1975.

151. **Andrews, H. J. and Mair, N. S.,** Outbreak of *Y. pseudotuberculosis* infection at a boy's boarding school, *Com. Dis. Rep.,* 34, 1976.

152. **Winblad, S.,** The epidemiology of human infections with *Yersinia pseudotuberculosis* and *Yersinia enterocolitica* in Scandinavia, in *Int. Symp. Pseudotuberculosis,* Regamey, R. H., Ed., S. Karger, Basel, 1968, 133.

153. **Daniels, J. J. H. M.,** Enteric infection with *Yersinia pseudotuberculosis,* in *Contributions to Microbiology and Immunology,* Vol. 2, Winblad, S., Ed., S. Karger, Basel, 1973, 210.

154. **Flamm, H. and Kovac, W.,** Pathogenesis of pseudotuberculosis lymphadenitis, in *Int. Symp. Pseudotuberculosis,* Regamey, R. H., Ed., S. Karger, Basel, 1968, 9.

155. **Mair, N. S., Fox, E., and Thal, E.,** Biochemical, pathogenicity and toxicity studies of group III *Y. pseudotuberculosis* strains, *Contrib. Microbiol. Immunol.,* in press.

156. **Marlon, A., Gentry, L., and Merigan, T. C.,** Septicemia with *Pasteurella pseudotuberculosis* and liver disease, *Arch. Intern. Med.,* 127, 947, 1971.

157. **Bradley, J. M. and Skinner, J. I.,** Isolation of *Y. pseudotuberculosis* serotype V from the blood of a patient with sickle-cell anaemia, *J. Med. Microbiol.,* 7, 383, 1974.

158. **Conn, H. O.,** Spontaneous peritonitis and bacteremia in Laennec's cirrhosis caused by enteric organisms. A relatively common but rarely recognized syndrome, *Ann. Intern. Med.,* 60, 568, 1964.

159. **Ignatovich, V. O., Vishnyakov, A. K., Znamensky, V. A., and Zalmover, I. Y.,** Epidemiology of pseudotuberculosis (Far Eastern scarlatina-like fever), *Zh. Mikrobiol. Epidemiol. Immunobiol.,* 44, 24, 1967.

160. **Zalmover, I. Y.,** Some results of an eight-year study of the clinical picture of Far-Eastern scarlatina-like fever, *Sov. Med.,* 32, 93, 1969.

161. **Winblad, S.,** *Contributions to Microbiology and Immunology,* Vol. 2, Grumbach, Ed., S. Karger, Basel, 1973, 129.

162. **Masshoff, W.,** Eine neuartige Form der mesenterialen Lymphadenitis, *Dtsch. Med. Wochenschr.,* 78, 532, 1953.

163. Informal survey of hospitals in greater metro Vancouver area of British Columbia, 1978.

164. **Hubbert, W. T.,** Yersiniosis in mammals and birds in the United States. Case reports and review, *Am. J. Trop. Med. Hyg.,* 21, 458, 1972.

165. **Kunz, L. L. and Hutton, G. M.,** Diseases of the laboratory guinea pig, *Vet. Scope,* 16, 12, 1971.

166. **Bankier, J. C. and Humphries, F. A.,** Laboratory of Animal Pathology, British Columbia Department of Agriculture, Vancover, unpublished data, 1953.

167. **Langford, E. V.,** *Y. enterocolitica* isolated from animals in the Fraser Valley of British Columbia, *Can. Vet. J.,* 13, 109, 1972.

168. **Collet, P., Renault, L., and Valentin, F.,** Pseudotuberculose hepatique a bacille de Malassez et Vignal chez le chien, *Bull. Soc. Sci. Vet. Lyon,* 57, 307, 1955.

169. **Mair, N. S.,** Yersiniosis in wildlife and its public health implications, *J. Wildl. Dis.,* 9, 64, 1973.

170. **Morita, M., Nakamatsu, M., and Goto, M.,** Pathology of pseudotuberculosis in mice experimentally infected with *Y. pseudotuberculosis, Jpn. J. Vet. Sci.,* 38, 471, 1976.

171. **Pilet, C., Valette, L., Labie, C., and Fontaine, M.,** Pseudotuberculosis in nutria, *Bull. Acad. Vet. Fr.,* 31, 299, 1958.

172. **Truche, G. and Isnard, I.,** Un nouveau cas de pseudotuberculose chez la poule, *Bull. Acad. Vet. Fr.,* 10, 38, 1937.

173. **Stovell, P. L. and Avery, R. J.,** unpublished data concerning pseudotuberculosis in chickens in Alberta, 1960.

174. **Krynski, S.,** *Int. Symp. Pseudotuberculosis,* Regamey, R. H., Ed., S. Karger, Basel, 1968, 7.

175. **Krynski, S. and Machel, M.,** Infection a *Y. pseudotuberculose* chez les tiques *Ornithodorus moubata* (Murray). I. Infection dans le coelome des tiques adultes, *Arch. Inst. Pasteur Tunis,* 49, 43, 1972.

176. **Machel, M.,** The influence of temperature on the course of experimental infection of *Ornithodorus moubata* (Murray) due to *Y. pseudotuberculosis, Wiad. Parazytol.,* 18, 591, 1972.

177. **Machel, M.,** Method of intraoral infection of *Ornithodorus moubata* (Murray) ticks by feeding on guinea-pig injected subcutaneously with bacterial suspension, *Z. Angew. Zool.,* 5, 161, 1972.

178. **Timofeeva, L.,** *Int. Symp. Pseudotuberculosis,* Regamey, R. H., Ed., S. Karger, Basel, 1968, 233.

179. **Blanc, G. and Baltazard, M.,** Behaviour of pathogenic organisms in bloodsucking insects, *Arch. Inst. Pasteur Maroc.,* 3, 121, 1944.

180. **Steele, J. H.,** *The Theory and Practice of Public Health,* 4th ed., Hobson, W., Ed., Oxford University Press, 1975, 304.

181. **Karlsson, K. A. and Thal, E.,** *Int. Symp. Pseudotuberculosis,* Regamey, R. H., Ed., S. Karger, Basel, 1968, 187.

182. **Goldenberg, M. and Hudson, B. W.,** *Int. Symp. Pseudotuberculosis,* Regamey, R. H., Ed., S. Karger, Basel, 1968, 303.

183. **Sizaret, P. and Mollaret, H. H.,** *Int. Symp. Pseudotuberculosis,* Regamey, R. H., Ed., S. Karger, Basel, 1968, 197.

184. **Zaremba, M. and Kaczmarski, W.,** The passive haemagglutination inhibition test in the detection of *Y. pseudotuberculosis* antigens in infected materials, *Arch. Immunol. Ther. Exp.*, 22, 61, 1974.

185. **Andrew, J. H., Weedon, D., and Mair, N. S.,** Terminal ileitis mesenteric lymphadenitis and appendicitis due to *Y. pseudotuberculosis* type VA: case report, *Pathology*, 8, 189, 1976.

186. **Tsubokura, M., Itagaki, K., and Kiyatani, K.,** Studies on *Y. pseudotuberculosis.* III. A method for isolation of *Y. pseudotuberculosis* from feces, *Jpn. J. Vet. Sci.*, 35, 33, 1973.

187. **Wetzler, T. F.,** *Diagnostic Procedures for Bacterial Mycotic & Parasitic Infections*, Bodily, H. L. and Updyke, E. L., Eds., American Public Health Association, New York, 1970, 449.

188. **Chen, T. H. and Elberg, S. S.,** Scanning electron microscopic study of virulent *Y. pestis* and *Y. pseudotuberculosis* type I, *Infect. Immun.*, 15, 972, 1977.

189. **Darland, G., Ewing, W. H., and Davis, B. R.,** The biochemical characteristics of *Y. enterocolitica* and *Y. pseudotuberculosis*, U.S. Department of Health, Education and Welfare, Publication No. (CDC) 75—8294, 21, 1975.

190. **Mair, N. S., White, G. D., Schubert, F. K., and Harbourne, J.,** *Y. enterocolitica* infection in the bush-baby, *Vet. Rec.*, 86, 69, 1970.

191. **Brenner, D. J., Steigerwaltz, A. G., Falcao, D. F., Weaver, R. E., and Fanning, G. R.,** Characterization of *Y. enterocolitica* and *Y. pseudotuberulosis* by deoxyribonucleic acid hybridization and by biochemical reactions, *Abs. Hyg.*, 51, 1188, 1976.

192. **Maiskii, V. G. and Lalazarova, I. G.,** A method of differentiation of plague and pseudotuberculosis organisms by adenosine deaminase, *Zh. Mikrobiol. Epidemiol. Immunobiol.*, 10, 124, 1973.

193. **Merka, V. and Splino, M.,** Sensitivity of *Y. pseudotuberculosis* in vitro, *Zentralbl. Bakteriol. Parasitenkd. Infektionskr. Hyg. Abt. 1: Orig. Reihe A*, 219, 407, 1972.

194. **Hausnerova, S., Hausner, O., and Pauckova, V.,** Antibiotic sensitivity of *Y. enterocolitica* strains isolated in two regions of Czechoslovakia, *Contrib. Microbiol. Immunol.*, 2, 76, 1973.

195. **Kanazawa, Y. and Kuramata, T.,** Difference in susceptibility to benzylpenicillin between *Y. enterocolitica* and *Y. pseudotuberculosis*, *Jpn. J. Microbiol.*, 18, 483, 1974.

196. **Brzin, B.,** *Int. Symp. Pseudotuberculosis*, Regamey, R. H., Ed., S. Karger, Basel, 1968, 207.

197. **Borowski, J. and Zaremba, M.,** Some problems connected with *Y. pseudotuberculosis* resistance to antibiotics, *Contrib. Microbiol. Immunol.*, 2, 196, 1973.

198. **Joubert, L., Bonnod, J., and Oudar, J.,** Une enzootie de pseudotuberculose du cobaye d'elevage a destination scientifeque. Depistage par le test a l'aureomycine de H. Mollaret, *Rev. Serv. Biol. Vet. Armees*, 15, 10, 1962.

199. **Currie, J. A., Marshall, J. D., and Crozier, D.,** The detection of *pasteurella pseudotuberculosis* antibodies by the microhemagglutination test, *J. Infect. Dis.*, 116, 117, 1965.

200. **Joubert, L.,** Role epidemiologique des oiseaux dans la pseudotuberculose humaine, *13th World Vet. Congr. Paris*, Vol. 1, 247, 1967.

201. **Diaz, R.,** Antigenic relationship of *Y. enterocolitica*, *Contrib. Microbiol. Immunol.*, 2, 157, 1973.

202. **Hallstrom, K. A. and Paltemaa, S.,** A precipitation arc in immunoelectrophoresis specific to *Y. pseudotuberculosis* serotype 2, *Contrib. Microbiol. Immunol.*, 2, 203, 1973.

203. **Thal, E. and Wellmann, G.,** *Int. Symp. Pseudotuberculosis*, Regamey, R. H., Ed., S. Karger, Basel, 1968, 211.

204. **Goebel, H. H. and Masshoff, W.,** *Int. Symp. Pseudotuberculosis*, Regamey, R. H., Ed., S. Karger, Basel, 1968, 23.

205. **Murray-Pullar, F.,** Pseudotuberculosis of sheep due to *B. pseudotuberculosis rodentium* (so-called "pyaemic hepatitis"), *Aust. Vet. J.*, 8, 181, 1932.

206. **Steele, J. H.,** personal communication, 1978.

207. **Daniels, J. J. H. M.,** Enteral infection with *Pasteurella pseudotuberculosis:* the isolation of the organism from human faeces, *Br. Med. J.*, 2, 997, 1961.

208. **Weisman, J. and Singer, N.,** Isolation of *Yersinia (Pasteurella) pseudotuberculosis* from the palm dove *(Streptopelia senegalensis)*, *Avian Dis.*, 20, 202, 1976.

209. **Hamilton, D. W.,** *Pasteurella pseudotuberculosis* as a cause of supperative mesenteric lymphadenitis, *Med. J. Aust.*, 1, 1156, 1970.

YERSINIOSIS *(YERSINIA ENTEROCOLITICA)*

L. G. Staley

Yersinia enterocolitica is the etiologic agent of a number of syndromes in man. Enterocolitis is the most frequently reported although pseudoappendicitis and terminal ileitis are the most dramatic. There appears to be a relationship between infection with *Y. enterocolitica* and the occurrence of nonsupperative arthritis and certain thyroid disorders. A number of unusual and miscellaneous infections have also been reported. There are a number of serotypes, some more frequently associated with human disease than others. The organism has been isolated from man, animals, and the environment. Isolation techniques are not unusual, but colony identification requires skill. *Y. enterocolitica* responds to antibiotics typically used in treating enteric disease. Epidemiology and strain pathogenicity remain unsolved at this time.

CLINICAL DISEASE

Enterocolitis typically results in a combination of symptoms including fever, abdominal pain, diarrhea, nausea, and headache. The percentage of patients exhibiting such symptoms varies between disease outbreaks within a country and between countries. Asakawa et al.[5] compared two outbreaks in Japan in which the percentage of cases with diarrhea varied from 32.4 to 60.1%. Gutman et al.,[21] summarizing cases in the U.S., noted that 69% of the cases exhibited diarrhea, while Rakovsky and co-workers[42] noted that 80.9% of the cases in Czechoslovakia manifest diarrhea.

Seasonal fluctuation of case loads has been observed. Winblad[66] stated that year after year in Sweden the number of cases of enterocolitis (as well as total enterocolitica cases) increases during the summer months and peaks in November. This observation has been repeated in other European and Scandinavian countries. Age group attack rates for this syndrome have been evaluated. Generally speaking, children aged 7 years or less appear to be more frequently affected.[63] However, there appear to be geographic differences. Winblad[66] suggested that 50% of the enterocolitis cases appear in persons 30 years of age or younger in Sweden. Vandepitte et al.[57] stated that the vast majority of enterocolitis cases in Belgium occur in persons 4 years of age or less.

The pseudoappendicitis syndrome (terminal ileitis, mesenteric lymphadenitis) appears to share the seasonal prevalence previously mentioned. Clinical symptoms closely parallel those of appendicitis. Fever (39°C ±), elevated pulse rate, rebounding tenderness in the right iliac fossa, elevated WBC with neutrophilia, and a combination of nausea, vomiting, and diarrhea are typical.[20,46]

Cases of this nature may occur as isolated incidents or a portion of a community outbreak. In several documented community outbreaks of *Y. enterocolitica* infection, a few cases in each were hospitalized as suspect appendicitis.[5] In a recent outbreak in New York State, 33 of 218 clinically ill students were hospitalized with pseudoappendicitis caused by this agent.[59] Age group prevalence again seemed to vary geographically. Winblad[66] suggested that in Sweden the majority of cases are persons 30 years of age or younger with the peak incidence rate occurring in those 10 years of age or younger. Vandepitte and associates[57] stated that in Belgium this syndrome peaks in the 10 to 19 years of age group. The period of incubation for enteric forms of the disease is variable; observations range from 2 days[14] to 10 days.[50]

Individuals recovering from *Yersinia enterocolitica* infections of the G.I. tract are occasionally confronted with nonsupperative arthritis as a sequela. Ahvonen and

Rossi[2] reported a family outbreak of gastroenteritis due to *Yersinia enterocolitica*; six persons were involved. Four of the the six developed nonsupperative arthritis following recovery from the intestinal syndrome. All six were serologically positive for *Y. enterocolitica*. Winblad[67] reported 74 cases of nonsupperative arthritis (during a 6-year period) that were serologically diagnosed as complicated *Yersinia enterocolitica* infections. Of those 74 patients, 18 were feces-culture positive to the same serotype identified serologically.

There may be an association between *Y. enterocolitica* infection and the occurrence of selected thyroid syndromes, specifically Graves' disease and diffuse nontoxic goiter. In Denmark, a study by Bech et al.[6] revealed that 59.5% of Graves' disease patients demonstrated *Y. enterocolitica* serotype 3 antibodies as compared to 16.6 and 27.7% for two control groups ($P < 0.0005$).

Atypical infections due to *Y. enterocolitica* are increasingly reported as awareness of the existence of the organism increases within the clinical medical community. The WHO Collaborating Centre for *Yersinia pseudotuberculosis*[63] pointed out that uncommon infections of *Y. enterocolitica* have resulted in erythema nodosum, septicemia, pyuria, Reiter's syndrome, and wound infections. Leino and Kalliomaki[32] reported on 56 patients with elevated antibody titers for *Y. enterocolitica*. Carditis was diagnosed in one patient, while several others exhibited ECG abnormalities of various types. Several urinary abnormalities were attributed to *Y. enterocolitica*. Chin and Noble[12] reported on ocular infection caused by *Y. enterocolitica* in a 77-year-old woman. Hepatosplenic abscesses[39] and lung abscesses with osteomylitis[45] have been reported. Bottone et al.[8] discussed 13 isolates of *Y. enterocolitica*, 9 of which were from atypical infection sites. Bissett[7] reported 24 human isolates, a number of which were recovered from patients with chronic conditions felt to be contributory to the infection such as Crohn's disease, heroin addiction, and carcinoma of the colon.

Infections caused by *Y. enterocolitica* have been reported from numerous countries. The prevalence of infection (all syndromes) varies greatly from region to region and country to country. Such a phenomenon is probably due to a multitude of factors relating to the agent, host, and environment; interest and awareness also play a role. A Montreal hospital reported no *Y. enterocolitica* cases or isolates prior to 1966. During the following 7 years or so, 108 cases were identified.[15] Another Canadian hospital for children reported 36 cases between 1972 and 1974.[41]

It has been suggested that the incidence of infection caused by this agent is rising and that the disease is spreading.[63] In Finland from 1969 to 1971, Toivanen et al.[51] compared sera from blood donors and healthy mothers in a maternity hospital against similar sera collected in 1973* and found titers in excess of 1:160 in the 1973 sample population, nearly a tenfold increase.

Questions regarding incidence and prevalence, geographic differences, and age groups affected within a population will undoubtedly be better answered as clinical awareness becomes more widespread.

THE ORGANISM

Credit for the first isolation of the bacterium presently referred to as *Y. enterocolitica* is given to Schleifstein and Coleman, as published in the *New York State Journal of Medicine*** in 1939.[7,34] Prior to 1964, the organism was referred to by a number of names including *Pasteurella pseudotuberculosis b, P. pseudotuberculosis*-like orga-

---

*   Including sera from hospital personnel composing approximately 27% of the 1973 sample.
** Volume 39, 1749 — 1753.

nisms, *Pasteurella Y.*, and *Pasteurella X.* In 1964, Fredericksen proposed adoption of the current terminology, *Yersinia enterocolitica.*[28]

Knapp and Thal[28] were confronted by Professor K. F. Meyer (Thal being a former student of Meyer's) in the early 1950s with "cerebral sticks" as only he could employ. Subsequent investigations by Knapp and Thal established that what is now called *Y. enterocolitica* was not a variant of the then *Pasteurella pseudotuberculosis* (now *Y. pseudotuberculosis*) but a distinct entity. The original isolates were of animal origin. Human isolations followed infrequently. Isolations from human, animal, and environmental sources have increased markedly during the last 10 years.

Y. enterocolitica, considered a member of the Enterobacteriaceae, is a Gram-negative, facultative anaerobe. Cells are ovoid or rod shaped and motile at room temperature (below 30°C).[34] This organism may well be considered a psychrophile since it grows at $+4°C$ (approximately 40°F) while most enteric organisms do not; it grows slowly at 37°C. In meats, 60°C applied for a few minutes kills the organism.[58]

The species *enterocolitica* is composed of a heterologous group of organisms that can be biochemically separated into groups (biotypes or chemotypes); each biotype is composed of one or more serotypes. Such typing schemes have been developed by both Nilehn[36] and Wauters.[47] Table 1 depicts the biochemical typing scheme developed by Wauters.

Serotyping systems utilizing O or H antigens or combinations of both have been developed and are employed in various countries and geographic areas. Phage typing has also been developed, although limited in spectrum, and is employed in specific areas.[35] Table 2 shows the interrelationship between biotypes and serotypes as presented by Wauters.[60]

It is worth noting that there exists considerable cross-reaction between *Y. enterocolitica* antigen and antisera to other bacterial genera. Of specific interest is the cross-reaction between *Brucella abortus* antisera and the antigen of *Y. enterocolitica* serotype 9.[13] This may well result in complications and reevaluation of brucellosis testing programs in those areas where *Y. enterocolitica* serotype 9 is prevalent.

At present, 34 specific *Y. enterocolitica* serotypes are recognized based on serologic identification procedures that use O antigens. Nonetheless, strains are isolated periodically that are not typable using these antisera.[35,60,62] Criteria for classification of *Y. enterocolitica* isolates may be modified as the number of atypical strains isolated increases.

A number of protocols for isolation and identification of *Y. enterocolitica* have been established. Laboratory specimens may be subjected to a cold-enrichment procedure, as deemed necessary, utilizing sterile saline, Rappaport's medium, buffered phosphate solution, or 0.1% peptone broth. Incubation temperature of 4°C for 2 to 5 days significantly increases strain isolation,[16] and incubation for as long as several weeks has been suggested.[35] Suggested isolation media include SS, MacConkey's (pH 7.2 to 7.4),[52] MacConkey-Tween-80®,[31] and bismuth sulfite.[58] Plates should be incubated at room temperature for 24 to 48 hr or longer.

The search for suspect colonies is facilitated by use of an obliquely or indirectly illuminated colony scope. The colonies are clear or grayish, tiny (< 1.0 to 2.5 mm), and nonlactose fermenting; on bismuth sulfite, they are black. Colony morphology has been described as smooth[34] to granular in appearance.[61] Personal experience with ATCC 23715 indicates that colonies have a faint "cottonish" appearance on MacConkey's medium and appear smooth and metalic black on bismuth sulfite. A reference strain may be helpful to the investigator who is unfamiliar with *Y. enterocolitica* colony morphology.

Suspect isolates may be screened in TSI, motility agar, and urea agar. Typical reac-

Table 1
BIOCHEMICAL TYPING SCHEME FOR
YERSINIA ENTEROCOLITICA

	Biochemical types				
Tests	1.	2	3	4	5
Lecithinase	+	−	−	−	−
Indol	+	(+)[a]	−	−	−
Lactose (oxyd) (48 hr)	+	+	+	−	−
Xylose (48 hr)		+	+	−	−
Nitrate	+	+	+	+	−
Trehalose	+	+	+	+	−
Ornithine decarboxylase	+	+	+	+	−
β-Galactosidase	+	+	+	+	−

[a] (+) = 29°C.

From Sonnenwirth, A. C., *Manual of Clinical Microbiology*, 2nd ed., Lennette, E. H., Spaulding, E. H., and Truant, J. P., Eds., American Society for Microbiology, Washington, D.C., 1974, 227. With permission.

Table 2
BIOTYPE AND SEROTYPE
RELATIONSHIPS FOR
YERSINIA ENTERO
COLITICA

Biochemical type	Serological group
3	1
5	2
4	3, 15
2	5$_B$, 9
1	Most others

From Wauters, G., *Yersinia, Pasteurella, and Francisella, Proc. Int. Symp., Malmo 1972*, Winblad, S., Ed., S. Karger, Basel, 1973, 39. With permission.

tions are as follows: TSI — acid slant, acid butt, no gas, and no H$_2$S; motile at room temperature but not at 36°C; urea positive. Characterization of *Y. enterocolitica* may be accomplished by employing the tests listed in Table 3 on those isolates that exhibit typical reactions during the screening tests.[35] All tests require 24-hr incubation at 36°C, except motility tests that are incubated at temperatures mentioned previously.[47] It is noted that room temperature incubation, except with motility tests, provides comparable results with few exceptions.[23]

ISOLATIONS

Of the 34 serotypes of *Y. enterocolitica*, a majority have been isolated from animals of various species and the environment. Table 4 documents a number of such isolates. Isolates from human cases as documented by various investigators are presented in

Table 3
BIOCHEMICAL REACTIONS OF
YERSINIA ENTEROCOLITICA

Tests	Results
Oxidase	−
Christensen's urea	+
Lactose	− (Enteric base media)
Maltose	+ (L)ᵃ
Sucrose	+
Simmon's citrate	−
Arginine dihydrolase	−
Lysine decarboxylase	−
Ornithine decarboxylase	+
Phenylalanine deaminase	−

ᵃ Late.

Based on Morris, G. K. and Feeley, J. C., *Bull. W.H.O.*, 54, 82, 1976. With permission.

Table 5. Several entries in both tables are laboratory summaries and thus represent data accumulated over a number of years.

Y. enterocolitica seems to be a ubiouitous organism. Most serotypes appear to be capable of producing human illness, given appropriate circumstances. Yet, the vast majority of human illnesses appear to be caused by a limited number of serotypes. Serotype 3 is the dominant cause of human illness in Europe, Japan, and Canada. Serotype 9 is the common cause of human illness in Finland, Belgium, and the Netherlands. Serotype 8 is a major cause of human illness in the U.S.[66]

RESERVOIRS AND MODES OF TRANSMISSION TO MAN

There is a great deal of speculation regarding the epidemiology of *Y. enterocolitica* and its ability to cause disease in man. Asakawa et al.,[5] in evaluating several large outbreaks in schools in Japan, concluded that food or water was the most probable source of infection. Each outbreak exhibited a fairly typical point source case pattern. Zen-Yoji et al.[68] found the same serotype (serotype 3) in swine in Japan that was recovered from the above outbreaks. Although hardly conclusive, contaminated pork could conceivably serve as a source of infection for man. Recently, isolations that coincide with serotypes isolated from human cases were made from several foods (see Tables 4 and 5).

In Czechoslovakia, serotype 3 is a frequent cause of human illness and has also been isolated from swine. In the rural regions, human infections peak during the winter season (December through March). This peak coincides with the period of home slaughter of swine and suggests that pork products and swine may act as sources of human infection.[42]

Wilson et al.[64] described a nonenteric infection in a 4-month-old infant. *Y. enterocolitica* serotype 20 was cultured from the child (lymphnode aspirate) as well as from three puppies (rectal swabs) in the household and dried dog feces from the yard. It is tempting to incriminate the dogs as the source of infection. Chocolate milk was found to be the source of infection in an outbreak in New York State as reported by Wakelee et al.[59]

In a hospital outbreak described by Toivanen et al.,[50] several nurses became infected

Table 4
NONHUMAN ISOLATES

Location	Source of isolates	Number of samples	Number positive	Serotype	Biotype (Wauters)	Ref.
Finland	Pigs	205	1	3	4	3
	Dogs	296	3	3	4	3
				9	2	3
	Cats	46	1	9	2	3
Canada	Milk	1	1	NA[a]	—	14
Rotterdam	Swine feces (diarrhea)	641	39	3	4	17
			14	9	2	17
Norway	Dog	—	1	3	4	18
Texas	Meat (vacuum packed)	147	1	22	1	23
			2	17	1	23
			9	NT[b]	—	23
California	Water	34	1	16	1	24
			9	NT[b]	—	24
Japan	Beef	61	15	15	4	26
				22	1	26
				30	1	26
				31	1	26
				NT	—	26
Norway	Goats	—	—	2	5	29
	Water	50	1	13	1	30
			1	7	1	30
			9	Variants or NT	—	30
U.S.	Monkeys	3	3	NT	—	33
Japan	Monkey feces	154	30	12	1	37
			1	5	1	37
			1	6	1	37
			1	14	1	37
Colorado	Water	125 rivers; 26 reservoirs; 563 wells	47%	52% NT	—	44
			11%	4% 1, 7	1	44

Location	Source	No.	1%	10% 4, 33 / Others / Unknown		Ref.
Ontario	Dogs and cats	251	1	5, 27	1	44
	Goose	1	1	3	0	44
	Water	100	1	4, 32	1	52
			1	14	1	52
			1	16	1	52
			1	17	1	52
			3	NT	—	52
Canada	Swine cecum	544	10	3	4	52
			5	5	1	53
			1	6	1	53
			1	7	1	53
			1	8	1	53
			1	14	1	53
				Unknown	—	53
Japan	Dog	115	2	3	4	55
	Chicken meat	40	1	4	1	55
	Rat cecum	65	4	4	1	55
				4	1	55
				5	1	55
				7	1	55
				12	—	55
	Swine cecum	299	4	20	4	56
			5	3	1	56
			1	5	1	56
			1	10	1	56
			2	12	—	56
Belgium	Chinchilla	—	6	NT	3	57
	Hare	—	3	1	5	57
	Pig	—	9	2	4	57
			1	3	1	57
			3	4	1	57
	Cow	—	1	5	1	57
			1	6	1	57
	Canary	—	1	5	1	57
			2	6	1	57

Table 4 (continued)
NONHUMAN ISOLATES

Location	Source of isolates	Number of samples	Number positive	Serotype	Biotype (Wauters)	Ref.
U.S.	Dogs	4	3	20	1	64
Japan	Swine cecum and mesenteric lymph nodes	2713	137	3	4	68
			4	5a	1	68
			23	5b	2	68
			5	6	1	68
			3	7	1	68
			51	12	1	68
			8	NT	—	68
	Rat cecum	165	10	5a	1	68
			25	6	1	68
			16	7	1	68
			1	8	1	68
			3	14	1	68
			2	16	1	68
			5	25	1	68
			13	NT	—	68

Table 5
HUMAN ISOLATES

Location	Number of samples	Number positive	Serotype	Biotype (Wauters)	Ref.
Finland	—	127	3	4	1
	6	4	3	4	2
Germany	—	6	3	4	4
		3	9	2	4
Japan	1526	187	3	4	5
California	—	6	8	1	7
		5	5	1	7
		2	11	1	7
		1	16	1	7
		2	10	1	7
		1	3	4	7
		2	6	1	7
		1	10	1	7
		2	1	3	7
		3	13(7)	1	7
New York State	—	1	8	1	8
		12	17	1	8
Kentucky	1	1	NA[a]	—	12
North Carolina	21	16	8	1	21
Finland	—	43	3	4	32
		13	9	2	32
		90%	3	4	36
		7%	9	2	36
South Africa	1	1	3	4	39
	—	34	3	4	40
Canada	—	Majority (36) of remainder	3	4	41
			8	1	41
Hungary	—	3	9	2	49
		55	3	4	49
Finland	—	8	9	2	50
Ontario	—	1	5	2	54
		1	3	4	54
Belgium	—	599	3	4	57
		40	9	2	57
		1	1	3	57
		3	5	1	57
		1	6	1	57
		3	10	1	57
		1	13	1	57
		1	14	1	57
		1	16	1	57
New York State	—	27	8	1	59
		1	5	1	59
		5	Not serotyped	—	59
U.S.	—	14	8	1	62
		3	5	1	62
		1	1	3	62
		1	2	5	62
		1	11	1	62
		1	13	1	62
		1	15	4	62

[a] Not applicable.

Table 5 (continued)
HUMAN ISOLATES

Location	Number of samples	Number positive	Serotype	Biotype (Wauters)	Ref.
U.S.		1	16	1	62
		4	NT[b]	—	62
	8	1	20	1	64
		4	6	1	64
Sweden	—	74 serologic	/	4	67
		18 fecal	/	4	67
Sweden	—	Total — 718 (serologic and bacterial)	3	4	66

[b]   Not typable.

through contact with a hospitalized index case. Two family members of the nurses, who had no patient contact, also developed clinical illness. Serotype 9 was the common isolate in all cases. Person-to-person transmission was strongly suggested by the author and seems quite reasonable.

Efforts to experimentally establish a carrier state in the dog have met with mixed success. Gray,[19] using a serotype 8 strain isolated in Missouri in 1968, was unable to establish infection. Oral and intraperitoneal doses as great as 4.9×10^9 organisms were administered. Lack of infection was verified by stool culture, serologic evaluation, and necropsy tissue culture.

Unpublished work at Walter Reed Army Medical Center was more successful.[43] A recent field isolate of known human virulence was used.* An oral dose of 10^{12} organisms given to four young beagles resulted in periodic fecal shedding (as long as 52 days), minimal antibody titers, no clinical illness, and recovery of the organism from mesenteric lymph nodes and other tissues at necropsy. Recovered organisms were lethal to gerbils.

The epidemiologic picture is not complete. Nonetheless, it appears prudent to state that animals may act as a reservoir for *Y. enterocolitica* and foods may act as a source of infection (particularly those of animal origin). Person-to-person transmission appears possible but not common, and fomites may be involved

MECHANISM OF INFECTION AND PATHOGENICITY

Recent work by Kanamori[27] in Japan may shed light on the subject. *Y. enterocolitica* isolates from human patients were used: serotype 3 from an enteritis case and serotype 9 from an arthritis case. Lipopolysaccharide (LPS) and Boivin-type endotoxin were extracted. These were evaluated for pyogenicity (rabbits), Shwartzman reactivity (rabbits), and lethality (mice). There was little or no difference in biological activity of the LPS extracted from the two strains. However, the endotoxins varied in their composition, and serotype 3 (from the enteritis case) endotoxin demonstrated biological activity remarkably greater than that shown by the endotoxin from serotype 9.

The speculation follows that virulence and mechanism of infection may be related to endotoxin composition.

Pathogenicity studies have long been attempted with little success. An isolate de-

*   Brewer strain, provided by T. J. Quan, Center for Disease Control, Atlanta, 1973.

scribed by Carter and co-workers,[11] now known as ATCC 27729, was found to be pathogenic for mice by oral and intravenous routes. For CD-1 mice, the intravenous LD_{50} is 2.4×10^2; the oral LD_{50} is 2×10^8 organisms. This isolate of Y. $enterocolitica$ was recovered from a human case (as well as a water source) and is serotype 8.

Using the same isolate and strain of mice, Carter[9] produced disease with a $0.5\ LD_{50}$ dose given orally. The pathology produced in the mice virtually duplicated that observed in persons with enteritis, terminal ileitis, and mesenteric lymphadenitis caused by Y. $enterocolitica$.

It has also been established that ATCC 27729 demonstrates greater virulence for CD-1 mice when cultured at 25°C rather than 37°C. Following intravenous injection, organisms grown at 25°C maintained septicemia for longer time periods and exhibited resistance to phagocytosis and intracellular killing.[10] This phenomena may contribute to seasonal case peaks in cold months as reported by a number of previously mentioned investigators.

Fourteen isolates from North America were screened for pathogenicity using NIH general-purpose mice and gerbils. Subcutaneous and intraperitoneal injection routes were used. Ten of the isolates produced mortality or morbidity in mice. Serotypes represented included 3, 4, and 8 as well as several nontypable isolates. Gerbils appeared to be extremely sensitive since as few as 250 organisms injected intraperitoneally produced mortality.[38]

As a final example of pathogenicity, a human volunteer received an oral dose of 3.5×10^9 organisms. Although the serotype was not reported, it was probably serotype 3 since it constituted the vast majority of the isolates reported by the investigators. Clinical enteritis was dramatic and the individual remained symptomatic for 4 weeks. During the course of the illness, the organism was cultured from the stool in nearly pure culture.[49]

PATHOLOGY

Lesions resulting from Y. $enterocolitica$ infection are determined by a multitude of factors including site of infection, predisposing host factors, and possibly virulence factors of the organisms that are not yet firmly established.

Pathologic lesions of G.I. tract infections are nearly identical in animals and man. They include ulceration of the mucosal lining of the gut (occasionally involving the stomach), microabscesses within Peyer's patches, and micro- and macroabscesses of the liver and spleen. Abscesses in the lungs may also occur, depending upon the duration of the clinical episode. Abscesses are usually small and yellowish-white. Neutrophils predominate in abscesses except in lung lesions where plasma cells may predominate mediastinal lymph node architecture. Elevated WBC is typical and variable in degree with neutrophilia and left shift.[9,22,33,39,48] Isolations have also been made from numerous clinically normal humans and animals.

ANTIBIOTIC SENSITIVITY

Y. $enterocolitica$ generally responds satisfactorily to those antibiotics used in treating diseases caused by Gram-negative rods. Tetracycline, chloramphenicol, neomycin, gentamicin, and streptomycin are typical examples. Penicillin and its semi-synthetic broad-spectrum derivatives are ineffective at practical dose levels.[25] Due to the large number of serotypes and organism ubiquity, antibiotic sensitivity testing of clinical isolates seems prudent. Dramatic septicemic cases have been documented that are refractory to treatment. Rabson et al.[39] described such a case; the isolate was sensitive to oxytetracycline, yet the patient expired. Such occurrences may be due to toxin production by the organism, as alluded to previously.

CONCLUSION

Y. enterocolitica appears to be capable of producing clinical illness with a wide range of syndromes. Intestinal disease seems to be most consistently associated with infection, but this may be due to clinical awareness. Selected serotypes, specifically 3, 8, and 9, can be considered zoonotic with some certainty. Means of transmission for the infectious agent seems to be unlimited with ingestion offering the best chance for establishing disease. Recovery of the organism from clinical and environmental specimens is enhanced by incubation at 4°C prior to isolation efforts. Recognition of the colonies on isolation media requires practice; known strains for reference may be of value.

This organism appears to be truely ubiquitous. The pathogenicity of many strains and isolates remains a mystery at this time, thus their public health significance remains unknown. Continued compilation of data regarding clinical isolations, increased clinical and laboratory awareness, and a standard method for evaluating strain pathogenicity are needed.

There is growing interest throughout the medical and scientific community regarding this organism and its pathogenicity as evidenced by (1) the International Symposium on Yersinia, Pasteurella, and Francisella, held in Malmo, Sweden, in 1972, (2) the Annual Meeting of the American Society of Microbiologists, New Orleans, May 1977, and (3) the International Symposium on Yersinia, held in Montreal in September 1977.

REFERENCES

1. **Ahvonen, P.,** *Yersinia enterocolitica* infections in Finland, in *Yersinia, Pasteurella, and Franciscella, Proc. Int. Symp., Malmo 1972,* Winblad, S., Ed., S. Karger, Basel, 1973, 133.
2. **Ahvonen, P. and Rossi, T.,** Familial occurrence of *Yersinia enterocolitica* and acute arthritis, *Acta Pediatr. Scand. Suppl.,* 206, 121, 1970.
3. **Ahvonen, P., Thal, E., and Vasenius, H.,** Occurrence of *Yersinia enterocolitica* in animals in Finland and Sweden, in *Yersinia, Pasteurella, and Francisella, Proc. Int. Symp., Malmo 1972,* Winblad, S., Ed., S. Karger, Basel, 1973, 135.
4. **Aleksic, S., Rohde, R., and Mihajlovic, L.,** Diagnosis of infections by *Yersinia enterocolitica, Infection,* 2(1), 40, 1974.
5. **Asakawa, Y., Akahane, S., Kagata, N., Noguchi, M., Sakazaki, R., and Tamura, K.,** Two community outbreaks of human infections with *Yersinia enterocolotica, J. Hyg.* (Cambridge), 71, 715, 1973.
6. **Bech, K., Nerup, J., and Larsen, J. H.,** *Yersinia enterocolitica* infection and thyroid diseases, *Acta Endocrinol.,* 84, 87, 1977.
7. **Bissett, M. L.,** *Yersinia enterocolitica* isolates from humans in California, 1968-1975, *J. Clin. Microbiol.,* 4(2), 137, 1976.
8. **Bottone, E. J., Chester, B., Malowany, M. S., and Allerhand, J.,** Unusual *Yersinia enterocolitica* isolates not associated with mesenteric lymphadenitis, *Appl. Microbiol.,* 27(5), 858, 1974.
9. **Carter, P. B.,** Pathogenicity of *Yersinia enterocolitica* for mice, *Infect. Immun.,* 11, 164, 1975.
10. **Carter, P. B. and Collins, F. M.,** Experimental *Yersinia enterocolitica* infection in mice: kinetics of growth, *Infect. Immun.,* 9, 851, 1974.
11. **Carter, P. B., Varga, C. F., and Keet, E. E.,** New strains of *Yersinia enterocolitica* pathogenic for rodents, *Appl. Microbiol.,* 26(6), 1016, 1973.

12. **Chin, G. N. and Noble, R. C.**, Ocular involvement in *Yersinia enterocolitica* infection presenting as Parinaud's oculoglandular syndrome, *J. Ophthalmol.*, 83(1), 19, 1977.

13. **Corbel, M. J.**, Immunological properties of an antigen from *Yersinia enterocolitica* serotype 9 crossreacting with *Brucella* species agglutinogens, in *Yersinia, Pasteurella, and Francisella*, Proc. Int. Symp., Malmo 1972, Winblad, S., Ed., S. Karger, Basel, 1973, 150.

14. **deGrace, M., Laurin, M. F., Belanger, C., Rolland, P. E., Blais, R., Breton, J. P., and Martineau, B.**, *Yersinia enterocolitica* gastroenteritis outbreak — Montreal, *Can. Dis. Weekly Rep.*, 2(11), 41, 1976.

15. **Delorme, J., Laverdiere, M., Martineau, B., and Lafleur, L.**, Yersiniosis in children, *Can. Med. Assoc. J.*, 110, 281, 1974.

16. **Eiss, J.**, Selective culturing of *Yersinia enterocolitica* at a low temperature, *Scand. J. Infect. Dis.*, 7(4), 249, 1975.

17. **Esseveld, H. and Goudzwaard, C.**, On the epidemiology of *Y. enterocolitica* infections: pigs as the source of infections in man, in *Yersinia, Pasteurella, and Francisella, Proc. Int. Symp., Malmo 1972*, Winblad, S., Ed., S. Karger, Basel, 1973, 99.

18. **Forstad, L., Londsverk, T., and Lassen, J.**, Isolation of *Yersinia enterocolitica* from a dog with chronic enteritis, *Acta Vet. Scand.*, 17(2), 261, 1976.

19. **Gray, J. R.**, A Study to Determine Canine Susceptibility to Infection with *Yersinia enterocolitica*, Master's thesis, University of Texas, Health Science Center at Houston, School of Public Health, No. T313.

20. **Gurry, J. F.**, Acute terminal ileitis and yersinia infection, *Br. Med. J.*, 2, 264, 1974.

21. **Gutman, L. T., Ottesen, E. A., Quan, T. J., Noce, P. S., and Katz, S. L.**, An inter-familial outbreak of *Yersinia enterocolitica* enteritis, *N. Engl. J. Med.*, 288, 1372, 1973.

22. **Hacking, M. A. and Sileo, L.**, *Yersinia enterocolitica* and *Yersinia pseudotuberculosis* from wildlife in Ontario, *J. Wildl. Dis.*, 10, 452, 1974.

23. **Hanna, M. O., Zink, D. L., Carpenter, Z. L., and Vanderzant, Z.**, *Yersinia enterocolitica*-like organisms from vacuum packaged beef and lamb, *J. Food Sci.*, 41, 1254, 1976.

24. **Harvey, S., Greenwood, J. R., Pickett, M. J., and Mah, R. A.**, Recovery of *Yersinia enterocolitica* from streams and lakes of California, *Appl. Environ. Microbiol.*, 32(3), 352, 1976.

25. **Hausnerova, S., Hausner, O., and Pauckova, V.**, Antibiotic sensitivity of *Yersinia enterocolitica* strains isolated in two regions of Czechoslovakia, in *Yersinia, Pasteurella, and Francisella, Proc. Int. Symp., Malmo 1972*, Winblad, S., Ed., S. Karger, Basel, 1973, 76.

26. **Inoue, M. and Kurose, M.**, Isolation of *Yersinia enterocolitica* from cow's intestinal contents and beef meat, *Jpn. J. Vet. Sci.*, 37, 213, 1975.

27. **Kanamori, M.**, Biological activities of endotoxins from *Yersinia enterocolitica*, *Jpn. J. Microbiol.*, 20(4), 273, 1976.

28. **Knapp, W. and Thal, E.**, Differentiation of *Yersinia enterocolitica* by biochemical reactions, in *Yersinia, Pasteurella, and Francisella, Proc. Int. Symp., Malmo 1972*, Winblad, S., Ed., S. Karger, Basel, 1973, 10.

29. **Krogstad, O.**, *Yersinia enterocolitica* infection in goats. A serological and bacteriological investigation, *Acta Vet. Scand.*, 15(4), 597, 1974.

30. **Lassen, J.**, *Yersinia enterocolitica* in drinking water, *Scand. J. Infect. Dis.*, 4, 125, 1972.

31. **Lee, W. H.**, Two modified media for the isolation of *Yersinia enterocolitica*, in *Abstr. Annu. Meet. Am. Soc. of Microbiologists*, Abstract Code No. P16, American Society for Microbiology, Washington, D.C., 1975, 202.

32. **Leino, R. and Kalliomaki, J. L.**, Yersiniosis as an internal disease, *Ann. Intern. Med.*, 81, 458, 1974.

33. **McClure, H. M., Weaver, R. E., and Kaufmann, A. F.**, Pseudotuberculosis in nonhuman primates: infection with organisms of the *Yersinia enterocolitica* group, *Lab. Anim. Sci.*, 21(3), 376, 1971.

34. **Mollaret, H. H. and Thal, E.**, *Yersinia*, in *Bergey's Manual of Determinative Bacteriology*, 8th ed., Williams & Wilkins, Baltimore, 1974, 330.

35. **Morris, G. K. and Feeley, J. C.**, *Yersinia enterocolitica*: a review of its role in food hygiene, *Bull. W.H.O.*, 54, 79, 1976.

36. **Nilehn, B.**, Studies on *Yersinia enterocolitica*, *Acta Pathol. Microbiol. Scand. Suppl.*, 206, 1, 1969.

37. **Otsuki, K., Tsubokura, M., Itagaki, K., Hirai, K., and Nigi, H.**, Isolation of *Yersinia enterocolitica* from monkeys and deer, *Jpn. J. Vet. Sci.*, 35, 447, 1973.

38. **Quan, T. J., Meek, J. L., Tsuchiya, K. R., Hudson, B. W., and Barnes, A. M.**, pathogenicity of recent North American isolates of *Yersinia enterocolitica*, *J. Infect. Dis.*, 129(3), 341, 1974.

39. **Rabson, A. R., Koornhof, H. J., Notman, J., and Maxwell, W. G.**, Hepatosplenic abscesses due to *Yersinia enterocolitica*, *Br. Med. J.*, 4, 341, 1972.

40. **Rabson, A. R. and Koornhof, H. J.,** *Yersinia enterocolitica* infections in South Africa, in *Yersinia, Pasteurella, and Francisella, Proc. Int. Symp., Malmo 1972,* Winblad, S., Ed., S. Karger, Basel, 1973, 102.
41. **Randall, C.,** Experience with *Yersinia enterocolitica* at the Hospital for Sick Children, *Can. Med. Assoc. J.,* 113, 542, 1975.
42. **Rakovsky, J., Pauckova, V., and Aldova, E.,** Human *Yersinia enterocolitica* infections in Czechoslovakia, in *Yersinia, Pasteurella, and Francisella, Proc. Int. Symp., Malmo 1972,* Winblad, S., Ed., S. Karger, Basel, 1973, 93.
43. **Reardon, M.,** Department of Veterinary Pathology, Division of Pathology, Walter Reed Army Institute of Research, Walter Reed Army Medical Center, Washington, D.C., personal communication, 1977.
44. **Saari, T. N and Quan, T. J.,** Waterborne Yersinia enterocolitica in Colorado, in Abst. Annu. Meet. Am. Soc. Microbiologists, Abstract Code No. C119, American Society for Microbiology, Washington, D. C., 1976, 45. C119.
45. **Sebes, J. I.,** Lung abscess and osteomylitis of rib due to *Yersinia enterocolitica, Chest,* 69(4), 546, 1976.
46. **Sjostrom, B.,** Surgical aspects of infection with *Yersinia enterocolitica,* in *Yersinia, Pasteurella, and Francisella, Proc. Int. Symp., Malmo 1972,* Winblad, S., Ed., S. Karger, Basel, 1973, 137.
47. **Sonnenwirth, A. C.,** *Yersinia,* in *Manual of Clinical Microbiology,* 2nd ed., Lennette, E. H., Spaulding, E. H., and Truant, J. P., Eds., American Society for Microbiology, Washington, D.C., 1974, 227.
48. **Sternby, N. H.,** Morphologic findings in appendix in human *Yersinia* enterocolitic infection, in *Yersinia, Pasteurella, and Francisella, Proc. Int. Symp., Malmo 1972,* Winblad, S., Ed., S. Karger, Basel, 1973, 141.
49. **Szita, J., Kali, M., and Redey, B.,** Incidence of *Yersinia enterocolitica* infection in Hungary, in *Yersinia, Pasteurella, and Francisella, Proc. Int. Symp., Malmo 1972,* Winblad, S., Ed., S. Karger, Basel, 1973, 106.
50. **Toivanen, P., Oikkonen, L., and Aantas, S.,** Hospital outbreak of *Yersinia enterocolitica* infection *Lancet,* 1, 801, 1973.
51. **Toivanen, P., Oikkonen, L., and Aantaa, S.,** Is the incidence of *Yersinia enterocolitica* increasing?, *Acta Pathol. Microbiol. Scand. Sect. B,* 82, 303, 1974.
52. **Toma, S.,** Survey on the incidence of *Yersinia enterocolitica* in the province of Ontario, *Can. J. Public Health,* 64, 477, 1973.
53. **Toma, S.,** Isolation of *Yersinia enterocolitica* from swine, *J. Clin. Microbiol.,* 2(6), 478, 1975.
54. **Toma, S., Lior, H., Quinn-Hill, M., Sher, N., and Walker, W. A.,** *Yersinia enterocolitica* infection: report of two cases, *Can. J. Public Health,* 63, 433, 1972.
55. **Tsubokura, M., Fukuda, T., Otsuki, K., Kubota, M., Itagaki, K., and Tanamachi, S.,** Isolation of *Yersinia enterocolitica* from some animals and meats, *Jpn. J. Vet. Sci.,* 37, 213, 1975.
56. **Tsubokura, M., Otsuki, K., and Itagaki, K.,** Studies on *Yersinia enterocolitica.* I. Isolation of *Y. enterocolitica* from swine, *Jpn. J. Vet. Sci.,* 35, 419, 1973.
57. **Vanderpitte, J., Wauters, G., and Isebaert, A.,** Epidemiology of *Yersinia enterocolitica* infections in Belgium, in *Yersinia, Pasteurella, and Fransicella, Proc. Int. Symp., Malmo 1972,* Winblad, S., Ed., S. Karger, Basel, 1973, 111.
58. **Vanderzant, C.,** Professor, Department of Animal Science, Texas A & M University, College Station, Tex., personal communication, 1977.
59. **Wakelee, A., MacLeod, K. I. E., Mellon, W., Moldt, M., Paul, L., Bacorn, R. W., Lyman, D. O., Medvesky, M., Shavegani, M., and Toly, M. H.,** *Yeserinia enterocolitica* outbreak — New York, Morbidity and Mortality Weekly Report, U.S. Department of Health, Education, and Welfare, Public Health Service, Center for Disease Control, Atlanta, 26(7), 53, 1977.
60. **Wauters, G.,** Correlation between ecological, biochemical behavior and antigenic properties of *Yersinia entercolitica,* in *Yersinia, Pasteurella, and Francisella, Proc. Int. Symp., Malmo 1972,* Winblad, S., Ed., S. Karger, Basel, 1973, 38.
61. **Wauters, G.,** Improved methods for isolation and recognition of *Yersinia enterocolitica,* in *Yersinia, Pasteurella, and Francisella, Proc. Int. Symp., Malmo 1972,* Winblad, S., Ed., S. Karger, Basel, 1973, 68.
62. **Weaver, R. E. and Jordan, J. G.,** Recent human isolates of *Yersinia enterocolitica* in the United States, in *Yersinia, Pasteurella, and Francisella, Proc. Int. Symp., Malmo 1972,* Winblad, S., Ed., S. Karger, Basel, 1973, 120.
63. WHO Collaborating Centre for Yersinia Pseudotuberculosis, Worldwide spread of infections with *Yersinia enterocolitica, W.H.O. Chron.,* 30, 494, 1976.

64. **Wilson, H. D., McCormick, J. B., and Feeley, J. C.,** *Yersinia enterocolitica* infection in a four month old infant associated with infection in household dogs, *J. Pediatr.*, 89(5), 767, 1976.

65. **Winblad, S.,** Studies on the O-serotypes of *Yersinia enterocolitica,* in *Yersinia, Pasteurella, and Francisella, Proc. Int. Symp., Malmo 1972,* Winblad, S., Ed., S. Karger, Basel, 1973, 27.

66. **Winblad, S.,** The clinical panorama of human yersiniosis enterocolitica, in *Yersinia, Pasteurella, and Francisella, Proc. Int. Symp., Malmo* 1972, Winblad, S., Ed., S. Karger, Basel, 1973, 129.

67. **Winblad, S.,** Arthritis associated with *Yersinia enterocolitica* infections, *Scand. J. Infect. Dis.,* 7(3) 191, 1975.

68. **Zen-Yoji, H., Sakai, S., Maruyama, T., and Yanagawa, Y.,** Isolation of *Yersinia enterocolitica* and *Yersinia pseudotuberculosis* from swine, cattle, and rats at an abbattoir, *Jpn. J. Microbiol.,* 18(1), 103, 1974.

EDITORIAL COMMENT

Recently at the 3rd International Symposium on Yersinia that was held in Montreal, Canada and Saranac Lake, New York, September 1977, some very interesting papers were presented that are to be published at a later date. Hence, we are taking this opportunity to abstract them.

The first is in regard to the "Canadian Experience with *Yersinia enterocolitica* (1966 to 1977)" by S. Toma, L. Lafleur, and V. R. Deidrick. In their paper they point out that they have collected data on 1219 cultures of *Yersinia enterocolitica* that were isolated in Canada. Of these, 977 cultures were isolated from humans. *Y. enterocolitica* serotype 0:3, biotype 4, phage type IXb was the most predominant type in Ontario, Quebec and the four Eastern Provinces. In the Western Provinces, the predominant strains were indole positive, serotypes 0:8; 5,27 and 4,32. Most of the 242 cultures of nonhuman origin, except those isolated from swine and a few isolated from wild animals, were indole positive, biochemically atypical, and serologically nontypable or belonging to different serotypes that have seldom been found in human infections.

Of the nonhuman isolates, 242 cultures were divided as follows: 114 were isolated from milk, 45 from water, and 21 from food productions (hamburger, sausage, mushroom salad, oysters, fish). The great majority of these cultures were indole positive, biochemically atypical, and serologically either nontypable or belonging to different serotypes that were seldom encountered in human infections. The following 62 cultures were isolated: swine (34), pets (2), poultry (3), beavers (5), chinchillas (9), monkeys (2), a guinea pig, raccoon, Pekin robin, Canada goose, and pigeon droppings. There were 21 *Y. enterocolitica* cultures isolated from cecal content of slaughtered animals that belonged to serotypes that were frequently isolated from human yersiniosis, i.e., 13 were serotype 0:3, biotype 4 and phage type IXb, and 2 cultures isolated from a monkey with diarrhea and a second monkey contact of the index case were serotype 0:9. Eight cultures isolated from chinchillas were serotype 0:5,27. Indole-positive cultures that were phage-typed belonged to different subgroups of the phage group X.

The majority of cultures were isolated from two provinces only — Quebec and Ontario, i.e., 1126 out of 1219 cultures, or 894 out of the total of 977 human cultures. This represents an isolation rate approximately eight times greater in these two provinces than in the remaining Canadian provinces. The higher incidence of *Y. enterocolitica* isolation in these two provinces reflects, most probably, a greater awareness of this bacterial species by physicians and laboratory workers rather than a higher rate of occurrence of this infection.

In humans, 848 cultures were isolated from fecal specimens which represents 95% of 895 cultures that had the source of isolation stated.

Yersinia enterocolitica serotype 0:3, biotype 4 was the most predominant human serotype in Canada (80%,) followed by serotypes 5,27 (4.4%); 8 (3.2%); 6,30 (2.6%); 4,32 (1%); other different serotypes (3.9%), and nontypable cultures (5%). The predominance of *Y. enterocolitica,* serotype 0:3, in human infections in Canada represents the same pattern found in those European and African countries that have isolated *Yersinia,* and also in Japan, Israel, and Brazil.

Y. enterocolitica serotypes isolated in the Western Provinces of Canada were different from those isolated in other areas. They were mostly indole positive, serotypes 0:8 (39%); 5,27 (23%); 4,32 (13%); 6,30 (3.8%); 3 — indole negative — (3.8%); other different serotypes (7.6%); or nontypable strains (9.8%). This unusual prevalence of indole-positive *Y. enterocolitica* cultures in humans was found also in the U.S. Between 1972 and March 1977, *Y. enterocolitica* cultures from 60 human patients were serotyped at the Center for Disease Control, U.S. Public Health Service, Fort Collins,

Colorado. All of these cultures were indole positive, serotype 0:8 (33.3%), nontypable (21.6%), or distributed among 11 serotypic patterns (45.1%).

Serotype 0:9, the second most common human serotype in Europe, South Africa, and Japan, was isolated in Canada for the first time in 1975 from two monkeys and in 1976 from a human (Ontario). Four cultures of the same serotype were isolated in the U.S. from human and nonhuman sources.

The phage-type patterns of *Y. enterocolitica* were quite unusual. All but five *Y. enterocolitica* cultures, serotype 0:3, belonged to the Canadian phage type IXb. This phage type has not been reported, to date, from any other country. Five cultures, serotype 0:3, were phage type VIII, which is largely present in Europe, Japan, Brazil, Zaire, and Israel. Three patients who yielded phage type VIII had arrived from Europe where they probably acquired the infection, and one culture was isolated from a 2-month-old infant of unknown background. It is interesting to mention that three cultures of *Y. enterocolitica*, serotype 0:3, from the U.S. were phage type VIII; one was phage-typed in Paris and two in our laboratory.

Swine was the only nonhuman source that yielded consistently those bio-sero-phage types that are frequently isolated from humans. These human types of *Yersinia* were isolated only sporadically from other domestic or wild animals. Cultures isolated from water, milk, and other food productions were atypical, *Yersinia*-like organisms, differing from those isolated in human yersiniosis.

Another report described was "The Occurrence of *Yersinia enterocolitica* in the Throat of Swine" by K. B. Pedersen of the State Veterinary Serum Laboratory, Copenhagen, Denmark.

Knowledge about the epidemiology of human infections with *Y. enterocolitica* is still incomplete. However, in several reports swine have been incriminated as a possible source of human infections because of frequent isolates of human-pathogenic serotypes from pigs.

From November 1976 to July 1977 a total of 282 throat swabs and corresponding heart-blood samples were collected from bacon pigs at slaughterhouse. Each sample was enriched both in phosphate buffered saline (pH 7.6) and nutrient broth. For enrichment the cultures were stored at 4°C for 2 to 3 weeks. Direct plating was not attempted. From each such cold-enrichment culture two surface cultures were made on plates of either MacConkey agar or SS agar, one being incubated at 22°C, the other at 37°C, for 48 hr. Three-week-old cold-enrichment cultures were examined for *Y. enterocolitica* serotype 0:3 antigen by indirect fluorescent antibody technique using fluorescein-isothiocyanate labeled sheep anti-rabbit immunoglobulin (Institute Pasteur).

Y. enterocolitica serotype 0:3 was isolated from 84 (30%) of 282 throat swab samples. No other serotypes of *Y. enterocolitica* were isolated. After plating from PBS-enrichment cultures, 36 isolates were obtained and 50 from nutrient-broth-enrichment cultures. There were 22 specimens that were positive by culture from both types of enrichment medium. A further 20 samples that were indirect fluorescent antibody-(IFA) positive but negative by plating became positive by culture after repeated plating (8) or after repeated cold-enrichment in nutrient broth (12).

The agglutinin titer in most of the porcine sera was lower than 1:10. About 50% of the isolates of *Y. enterocolitica* serotype 0:3 were made from this group of pigs. In pigs with higher serum titers, a relationship seemed to exist between the titer level and the rate of isolation of the organism. Thus the bacterium was isolated from all of five pigs with a serum titer of 1:80 or higher. Of pigs with titers of 1:40 or higher, 78% were carriers of *Y. enterocolitica*. In man an agglutinin titer of 1:160 or higher is interpreted as significant, indicating actual infection. The agglutinin titers against *Y. enterocolitica* serotype 0:9 were low, none exceeding 1:20.

Although the actual significance of swine as a source of human infections is unknown, it is beyond dispute that an extensive reservoir of human-pathogenic serotypes of *Y. enterocolitica* exists in pigs. From this reservoir accidental transmission to man may occur. The organism seems to be harmless to swine and is apparently a common inhabitant of the throat of swine.

Another interesting paper from Europe was "The Isolation of Urease-Negative Strains of *Yersinia*" by O. Hausner and S. Hausnerova of the Regional Station of Hygiene, Ceske Budejeovice, Czechoslovakia.

Three urease-negative *Yersinia enterocolitica* strains of biotype 2 have been isolated from stool and urine of health persons. They were diagnosed on an isolation medium used routinely in the bacteriological laboratory of the Regional Station of Hygiene in Ceske Budejovice for isolation and diagnosis of Gram-negative facultatively anaerobic fermenting rods. An important characteristic was the smell of the culture, typical of all the indole-positive strains of *Yersinia enterocolitica*.

The author states that three strains of *Yersinia enterocolitica* are distinguished by the absence of an important biochemical feature — splitting of urea. Despite this circumstance they could be identified in routine processing of the materials by the characteristic smell of the cultures, not yet chemically specified. The smell of cultures was a guide for early microbiologists and is still made use of to determine a number of other Gram-negative rod-like bacterial species, such as *Hafnia, Serratia, Enterobacter, Providencia, Salmonella, Citrobacter, and Aeromonas*. Naturally, recourse to such an expedient is no longer a mechanical diagnosis for a tape-controlled apparatus, but rather an art inherent to man only.

"An Environmental Survey for *Yersinia enterocolitica* in Houston, Texas — Phase I: The Canine" was described by L. G. Staley, T. W. Huber, and J. H. Steele of the University of Texas Health Science Center, School of Public Health, Houston, Texas.

A total of 161 fecal specimens of canine origin from animals exhibiting clinical signs of gastroenteric illness and cecae obtained from necropsied animals were evaluated. One specimen was culture positive, serotype 0:5. A human case (study) was also encountered during this survey in which two isolates were identified as serotype 0:2,3, and the related canine specimen proved to be serotype 0:6. Two nontypable isolates were also recovered from this canine.

A number of isolates were made in the home and garden where the human case occurred. It is difficult to determine if there was any relation between the canine isolation and the human case.

The authors discuss the human case as being the first in the Houston area of serotype 0:2,3 that raises questions. Was it a pathogen, an opportunist, or a skin contaminant? What was the source of the organism for this patient?

The percentage of dogs infected with *Y. enterocolitica* appears to be very low, a 0.6% infection level. The serotypes of canine origin reported here (0:5, 0:6) correspond with serotypes isolated from a few U.S. human cases. This evidence, though limited in numbers, further suggests that the canine is capable of serving as a reservoir or source of infection for man with *Y. enterocolitica*. However, the small number of isolates of these two serotypes of human and canine origin further suggests that, if a reservoir/host relationship exists, it occurs very infrequently.

Another interesting paper was entitled "Speciation in *Yersinia*" by D. J. Brenner of the U.S. Public Health Service, Center for Disease Control. In this paper the deoxyribonucleic acid (DNA) relatedness among members of the genus *Yersinia* and the biochemical reactions of these organisms were compared. These data were used to reassess speciation within the genus *Yersinia*, and three new species were proposed.

This problem of speciation is very complicated. Hence, the editor feels that this must be reviewed by experts in the field.

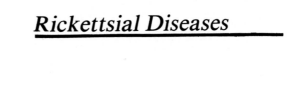

Rickettsial Diseases

THE SPOTTED FEVER-GROUP DISEASES

W. Burgdorfer

INTRODUCTION

Diseases of the spotted fever group include Rocky Mountain spotted fever, North Asian tick typhus, boutonneuse fever, rickettsialpox, and Queensland tick typhus. These zoonoses are caused by rickettsiae that share a soluble antigen that fixes complement in the presence of guinea pig antisera prepared against any member of the group. On the basis of cross-toxin-neutralization tests and other comparisons, the group has been divided into four subgroups: (1) *Rickettsia rickettsii,* the agent of Rocky Mountain spotted fever, and *R. sibirica,* the agent of North Asian tick typhus, (2) *R. conorii,* the agent of boutonneuse fever, and *R. parkeri* that causes infection in guinea pigs but not in man, (3) *R. akari,* the agent of rickettsialpox, and *R. australis,* the agent of Queensland tick typhus, and (4) *R. montana* that thus far has not been incriminated as a pathogen of man.[1]

During recent ecologic studies in the U.S. and Europe, rickettsiae were isolated that are antigenically related to the spotted fever group but appear to be distinct from those mentioned above.[2-4] Little is known about their ecology or potential pathogenicity for man. Those for which names have been proposed are (1) *R. rhipicephali,* a rickettsia isolated in various parts of the U.S. from the brown dog tick (*Rhipicephalus sanguineus*) and occasionally from the American dog tick (*Dermacentor variabilis*) and (2) *R. slovaca,* a rickettsial agent recovered from *D. marginatus* ticks in central Slovakia.[5,6] Recently, *R. texiana* was suggested as the etiologic agent of the syndrome referred to as "Bullis fever."[7] A summary of the salient epidemiologic features of the spotted fever-group diseases is presented in Table 1.

Man becomes infected with the spotted fever-group rickettsiae by accidental intrusion into the natural cycles of infection or by exposure to arthropod vectors transferred into his environment. With the exception of rickettsialpox that is caused by a mite-borne agent, spotted fever diseases are caused by tick-borne rickettsiae. In their acarine vectors, they produce a generalized infection in all tissues including the ovary — a phenomenon responsible for the transfer of rickettsiae via eggs to the progeny (transovarial infection).[8]

Spotted fever group rickettsiae grow well intracellularly (occasionally intranuclearly) in the endodermal cells lining the yolk sac of embryonated hen eggs as well as *in vitro* in chick embryo cells and in primary or established or mammalian and arthropod cell cultures.[9] Morphologically indistinguishable from each other, rickettsiae are pleomorphic, coccoidal or rod-shaped (0.3 to 0.7 by 1.5 to 2.0 μm), and bounded by a three-layered cell wall (Figure 1). They contain both RNA and DNA, multiply by binary fission, are Gram-negative, and stain weakly with aniline dyes. Staining methods most commonly used are the fluorescent antibody (FA) stain and those of Giménez, Macchiavello, and Giemsa.[10-12] FA stain differentiates the spotted fever-group agents from rickettsia-like microorganisms in certain tissues of arthropod vectors.

In their natural mammalian hosts, most spotted fever-group rickettsiae produce inapparent infections with rickettsemias. Virulent strains of *R. rickettsii,* however, are known to cause scrotal reactions in male meadow voles (*Microtus pennsylvanicus*).[13] In man, the diseases are characterized by fever, chills, headache, muscle pains, and rash. A primary lesion, absent in Rocky Mountain spotted fever, frequently develops at the site of the vector bite. Most spotted fever-group diseases are benign; deaths

Table 1
SPOTTED FEVER-GROUP RICKETTSIAE TRANSMITTED FROM ANIMALS TO MAN

Disease type	Etiologic agent	Geographic distribution	Natural cycle		Mode of transmission
			Vectors	Host animals	
Rocky Mountain spotted fever	Rickettsia rickettsii	North and South America	Dermacentor; Amblyomma; Rhipicephalus; Haemaphysalis; Ixodes (?) spp.	Small mammals (rodents, dogs, rabbits); birds (?)	Tick bite
North Asian tick typhus	R. sibirica	Siberia; central Asia; Mongolia; eastern Europe (?)	Dermacentor; Haemaphysalis; Rhipicephalus	Small mammals, mostly rodents; birds (?)	Tick bite
Boutonneuse fever	R. conorii	Countries bordering the Mediterranean Sea; countries bordering the Black Sea; Middle East; Africa; India	Rhipicephalus; Hyalomma; Amblyomma; Haemaphysalis; Dermacentor (?); Ixodes(?) spp.	Small mammals (rodents, dogs); birds (?)	Tick bite
Queensland tick typhus	R. australis	Australia	Ixodes holocyclus	Small marsupials and rodents	Tick bite
Rickettsialpox	R. akari	North America; U.S.S.R.; South Africa; Korea	Liponyssoides (Allodermanyssus) sanguineus	House mice; other commensal rodents (?)	Mite bite

Adapted from Hubbert, W., McCulloch, W. T., and Schnurrenberger, P. R., Eds., *Diseases Transmitted from Animals to Man* 6th ed., Charles C Thomas, Springfield, Ill., 1975, 384. With permission.

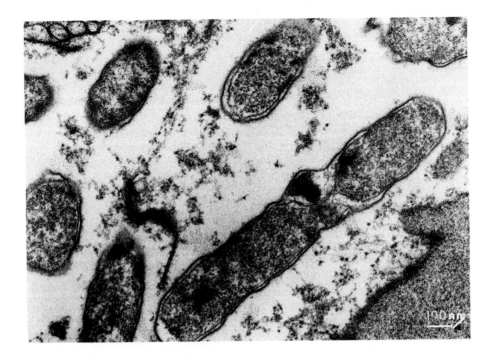

FIGURE 1.   The spotted fever agent, *R. rickettsii*, in salivary gland tissue of *Dermacentor andersoni*. (Courtesy of S. F. Hayes).

occur only among aged and debilitated patients. An exception is Rocky Mountain spotted fever, a relatively severe illness that has a mortality rate as high as 35% in untreated patients.[14]

Diagnosis of the spotted fever-group diseases on clinical grounds alone is difficult but should be considered if fever, chills, and headache are seen in patients who have a history of exposure to tick-infested areas and/or tick bite. Development of a primary lesion (eschar) at the site of an arthropod bite and the character of the rash are of diagnostic value early in the course of the disease. However, laboratory confirmation is based on isolation of the etiologic agent in test animals or demonstration of a rise in specific antibody titers during convalescence, or both.[15]

In their early stages, all spotted fever-group diseases can be cured with broad-spectrum antibiotics.[16] Prevention and control efforts include maintaining public awareness about a disease and its arthropod vectors, reduction and eradication of ticks and mites and their animal hosts, and application of prophylactic measures.[17,18]

In the following sections, clinical, epidemiological, and ecological features of each of the spotted fever-group diseases will be discussed. A separate section is devoted to laboratory diagnosis, treatment, prevention, and control. For additional reading, textbooks and reviews should be consulted.[19-24]

ROCKY MOUNTAIN SPOTTED FEVER

Disease

Rocky Mountain spotted fever is a relatively severe, self-limiting disease caused by a rickettsia transmitted to man by various species of ixodid ticks. It is characterized by fever, headache, bone and muscle pains, and a generalized rash that first appears on the wrists and ankles and frequently becomes hemorrhagic. Synonyms are spotted fever, American tick-borne typhus, mountain fever, Sao Paulo fever, Tobia fever, *fiebre manchada, fiebre petequial*, and *febre maculosa*.

History

There is little doubt that spotted fever occurred among the Indians of the northwestern U.S. before arrival of the white man. However, it was not until 1896 that Wood presented the first clinical data on cases in Idaho and considered spotted fever a distinct entity of unknown origin.[25] Maxey is given credit for the first complete clinical account, describing the disease as febrile with a centripetal rash in the form of reddish-purple black blotches.[26] At the invitation of the Montana State Board of Health, Wilson and Chowning[27,28] initiated investigations into the nature, cause, and prevention of this disease in the Bitter Root Valley of western Montana where mortality was as high as 90%. They advanced the hypothesis that spotted fever was caused by a piroplasma-like protozoon (*Piroplasma hominis*) occurring in ground squirrels and transmitted by ticks. In 1906, Ricketts evaluated this hypothesis but failed to detect piroplasma-like organisms in the blood of patients. However, he succeeded in infecting guinea pigs and monkeys with the blood of patients and proved that the wood tick, *Dermacentor andersoni,* was the vector.[29,30] His observations concerning transstadial and transovarial passage of the etiologic agent in ticks and the susceptibility of small rodents to this agent provided the foundation for future ecologic and epidemiologic studies.[31,32]

Although Ricketts noted and described the etiologic agent, he did not name it. This was done by Wolbach in 1919, who proposed the name *Dermacentroxenus rickettsi,* now known as *Rickettsia rickettsii.*[33]

Etiologic Agent

The etiologic agent, *R. rickettsii,* represents the prototype of the spotted fever-group rickettsiae. It was described for the first time in 1909 by Ricketts[34] as " . . . a bipolar staining bacillus of minute size. . ." in tick tissues and eggs. Morphologically, it appears in coccoidal, bacillary, or filamentous forms and measures 0.2 to 0.4 by 1.0 to 1.8 μm. Growth characteristics include intranuclear development, a phenomenon described for all spotted fever-group rickettsiae and recently for *R. canada,* a member of the typhus group.[35,36] *R. rickettsii* is propagated in nature in various species of mammals, particularly rodents and lagomorphs and their ticks. Isolates from naturally infected ticks, particularly of the Rocky Mountain region of the U.S., vary in virulence for male guinea pigs. Accordingly, four types (R, S, T, and U) have been described and are said to exist in nature independently of each other.[37]

True and Alternate Hosts

Despite Ricketts' early suggestion that the etiologic agent of Rocky Mountain spotted fever is maintained in nature in a cycle between ticks and one or more of their hosts, it was not until 1937 that the first rickettsial isolations were made from opossums and wild rabbits in Brazil.[38] In the U.S., *R. rickettsii* has been isolated from meadow voles (*Microtus pennsylvanicus*), a pine vole (*Pitymys pinetorum*), a white-footed mouse (*Peromyscus leucopus*), a cotton rat (*Sigmodon hispidus*), cottontail rabbits (*Sylvilagus floridanus*), an opossum (*Didelphis marsupialis virginiana*), a snowshoe hare (*Lepus americanus*), chipmunks (*Eutamias amoenus*), and golden-mantled ground squirrels (*Spermophilus lateralis tescorum*).[39-42] Serologic evidence of exposure to *R. rickettsii* has been recorded for many more mammals and birds serving as blood donors for tick vectors. In the eastern U.S. and South America, domestic pets such as dogs and, to lesser extent, cats play an important role as hosts for ticks. Only one isolation of *R. rickettsii* has thus far been reported from dogs.[43]

Distribution

Rocky Mountain spotted fever occurs only in North and South America. In the U.S., it was first described in Montana and thought to occur only in the Rocky Mountain regions.[26] Since 1930, however, the disease has also been recognized in the eastern and southeastern parts of the country.[44] Today, it is known to occur throughout the U.S., except in Alaska, Maine, Vermont, and Hawaii. More than 97% of all cases reported are from the eastern and southeastern states.[45] Spotted fever has also been reported from Canada (British Columbia, Alberta, and Saskatchewan), Mexico, Panama, Colombia, and Brazil.[46]

Disease in Animals

There is no evidence that clinical disease occurs in naturally infected host animals. When inoculated with *R. rickettsii,* most species experience rickettsemias of varying length and concentration without showing signs of disease. Scrotal swelling and reddening and occasional deaths have been recorded for meadow voles (*M. pennsylvanicus*) after inoculation with highly virulent strains.[13] Elevated temperatures lasting for 3 to 7 days occur in cottontails (*Sylvilagus* spp.) and dogs. Lassitude, anorexia, and cough may occur in puppies.[47,48]

Guinea pigs and voles are very susceptible to *R. rickettsii* and are the animals of choice for laboratory studies. Guinea pigs infected with a virulent strain of *R. rickettsii* develop fever (> 40°C) that may last from 5 to 14 days. On the third or fourth day of fever, the scrotum becomes edematous and erythematous and the testes can no longer be readily pushed into the abdominal cavity. The scrotal reaction develops as a result of vascular lesions and is characterized by edema, injection of vessels, and hemorrhages in the tunica vaginalis. Large quantities of rickettsiae can usually be seen in impression smears of this tissue. A macular rash develops on the scrotum, and lesions may then become necrotic. Necrosis and sloughing of ears and footpads are frequently seen. If the animal dies, death usually occurs on the sixth to eighth day of fever and, in most instances, is preceded by a sudden drop in rectal temperature.

Certain strains of *R. rickettsii,* although pathogenic for man, are nonpathogenic for guinea pigs and do not produce scrotal reactions and/or fever. In meadow voles, however, most strains of *R. rickettsii* produce hemorrhages in the tunica vaginalis.[49] Domestic rabbits rarely die from spotted fever although they do develop fever and their ears and scrotum often become affected. Primates are very susceptible to *R. rickettsii,* and the clinical disease in them is similar to that in man except that the rash is most frequently restricted to the limbs, head, lower back, and perineal regions.[50]

Disease in Man

Rocky Mountain spotted fever has an incubation period of 2 to 14 days. Onset is sudden with severe headache, chills, general aching, nausea, and fever. Body temperature may rise to 40°C by the second day, and fever may last until the end of the second week. The rash appears between the second and sixth day of fever and characteristically begins on the wrists, ankles, palms, soles, and forearms and extends to the buttocks, trunk, neck, and face. Initially macular, it becomes maculopapular and then petechial. Thrombocytopenia and coagulation disorders are common in almost 50% of patients. Neurologic signs such as agitation, insomnia, delirium, or coma usually are recorded at the end of the first week of fever. Complications include bronchopneumonia, otitis media, and parotitis caused by secondary bacterial infections. Occasionally, hemiplegia and peripheral neuritis occur. In untreated patients, thromboses of major blood vessels may lead to gangrene of the limbs. The elevated temperature begins to gradually decrease by the second week, but full recovery may take several weeks or months, especially in untreated patients. When the disease is fatal, death usually occurs near the end of the second week as a result of toxemia, vasomotor weakness, shock, or renal failure.

The pathology of Rocky Mountain spotted fever essentially consists of vascular lesions of capillaries, arterioles, and small arteries in practically all sites of the body although predilections are the CNS, skin, liver, heart, lung, and testes. Rickettsiae invade the capillary endothelium, multiply in numbers, and lead to cell swelling, proliferation, or necrosis. In addition to changes in the capillaries, smooth muscle cells are also invaded. Destruction of these cells is the most distinctive feature of spotted fever. With the death of these cells, necrosis occurs in the intima and the media of the blood vessels, causing thrombosis and extravasation of blood.

General Mode of Spread and Epidemiology

In the U.S., the adult wood tick, *Dermacentor andersoni,* and the adult American dog tick, *D. variabilis,* are the most important vectors of *R. rickettsii* for man.[51] Wood ticks are limited to the Rocky Mountain areas, whereas dog ticks occur in the eastern and southeastern parts of the country as well as in California and other western states.

The lone star tick, *Amblyomma americanum,* of which all stages readily attack man, has been incriminated as an effective vector.[52] As yet, there is no conclusive evidence that it is involved in maintaining and transmitting rickettsiae indistinguishable from *R. rickettsii.* In Mexico, the Cayenne tick, *A. cayennense,* and the brown dog tick, *Rhipicephalus sanguineus,* are vectors. *A. cayennense,* of which all stages bite man, also occurs in southern Texas and Florida and appears to be the principal vector in Brazil, Panama, and Colombia.[46]

Other species of ixodid ticks, such as *Haemaphysalis leporispalustris, D. parumapertus, Ixodes dentatus, I. brunneus,* and *I. texanus,* have been found naturally infected with *R. rickettsii* but are of no significance in the epidemiology of spotted fever since they rarely bite man.[53-56] However, in various parts of the U.S., rickettsial strains closely related or identical to *R. rickettsii* have been recovered recently from *D. occidentalis, I. scapularis, I. pacificus,* and *I. cookei.*[56-59] These ticks do attack man and must, therefore, be considered potential vectors of *R. rickettsii.*

Ticks become infected with *R. rickettsii* by feeding on rickettsemic host animals, particularly young rodents, and by passage of rickettsiae via eggs to progeny of infected female ticks. Infection depends upon the dose of rickettsiae ingested, i.e., the number of rickettsiae circulating in the peripheral blood of host animals.[60] This "minimum dosage requirement" reflects certain defense mechanisms — as yet undefined — commonly referred to as "gut barrier." These mechanisms cannot be overcome unless high concentrations of rickettsiae are ingested. Ticks that feed on animals with high concentrations of rickettsiae in their blood usually become infected, and rickettsial development takes place in all tick tissues. Presence of rickettsiae in germinal cells of female ticks results in the transfer of organisms from egg to offspring. The efficiency of this phenomenon, called transovarial infection, depends upon the degree of rickettsial development in ovarian tissues; the infection rate in filial ticks may be as high as 100%.[8]

Infection rates in ticks collected from nature are usually low, ranging from less than 1% to as high as 13.5% in *D. andersoni* from western Montana and from 0.3% to as high as 10.4% in *D. variabilis* from various eastern and southeastern states.[24]

Transmission of *R. rickettsii* to man usually occurs through the bite of an infected tick acquired during occupational or recreational activities in natural foci or brought

Table 2
ANNUAL INCIDENCE AND FATALITY RATES OF ROCKY MOUNTAIN SPOTTED FEVER IN THE WESTERN AND EASTERN U.S., 1960 TO 1976

Year	Total number of cases, U.S.	Western states[a]		Eastern states[b]		Nationwide case-fatality rate (%)
		Number of cases	% of total number of cases	Number of cases	% of total number of cases	
1960	204	23	11.2	181	88.8	5.4
1961	219	24	10.9	195	89.1	5.0
1962	240	28	11.6	212	88.4	5.0
1963	216	20	9.2	196	91.8	7.4
1964	277	24	8.6	253	91.4	6.1
1965	281	26	9.3	255	90.7	5.6
1966	268	12	4.4	256	95.6	7.8
1967	305	20	6.5	285	93.5	9.2
1968	288	11	3.8	277	96.2	7.3
1969	498	24	4.8	474	95.2	7.2
1970	380	12	.1	368	96.9	7.6
1971	432	13	3.0	419	97.0	8.3
1972	523	13	2.4	510	97.6	9.6
1973	668	20	2.9	648	97.1	5.7
1974	754	8	1.1	746	98.9	6.5
1975	844	13	1.5	831	98.5	3.4
1976	937	9	0.9	928	99.1	4.8

[a] States west of the 100th meridian.
[b] States included by and east of the 100th meridian.

near or into human dwellings by household pets, primarily dogs. Manual deticking of pet animals also may lead to contamination of conjunctivae or abraded skin with infectious fluids and tissues from crushed ticks.

Annual incidence of Rocky Mountain spotted fever is available for the U.S. only.[61] Since 1959, when the number of cases reported annually was at an all time low of fewer than 200, morbidity has gradually increased (Table 2). The 668 cases reported in 1973 represented the highest number recorded in a single year until that time. Since then, however, the incidence has continued to increase, reaching 754, 844, and 937 cases in 1974, 1975, and 1976, respectively. These figures probably do not represent the true incidence of spotted fever in the U.S. because, although it is a reportable disease, not all cases are brought to the attention of the Center for Disease Control (CDC).

Creation of new tick habitats through changes in land use (urbanization, creation of recreational parks, etc.) and increased recreational activities that bring more persons into contact with natural foci are some of the factors considered to be responsible for the increased incidence.[24] On the other hand, renewed awareness among physicians and the public, a result of recent research and educational programs about spotted fever and its tick vectors, may have led to improved surveillance and better reporting.[17]

Despite the availability of effective antibiotics, fatality rates of 5 to 7% are reported every year (Table 2).[45,61] Most deaths occur because patients do not seek medical care, the disease goes unrecognized (particularly in early stages), or specific treatment is delayed.

BULLIS FEVER

In the early 1940s, a disease syndrome called "Bullis fever" involved more than 1000 cases and 1 death among army personnel at Camp Bullis near San Antonio.[7]

Following an incubation period of 7 to 10 days, the disease started abruptly with chills and a fever ranging from 102 to 105°F and lasting from 4 to 14 days. Most patients complained of postorbital and occipital headache, lassitude, prostration, anorexia, and general weakness during the febrile stages. All patients had enlargement of some lymph glands although quite often there was a generalized lymphadenopathy. In about 10% of the cases, a maculopapular rash involving the trunk was noted.

All patients gave a history of having been bitten by the lone star tick, *Amblyomma americanum*. Rickettsia-like organisms indistinguishable from each other were isolated from patients, and ticks and were propagated in white mice and chick embryos. The organisms showed no relationship to spotted fever- or typhus-group rickettsiae or to *Coxiella burnetii*, the causative agent of Q fever.

Bullis fever is rarely referred to in the literature of rickettsial diseases because the true nature of the etiologic agent has never been established; and far more important, no additional cases have been reported since World War II.

In a recent retrospective review of evidence for a rickettsial etiology in Bullis fever, the name *R. texiana* was proposed for the agent of this almost forgotten syndrome.[7]

NORTH ASIAN TICK TYPHUS*

Disease

North Asian tick typhus is a benign, acute febrile rickettsial illness characterized by fever, a primary lesion at the site of the tick bite, regional lymphadenitis, and a roseolo-papular rash. Synonyms are Siberian tick typhus and North Asian tick-borne rickettsiosis.

History

During 1934 and 1935, Russian physicians in Primorye and the Far East (Ussura River, upper and central Amur) noted cases of a previously unknown disease characterized by severe headache, insomnia, high fever, and a roseolo-papular, occasionally petechial rash. It was soon established that the disease was caused by a rickettsia spread by various species of *Dermacentor* and *Haemaphysalis* ticks. The causative agent, isolated in 1938, was named *Dermacentroxenus rickettsii* var. *sibirica*.

Etiologic Agent

The etiologic agent, *D. rickettsi* var. *sibirica*, is highly pleomorphic ranging from coccoidal to bacillary and even thread-like forms. In the Western Hemisphere, it is referred to as *R. sibirica* and not *R. siberica*, as noted in many publications. Bacillary forms are 0.7 to 2.5 μm in length and average about 0.3 μm in width. Thread-like organisms may be as much as 27 μm long. Like all other spotted fever-group rickettsiae, *R. sibirica* develops intracellularly as well as intranuclearly. It grows well in yolk sac tissues of embryonated hen eggs and has been cultivated in a variety of primary and established tissue cultures. In its natural tick vectors, *R. sibirica* produces a generalized infection and is transmitted via eggs to the offspring. It also develops in lice (including the body louse, *Pediculus humanus humanus*) and other arthropods.[63] Al-

---

* A comprehensive review of available Russian literature has been translated into English and should be consulted for specific references.[62]

though monkeys, rabbits, hamsters, cotton rats, white rats, and white mice are very susceptible to *R. sibirica*, guinea pigs are the animals of choice for experimental studies.

True and Alternate Hosts

Wild rodents and their ticks are the most important hosts in the natural cycle of *R. sibirica*. Isolations have been reported from various animals, including house mice (*Mus musculus*), field mice (*Apodemus gregorius*), voles (*Microtus* spp.), rats (*Rattus norvegicus*), hamsters (*Cricetulus* spp.), chipmunks (*Eutamias* spp.), susliks (*Spermophilus* spp.), lemmings (*Lagurus* spp.), and European hares (*Lepus europaeus*).[62,64] The following species of ixodid ticks are recognized as efficient vectors: *D. nuttalli, D. marginatus, D. silvarum, H. punctata,* and *H. concinna*.[62] Additional ticks and hematophagous arthropods from which rickettsiae indistinguishable from *R. sibirica* have been recovered include *H. japonica douglasi, Hyalomma asiaticum, Rhipicephalus sanguineus,* mites of the genera *Nothrolopsis* and *Schoengastia,* gamasid mites, and fleas (*Neopsylla setosa* and *Ctenophthalmus arvalis*).

Distribution

North Asian tick typhus occurs in an area extending from islands in the Sea of Japan through the Pacific Far East and Siberia to the Mongolian, Kazakh, Kirgiz, and Armenian Republics. Natural foci probably exist throughout Asiatic Russia and the Soviet republics of central Asia and are associated closely with steppe landscapes.[62] Detection of *Rickettsia sibirica* in ticks of West Pakistan and Czechoslovakia suggests an even wider distribution of this zoonosis.[65,66]

Disease in Animals

Natural host animals become infected without developing signs of disease. Guinea pigs show fever for 4 to 7 days, periorchitis, hyperemia, and edema of the scrotum 3 to 4 days after inoculation. The scrotal reaction disappears when the fever subsides. At the peak of fever, the spleen is enlarged, adrenal glands are enlarged and hyperemic, and the brain and meninges are hyperemic. Pathologic changes are primarily caused by damage to the vascular endothelium. In rhesus monkeys (*Macacus rhesus*), fever, lymphadenitis, and rash occur after an incubation period of 3 to 10 days. The CNS may be affected (nuchal rigidity, rigidity of the lower extremities, prostration), and deterioration of cardiac function may cause death. Lesions of the lymphatic system, enlarged spleen and adrenals, infarcts in the lungs and spleen, serohemorrhagic effusions in peritoneal and pleural cavities, and cutaneous and subcutaneous hemorrhages are the most striking pathologic changes.

Unless inoculated intradermally, domestic rabbits have asymptomatic infections. A hemorrhagic inflammatory reaction appears 2 days after intradermal inoculation and subsides 7 to 8 days later with the formation of a scab. Rats are highly susceptible and, like guinea pigs, develop fever for as long as 10 days; scrotal edema and erythema are seen. Infection is rarely fatal in white rats, but it often kills young cotton rats after 3 to 7 days. Young hamsters infected with *R. sibirica* become sick within 2 to 5 days after inoculation and die 6 to 8 days later. Mice inoculated intranasally with *R. sibirica* die 28 to 96 hr later. Those inoculated intraperitoneally do not show clinical signs although rickettsiae are detectable in the mesothelial cells of the peritoneum.

Disease in Man

After an incubation period that rarely exceeds 1 week, the disease begins abruptly with chills and fever. Rarely, a 2- to 3-day prodromal period characterized by general malaise, pains, and loss of appetite may precede the onset. Body temperature gradually increases and reaches its peak by the 4th to the 6th day of illness; it becomes remittent thereafter, and recovery is usually complete by the 12th to 18th day. A primary lesion with regional lymphadenitis may develop at the site of the tick bite.

A rash in the form of bright pink roseolae and papulae of various sizes usually develops between the second and fifth day of illness. It is first seen on the exterior surface of the extremities and spreads over the trunk, buttocks, and sometimes the face. Petechiae develop only in severe cases, mostly in elderly patients. The rash usually fades slowly.

Mode of Spread and Epidemiology

R. sibirica is transmitted to man by tick bite; however, inhalation of infectious tick feces and contamination of abraded skin or mucous membranes with mashed tick tissues or blood of infected animals should be considered as possible modes of transmission. The most important vectors to man are *D. nuttalli, D. marginatus, D. silvarum, Haemaphysalis punctata,* and *H. concinna.*[62-64] Their larvae and nymphs feed on a large variety of small mammals, whereas adults feed on large wild and domestic animals, especially cattle and dogs. *Haemaphysalis* spp. also parasitize birds. With the exception of *D. nuttalli* and *H. concinna,* the nymphs of which are androphilic, only adults attack man.

North Asian tick typhus occurs primarily in agricultural areas where it affects persons engaged in field work. Domestic animals, mainly cattle, are important means by which ticks are brought near or into human dwellings. Infections are known to occur among urban populations but are usually associated with a person's temporary contact (field trips, vacation) with tick-infested areas. Appearance of North Asian tick typhus coincides with seasonal activities of adult tick vectors. The first cases are reported in April, with the highest incidence in May and June, a sharp drop during the summer, and a slight increase in September.

BOUTONNEUSE FEVER

Disease

Boutonneuse fever is a mild rickettsiosis characterized by an eschar (*tâche noire,* black spot) at the site of the tick bite, regional lymphadenitis, and a maculopapular rash covering the entire body, including palms and soles. Synonyms are *fièvre exanthé-matique de Marseilles,* Marseilles fever, and *fièvre escha-nodulaire.*

History

In 1910, Conor and Bruch[67] discovered a new clinical entity in and near Tunis and named it "boutonneuse fever" because of the button-like rash seen in most patients. The characteristically associated eschar was first studied by Pieri in Italy, who considered it to be the possible port of entry of the causative agent.[68] Association of cases with tick-infested dogs and formation of the *tâche noire* at the site of tick feeding suggested that the brown dog tick, *Rhipicephalus sanguineus,* was the vector. This was proven in 1930 by Durand and Conseil,[69] who produced the disease in man by injecting suspensions of *R. sanguineus* taken from a dog. In 1932, Brumpt[70] described the rickettsial nature of the pathogen and named it *Rickettsia conorii.*

Etiologic Agent

The etiologic agent, *R. conorii,* is related to *R. rickettsii* by virtue of a common soluble CF antigen, complete cross-protection in convalescent guinea pigs, and intracellular and intranuclear growth characteristics. These agents are distinguished from each other by the failure of *R. rickettsii* and *R. conorii* vaccines to provide cross-protection, by CF tests with washed antigens, and by the mouse toxin-neutralization test.[1] Like other spotted fever-group rickettsiae, *R. conorii* produces species-specific complement-fixing antibodies in adult Swiss mice. Morphologically, *R. conorii* is indistinguishable from other spotted fever-group agents. It grows well in guinea pigs and embryonated hen eggs and has been propagated in various mammalian, avian, and arthropod cell cultures.[9]

True and Alternate Hosts

Numerous strains of *R. conorii* have been recovered from tick vectors but relatively few have been recovered from mammalian hosts. Dogs are often considered to be the main source for infecting ticks, yet there are no quantitative data concerning susceptibility of dogs to this agent.[69] Small rodents, particularly rats, appear to be more important hosts. In South Africa, strains of *R. conorii* have been recovered from *Otomys irroratus* and *Rattus rattus* and, in Kenya, from *Arvicanthis niloticus*, *R. rattus*, *Mastomys natalensis*, *Otomys* sp., *Aethomys kaiseri*, *Lophuromys flavopunctatus*, and *Lemniscomys striatus*.[71,72] In Malaysia, presumptive isolations were made from *R. muelleri*, *R. whiteheadi*, *R. rattus argentiventer*, and *R. rattus diordi*.[73]

Distribution

Soon after its first description in Tunis, boutonneuse fever was reported from almost all Mediterranean countries of Europe, Asia, and Africa.[74] Clinical and serologic evidence suggests that similar diseases in South Africa (South African tick-bite fever), Kenya (Kenya tick typhus), Ethiopia, Republic of Congo, and India (Indian tick typhus) are caused by *R. conorii* or closely related rickettsial agents.[46-65,75-79]

Disease in Animals

Little is known about the clinical manifestations of boutonneuse fever in naturally infected animals. Dogs remain normal although their blood has been shown to be infectious.[69] Many species of wild rodents have inapparent infections. Exceptions are South African gerbils of the genus *Tatera* that often die with heavy rickettsial infections in the peritoneum.[80] Guinea pigs and meadow voles are probably the most useful animals for laboratory studies. Fever ($> 40°C$) of 4 to 6 days duration and pronounced scrotal swelling occur in guinea pigs 3 to 6 days after they are inoculated intraperitoneally with infectious material. Scrotal reactions also occur in meadow voles, and they have massive rickettsial infections in the tunica vaginalis.

Disease in Man

After an incubation period of 5 to 7 days, the disease starts abruptly with chills and a fever that may last from 1 to 2 weeks. Occasionally, a severe conjunctivitis may be the initial site of infection. Joint and muscle pains and often violent and persistent frontal, retroorbital, or general headaches are common symptoms. A primary eschar (*tache noire*) consisting of a small ulcer with a black, necrotic center can usually be found at the onset of disease. It may be on any part of the body and is usually associated with tender enlargement of the regional lymph nodes. On the third to fifth day of illness, a maculopapular rash develops, usually appearing first on the forearms. It rapidly spreads over the entire body, including palms, soles, and face, and may become hemorrhagic. After the fever subsides, the rash disappears without desquamation. Boutonneuse fever is a mild disease that causes practically no mortality.

Mode of Spread and Epidemiology

R. conorii is maintained and perpetuated in nature in two distinct cycles: (1) a primary cycle that involves a variety of small mammals and their ectoparasites, including ticks, and (2) a secondary or domestic cycle that involves dogs and their ticks.[81] As in Rocky Mountain spotted fever, dogs are not the primary source for infecting ticks but are merely important means by which infected ticks are brought into and maintained in man's environment. Such ticks not only become potential vectors to man but also become long-term reservoirs of *R. conorii* because they pass rickettsiae transovarially to their progeny.[82] This explains the focal nature of the disease and the occurrence of new cases for several successive years. Transmission of *R. conorii* to man occurs either by the bite of infected ticks or through dermal contact with rickettsiae during handling of infected ticks.

In countries along the Mediterranean coast, the brown dog tick, *Rhipicephalus sanguineus*, is considered to be the main vector. In France, other species of ixodid ticks — *I. ricinus, I. hexagonus, D. marginatus,* and *D. reticulatus* — are said to be involved in the natural cycle of *Rickettsia conorii*.[83,84] In South Africa, boutonneuse fever has been reported from urban areas among persons who own dogs infested with ticks, particularly *H. leachii* and all stages of *Rhipicephalus sanguineus*.

Nevertheless, the disease occurs more commonly among picnickers, farmers, and travelers in the veld where rodents and their ticks constitute the primary cycle of *Rickettsia conorii*. Naturally infected ticks include *Amblyomma hebraeum, R. appendiculatus, R. evertsi, H. leachii,* and *Hyalomma marginatus rufipes*.[71]

Primary cycles between rodents and their ticks in Kenya and Malaysia were also described.[72,73] In Kenya, *R. conorii* was recovered from various species of rats and mice (see above) as well as from immature *H. leachii* and *R. simus* parasitizing them. Other tick species found naturally infected include *A. variegatum, R. evertsi evertsi,* and *H. albiparmatum*. In Malaysia, *I. granulatus, Haemaphysalis* spp., and their hosts, rats (*Rattus* spp.) and shrews (*Tupaia glis*), are the important components of the primary cycle. Through occasional contact of these rodents with semidomesticated rats (*R. rattus jalorensis* and *R. exudans*), an exchange of ticks and rickettsiae takes place and results in the secondary domestic cycle involving animals closely associated with man (*Mus musculus, R. rattus argentiventer, R. rattus diordi,* and *Suncus murinus*).

A recent survey for rickettsiae among cattle ticks from Ethiopia has yielded numerous isolates of *Rickettsia conorii* or closely related agents from *R. simus, A. variegatum, A. cohaerens,* and *A. gemma*.[85]

QUEENSLAND TICK TYPHUS

Disease

Queensland tick typhus is a benign rickettsial disease characterized by general malaise, headache, fever, and regional lymphadenitis. Sometimes an eschar forms at the site of the tick bite, and a rash that varies greatly in character from case to case appears.

History

In 1946, Brody[86] described the first case of a boutonneuse fever-like illness in North Queensland. That same year, Andrew et al.[87] reported 12 additional cases among troops engaged in jungle warfare training on the Atherton Tableland, an area characterized by a dense population of marsupials and rodents and heavy tick infestation. Because the majority of patients were known to have been bitten by ticks, this new disease entity was named North Queensland tick typhus. It is occasionally referred to as "Queensland tick typhus," especially since 1948 when three cases occurred in South Queensland.[88]

Etiologic Agent

In 1946, a rickettsia was isolated in white mice from the blood of two patients and was subsequently identified as a new species of the spotted fever group. The organism was named *R. australis*.[89-91]

True and Alternate Hosts

Until recently, strains of *R. australis* had only been isolated from patients. History of tick exposure and occasional development of an eschar at the site of a tick bite suggested that this disease agent was tick-borne. The scrub tick, *I. holocyclus,* was incriminated as a vector because larval and adult specimens had frequently been removed from patients. The first isolations of *R. australis* from *I. holocyclus* and *I. tasmani* were reported in 1976.[92] As yet, no vertebrate hosts have been found to be sources for infecting ticks. Nevertheless, serologic surveys in areas where human cases occurred revealed antibodies in the short-nosed bandicoot (*Isoodon obesulus*), a long-nosed bandicoot (*Perameles nasuta*), Johnstone's oppossum (*Trichosurus vulpecula johnstonii*), rufous ratkangaroos (*Aepyprymnus rufescens*), and Atherton uromys (*Uromys sherrini*).[93]

Distribution

Queensland tick typhus is restricted to northern and southern Queensland.

Disease in Animals

Guinea pigs and Swiss mice are the animals of choice for experimental work with *R. australis*. Guinea pigs inoculated intraperitoneally with infectious material respond with fever (> 40°C) for 2 to 4 days and swelling and erythema of the scrotum. Killed at the height of the disease, these animals show inflammatory changes and, occasionally, exudates on the tunica vaginalis and testes. Infection in weaned Swiss mice causes slight splenomegaly and a peritoneal exudate in which few rickettsiae are seen. Suckling mice, on the other hand, invariably die as the result of massive rickettsial infection.

Disease in Man

The incubation period varies from 2 to 10 days. The disease starts gradually with general malaise, headache, and moderate continuous or remittent fever that subsides after 2 to 12 days. An eschar resembling that of scrub typhus may develop at the site of the tick bite, and the lymph nodes that drain the eschar become enlarged and painful. The rash appears 1 to 6 days after onset of illness and varies greatly in character; individual lesions may be small, scattered, erythematous macules and papules, or they may consist of large pink papules. In one patient, lesions became confluent on the trunk and formed large purplish blotches that involved the face, scalp, and palms. The rash disappears soon after defervescence.

Mode of Spread and Epidemiology

The endemic regions in Queensland are characterized as savannah country interspersed with dense belts of rain forests. These contain a dense marsupial and rodent fauna and are heavily infested with various species of ticks, of which the scrub tick, *Ixodes holocyclus,* is the most androphilic. Occurrence of disease in persons bitten by this tick and the recent recovery of *R. australis* from field-collected specimens leave no doubt that *I. holocyclus* is the main vector to man. Isolation of this agent from *I. tasmani*, however, suggests a more complex ecological cycle that needs further studies. Queensland tick typhus probably occurs more frequently than reported but is not recognized because it is mild and self-limited.[94]

RICKETTSIALPOX

Disease

Rickettsialpox is a mild, self-limited disease characterized by an eschar-like lesion, fever of 1 week duration, headache, backache, lymphadenopathy, leukopenia, and a generalized papulovesicular rash. Synonyms are Kew Garden spotted fever and vesicular and varioliform rickettsiosis.

History

The disease was first observed during the summer of 1946 when more than 80 cases occurred in the Kew Garden housing development of New York City.[95] Large numbers of mice in apartments or basement and storage rooms suggested that house mice (*Mus musculus*) and their hematophagous mites, *Liponyssoides* (*Allodermanyssus) sanguineus,* may have been the sources of a rickettsial agent that was first isolated from the blood of a patient.[96] A rickettsia identical with that isolated from the patient was soon recovered from both mites and mice and was named *R. akari*.[97,98]

Etiologic Agent

Although *R. akari* has antigens in common with the spotted fever agent *R. rickettsii,* it is more closely related to *R. australis,* from which it is readily distinguished by cross-complement-fixation tests with convalescent mouse sera.[99] Its morphology and intracellular and intranuclear growth characteristics are similar to those of the other spotted fever-group rickettsiae.

True and Alternate Hosts

Isolations from natural hosts have been reported from the house mouse, *M. musculus,* the Korean vole, *Microtus fortis pelliceus,* and the mite vector, *L. sanguineus*.[97,98,100] Mice, voles, guinea pigs, and embryonated hen eggs are all susceptible to experimental infection, but the Swiss mouse is the animal of choice for isolation purposes.

Distribution

From 1946 to 1949, more than 500 cases of rickettsialpox, all limited to metropolitan New York City, were reported. Since then, limited outbreaks have occurred in Boston, West Hartford (Conn.), Philadelphia, Cleveland, Utah, and Pittsburgh.[101] A disease indistinguishable from rickettsialpox has been described in the U.S.S.R. as vesicular rickettsiosis.[102] It is caused by the rickettsial agent *Dermacentroxenus murinus,* which has been shown to be the same agent as *R. akari.* Serologic and/or clinical evidence of rickettsialpox has been reported from French Equatorial Africa, South Africa, and Costa Rica.[71,103,104]

Disease in Animals

Strains of *R. akari* vary in their pathogenicity for mice and guinea pigs. Unlike house mice that are not adversely affected, Swiss mice develop lethargy, ruffled fur, labored breathing, and anorexia and may die between the 9th and 13th day after inoculation. Often, mice appear healthy but have axillary lymphadenopathy, increased amounts of peritoneal fluid, and an enlarged and congested spleen at necropsy. Serial passages of the organism in mice usually result in death 5 to 10 days after inoculation. Guinea pigs inoculated intraperitoneally become febrile 2 to 6 days later, and the fever lasts from 3 to 5 days. A scrotal reaction in the form of swelling and redness is seen on about the fifth day of fever. Chick embryos are very susceptible and support the growth of large quantities of *R. akari* in the amniotic sac and in yolk sac tissues.

Disease in Man

The first sign of rickettsialpox in more than 90% of patients is a lesion at the site of an infectious mite bite. It evolves into a central vesicle and then into an eschar. Because most patients are not aware of having been bitten by a mite, the incubation period is difficult to determine, but it is thought to vary between 10 and 24 days. The disease begins suddenly with chills, fever, sweating, headache, muscle pains, and backache. Within 1 to 4 days, a maculopapular rash appears over many areas of the body but never on the palms and soles. The rash becomes vesicular; vesicles resorb dry and form black crusts that desquamate within 1 week without producing eschars. Except for fever, rash, and enlarged and tender lymph nodes, there are no other clinical manifestations. Chills usually do not persist for more than 24 hr, and the week-long elevated temperatures gradually return to normal levels.

Mode of Spread and Epidemiology

Rickettsialpox is an urban disease associated with large numbers of domestic rodents, particularly house mice and their blood-sucking mites.[95,105] However, recovery of *R. akari* from the field vole, *M. fortis pelliceus,* in Korea and reports from South Africa where the infection has been contracted in the bush veld suggest the existence of rural cycles not involving commensal rodents.[71,100]

The only vector incriminated thus far is the rodent mite, *L. (Allodermanyssus) sanguineus,* the developmental stages of which (except the larva) are hematophagous and readily attack man, especially if its normal host has been reduced or eliminated by rodent control programs. The mites acquire *R. akari* by feeding on a rickettsemic mouse. They are not only efficient vectors but also reservoirs by virtue of their ability to pass rickettsiae transovarially to their progeny.[106]

Transmission to man occurs chiefly through the bite of an infected mite. Sometimes, especially among laboratory workers, the infection is acquired via the respiratory route.[107]

DIAGNOSIS, TREATMENT, PREVENTION, AND CONTROL OF THE SPOTTED FEVER-GROUP DISEASES

Laboratory Diagnosis

Laboratory diagnosis of the spotted fever-group zoonoses is based upon isolation of the etiologic agent in laboratory animals and demonstration of a rise in specific antibody titers during convalescence.[15]

Male guinea pigs, male meadow voles, and Swiss mice are the animals of choice for isolation of spotted fever-group rickettsiae pathogenic for man. Male guinea pigs respond to intraperitoneal inoculation of infected blood or vector tissues with fever and scrotal reactions characterized by swelling and reddening. Virulent strains of *R. rickettsii* produce a severe and often fatal infection that is associated with scrotal reactions appearing in the form of hemorrhagic and necrotic lesions; occasionally, these lesions also involve footpads and ears. On the other hand, many isolates of this agent are nonpathogenic for guinea pigs. Meadow voles have been shown to be susceptible to all spotted fever rickettsiae isolated to date and reveal infections characterized by rickettsial development in the tunica vaginalis.[108] Swiss mice are recommended for recovery of *R. akari* and *R. australis* that produce fatal infections in the macrophages of the peritoneum of adult and suckling mice, respectively.[109,110]

Embryonated hen eggs have long been used to isolate and cultivate rickettsiae from the blood or tissue of patients and laboratory animals. For this purpose, suspensions are inoculated via the yolk sac of 5- to 7-day-old eggs. Death of embryos 4 to 10 days after inoculation suggests rickettsial growth that may vary in density from one isolate to another.[111] In recent years, a variety of primary and established mammalian, avian, and arthropod cell cultures have been applied to rickettsial studies and have been found suitable for primary isolation of these organisms.[9]

Several procedures have been described for demonstrating specific antibodies in serums of patients or animals sick or convalescing from spotted fever-group diseases.[15,112] The Weil-Felix reaction and complement-fixation (CF) test are the most commonly used because required diagnostic reagents are commercially available. The far more sensitive agglutination and neutralization procedures use antigens that are difficult to prepare and commercially unavailable. With the exception of *R. akari,* all spotted fever-group agents elicit antibodies that in the Weil-Felix test may agglutinate OX-19 and, to a lesser exent, OX-2 strains of *Proteus vulgaris.* Paired sera, i.e., one taken soon after onset of the disease and another taken during convalescence, should be tested simultaneously. The test is considered positive if at least a fourfold increase in antibody titer is demonstrated in the convalescent serum. The Weil-Felix reaction is nonspecific and provides only presumptive evidence of a rickettsial infection. Similarly, a negative test does not always exclude rickettsial infection.

The CF test with soluble antigens to detect group-specific rickettsial antibodies that appear as early as 10 days after onset of illness is far more reliable. It is very specific for demonstrating antibodies to *R. akari* and *R. australis* in Swiss mice.[99] Nevertheless, for serologic differentiation of the spotted fever-group rickettsiae in patients and guinea pigs, type-specific antigens are required. These are commercially unavailable and have to be prepared by rather sophisticated methods, including differential centrifugation plus ether extraction, use of anion exchange resins in chromatographic columns, density-gradient zonal centrifugation, and Renografin density-gradient centrifugation.[113,114]

More sensitive than the CF test are the recently developed microagglutination (MA), microimmunofluorescence (micro-IF), and indirect hemagglutination tests.[115-117] The MA test is an adaptation of the microtiter technique; it is easy to perform but requires highly pure antigens unavailable in most laboratories. The micro-IF test, a widely used procedure for immunotyping trachoma inclusion conjunctivitis-lymphogranuloma venereum chlamydiae, appears equally promising in serotyping spotted fever-group rickettsiae. All spotted fever-group rickettsial species tested to date in weanling mice were found to produce antibodies readily identified by this procedure.[118] An additional advantage of the indirect micro-IF test is the fact that it permits detection of rickettsial agglutinins (IgM) present early in the course of an illness and of agglutinins (IgG) that persist long after convalescence. The indirect hemagglutination test is also said to be a sensitive procedure for detecting group-specific spotted fever antibodies; its routine application needs to be evaluated.

Treatment, Prevention, and Control

All pathogenic spotted fever-group rickettsiae are susceptible to broad-spectrum antibiotics;[16] tetracycline, oxytetracycline, and chlortetracycline are very effective. Headache and other toxic signs abate within 24 to 48 hr, the rash fades in 2 to 3 days, and defervescence occurs within 3 to 4 days. Therapeutic regimens depend upon the body weight of a patient. For a 70-kg adult, an initial dose of 2 g may be given, followed by an oral dose of 250 mg every 6 hr until defervescence is complete. Chloramphenicol is also effective, but because of the possibility of dangerous side effects (blood dyscrasias), it is not generally recommended.

Prevention and control of the spotted fever-group diseases are based on: (1) education of the public about the diseases and the arthropod vectors, (2) reduction and eradication of vectors and their rodent hosts, and (3) personal prophylactic measures.

In areas where a disease is highly endemic, the public should be periodically reminded (through pamphlets, newspapers, etc.) about the clinical manifestations and those arthropod vectors that transmit the etiologic agent.[17] Ticks and mites removed from patients should not be discarded but be submitted to qualified laboratories for examination. Ticks, for instance, can be readily examined for rickettsial agents by the hemolymph test. This involves examination of hemolymph obtained by amputating a portion of one or more tick legs.[119]

Where ticks infest homes and surroundings, control should be carried out by application of acaricides* in the form of dust, emulsions, and aqueous suspensions.[18] Domestic animals, including pets, should also be treated. In the U.S., "tick collars" have been found to be effective in controlling tick infestations of dogs and cats. In the case of rickettsialpox, control measures should be directed towards eradication of mite vectors as well as of their rodent hosts. Application of residual miticides to mice-infested areas should be used first to prevent dispersing mites deprived of their natural food supply.

Where application of acaricides is impractical, as in heavily wooded and brushy areas, tick infestations can be reduced or totally eliminated through land clearing, irrigation, cultivation, and periodically conducting programs to exterminate rodents. Feral dogs that play an important role in the epidemiology of several spotted fever-group diseases should be eliminated.

Proper clothing should be worn in tick-infested areas to reduce the chances of tick bite. Each outer garment should overlap the one above, e.g., trouser legs should be covered by socks and shirt tails should be tucked inside trousers. It is essential to repeatedly search the body and inside of clothing for ticks because they seldom attach immediately. Effective repellents, such as diethyltoluamide and dimethylphthalate, are recommended and should be applied to clothing and exposed parts of the body. Attached ticks should be removed immediately by pulling them off gently with the fingers or with broad-tongued forceps, taking care not to crush them. The bite wound should be treated with an antiseptic, and the hands, which may be contaminated with infectious tick fluids, should be washed thoroughly with soap and water.

Rocky Mountain spotted fever is the only disease of the spotted fever group for which a vaccine had been prepared.[22] Its use was recommended for persons living in areas where the disease is endemic. However, since this vaccine afforded limited protection only, it recently has been withdrawn from the market. A more effective vaccine is under investigation and may become available for distribution in the future.

---

* Because of national restrictions in the application of insecticides, it is suggested that local pesticide authorities or agricultural extension offices be consulted for products currently recommended.

REFERENCES

1. **Lackman, D. B., Bell, E. J., Stoenner, H. G., and Pickens, E. G.,** The Rocky Mountain spotted fever group of rickettsias, *Health Lab. Sci.,* 2, 135, 1965.
2. **Burgdorfer, W., Sexton, D. J., Gerloff, R. K., Anacker, R. L., Philip, R. N., and Thomas, L. A.,** *Rhipicephalus sanguineus:* vector of a new spotted fever group rickettsia in the United States, *Infect. Immun.,* 12, 205, 1975.
3. **Hughes, L. E., Clifford, C. M., Gresbrink, R., Thomas, L. A., and Keirans, J. E.,** Isolation of a spotted fever group rickettsia from the Pacific Coast tick, *Ixodes pacificus,* in Oregon, *Am. J. Trop. Med. Hyg.,* 25, 513, 1976.
4. **Brezina, R., Rehacek, J., Ac, P., and Majerska, M.,** Two strains of rickettsiae of Rocky Mountain spotted fever group recovered from *Dermacentor marginatus* ticks in Czechoslovakia. Results of preliminary serologic identification, *Acta Virol.,* 13, 142, 1968.
5. **Burgdorfer, W., Brinton, L. P., Krinsky, W. L., and Philip, R. N.,** *Rickettsia rhipicephali,* a new spotted fever group rickettsia from the brown dog tick, *Rhipicephalus sanguineus, Proc. 2nd Int. Symp. Rickettsiae and Rickettsial Diseases,* Kazar, Ormsbee, and Tarasevich, Eds., VEDA, Bratislava, 1978, 307.
6. **Urvolgyi, J. and Brezina, R.,** *Rickettsia slovaca:* a new member of spotted fever group rickettsiae, *Proc. 2nd Int. Symp. Rickettsiae and Rickettsial Diseases,* Kazar, Ormsbee, and Tarasevich, Eds., VEDA, Bratislava, 1978, 299.
7. **Anigstein, L. and Anigstein, D.,** A review of the evidence in retrospect for a rickettsial etiology in Bullis Fever, *Tex. Rep. Biol. Med.,* 33, 201, 1975.
8. **Burgdorfer, W. and Brinton, L. P.,** Mechanisms of transovarial infection of spotted fever rickettsiae in ticks, *Ann. N.Y. Acad. Sci.,* 266, 61, 1975.
9. **Gerloff, R. K.,** Tissue cultures and culture media for microorganisms of the tribe Rickettsieae, in *CRC Handbook Series in Nutrition and Food,* Rechcigl, M., Jr., Ed., CRC Press, Cleveland, in press.
10. **Giménez, D. F.,** Staining rickettsiae in yolk sac cultures, *Stain Technol.,* 39, 135, 1964.
11. **Macchiavello, A.,** Estudios sobre tifus exanthematico. III. Un nuevo metodo para tenir *Rickettsia, Rev. Chil. Hig. Med. Prev.,* 1, 101, 1937.
12. **Burgdorfer, W.,** Evaluation of the fluorescent antibody technique for the detection of Rocky Mountain spotted fever rickettsiae in various tissues, *Pathol. Microbiol.,* 24(Suppl.), 27, 1961.
13. **Jellison, W. L.,** Rocky Mountain spotted fever. The susceptibility of mice, *Public Health Rep.,* 49, 363, 1934.
14. **Beeson, P. B. and McDermott, W.,** Rickettsial diseases, in *Cecil-Loeb Textbook of Medicine,* Vol. 1, 13th ed., W. B. Saunders, Philadelphia, 1971, 470.
15. **Elisberg, B. L. and Bozeman, F. M.,** Rickettsiae, in *Diagnostic Procedures for Viral and Rickettsial Infections,* Lennette, E. H. and Schmidt, N. J., Eds., American Public Health Association, New York, 1969, 826.
16. **Ley, H. L., Jr. and Smadel, J. E.,** Antibiotic therapy of rickettsial diseases, *Antibiot. Chemother.* (Washington, D.C.), 4, 792, 1954.
17. **Burgdorfer, W., Adkins, T. R., Jr., and Priester, L. E.,** Rocky Mountain spotted fever (tick-borne typhus) in South Carolina: an educational program and tick/rickettsial survey in 1973 and 1974, *Am. J. Trop. Med. Hyg.,* 24, 866, 1975.
18. **Grothaus, R. H. and Weidhaas, D. E.,** Control of arthropods of medical importance, in *Tropical Medicine,* Hunter, G. W., Swartzwelder, J. C., and Clyde, D. F., Eds., W. B. Saunders, Philadelphia, 1976, 783.
19. **Moulder, J. W.,** *The rickettsias,* in *Bergey's Manual of Determinative Bacteriology,* 8th ed., Williams & Wilkins, Baltimore, 1974, 882.
20. **Ormsbee, R. A.,** Rickettsiae (as organisms), *Annu. Rev. Microbiol.,* 23, 275, 1969.
21. **Zdrodovskii, P. F. and Golinevich, H. M.,** *The Rickettsial Diseases,* Pergamon Press, New York, 1960.
22. **Woodward, T. E. and Jackson, E. B.,** Spotted fever rickettsiae, in *Viral and Rickettsial Infections of Man,* 4th ed., Horsfall, F. L., Jr. and Tamm, I., Eds., Lippincott, Philadelphia, 1965, 1095.
23. **Hoogstraal, H.,** Ticks in relation to human diseases caused by *Rickettsia* species, *Annu. Rev. Entomol.,* 12, 377, 1967.
24. **Burgdorfer, W.,** A review of Rocky Mountain spotted fever (tick-borne typhus), its agent, and its tick vectors in the United States, *J. Med. Entomol.,* 12, 269, 1975.
25. **Wood, M. W.,** Spotted fever as reported from Idaho, *Rep. Surg. Gen. U.S. Army,* 60, 1896.
26. **Maxey, E. E.,** Some observations on the so-called "spotted fever" of Idaho, *Med. Sentinel* (Portland), 7, 433, 1899.

27. Wilson, L. B. and Chowning, W. M., The so-called "spotted fever" of the Rocky Mountains: a preliminary report to the Montana State Board of Health, *JAMA*, 39, 131, 1902.

28. Wilson, L. B. and Chowning, W. M., Studies in *Pyroplasmosis hominis* ("spotted fever" or "tick fever") of the Rocky Mountains, *J. Infect. Dis.*, 1, 31, 1904.

29. Ricketts, H. T., The study of "Rocky Mountain spotted fever" (tick fever?) by means of animal inoculation, *JAMA*, 47, 33, 1906.

30. Ricketts, H. T., The transmission of Rocky Mountain spotted fever by the bite of the wood tick (*Dermacentor occidentalis*), *JAMA*, 47, 358, 1906.

31. Ricketts, H. T., Further experiments with the wood tick in relation to Rocky Mountain spotted fever, *JAMA*, 49, 1278, 1907.

32. Ricketts, H. T., The role of the wood tick (*Dermacentor occidentalis*) in Rocky Mountain spotted fever, and the susceptibility of local animals to this disease, *JAMA*, 49, 24, 1907.

33. Wolbach, S. B., Studies on Rocky Mountain spotted fever, *J. Med. Res.*, 41, 1, 1919.

34. Ricketts, H. T., A micro-organism which apparently has a specific relationship to Rocky Mountain spotted fever, *JAMA*, 52, 379, 1909.

35. Wisseman, C. L., Jr., Edlinger, E. A., Waddell, A. D., and Jones, M. R., Infection cycle of *Rickettsia rickettsii* in chicken embryo and L-929 cells in culture, *Infect. Immun.*, 14, 1052, 1976.

36. Burgdorfer, W. and Brinton, L. P., Intranuclear growth of *Rickettsia canada*, a member of the typhus group, *Infect. Immun.*, 2, 112, 1970.

37. Price, W. H., Variation in virulence of *Rickettsia rickettsii* under natural and experimental conditions, in *The Dynamics of Virus and Rickettsial Infections,* Hartman, F. W., Horsfall, F. L., Jr., and Kidd, J. G., Eds., Blakiston, New York, 1954, 164.

38. Travassos, J., Studies on rickettsial diseases in Brazil, in *Proc. 4th Int. Congr. Tropical Medicine: Malaria,* Vol. 1, Publication No. 3246, U.S. Department of State, Washington, D.C., 1948, 414.

39. Gould, D. J. and Miesse, M. L., Recovery of a rickettsia of the spotted fever group from *Microtus pennsylvanicus* from Virginia, *Proc. Soc. Exp. Biol. Med.*, 85, 558, 1954.

40. Shirai, A., Bozeman, F. M., Perri, S., Humphries, J. W., and Fuller, H. S., Ecology of Rocky Mountain spotted fever. I. *Rickettsia rickettsii* recovered from a cottontail rabbit from Virginia, *Proc. Soc. Exp. Biol. Med.*, 107, 211, 1961.

41. Burgdorfer, W., Newhouse, V. F., Pickens, E. G., and Lackman, D. B., Ecology of Rocky Mountain spotted fever in western Montana. I. Isolation of *Rickettsia rickettsii* from wild mammals, *Am. J. Hyg.*, 76, 293, 1962.

42. Bozeman, F. M., Shirai, A., Humphries, J. W., and Fuller, H. S., Ecology of Rocky Mountain spotted fever. II. Natural infection of wild mammals and birds in Virginia and Maryland, *Am. J. Trop. Med. Hyg.*, 16, 48, 1967.

43. de Magalhaes, O. and Rocha, A., Tifo exanthematico do Brazil; papel do cao (*C. familaris*) na constituicao dos focos da molestia, *Bras. Med.*, 56, 370, 1942.

44. Rumreich, A., Dyer, R. E., and Badger, L. F., The typhus-Rocky Mountain spotted fever group. An epidemiological and clinical study in the eastern and southeastern states, *Public Health Rep.*, 46, 470, 1931.

45. Hattwick, M. A. W., Peters, A. H. H., Gregg, M. B., and Hanson, B., Surveillance of Rocky Mountain spotted fever, *JAMA*, 225, 1338, 1973.

46. Cox, H., The spotted fever group, in *Viral and Rickettsial Infections of Man,* 3rd ed., Rivers, T. M. and Horsfall, F. L., Jr., Eds., Lippincott, Philadelphia, 1959, 828.

47. Badger, L. F., Rocky Mountain spotted fever: susceptibility of the dog and sheep to the virus, *Public Health Rep.*, 48, 791, 1933.

48. Sexton, D. J., Burgdorfer, W., Thomas, L., and Norment, B. R., Rocky Mountain spotted fever in Mississippi: survey for spotted fever antibodies in dogs and for spotted fever group rickettsiae in dog ticks, *Am. J. Epidemiol.*, 103, 192, 1976.

49. Burgdorfer, W., unpublished data.

50. Saslaw, S. and Carlisle, H. N., Aerosol infection of monkeys with *Rickettsia rickettsii*, *Bacteriol. Rev.*, 30, 636, 1966.

51. Burgdorfer, W., Ecology of tick vectors of American spotted fever, *Bull. W.H.O.*, 40, 375, 1969.

52. Parker, R. R., Kohls, G. M., and Steinhaus, E. A., Rocky Mountain spotted fever: spontaneous infection in the tick *Amblyomma americanum*, *Public Health Rep.*, 58, 721, 1943.

53. Parker, R. R., Pickens, E. G., Lackman, D. B., Bell, E. J., and Thrailkill, F. B., Isolation and characterization of Rocky Mountain spotted fever rickettsiae from the rabbit tick *Haemaphysalis leporispalustris* Packard, *Public Health Rep.*, 66, 455, 1951.

54. Philip, C. B. and Hughes, L. E., Disease agents found in the rabbit tick, *Dermacentor parumapertus*, in the southwestern United States, *Atti. Congr. Int. Microbiol.*, 5, 541, 1955.

55. **Parker, R. R., Bell, J. F., Chalgren, W. S., Thrailkill, F. B., and McKee, H. T.**, The recovery of strains of Rocky Mountain spotted fever and tularemia from ticks of the eastern United States, *J. Infect. Dis.*, 91, 231, 1952.

56. **Bozeman, F. M. and Sonenshine, D. E.**, personal communication, 1970.

57. **Bell, E. J.**, personal communication, 1970.

58. **Burgdorfer, W. and Lancaster, J. L., Jr.**, unpublished data.

59. **Hughes, L. E., Clifford, C. M., Gresbrink, R., Thomas, L. A., and Keirans, J. E.**, Isolation of a spotted fever group rickettsia from the Pacific Coast tick, *Ixodes pacificus*, in Oregon, *Am. J. Trop. Med. Hyg.*, 25, 513, 1976.

60. **Burgdorfer, W., Friedhoff, K. T., and Lancaster, J. L., Jr.**, Natural history of tick-borne spotted fever in the USA. Susceptibility of small mammals to virulent *Rickettsia rickettsii*, *Bull. W.H.O.*, 35, 149, 1966.

61. Center for Disease Control, Morbidity and Mortality Weekly Reports, Annual Supplements, Department of Health, Education, and Welfare, Atlanta, 1946 to 1975.

62. **Lyskovtsev, M. M.**, Tick-borne rickettsiosis, *Misc. Publ. Entomol. Soc. Am.*, (English translation), 6, 41, 1968.

63. **Weyer, F.**, Beobachtungen bei der Übertragung von brasilianischem Fleckfieber und sibirischem Zeckenbiss Fieber auf die Kleiderlaus, *Z. Tropenmed. Parasitol.*, 9, 174, 1958.

64. **Zdrodovskii, P. F. and Golinevich, H. M.**, *The Rickettsial Diseases*, Pergamon Press, New York, 1960, 311.

65. **Robertson, R. G. and Wisseman, C. L., Jr.**, Tick-borne rickettsiae of the spotted fever group in West Pakistan. II. Serological classification of isolates from West Pakistan and Thailand. Evidence for two new species, *Am. J. Epidemiol.*, 97, 55, 1973.

66. **Rehacek, J., Zupancicova, M., Ac, P., Brezina, R., Urvölgyi, J., Kovacova, E., Tarasevic, I. V., Jablonskaya, V. A., Pospisil, R., and Baloghova, D.**, Rickettsioses studies. II. Natural foci of rickettsioses in east Slovakia, *Bull. W.H.O.*, 53, 31, 1976.

67. **Conor, A. and Bruch, A.**, Une fièvre éruptive observée en Tunisie, *Bull. Soc. Pathol. Exot.*, 3, 492, 1910.

68. **Pieri, J.**, *La Fièvre Exanthématique du Littoral Méditerraneen ou Fièvre Boutonneuse*, Doin, Paris, 1933.

69. **Durand, P. and Conseil, E.**, Transmission experimentale de la fievre boutonneuse par *Rhipicephalus sanguineus*, *C. R. Acad. Sci.*, 190, 1244, 1930.

70. **Brumpt, E.**, Longevité du virus de la fièvre boutonneuse (*Rickettsia conori* n. sp.) chez la tique *Rhipicephalus sanguineus*, *C. R. Soc. Biol.*, 110, 1199, 1932.

71. **Gear, J.**, The rickettsial diseases of Southern Africa, *S. Afr. J. Clin. Sci.*, 5, 158, 1954.

72. **Heisch, R. B., Grainger, W. E., Harvey, A. E. C., and Lister, G.**, Feral aspects of rickettsial infections in Kenya, *Trans. R. Soc. Trop. Med. Hyg.*, 56, 272, 1962.

73. **Marchette, N. J.**, Rickettsioses (tick typhus, Q fever, urban typhus) in Malaya, *J. Med. Entomol.*, 2, 339, 1966.

74. **Olmer, D. and Olmer, J.**, Epidémie des rickettsioses sur le littoral Méditerranéen; la fièvre boutonneuse, *Rev. Pathol. Gen. Comp.*, 56, 80, 1956.

75. **Sant Anna, J. F.**, On a disease in man following tick-bites and occurring in Lourenço Marques, *Parasitology*, 4, 87, 1911.

76. **Pijper, A. and Crocker, C. G.**, Rickettsioses of South Africa, *S. Afr. Med. J.*, 12, 613, 1938.

77. **Anderson, G. V. W.**, Notes from several cases of pseudo or para typhus, *Kenya Med. J.*, 2, 42, 1925.

78. **Megaw, J. W. D.**, A typhus-like fever in India, possibly transmitted by ticks, *Indian Med. Gaz.*, 56, 361, 1921.

79. **Philip, C. B., Hughes, L. E., Rao, K. N. A., and Kalra, S. L.**, Studies on "Indian Tick Typhus" and its Relation to Other Human Typhus-like Rickettsioses, paper presented at the Fifth Int. Congr. Microbiology, Rio de Janeiro, Aug. 17 to 24, 1950, 115.

80. **Gear, J. and Davis, D. H. S.**, The susceptibility of the South African gerbils (genus *Tatera*) to rickettsial diseases and their use in the preparation of anti-typhus vaccine, *Trans. R. Soc. Trop. Med. Hyg.*, 36, 1, 1942.

81. **Camicas, J. L.**, Conceptions actuelles sur l'épidémiologie de la fièvre boutonneuse dans la région Ethiopienne et la Sous-Région Europeenne Méditerranéene, *Cah. O.R.S.T.O.M. Ser Entomol. Med. Parasitol.*, 13, 229, 1975.

82. **Blanc, G. and Caminopetros, J.**, Etudes épidémiologiques et expérimentales sur la fièvre boutonneuse, faites à l'Institut Pasteur d'Athènes, *Arch. Inst. Pasteur Tunis*, 20, 343, 1932.

83. **Giroud, P., Capponi, M., Dumas, N., and Rageau, J.**, Les *Ixodes ricinus* et *hexagonus* de France contiennent des agents rickettsiens ou proches, *C. R. Acad. Sci.*, 260, 4874, 1965.

84. **Giroud, P., Capponi, M., Dumas, N., Colas Belcour, J., and Masson, R.,** Mise en évidence d'une façon presque constante sur les tiques de l'Est de la France de l'antigène de groupe boutonneux pourpré et isolement de souches, *C. R. Acad. Sci.,* 255, 611, 1962.
85. **Burgdorfer, W., Ormsbee, R. A., Schmidt, M. L., and Hoogstraal, H.,** A search for the epidemic typhus agent in Ethiopian ticks, *Bull. W.H.O.,* 48, 563, 1973.
86. **Brody, J.,** A case of tick typhus in North Queensland, *Med. J. Aust.,* 1, 511, 1946.
87. **Andrew, R., Bonnin, J. M., and Williams, S.,** Tick typhus in North Queensland, *Med. J. Aust.,* 2, 253, 1946.
88. **Streeten, G. E. W., Cohen, R. S., Gutteridge, N. M., Wilmer, N. B., Brown, H. E., Smith, D. J. W., and Derrick, E. H.,** Tick typhus in South Queensland: report of three cases, *Med. J. Aust.,* 1, 372, 1948.
89. **Plotz, H., Smadel, J. E., Bennett, B. L., Reagan, R. L., and Snyder, M. J.,** North Queensland tick typhus. Studies of the aetiological agent and its relation to other rickettsial diseases, *Med. J. Aust.,* 2, 263, 1946.
90. **Lackman, D. and Parker, R. R.,** The serological characterization of North Queensland tick typhus, *Public Health Rep.,* 63, 1624, 1948.
91. **Philip, C. B.,** Miscellaneous human rickettsioses, in *Communicable Diseases,* Pullen, R. L., Ed., Lea & Febiger, Philadelphia, 1950, 781.
92. **Campbell, R. W. and Domrow, R.,** Rickettsioses in Australia: ecology of *Rickettsia tsutsugamushi* and *Rickettsia australis, Proc. 2nd Int. Symp. Rickettsiae and Rickettsial Diseases,* Kazar, Ormsbee, and Tarasevich, Eds., VEDA, Bratislava, 1978, 505.
93. **Fenner, F.,** The epidemiology of North Queensland tick typhus: natural mammalian hosts, *Med. J. Aust.,* 2, 666, 1946.
94. **Knyvett, A. F. and Sandars, D. F.,** North Queensland tick typhus: a case report defining a new endemic area, *Med. J. Aust.,* 2, 592, 1964.
95. **Greenberg, M., Pellitteri, O. J., and Jellison, W. L.,** Rickettsialpox — a newly recognized rickettsial disease. III. Epidemiology, *Am. J. Public Health,* 37, 860, 1947.
96. **Huebner, R. J., Stamps, P., and Armstrong, C.,** Rickettsialpox — a newly recognized rickettsial disease. I. Isolation of the etiologic agent, *Public Health Rep.,* 61, 1605, 1946.
97. **Huebner, R. J., Jellison, W. L., and Pomerantz, C.,** Rickettsialpox — a newly recognized rickettsial disease. IV. Isolation of a rickettsia apparently identical with the causative agent of rickettsialpox from *Allodermanyssus sanguineus,* a rodent mite, *Public Health Rep.,* 61, 1677, 1946.
98. **Huebner, R. J., Jellison, W. L., and Armstrong, C.,** Rickettsialpox — a newly recognized rickettsial disease. V. Recovery of *Rickettsia akari* from a house mouse (*Mus musculus*), *Public Health Rep.,* 62, 777, 1947.
99. **Pickens, E. G., Bell, E. J., Lackman, D. B., and Burgdorfer, W.,** Use of mouse serum in identification and serologic classification of *Rickettsia akari* and *Rickettsia australis, J. Immunol.,* 94, 883, 1965.
100. **Jackson, E. B., Danauskas, J. X., Coale, M. C., and Smadel, J. E.,** Recovery of *Rickettsia akari* from the Korean vole, *Microtus fortis pelliceus, Am. J. Hyg.,* 66, 301, 1957.
101. **Lackman, D. B.,** a review of information on rickettsialpox in the United States, *Clin. Pediatr.* (Philadelphia), 2, 296, 1963.
102. **Zdrodovskii, P. F. and Golinevich, H. M.,** *The Rickettsial Diseases,* Pergamon Press, New York, 1960, 340.
103. **Le Gac, P.,** Research on rickettsialpox in Oubangui-Chari, *West Afr. Med. J.,* 2, 42, 1953.
104. **Peacock, M. G., Ormsbee, R. A., and Johnson, K. M.,** Rickettsioses of Central America, *Am. J. Trop. Med. Hyg.,* 20, 941, 1971.
105. **Nichols, E., Rindge, M. E., and Russell, G. G.,** The relationship of the habits of the house mouse and the mouse mite (*Allodermanyssus sanguineus*) to the spread of rickettsialpox, *Ann. Intern. Med.,* 39, 92, 1953.
106. **Kiselev, R. J. and Volchanetskaia, G. I.,** Importance of the mite *Allodermanyssus sanguineus* in the epidemiology of variola-similar rickettsiosis, in *Natural Nidus of Human Diseases,* Pavlovsky, E. N., Ed., Medgiz, Leningrad, 1955, 248.
107. **Sulkin, S. E.,** Laboratory-acquired infections, *Bacteriol. Rev.,* 25, 203, 1961.
108. **Burgdorfer, W.,** unpublished data.
109. **Rose, H. M.,** The clinical manifestations and laboratory diagnosis of rickettsialpox, *Ann. Intern. Med.,* 31, 871, 1949.
110. **Campbell, R. W. and Pope, J. H.,** The value of newborn mice as a sensitive host for *Rickettsia australis, Aust. J. Sci.,* 30, 324, 1968.
111. **Stoenner, H. G., Lackman, D. B., and Bell, E. J.,** Factors affecting the growth of rickettsias of the spotted fever group in fertile hens' eggs, *J. Infect. Dis.,* 110, 121, 1962.

112. **Ormsbee, R. A.**, Rickettsiae, in *Manual of Clinical Microbiology,* 2nd ed., Lennette, E. H., Spaulding, E. H., and Truant, J. P., Eds., American Society of Microbiology, Washington, D.C., 1974, 805.
113. **Anacker, R. L., Gerloff, R. K., Thomas, L. A., Mann, R. E., Brown, W. R., and Bickel, W. D.,** Purification of *Rickettsia rickettsi* by density-gradient zonal centrifugation, *Can. J. Microbiol.,* 20, 1523, 1974.
114. **Weiss, E., Coolbaugh, J. C., and Williams, J. C.,** Separation of viable *Rickettsia typhi* from yolk sac and L cell host components by Renografin density gradient centrifugation, *Appl. Microbiol.,* 30, 456, 1975.
115. **Fiset, P., Ormsbee, R. A., Silberman, R., Peacock, M., and Spielman, S. H.,** A microagglutination technique for the detection and measurement of rickettsial antibodies, *Acta Virol.,* 13, 60, 1969.
116. **Philip, R. N. and Casper, E. A.,** Serotyping spotted fever-group rickettsiae with mouse antisera by microimmunofluorescence. A preliminary report, in *Proc. 2nd Int. Symp. Rickettsiae and Rickettsial Diseases,* Kazar, Ormsbee, and Tarasevich, Eds., VEDA, Bratislava, 1978, 269.
117. **Shirai, A., Dietel, J. W., and Osterman, J. V.,** Indirect hemagglutination test for human antibody to typhus and spotted fever group rickettsiae, *J. Clin. Microbiol.,* 2, 430, 1975.
118. **Philip, R.N., Casper, E. A., Ormsbee, R. A., Peacock, M. G., and Burgdorfer, W.,** Microimmunofluorescence test for the serological study of Rocky Mountain spotted fever and typhus, *J. Clin. Microbiol.,* 3, 51, 1976.
119. **Burgdorfer, W.,** Hemolymph test. A technique for detection of rickettsiae in ticks, *Am. J. Trop. Med. Hyg.,* 19, 1010, 1970.

ADDENDUM

In two 1977 publications,[1,2] it was concluded that the dog can be readily infected with *R. rickettsii*, develops an ensuing high and persistent rickettsemia, and therefore may be a ready source of infection for ticks. These conclusions were based on experiments in which 26 adult beagles were inoculated intravenously with 1.0 mℓ of chick-embryo yolk sac suspensions containing 10^2 to $10^{7.25}$ guinea pig ID_{50} of *R. rickettsii*. All of the animals developed a clinical syndrome that varied in severity with the dose of inoculum. Of 20 dogs inoculated with at least 10^5 guinea pig ID_{50}, 15 died and most of the survivors were rickettsemic for at least 14 days. Rickettsial concentrations in their blood exceeded 10^2 guinea pig ID_{50} from day 2 to day 10 after inoculation of at least 10^4 guinea pig ID_{50}. Lower levels of rickettsemia were detected in a single dog that had been inoculated with only 10^2 guinea pig ID_{50}.

These highly tentative results do not reflect the pathogenicity of the spotted-fever agent, *R. rickettsii*, in dogs infected under natural conditions, and they do not justify the authors' conclusions. It has been known since the 1930s that dogs are susceptible to *R. rickettsii*, but they usually develop an inapparent or mild transient illness characterized by elevated temperature, lassitude, anorexia, cough, and a mild rickettsemia that may last from 4 to 6 days.[3,4] The concentration of rickettsiae circulating during that time is generally low although it may be sufficient to infect a low percentage of simultaneously feeding normal ticks.[4] Dogs rarely die from spotted fever.

Recent observations[5] also do not support the conclusions of Keenan et al.[1] During a 2-year study involving 6000 dogs in Massachusetts, 300 to 450 dogs were found to have antibodies to Rocky Mountain spotted fever (RMSF) group antigen. (Presumably, the positive number depended on the titer considered significat of infection.) Only 13 dogs had an illness suggestive of spotted fever and all had significant rises in antibody titer. According to their owners, the rest of the seropositive dogs were never sick. It was speculated that few RMSF strains in nature are pathogenic for dogs.

REFERENCES

1. **Keenan, K. P., Buhles, W. C., Jr., Huxsoll, D. L., Williams, R. G., Hildebrandt, P. K., Campbell, J. M., and Stephenson, E. H.,** Pathogenesis of infection with *Rickettsia rickettsii* in the dog: a disease model for Rocky Mountain spotted fever, *J. Infect. Dis.,* 135, 911, 1977.
2. **Keenan, K. P., Buhles, W. C., Jr., Huxsoll, D., L., Williams, D. and Hildebrandt, P. K.,** Studies on the pathogenesis of *Rickettsia rickettsii* in the dog: clinical and clinicopathologic changes of experimental infection, *Am. J. Vet. Res.,* 38, 851, 1977.
3. **Badger, L. F.,** Rocky Mountain spotted fever: susceptibility of the dog and sheep to the virus, *Public Health Rep.,* 48, 491, 1933.
4. **Price, W. H.,** The epidemiology of Rocky Mountain spotted fever. II. Studies on the biological survival mechanism of *Rickettsia rickettsii, Am. J. Hyg.,* 60, 292, 1954.
5. **Murray, E. S.,** Contribution in case records of the Massachusetts General Hospital, *N. Engl. J. Med.,* 298, 1076, 1978.

SCRUB TYPHUS

R. N. Philip

DISEASE

Scrub typhus is a rickettsial disease caused by *Rickettsia tsutsugamushi* and transmitted by larval trombiculid mites (chiggers) indigenous to southeast Asia. The disease is characterized by fever, headache, lymphadenopathy, and rash. An eschar often develops at the site of the infected chigger bite. *R. tsutsugamushi* is maintained in mites of the subgenus *Leptotrombidium* and their murid hosts, particularly of the genus *Rattus*. Mite infestation occurs in moist, warm terrain consisting of secondary vegetation that provides good harborage to field rodents. Man is an accidental host who acquires the disease when he intrudes into often sharply localized foci colonized by infected mites. Synonyms are tsutsugamushi disease, mite-borne typhus, and chigger-borne typhus.

ETIOLOGIC AGENT

R. tsutsugamushi (R. orientalis) resembles other rickettsiae morphologically. The organisms are rods, usually about 0.4 × 1.2 μm in size, that stain deep purple by the method of Giemsa and characteristically occur in perinuclear clusters in the cytoplasm of infected cells. Electron microscopically, they also resemble other rickettsiae in that they possess a trilamellar cell wall and plasma membrane enclosing the cytoplasm in which dense ribosome-like granules and DNA-like strands may be observed.[1] These rickettsiae are similar to bacteria because they contain both DNA, RNA, and muramic acid, a characteristic component of the cell walls of Gram-negative bacteria.[2,3] The organisms replicate by transverse binary fission, and multiplication in cell culture is about threefold in 24 hr.[4,5] Once established, *R. tsutsugamushi* grows well in chick-embryo yolk sacs and several kinds of vertebrate cell cultures.

Scrub typhus rickettsiae are less stable than other rickettsiae in an extracellular environment. Viability is lost after heating rickettsiae at 56°C for 30 min, by ultraviolet irradiation for 5 min, or by 0.1% formalin at 23°C for 15 min.[6] Active purified preparations suitable for biochemical study have been difficult to obtain because rickettsiae are labile and rather tightly bound to host-cell constituents. Some factors affecting viability and penetration of rickettsiae into cells have been defined.[6] Glutamate and related substrates are oxidized by rickettsiae and help to maintain viability and infectivity. Compounds such as 2,4-dinitrophenol that are metabolic inhibitors in the normal pathway of glutamate oxidation are deleterious to viability of rickettsiae. Protein, such as bovine serum albumin, protects viability by a mechanism as yet unknown, and divalent cations in the suspending fluid enhance attachment of rickettsiae to host cells by electrostatic binding.

All strains of *R. tsutsugamushi* possess one or more antigens in common as evidenced by the ability of one strain to protect against another during cross-immunity tests in experimental animals. Nevertheless, there exists greater antigenic heterogeneity among strains than is encountered in other groups of rickettsiae. This has been established by various immunologic techniques including complement-fixation (CF), toxin-neutralization, vaccination-challenge, serum-neutralization, and direct immunofluorescence.[7-13]

Three major antigenic groups of strains of *R. tsutsugamushi* are recognized, the prototypes of which are Gilliam, Karp, and Kato.[14] In Japan, most newly isolated strains can be classified into one of these three serotypes. Most of 77 isolates from Thailand appear to be antigenically related to Gilliam, Karp, and Kato, but many cannot be placed into a single category.[15] Five isolates are antigenically distinctive and, therefore, possible candidates for new prototypes. It is possible that other antigenically distinct types of scrub typhus rickettsiae exist in highly endemic areas.

It has been suggested that antigenic heterogeneity of strains is less in the periphery than in the epicenter of the scrub typhus region, that serotypes are genetically stable, and that new geographic variants resulting from antigenic drift are infrequent.[12] In contrast to findings in Thailand where scrub typhus is widely endemic, all of the 79 strains of *R. tsutsugamushi* isolated in Pakistan cross-reacted with at least one of the three prototype strains (Gilliam, Karp, and Kato) and most reacted only with the Karp serotype.[12]

In Japan, there is a relationship between a particular strain serotype and geographic origin of the rodent host, severity of the disease, and mite vector.[16] This could not be demonstrated in Thailand or West Pakistan.[12,17]

TRUE AND ALTERNATE HOSTS

Invertebrate

Mites of the subgenus *Leptotrombidium* are incriminated or suspected of being major vectors of *R. tsutsugamushi* wherever outbreaks of scrub typhus occur.[18] Since only larval forms are parasitic and usually feed only once, and transovarial and transstadial transmission of rickettsiae has been demonstrated in *Leptotrombidium*, these mites are also considered to be true hosts of scrub typhus rickettsiae. The most important vector species are *L. deliense, L. akamushi, L. fletcheri, L. arenicola, L. pallidum, L. scutellare*, and *L. pavlovskyi*.[18]

The evidence incriminating *L. deliense* as a vector of *R. tsutsugamushi* is so impressive that wherever this mite occurs, the presence of scrub typhus should be suspected. This species has been found infected in Burma, China, India, Malaya, New Guinea, Pakistan, the Pescadores and Philippine Islands, Taiwan, Thailand, and Australia.[18,19] *L. akamushi* is the classical vector of tsutsugamushi disease along the Japanese rivers of Niigata, Akita, and Yamagata Prefectures, Honshu.[20] *L. fletcheri*, a form closely related to *L. akamushi,* is an important vector of scrub typhus rickettsiae in Malaya, New Guinea, the Philippines, and Indonesia.[18] *L. arenicola* is believed to be a vector of *R. tsutsugamushi* on the beaches of Malaya.[18] *L. pallidum* has been incriminated as an occasional vector in scattered areas of Japan from autumn to spring.[20] It is also considered to be a source of intrazootic infection in Korea and the Primorye region of the U.S.S.R.[21,22] However, *L. pavlovskyi* is thought to be the principal vector of *R. tsutsugamushi* in that Russian region.[22] *L. scutellare* is the source of tsutsugamushi disease in the Mt. Fuji area and Izu-Shichito Islands of Japan in late autumn.[20]

Other species of *Leptotrombidium* considered to be possible vectors, based on incomplete information, include *L. papale, L. tosa, L. orientale, L. fuji*, and *L. kawamurai*.[18] Present evidence indicates that other genera of mites are not important vectors of *R. tsutsugamushi*.

Vertebrate

Most warm-blooded vertebrates are susceptible to infection by *R. tsutsugamushi*. Furthermore, the major chigger vectors will parasitize most vertebrates that intrude into foci of mite infestation. Between 56 and 59 species of mammals and from 27 to 30 genera have been found to be naturally infected with *R. tsutsugamushi*.[18] Certain genera are more important than others. Murids, particularly of the genus *Rattus*, are the principal hosts of vector mites in Southeast Asia.[23] About three fourths of reported isolations of *R. tsutsugamushi* from vertebrates have been obtained from field rats and related genera, such as *Apodemus*.[18] Most of the 60 or so species of *Rattus* are found in the Indo-Malaysian region that is also the center of scrub typhus activity.[24] *R. rattus* is the largest species of the genus. It comprises well over 100 forms, the local field-dwelling members of which are important in a particular focus of infection. Commensal rats are not involved in the epidemiology of scrub typhus.

Voles and field mice are the principal hosts of vector chiggers in northern latitudes, particularly northern Japan where field rats are not found.[24] *Microtus montebelli* is the classical rodent host of *R. tsutsugamushi* in northwestern Honshu.[20]

Less important small mammalian hosts of *R. tsutsugamushi* include tree shrews in Southeast Asia, bandicoots in Australia, gerbils in Ceylon, and many others from which rickettsiae have been isolated infrequently.[18] Larger mammals may be infected but they play no direct role in the maintenance of natural infection.

The importance of birds as hosts of *R. tsutsugamushi* is poorly defined. In some areas of Southeast Asia, ground-dwelling birds with limited range are heavily infested with *Leptotrombidium* and are considered to be important in maintaining mite colonies.[23] Birds with wider ranges may help to disperse chiggers from one focus to another. Although some species of birds have been shown to be susceptible to experimental infection, attempts to recover *R. tsutsugamushi* from naturally infected birds have been unsuccessful until recently.[25,26]

DISTRIBUTION

More species of *Rattus* are found in the Indo-Malaysian area than anywhere else.[24] It has been suggested that these rodents originated there and spread peripherally in various evolving forms. Since rats are also major maintaining hosts of trombiculid mites, Southeast Asia became the epicenter for scrub typhus.

The scrub typhus region encompasses a land area of more than 5 million square miles and ranges from approximately 20° S to 45° N latitude.[23] Roughly, this region is bounded on the east by Japan, the Philippines, New Guinea, and the Solomon and New Hebrides Islands; on the south by northern Queensland, Australia; on the west by the Chagos Archipelago and Maldive Islands, Ceylon, India, Pakistan, and Tadzhikistan, U.S.S.R.; and on the north by Tibet, southern China, South Korea, the maritime territory of the U.S.S.R., Sakhalin, and several of the Kurile Islands.[21,23]

Distribution of scrub typhus within this region is determined by climatic and environmental conditions favorable to maintenance of mite vectors of *R. tsutsugamushi* and their vertebrate hosts. All developmental stages of the major vectors commonly require moist habitat (optimum relative humidity of 85% or greater at ground level) and moderate to high ambient temperatures (about 22 to 35°C).[23] In much of southeast Asia where climatic conditions are favorable throughout the year, populations of mites and maintaining hosts may be high and endemic areas extensive. Seasonal variations in climatic conditions are influential (particularly toward the periphery of the scrub typhus region), and endemic areas are scattered.

Examples of exceptional conditions include parts of Japan where *L. scutellare* and *L. pallidum* are vectors of *R. tsutsugamushi* during the fall, winter, and spring months, occurrence of endemic areas in Korea and eastern Siberia where winter temperatures sometimes reach −30°C, and "oases" of scrub typhus in subarctic conditions at elevations of 10,500 ft in the western Himalaya Mountains of Pakistan.[20,21,27]

Foci of infection that Audy[23] has termed "typhus islands" are often sharply localized and irregularly scattered within endemic areas. The circumscribed nature of such foci is related to the limited range of vector mites and their maintaining hosts. In hot, humid areas where ecologic conditions are especially suitable for supporting dense field rodent populations, there may be tremendous build-up in mite colonies. Typhus islands are established when chiggers that are congenitally infected with *R. tsutsugamushi* are introduced into these foci.[18]

Foci of infection usually occur in terrain covered by secondary or transitional forms of vegetation that may be classified as man-made wasteland, water-meadows, or fringe habitat.[23] Man's modification of his environment by removal of primary forests, practice of shifting cultivation, abandonment of fields, plantations, and village sites during conflict, neglect of garden plots in and around villages, etc. has profoundly influenced occurrence of scrub typhus. Grassy, moist terrain along rivers and streams in certain endemic areas has long been recognized as scrub typhus locale. Fringe habitat includes hedgerows and scrub terrain bordering cultivated land that offer good habitat for small mammals.

DISEASE IN ANIMALS

Isolates of *R. tsutsugamushi* vary in virulence for experimental animals from those that have no clinical effect and are difficult to establish to those that are lethal on primary passage. Once established, isolates may retain original characteristics or may change in pathogenicity on subpassage. The level of virulence for one species of animal may not follow the same pattern in other experimental hosts.[28]

Persistence of hyperendemic foci of scrub typhus and the high proportion of animals in such foci that have antibodies to *R. tsutsugamushi* are evidence that infection has little effect upon population fluctuations of natural hosts. *R. tsutsugamushi* can readily be recovered from a wide variety of mammals in scrub typhus areas. During a 3-year survey in Malaya, rickettsiae were isolated from more than 30 species, and isolation rates from certain kinds of ground-dwelling and semiarboreal rodents ranged as high as 50%.[29] Prevalence of antibodies to *R. tsutsugamushi* in these species was even higher. Even in northern areas such as Korea, rickettsiae may sometimes be present in a high proportion of field rodents.[21] Scrub typhus was infrequent among United Nations troops during the Korean War, yet 17% of field mice (*Apodemus agrarius*) collected from several localities in South Korea were found to be infected with *R. tsutsugamushi*.

The dynamics of scrub typhus infection in natural hosts are not well known. Early Japanese investigators demonstrated that voles (*Microtus montebelli*) from nontyphus areas were susceptible to experimental infection with *R. tsutsugamushi* but did not develop manifestations of disease.[30] Laboratory-reared *Rattus annandalei*, important rodent hosts in Malaya, were as susceptible to experimental infection with the Karp strain of *R. tsutsugamushi* as Swiss mice, but mortality from disease was very low even when 10^7 mouse LD_{50} was given.[29]

Experimental animals that have been used in the laboratory and found susceptible to infection by *R. tsutsugamushi* include monkeys and apes, rabbits, guinea pigs, white rats, hamsters, gerbils, cotton rats, and Swiss mice. Transmission studies by early Japanese workers made use of several species of monkeys, of which the short-tailed macaque (*Macacus fuscatus*) native to Japan was particularly susceptible.[31] Disease clinically resembling scrub typhus in man was induced by exposure of these monkeys to infected mites and by inoculation of infectious materials. The incubation period was commonly 6 or 7 days. Eschars accompanied by regional lymphadenopathy were produced after exposure to infected mites or intracutaneous inoculation of rickettsiae. The disease was usually milder in monkeys than in man, and cutaneous eruptions were never observed. Illness persisted 5 to 15 days, deaths were infrequent, and immunity to reinfection was durable.

Guinea pigs can be infected with *R. tsutsugamushi*, but the clinical response is variable and some strains of rickettsiae are difficult to maintain in this animal. Fever may be produced, but scrotal reactions are absent.[31]

Rabbits also show a variable clinical response to scrub typhus rickettsiae inoculated by the usual experimental routes of infection. If rickettsiae are injected into the anterior chamber of the eye of nonimmune animals, infection of Descemets membrane occurs, and keratitis with pannus and iritis follow.[32] The disease subsides after several weeks, leaving no residual scarring. The affected eye is usually refractory to reinfection by the homologous strain of rickettsiae. Strains of scrub typhus rickettsiae can also be maintained in rabbits by intratesticular inoculation.[31]

Gerbils, hamsters, white rats, and cotton rats were used in early studies of *R. tsutsugamushi*. These experimental animals are quite susceptible to infection by *R. tsutsugamushi*, but they offer no advantages over mice as experimental animals.

White mice are widely used. Clinical manifestations resulting from intraperitoneal inoculation of virulent rickettsiae usually appear at the end of the first week and include ruffling of the fur, swelling of the abdomen, and dyspnea.[31] Death usually occurs 24 to 48 hr after onset of the disease. Post-mortem examination reveals hyperemia of the inguinal and axillary lymph nodes, serofibrinous exudate in the peritoneal and pleural cavities, enlargement of the spleen, and hemorrhagic infiltrates in the lungs. Rickettsiae may be observed in mononuclear cells in appropriately stained smears of peritoneal exudate.   The clinical response of mice to experimental infection by *R. tsutsugamushi* is determined by virulence of the strain, route of inoculation, and number of viable rickettsiae inoculated.[33] Infection with virulent strains by intraperitoneal, intravenous, and intracerebral routes often results in 100% fatality, i.e., the infectious dose is equivalent to the lethal dose. With less virulent strains such as Gilliam, the lethal dose may be 1000 times greater than the infectious dose by the intraperitoneal route. However, even the virulent Karp strain, injected in doses that are lethal by the intraperitoneal route, is nonlethal by subcutaneous and intracutaneous routes. Some strains are nonlethal for mice under any condition.

R. tsutsugamushi characteristically persists for long intervals in tissues of sublethally infected hosts. After infection of field rats (*Rattus annandalei*) with the Karp strain, rickettsiae were isolated from kidneys of 94% of the animals at 2 months and 44% at 4 months.[29] *R. tsutsugamushi* persisted for as long as 75 days in blood and 99 days in brains of infected white rats.[34] Rickettsiae were isolated from blood of cotton rats infected with *R. tsutsugamushi* 102 days later and from brains for as long as 269 days.[35] Rickettsiae persisted in various tissues of infected white mice for at least 610 days, at which time the experiment was terminated.[35] Highest titers of rickettsiae in persistent infections are usually found in the kidney.[29,35] Several attempts to recover rickettsiae from bladder urine of infected animals were unsuccessful.[35]

Even though *R. tsutsugamushi* may persist for long periods, sublethally infected mice show early antibody responses (CF and neutralizing antibodies) and may be resistant to lethal challenge with antigenically related organisms for at least 6 months.[28] However, superinfection with rickettsemia in the absence of disease can be induced in chronically infected mice.[36] Such a phenomenon may help to explain the high prevalence of *R. tsutsugamushi* in murid hosts in hyperendemic areas.

DISEASE IN MAN

After an incubation period of about 10 to 12 days, scrub typhus usually begins with chilly sensations, fever, headache, generalized aches, malaise, and anorexia.[31] A primary lesion at the site of the chigger bite, usually single but occasionally multiple, may be noted as early as 5 days before onset of systemic symptoms. Sites are often on the lower part of the body. The primary lesion commonly begins as a small papule surrounded by a red aureola 2 to 6 mm wide that ulcerates after a few days, is accompanied by regional adenitis, and becomes encrusted (eschar). Generalized lymphodenopathy usually occurs, and the spleen may become palpable. The nonremissive fever increases during the first few days of disease, and a macular or maculopapular rash may appear upon the trunk and spread peripherally near the end of the first week. The rash varies in intensity, is almost never petechial, and may persist only a few hours to several days. Bronchitis and pneumonia may be present in severe cases. CNS involvement, myocarditis, transient deafness, and vascular disturbances, such as thrombophlebitis, are occasional complications. Convalescence in untreated cases commonly begins late in the second week of illness, and recovery is usually complete without sequelae. Death, which is infrequent even in untreated cases, usually occurs from pneumonia or circulatory failure during the second or third week.

Tetracycline and chloramphenicol are regularly effective in treatment of scrub typhus.[37-39] Tetracycline is given each day at 6-hr intervals in equally divided doses totaling 25 mg/kg of body weight. Chloramphenicol is given in daily doses of 50 mg/kg of body weight. Therapy should be continued for at least 7 to 10 days.[39] Most patients will become afebrile within 48 hr after start of treatment. These antibiotics are primarily rickettsiostatic, and ultimate cure depends upon development of an adequate immunologic response.[40-42] Relapses may occur if therapy is discontinued too soon. In one series of cases, 2 of 68 patients treated with tetracycline for 7 to 10 days relapsed 4 days after treatment was discontinued.[39] Such recurrences are readily controlled with antibiotics.

Variations in clinical manifestations of scrub typhus may be influenced by factors such as virulence of infecting strains, criteria used for diagnosis, incomplete immunity from earlier infection, race, age, specific treatment, and physiologic state of the patient at time of infection. Before specific antibiotic therapy was available, reported case fatality ratios varied from 0 to 65%.[23] In the classic focus of tsutsugamushi disease in Niigata Prefecture, Japan, 35% of more than 2000 cases reported between 1917 and 1952 were fatal.[20] However, on the Izu-Shichito Islands, Japan, there were no fatalities among 780 cases. Japanese investigators attribute this striking difference partly to variations in virulence of infecting strains. Likewise, variable case fatality ratios were found in scrub typhus outbreaks among allied forces in the South Pacific and Indo-Burma theaters of operation during World War II.[43] The physical condition of some patients under stress of combat influenced the outcome of the disease; however, variations were also attributed to differences in strain virulence.

The eschar is an important diagnostic sign, but it is not always present in scrub typhus. Early Japanese investigators reported that eschars were always present in tsutsugamushi disease. In Malaya, eschars were usually found in European patients but were often absent among Malayan natives.[31] This was partly attributed to lack of recognition because of differences in pigmentation of skin. Eschars were infrequently observed in more recent investigations based upon laboratory diagnoses. Thus, primary lesions were noted in only 23 of 53 Australian cases of scrub typhus diagnosed by isolation of rickettsiae or rise in Proteus OXK agglutinins.[38] Eschars confirmed by laboratory methods were found in only 46% of scrub typhus cases among American servicemen hospitalized for febrile illness in South Vietnam.[39]

Frequency of rash has also varied. Rash was noted in 65% or more of the cases among armed forces in World War II.[31] It was often used as a clinical criterion for diagnosis of scrub typhus. Rash was observed in only 45% and 34% of Australian and Vietnamese cases diagnosed by laboratory methods, respectively.[38,39] Some of these patients may have received antibiotic therapy before the anticipated appearance of rash. In Vietnam, clinical diagnosis of scrub typhus was more often considered in patients with a rash and eschar than in laboratory-confirmed cases without these manifestations.

Clinical laboratory findings may not be helpful in diagnosis of scrub typhus. Leukocyte counts usually range between 5,000 and 10,000 cells per mm³ of blood, but often during the second week there is an increase in lymphocytes, some of which are atypical in appearance.[31,39] Urinalysis does not show abnormalities except occasional proteinuria. Total serum protein levels are unchanged during the course of the disease, but serum albumin may decline and globulin may increase during the second and third weeks. Plasma fibrinogen levels may drop conspicuously in severe cases.[31]

Fluorescent antibodies and Proteus OXK agglutinins generally appear at the end of the first week of illness in untreated patients and reach maximum levels by the end of the third week.[31,39] Antibiotic therapy initiated during the first several days of illness may suppress or delay antibody responses.[42]

In fatal cases, the histopathology is basically disseminated focal vasculitis and perivasculitis, particularly in vessels of the skin, lungs, heart, and brain.[31] Endovasculitis, thrombosis, and focal hemorrhage may be present but are less prominent than those same signs observed in Rocky Mountain spotted fever and epidemic typhus. The inflammatory response in vascular walls and perivascular tissues consists of large mononuclear cells, plasma cells, and lymphocytes accompanied by focal edema. Lesions may extend to the parenchyma of various organs. In the heart, there is often interstitial myocarditis and focal necrosis of muscle fibers. Interstitial pneumonia with thickening of the septa in alveolar walls and foci of alveolar exudate are usually present. Perivascular proliferation of glial cells may be evident in the brain. Perivascular lesions are sometimes also present in the liver, kidneys, and testes. The G.I. tract may show petechial necrosal hemorrhages and enlargement of lymph follicles. Infarcts are occasionally found in the lungs, spleen, and kidneys.

Specific immunity against *R. tsutsugamushi* develops during convalescence from scrub typhus.[44] Second attacks of a disease clinically resembling scrub typhus are not uncommon in hyperendemic areas, but laboratory confirmation during both episodes is lacking. Multiple attacks are ascribed to infection by antigenically unrelated strains. During studies of scrub typhus in the late 1940s, volunteers infected with the Karp or Gilliam strain of *R. tsutsugamushi* were shown to be immune to disease when challenged with homologous strains 14 months later.[42,45] On the other hand, some subjects challenged with heterologous strains as early as 1 month after initial infection developed scrub typhus.

Preliminary results suggest that cell-mediated immunity may be important in scrub typhus. Years ago it was observed that *R. tsutsugamushi* infection in one eye of rabbits gave rise to solid immunity against reinfection in the same eye but only partial immunity to reinfection in the contralateral eye.[30] Recently, Shirai et al.[46] showed that passive transfer of spleen cells from inbred mice immunized with the Gilliam strain of *R. tsutsugamushi* protected nonimmunized recipient mice against lethal challenge with the Karp strain.

Recrudescent scrub typhus, similar to Brill-Zinsser disease in epidemic typhus, has not been reported. However, Smadel et al.[47] isolated *R. tsutsugamushi* from a lymph node of 1 of 12 asymptomatic persons in Malaya who had had scrub typhus during chemoprophylaxis field trials 1 to 2 years earlier; Hyashi and Watanabe[48] demonstrated rickettsemia after intravenous injection of typhoid vaccine into a patient 4 to 8 weeks after he had recovered from scrub typhus. Recrudescent scrub typhus, if it occurs, is difficult to distinguish from primary disease.

GENERAL MODE OF SPREAD

R. tsutsugamushi is transmitted to man and murid hosts by larval trombiculid mites of the genus *Leptotrombidium*. Other than infection occasionally acquired during laboratory study of rickettsiae, no other mode of transmission is known.

EPIDEMIOLOGY

The epidemiology of scrub typhus is a four-factor complex involving causative rickettsiae, vector chigger mites, vertebrate hosts that maintain the mites and serve as temporary reservoirs of *R. tsutsugamushi*, and man, who by modifying the environment influences the ecology of reservoir hosts and is an occasional victim of the disease.[23]

Since trombiculid mites serve both as principal reservoirs and vectors of rickettsiae, much attention has been directed to the bionomics of important vector species. These mites are parasitic only during larval stages and, as a rule, feed on their vertebrate hosts only once. A general description of the life cycle follows.[18] Several days after emergence from ova, larvae cluster on debris within several centimeters of the soil surface, awaiting any convenient warm-blooded host. They settle in loci on the host that are characteristic for the vector species and feed on tissue juices for 2 to 5 days until engorged. When replete, larvae drop onto the soil and transform into nymphs after a few days. The nymphs, as well as adults, feed on eggs of arthropods or dead soft-bodied insects. After several weeks, they again enter into a pupa-like stage from which the mites emerge as sexually mature adults. Adults may live 15 months or longer in soil within a few centimeters of the sites where they dropped as larvae. Stalked spermatophores deposited by males are collected by females. Egg laying commences after several weeks, and females deposit about 400 eggs during a 3- to 5-month period. The entire life cycle may take only 2 to 3 months, and in favorable areas as many as four generations of mites may be produced in 1 year.[23]

Transovarial transmission of *R. tsutsugamushi* has been demonstrated for *L. deliense, L. fletcheri, L. akamushi, L. arenicola, L. pallidum,* and *L. scutellare.*[18] Rapmund and associates[49] demonstrated transovarial transmission of rickettsiae by 98% of infected females; the infection rates among offspring were usually 100% in a colony of *L. fletcheri* studied for five generations. In contrast, they found a much lower efficiency of transmission through two generations of *L. arenicola* reared in the laboratory.[50] Studies on transovarial transmission of *R. tsutsugamushi* in a colony of *L. deliense* by Krishnan et al.[51] indicated that infection died out in the fourth generation. Likewise, Audy[23] reported sporadic infection in several generations of *L. deliense* derived from a single infected female. These observations suggest that transovarial transmission of rickettsiae may be highly efficient in some family lines of vector mites but inefficient in others,[18] possibly explaining the spotty distribution of infected mite foci.

Even though prevalence rates of *R. tsutsugamushi* may be high among small mammals in hyperendemic areas, the role of these animals as reservoirs of infection is uncertain. Chiggers fed on infected hosts can acquire rickettsiae, but true infection, judged by transovarial transmission following such feeding, has not been definitely demonstrated.[18] Audy[23] suggested that impermeability of gut epithelium limits generalized infection of the tissues of mites and transmission to subsequent generations. However, even if true infection of mites occurs infrequently after feeding on infected hosts, this mechanism could be important in maintaining *R. tsutsugamushi* in areas where infection of vertebrate hosts is frequent.[18]

Occurrence of scrub typhus in man is caused by fortuitous exposure to infected mites. Risk of disease is highest among individuals who by occupation or other activity, are most likely to encounter foci where infected mites occur. Morbidity in most endemic areas is usually greatest among young adult males. Exceptions are the Izu-Shichito Islands, Japan, and Taiwan where most cases occur among children.[20] This unusual age distribution is attributed to location of foci close to human habitation. In these localities, the disease is particularly mild and case fatality low, partly due to the fact that scrub typhus is less severe in children than adults.[23]

DIAGNOSIS

Specific diagnosis of scrub typhus is based upon isolation of rickettsiae or demonstration of antibody response to *R. tsutsugamushi*.[52] Blood obtained during febrile stages of illness is injected into laboratory mice that are observed for illness and death. Impression smears of spleen or peritoneum from mice dying after the fifth day are examined for rickettsia-like organisms. If deaths do not occur, mice are sacrificed on the 14th day, and subpassages are made of spleen homogenates. Mice surviving subpassage are challenged after several weeks with lethal doses of virulent *R. tsutsugamushi* such as Karp. Lethal isolates are identified by protecting infected mice with chloramphenicol (2.5 mg/mℓ of drinking water) and challenging them with virulent *R. tsutsugamushi* several weeks later. Mice that survive challenge are considered to have been infected with scrub typhus rickettsiae.

The Weil-Felix test for agglutinins against the OXK strain of *Proteus mirabilis* has been widely used for serodiagnosis. During early investigations, it was reported that most scrub typhus patients developed Proteus-OXK antibodies. However, more recent studies in Australia and Vietnam, using other diagnostic procedures, showed development of Proteus-OXK antibodies in less than 50% of patients with scrub typhus.[38,39] Occasionally, false-positive reactions were detected in patients with leptospirosis or relapsing fever.[28,53]

The CF test has been used in seroepidemiologic studies in Japan, but because of test insensitivity and antigenic heterogeneity of rickettsial strains, it is of limited value for serodiagnosis of scrub typhus.[54]

An indirect immunofluorescence test developed by Bozeman and Elisberg[55] is very useful for serologic diagnosis of scrub typhus. Strains representing various antigenic types of *R. tsutsugamushi* are grown in chick-embryo yolk sac. Preparations of active rickettsiae may be used individually or as pooled polyvalent antigens in tests of sera for fluorescent antibodies. The test is both specific and sensitive. In Vietnam, all 32 patients from whom rickettsiae were isolated also developed four-fold or greater rises in fluorescent antibody titers against *R. tsutsugamushi*.[39] Conversely, rickettsiae were recovered from all but 3 of 35 patients with antibody responses.

PREVENTION AND CONTROL

Attempts to develop immunogenic, inactivated rickettsial vaccines against scrub typhus shortly after World War II were unsuccessful. Vaccines induced immunity in mice against strains of *R. tsutsugamushi* homologous to those contained in vaccines but were ineffectual in protecting man against scrub typhus in Southeast Asia and Japan.[56,57] Failure was attributed in part to the antigenic heterogeneity of *R. tsutsugamushi*.

In a series of volunteer studies in Malaya, immunity comparable to that obtained from disease was induced by infection with scrub typhus rickettsiae controlled by antibiotic prophylaxis.[42,45] The Gilliam strain of *R. tsutsugamushi* was used initially in the hope that it would have minimal clinical effect because of its low pathogenicity for laboratory mice. However, the disease produced was comparable in severity to that acquired naturally. When appropriate doses of chloramphenicol were given prophylactically at 4-day intervals for 4 weeks, immunity against homologous disease was produced that persisted for at least 14 months. This procedure was also effective when virulent Karp rickettsiae were used as infecting organisms. For obvious reasons, immunochemoprophylaxis is not a practicable control measure.

Chemoprophylaxis may be used in circumstances where intense but transient exposure to *R. tsutsugamushi* is antcipated. Chloramphenicol or tetracycline given in adequate doses at short intervals for a month after exposure to rickettsiae will prevent disease.[58] However, risks from morbidity must be weighed against possible side effects from the antibiotics.

Control measures to prevent scrub typhus are directed particularly at vector mites and include use of repellents to protect the individual and elimination of mite foci by area control.[59] Miticidal chemicals effectively used for protection of personnel during World War II include dimethylphthalate, dibutylphthalate, and benzyl benzoate applied to clothing directly by hand or by dipping.[43] High cost, low availability, and inconvenience of application have limited the use of these repellents by residents of endemic localities.

Area control may be particularly effective in foci of infection close to sites of human habitation where exposure is high.[59] Procedures are aimed at removal of vegetative ground cover so that surface soils are exposed for drying. Clearing also eliminates suitable habitat for vertebrate hosts. Residual and toxicant side effects contraindicate a general use of herbicides.

Several long-acting chlorinated hydrocarbons are effective in eliminating vector mites. Benzene hexachloride and lindane have been used in Japan against *L. scutellare*.[59] Dieldrin, when applied to the ground at a rate of 2.5 lb/acre, was shown to be particularly effective in controlling mites of the *L. deliense* group for at least 2 years.[60] Advantages of residual insecticides must be weighed against the undesirable effects on other elements of the biotic environment. Some organophosphorous compounds and carbamates are miticidal and have little residual effect. Short-term acaricides may be acceptable in areas such as Japan where scrub typhus is seasonal.

Control measures may also be aimed at eliminating the harborage and sustenance for the maintaining hosts of chiggers. Rodent control campaigns should not be initiated until measures to eliminate the vector mite have been started. Pesticides, because of toxicity for other vertebrates, should not be used indiscriminately.

REFERENCES

1. **Anderson, D. R., Hopps, H. E., Barile, M. F., and Bernheim, B. C.,** Comparison of the ultrastructure of several rickettsiae, ornithosis virus, and *Mycoplasma* in tissue culture, *J. Bacteriol.,* 90, 1387, 1965.
2. **Allison, A. C. and Burke, D. C.,** The nucleic acid content of viruses, *J. Gen. Microbiol.,* 27, 181, 1962.
3. **Perkins, H. R. and Allison, A. C.,** Cell-wall constituents of rickettsiae and psittacosis-lymphogranuloma organisms, *J. Gen. Microbiol.,* 30, 469, 1963.
4. **Schaechter, M., Bozeman, F. M., and Smadel, J. E.,** Study on the growth of rickettsiae. II. Morphologic observations of living rickettsiae in tissue culture cells, *Virology,* 3, 160, 1957.

5. Bozeman, F. M., Hopps, H. E., Danauskas, J. X., Jackson, E. B., and Smadel, J. E., Study on the growth of rickettsiae. I. A tissue culture system for quantitative estimations of *Rickettsia tsutsugamushi*, *J. Immunol.*, 76, 475, 1956.

6. Cohn, Z. A., Bozeman, F. M., Campbell, J. M., Humphries, J. W., and Sawyer, T. K., Study on growth of rickettsiae. V. Penetration of *Rickettsia tsutsugamushi* into mammalian cells *in vitro*, *J. Exp. Med.*, 109, 271, 1959.

7. Bengtson, I. A., Apparent serological heterogeneity among strains of tsutsugamushi disease (scrub typhus), *Public Health Rep.*, 60, 1483, 1945.

8. Kitaoka, M. and Tanaka, Y., Rickettsial toxin and its specificity in 3 prototype strains, Karp, Gilliam and Kato, of *Rickettsia orientalis*, *Acta Virol.*, 17, 426, 1973.

9. Rights, F. L., Smadel, J. E., and Jackson, E. B., Studies on scrub typhus (tsutsugamushi disease). III. Heterogeneity of strains of *R. tsutsugamushi* as demonstrated by cross-vaccination studies, *J. Exp. Med.*, 87, 339, 1948.

10. Bennett, B. L., Smadel, J. E., and Gauld, R. L., Studies on scrub typhus (tsutsugamushi disease). IV. Heterogeneity of strains of *R. tsutsugamushi* as demonstrated by cross-neutralization tests, *J. Immunol.*, 62, 453, 1949.

11. Fox, J. P., The neutralization technique in tsutsugamushi disease (scrub typhus) and the antigenic differentiation of rickettsial strains, *J. Immunol.*, 62, 341, 1949.

12. Shirai, A. and Wisseman, C. L., Serological classification of scrub typhus isolates from Pakistan, *Am. J. Trop. Med. Hyg.*, 24, 145, 1975.

13. Shishido, A., Kohno, S., Hikita, M., Iida, T., Kawashima, H., and Kawamura, A., Complement fixation and direct immunofluorescence for typing of tsutsugamushi disease rickettsia, *Acta Med. Biol. Suppl.* (Niigata), 15, 87, 1967.

14. Shishido, A., Identification and serological classification of the causative agent of scrub typhus in Japan, *Jpn. J. Med. Sci. Biol.*, 15, 308, 1962.

15. Elisberg, B. L., Campbell, J. M., and Bozeman, F. M., Antigenic diversity of *Rickettsia tsutsugamushi*: epidemiologic and ecologic significance, *J. Hyg. Epidemiol. Microbiol. Immunol.*, 12, 18, 1968.

16. Kitaoka, M., Okubo, K., and Asanuma, K., Epidemiological survey by means of complement fixation test on scrub typhus in Japan, *Acta Med. Biol. Suppl.* (Niigata), 15, 69, 1967.

17. Elisberg, B. L., Sangkasiwana, V., Campbell, J. M., Bozeman, F. M., Bodhidatta, P., and Rapmund, G., Physiogeographic distribution of scrub typhus in Thailand, *Acta Med. Biol. Suppl.* (Niigata), 15, 61, 1967.

18. Traub, R. and Wisseman, C. L., Jr., The ecology of chigger-borne rickettsiosis (scrub typhus), *J. Med. Entomol.*, 11, 237, 1974.

19. Campbell, R. W. and Domrow, R., Rickettsioses in Australia: isolation of *Rickettsia tsutsugamushi* and *R. australis* from naturally infected arthropods, *Trans. R. Soc. Trop. Med. Hyg.*, 68, 397, 1974.

20. Sasa, M., Comparative epidemiology of tsutsugamushi disease in Japan, *Jpn. J. Exp. Med.*, 24, 335, 1954.

21. Jackson, E. B., Danauskas, J. X., Smadel, J. E., Fuller, H. S., Coale, M. C., and Bozeman, F. M., Occurrence of *Rickettsii tsutsugamushi* in Korean rodents and chiggers, *Am. J. Hyg.*, 66, 309, 1957.

22. Kulagen, S. M., Tarasevic, I. V., Kudryasova, N. I., and Plotnikova, L. F., The investigation of scrub typhus in the USSR, *J. Hyg. Epidemiol. Microbiol. Immunol.*, 12, 257, 1968.

23. Audy, J. R., The ecology of scrub typhus, in *Studies in Disease Ecology*, May, J. M., Ed., Hafer, New York, 1961, 389.

24. Harrison, J. L. and Audy, J. R., Hosts of the mite vector of scrub typhus. II. An analysis of the list of recorded hosts, *Ann. Trop. Med. Parasitol.*, 45, 186, 1951.

25. Philip, C. B., Scrub typhus, or tsutsugamushi disease, *Sci. Mon.*, 69, 281, 1949.

26. Somov, G. P. and Polivanov, V. M., Isolation of strains of *Rickettsia tsutsugamushi* from the organs of migrant birds in the Primorye, *Zh. Mikrobiol. Epidemiol. Immunol.*, 49, 6, 1972.

27. Traub, R., Wisseman, C. L., Jr., and Ahmad, N., The occurrence of scrub typhus infection in unusual habitats in West Pakistan, *Trans. R. Soc. Trop. Med. Hyg.*, 61, 23, 1967.

28. Carley, J. G., Doherty, R. L., Derrick, E. H., Pope, J. H., Emanuel, M. L., and Ross, C. J., The investigation of fevers in North Queensland by mouse inoculation, with particular reference to scrub typhus, *Australas. Ann. Med.*, 4, 91, 1955.

29. Walker, J. S., Gan, E., Chye, C. T., and Muul, I., Involvement of small mammals in the transmission of scrub typhus in Malaysia: Isolation and serological evidence, *Trans. R. Soc. Trop. Med. Hyg.*, 67, 838, 1973.

30. Kitashima, T. and Miyajima, M., Studien uber die Tsutsugamushi Krankheit, *Kitasato Arch. Exp. Med.*, 2, 237, 1918.

31. **Blake, F. G., Maxcy, K. F., Sadusk, J. F., Jr., Kohls, G. M., and Bell, E. J.**, Studies on tsutsuga-mushi disease (scrub typhus, mite-borne typhus) in New Guinea and adjacent islands: epidemiology, clinical observations, and etiology in the Dobadura area, *Am. J. Hyg.*, 41, 243, 1945.
32. **Nagayo, M., Tamiya, T., Mitamura, T., and Sato, S.**, On the virus of tsutsugamushi disease and its demonstration by a new method, *Jpn. J. Exp. Med.*, 8, 309, 1930.
33. **Smadel, J. E. and Elisberg, B. L.**, Scrub typhus rickettsia, in *Viral and Rickettsial Infections of Man*, 4th ed., Horsfall, F. L. and Tamm, I., Eds., Lippincott, Philadelphia, 1965, 1130.
34. **Kohls, G. M., Armbrust, C. A., Irons, E. N., and Philip, C. B.**, Studies on tsutsugamushi disease (scrub typhus, mite-borne typhus) in New Guinea and adjacent islands, *Am. J. Hyg.*, 41, 374, 1945.
35. **Fox, J. P.**, The long persistence of *Rickettsia orientalis* in the blood and tissues of infected animals, *J. Immunol.*, 59, 109, 1948.
36. **Kuwata, T.**, Analysis of immunity in experimental tsutsugamushi disease, *J. Immunol.*, 68, 115, 1952.
37. **Smadel, J. E., Woodward, T. E., Ley, H. L., Jr., and Lewthwaite, R.**, Chloramphenicol (chloro-mycetin) in the treatment of tsutsugamushi disease (scrub typhus), *J. Clin. Invest.*, 28, 1196, 1949.
38. **Doherty, R. L.**, A clinical study of scrub typhus in North Queensland, *Med. J. Aust.*, 2, 212, 1956.
39. **Berman, S. J. and Kundin, W. D.**, Scrub typhus in South Vietnam. A study of 87 cases, *Ann. Intern. Med.*, 79, 26, 1973.
40. **Smadel, J. E., Traub, R., Ley, H. L., Jr., Philip, C. B., Woodward, T. E., and Lewthwaite, R.**, Chloramphenicol (chloromycetin) in the chemoprophylaxis of scrub typhus (tsutsugamushi disease). II. Results with volunteers exposed in hyperendemic areas of scrub typhus. *Am. J. Hyg.*, 50, 75, 1949.
41. **Smadel, J. E., Bailey, C. A., and Kiercks, F. H.**, Chloramphenicol (chloromycetin) in the chemopro-phylaxis of scrub typhus (tsutsugamushi disease). IV. Relapses of scrub typhus in treated volunteers and their prevention, *Am. J. Hyg.*, 51, 229, 1950.
42. **Smadel, J. E.**, Influence of antibiotics on immunologic responses in scrub typhus, *Am. J. Med.*, 17, 246, 1954.
43. **Philip, C. B.**, Tsutsugamushi disease (scrub typhus) in World War II, *J. Parasitol.*, 34, 169, 1948.
44. **Smadel, J. E., Ley, H. L., Jr., Diercks, F. H., and Traub, R.**, Immunity in scrub typhus: resistance to induced reinfection, *Arch. Pathol.*, 50, 847, 1950.
45. **Smadel, J. E., Ley, H. L., Jr., Diercks, F. H., Paterson, P. Y., Wisseman, C. L., Jr., and Traub, R.**, Immunization against scrub typhus: duration of immunity in volunteers following combined liv-ing vaccine and chemoprophylaxis, *Am. J. Trop. Med. Hyg.*, 1, 87, 1952.
46. **Shirai, A., Catanzaro, P. J., Phillips, S. M., and Osterman, J. V.**, Host defenses in experimental scrub typhus: role of cellular immunity in heterologous protection, *Infect. Immun.*, 14, 39, 1976.
47. **Smadel, J. E., Ley, H. L., Jr., Diercks, R. H., and Cameron, J. A. P.**, Persistence of *Rickettsia tsutsugamushi* in tissues of patients recovered from scrub typhus, *Am. J. Hyg.*, 56, 294, 1952.
48. **Hayashi, H. and Watanabe, M.**, On the possibility of appearance of rickettsiae in the circulating blood after the recovery of rickettsiosis, *Kitasato Arch. Exp. Med.*, 21, 135, 1948.
49. **Rapmund, G., Upham, R. W., Sr., Kundin, W. D., Manikumaran, C., and Chan, T. C.**, Transovar-ian development of scrub typhus rickettsiae in a colony of vector mites, *Trans. R. Soc. Trop. Med. Hyg.*, 63, 251, 1969.
50. **Rapmund, G., Dohany, A. L., Manikumaran, C., and Chan, T. C.**, Transovarial transmission of *Rickettsia tsutsugamushi* in *Leptotrombidium* (*Leptotrombidium*) *arenicola* Traub (Acarina: Trom-biculidae), *J. Med. Entomol.*, 9, 71, 1972.
51. **Krishnan, K. V., Smith, R. O. A., Bose, R. N., Neogy, K. N., Roy, B. K. G., and Ghosh, M.**, Transmission of *Rickettsia orientalis* by the bite of the larvae of *Trombicula deliensis*, *Indian Med. Gaz.*, 84, 41, 1949.
52. **Elisberg, B. L. and Bozeman, F. M.**, Rickettsiae, in *Diagnostic Procedures for Viral and Rickettsial Infections*, 4th ed., Lennette, E. H. and Schmidt, N. J., Eds., American Public Health Association, New York, 1969, 826.
53. **Zarafonetis, C. J. D., Ingraham, H. S., and Berry, J. F.**, Weil-Felix and typhus complement-fixation tests in relapsing fever, with special reference to *B. proteus* OX-K agglutination, *J. Immunol.*, 52, 189, 1946.
54. **Kitaoka, M., Asanuma, K., and Ishimaru, M.**, Seroepidemiology of scrub typhus, *J. Med. Entomol.*, 9, 594, 1972.
55. **Bozeman, F. M. and Elisberg, B. L.**, Serological diagnosis of scrub typhus by indirect immunoflu-orescence, *Proc. Soc. Exp. Biol. Med.*, 112, 568, 1963.
56. **Card, W. L. and Walker, J. M.**, Scrub typhus vaccine. Field trial in southeast Asia, *Lancet*, 1, 481, 1947.
57. **Berge, T. O., Gauld, R. L., and Kitaoka, M.**, A field trial of a vaccine prepared from the Volner strain of *Rickettsia tsutsugamushi*, *Am. J. Hyg.*, 50, 337, 1949.

58. **Smadel, J. E., Traub, R., Frick, L. P., Diercks, F. H., and Bailey, C. A.,** Chloramphenicol (chloromycetin) in the chemoprophylaxis of scrub typhus (tsutsugamushi disease). III. Suppression of overt disease by prophylactic regimens of four-week duration, *Am. J. Hyg.,* 51, 216, 1950.
59. **Traub, R. and Wisseman, C. L., Jr.,** Ecological considerations in scrub typhus. III. Methods of area control, *Bull. W.H.O.,* 39, 231, 1968.
60. **Traub, R. and Dowling, M. A. C.,** The duration of efficacy of the insecticide dieldrin against the chigger vectors of scrub typhus in Malaya, *J. Econ. Entomol.,* 54, 654, 1961.

TYPHUS-GROUP RICKETTSIAE

R. N. Philip

Typhus-group rickettsiae are more closely related to rickettsiae of the spotted-fever group than those of other groups.[1] Nevertheless, the typhus and spotted-fever groups are genetically distinct as confirmed by slight but significant differences in DNA base composition.[2] Thus, molar percentages of guanine plus cytosine for the three species of rickettsiae in the typhus group are about 30, whereas they are about 32.5 for members of the spotted-fever group. Phenotypic differences are evident in antigenic composition and certain other biologic characteristics, e.g., growth in embryonated eggs.[1] Typhus- and spotted fever-group rickettsiae share antigens to some extent as indicated by occasional crossing of serologic responses that occurs in certain host species.[3] However, antigenic differences are more impressive than the similarities.

The three species of rickettsiae comprising the typhus group include: *Rickettsia prowazekii*, the etiologic agent of epidemic typhus; *R. typhi*, the cause of murine typhus; and *R. canada*, a rickettsia that has not yet been definitely incriminated as a cause of human disease. In many biologic respects, these rickettsiae are similar to each other, and most morphological and biochemical characteristics, as well as growth requirements described below for *R. typhi*, apply equally to other members of the group. They all share one or more antigens that are distinctive for the typhus group; but, in addition, they each possess one or more antigens that are unique to the species. Pathogenicity for experimental animals varies somewhat, and the ecologies of the three species are quite different.

For many years, it has been debated whether *R. typhi* and *R. prowazekii* are merely unstable phenotypic variations of the same organism conditioned by the circumstances under which they are naturally maintained, or whether they are genetically distinct. All experimental attempts to change the characteristics of *R. typhi* into those of *R. prowazekii*, or vice versa, have been unsuccessful. For example, *R. typhi* has been maintained by several investigators through as many as 89 passages in human body lice without biologic or antigenic change, and *R. prowazekii* has been passed several times in fleas without developing any characteristics of *R. typhi*.[4-6] Thus, it appears that biologic differences in the two organisms are stable genetic characteristics.

The reservoir of *R. prowazekii* infection is man. At present, epidemic typhus is not considered to be a true zoonosis. Therefore, this disease will not be discussed in detail. Remarks will be directed mainly to recent findings of epidemic typhus-like rickettsiae in flying squirrels, the epidemiologic significance of which remains to be defined. Discussion of *R. canada* will also be brief. There is little evidence that this organism is an important pathogen either for man or lower animals. Murine typhus is an important zoonosis and will, therefore, be described in detail.

MURINE TYPHUS

Disease

Murine typhus is an acute, febrile, exanthematic disease that occurs sporadically in warmer regions of the world and is seldom fatal. The causative agent is *R. typhi*, maintained in nature by a cycle that involves the commensal rat as the principal reservoir host and the oriental rat flea, *Xenopsylla cheopis*, as the major vector. Man becomes an incidental host when bitten by rat fleas and the wounds become contaminated with infected flea feces. Synonyms are endemic typhus, flea-borne typhus, and urban typhus.

Etiologic Agent

The morphologic and biochemical characteristics of *R. typhi* (*R. mooseri*) resemble those of other typhus- and spotted fever-group organisms. The rickettsiae are somewhat pleomorphic occurring usually as short rods measuring about 0.3 by 1.4 μm during the log phase of growth. They are Gram-negative and stain red by the Gimenez method.[7] Rickettsiae are readily cultivated in chick-embryo yolk sac and in a variety of avian, mammalian, and arthropod cell cultures, but they have not been grown in media free of living cells. They multiply by binary fission and grow profusely in the cytoplasm, but unlike spotted fever-group rickettsiae, they are not found in the nuclei of host cells.

The fine structure of typhus rickettsiae observed by electron microscopy includes an outer capsular layer easily lost during purification procedures, a five-layered cell wall, and a trilaminar cytoplasmic membrane surrounding protoplasm containing ribosome-like granules and DNA-like strands.[8-10]

Typhus rickettsiae contain both DNA and RNA. Cell walls resemble those of Gram-negative bacteria in chemical composition[11-13] and contain both muramic and diaminopimelic acid. They also contain polysaccharide, lipid, and protein complexes that exert biological properties similar to those of endotoxin from Gram-negative bacteria.[11,13]

Typhus rickettsiae have moderately active metabolic activity independent of the host cell. Energy is produced by oxidation of glutamate through a series of steps involving dicarboxylic acids of the Krebs cycle.[14,15] Incorporation of radiolabeled precursors has indicated some protein, lipid, and polyribonucleotide synthetic activity by rickettsiae, and various enzyme reactions have been demonstrated.[11,16]

Typhus rickettsiae are relatively unstable when separated from the host cell. This phenomenon is thought to be partially due to injury of the plasma membrane during purification procedures.[16] The organisms are inactivated by heating at 56°C for 30 min and are quite susceptible to chemical inactivation. Glutamate is an important substrate for maintaining extracellular viability of rickettsiae.[17] Divalent cations, potassium, sucrose, adenosine triphosphate and other nucleotides, and supplemental protein are also stabilizing agents.[16-18]

Rickettsiae actively penetrate host cells. This energy-requiring property is dependent upon metabolic integrity of the organisms and is enhanced by metabolic substrates such as glutamate in the suspending medium.[19] Nonviable as well as viable rickettsiae may be phagocytized by leukocytes.[20] Phagocytosis is enhanced by opsonins and cytophilic antibody.[20,21] In the absence of antibody, virulent typhus rickettsiae will multiply in human monocyte-derived macrophages and eventually destroy these phagocytes.[22] However, rickettsiae opsonized with antibody are localized in vacuoles in the cytoplasm of professional phagocytes and destroyed.[23] Cytophilic antibody facilitates phagocytosis but does not aid in destruction of the organisms.[24] Growth of rickettsiae in the cytoplasm of nonphagocytic cells is not dependent upon integrity of the cell nucleus.[25]

Although convalescent sera from typhus patients will solidly protect animals against virulent challenge with the homologous organism, antibodies are not directly rickettsicidal. Thus, antibody-bound typhus rickettsiae can penetrate the host cell and multiply unimpeded in cultures of chick-embryo fibroblasts.[26] Immunity appears to depend upon antibody and phagocytes acting in concert, as neither component is able to destroy rickettsiae independently of the other. These observations help to clarify the reasons for nonsterile immunity, relapses after early treatment, and recrudescences that are characteristic of typhus infections in man.

R. typhi possesses at least one antigen common to all rickettsiae in the typhus group and at least one that distinguishes this organism from all other members of the group.[27,28] The group antigen is loosely associated with surface structures and is released into the aqueous phase of the suspending medium by ether extraction of rickettsiae. The species-specific antigen(s) is firmly bound to the washed rickettsial cell.

Most immunogenic and serologic activities of *R. typhi* are associated with the cell wall. Cell walls from rickettsiae disrupted mechanically, or chemically with sodium deoxycholate, (1) protect guinea pigs against infectious challenge, (2) protect mice against toxic challenge, (3) evoke complement-fixing antibodies in guinea pigs, (4) manifest typhus-group complement-fixing and hemagglutination (human type O cells) reactivity, and (5) elicit delayed hypersensitivity in man after recovery from murine typhus.[12,29] Protoplasmic components of rickettsiae show none of these antigenic properties.[29] It is presumed that species-specific antigens are also located in the cell wall although this has not been directly demonstrated.

True and Alternate Hosts

During early investigations of typhus in Mexico, it was observed that some patients with mild disease were free of body lice (cited by Mooser).[30] Rickettsiae isolated from these persons produced scrotal reactions in guinea pigs that distinguished the organisms from European louse-borne typhus rickettsiae.[31] In a classical epidemiologic study of typhus endemic in the southeastern U.S., Maxcy[32] (1926) hypothesized that the causal agent was maintained in rats or mice and was transmitted to man by a parasitic arthropod. In 1931, Mooser et al.[33] isolated typhus rickettsiae from the brains of naturally infected rats in Mexico City, and Dyer et al.[34] recovered rickettsiae from fleas collected from rats in Baltimore. These were the first of many studies that established the primary importance of commensal rats and *X. cheopis* in the natural maintenance of *R. typhi*, thus confirming Maxcy's hypothesis.

Vertebrate Hosts

Wherever cases of murine typhus are frequent, commensal rats are also abundant, *R. typhi* can be isolated readily from rat tissues, and complement-fixing antibodies can be demonstrated in a high percentage of trapped rats. As exemplified in the U.S., successful rat-control campaigns are accompanied by a dramatic decrease in incidence of murine typhus.

Nevertheless, other small mammals may be incidental hosts of *R. typhi* and perhaps rarely even participate in the natural maintenance cycle. Vertebrates in the U.S. that have been shown to be naturally infected or susceptible to infection by *R. typhi* are listed in Table 1.

A sharp increase in the number of reported cases of murine typhus from 1930 to 1944 was accompanied by an apparent shift in disease pattern from urban to rural areas in the southeastern states.[44] There was concern that feral animals might be involved in the disease cycle. Consequently, serologic surveys of wildlife were conducted at various times in several southeastern states and California, and the susceptibility of various species to experimental infection by *R. typhi* was determined.[35-43] Antibodies were detected in 30 to 60% of rats trapped during the mid-1940s when typhus was still frequent.[45,46] Prevalence and titers of antibody were equally high in the two species of rats obtained from rural premises and urban centers, *Rattus rattus* and *R. norvegicus*. In contrast, typhus antibodies were infrequently detected among feral animals, and titers were usually low. Prevalence rates in feral species, represented by more than 100 animals, never exceeded 3%[36,45] *Mus musculus* often shares an ecologic niche with domestic rats, but its range is less restricted. Only mice obtained in or near dwellings in southeastern Texas were seropositive; those obtained farther afield were uniformly negative.[35] Antibody prevalence rates were much lower in domestic mice than in rats from the same urban environment.

Table 1
NATURALLY OCCURRING VERTEBRATES IN THE U.S. SHOWN TO BE INFECTED OR SUSCEPTIBLE TO INFECTION BY *RICKETTSIA TYPHI*

Vertebrate host			Natural infection		Experimental infection — isol.[a]	Ref.
Order	Family	Genus and species	Isol.[a]	Serol.[b]		
Rodentia	Muridae	*Rattus norvegicus* (brown rat)[c]	+	+	+	Numerous
		R. rattus (roof rat)[c]	+	+	+	Numerous
		Mus musculus (house mouse)	+	+	+	35—37
	Cricetidae	*Sigmodon hispidus* (cotton rat)		+	+	35, 36, 38—40
		Oryzomys palustris (rice rat)		+	+	36, 38, 40
		Neotoma floridana (wood rat)		+	+	35, 38, 40
		Peromyscus polionotus (old field mouse)	+	+	+	36, 38
		P. gossypinus (cotton mouse)		+	+	36, 38
		P. leucopus (white-footed mouse)			+	37
		Ochrotomys nuttalli (golden mouse)			+	38
		Microtus pennsylvanicus (meadow mouse)			+	37
	Sciuridae	*Sciurus niger* (fox squirrel)		+	+	36, 41
		S. carolinensis (gray squirrel)			+	40, 41
		Glaucomys volans (flying squirrel)			+	38
		Citellus beecheyi (ground squirrel)			+	42
		Tamias striatus (chipmunk)			+	41
		Marmota monax (woodchuck)			+	37
Lagomorpha	Leporidae	*Sylvilagus floridanus* (cottontail rabbit)		+	+	36,41
		S. aquaticus (swamp rabbit)			+	41
Marsupialia	Didelphidae	*Didelphis marsupialis* (opossum)	+	+	+	35, 36, 38, 40, 43
Carnivora	Mustelidae	*Mustela novaboracensis* (southern weasel)		+		36
		Mephitis mephitis (striped skunk)		+	+	36, 41, 43

Canidae	Canis familiaris (domestic dog)	+	+	36
Felidae	Felis domestica (domestic cat)		+	38

a Isolation of rickettsiae.
b Complement-fixing antibody titers ≥ 1:4.
c Primary hosts.

Results of surveys elsewhere have also emphasized the localization of infection to human habitation. Antibodies occurred more frequently in rats obtained from cities and towns than in those from rural areas of Kenya and Malaya.[47,48] Antibodies were seldom detected among feral animals including the many forms of field rats found in Malaya.

Despite the predominance of commensal rats in the natural maintenance of typhus, most small mammals from the U.S. that have been tested are experimentally susceptible to infection by *R. typhi* (Table 1). A vertebrate other than the rat appeared to be involved in the infection cycle in at least one instance. Recent cases of murine typhus in southern California occurred in foothill areas where rats and their ectoparasites are absent. The infection cycle in this instance was thought to involve opossums as the probable host.[43]

Vectors

The oriental rat flea, *X. cheopis*, is the most important vector of *R. typhi* in rat-to-rat as well as rat-to-human transmission. It is an abundant ectoparasite of commensal rats in warmer regions throughout the world. Wherever murine typhus is frequent, this flea is found. Typhus rickettsiae have been recovered repeatedly from *X. cheopis* in endemic areas, and studies of experimental infection of *X. cheopis* and transmission of *R. typhi* to susceptible guinea pigs and rats have indicated high vector efficiency.[49]

Rat ectoparasite surveys were conducted in the southeastern U.S. in the 1940s to determine the most important ectoparasites and their relation to transmission of typhus. Four species comprised 95% of the 270,000 ectoparasites collected between 1946 and 1949 from 20,000 rats in three southeastern Georgia counties.[50] They included (1) *X. cheopis*, (2) *Leptopsylla segnis*, mouse flea, (3) *Bdellonyssus bacoti*, tropical rat mite, and (4) *Polyplax spinulosa*, common rat louse. For typhus control, DDT dusting of rat harborages was done in two of the three counties early in the study. Incidence of typhus in man and prevalence of typhus antibodies among rats decreased dramatically in dusted counties during the next 2 years but dropped very little in the untreated county. Dusting strikingly reduced flea populations, but it had little or no effect on mite and louse infestation. Thus, control of fleas presumably eliminated the major element in disease transmission.

In Texas as well as Georgia, *X. cheopis* and, to a lesser extent, *L. segnis* were more often found on rats with typhus antibodies than on those without antibody.[50,51] Seropositive and seronegative rats were infested to a similar degree with *B. bacoti* and *P. spinulosa*.[50]

Seasonal abundance of *X. cheopis* on rats, particularly those obtained from rural premises, corresponded to seasonal occurrence of murine typhus and prevalence of typhus antibodies in rats.[51,52] These relationships were not evident for *L. segnis*, *B. bacoti*, or *P. spinulosa*.

Table 2 lists ectoparasites of rats found in the U.S. that have been shown to be naturally infected or susceptible to infection by *R. typhi* or have transmitted infection to experimental animals. Mooser et al.[61] showed that *P. spinulosa* could be infected by their feeding on infected rats. Rickettsiae multiplied within epithelial cells of the gut were shed in the feces and were transmitted from rat to rat by the louse. However, there is no epidemiologic information to substantiate experimental evidence that this abundant rat ectoparasite is an important vector of infection among rats. The rat louse is host-specific and does not bite man.

Dove and Shelmire[58] reported that *B. bacoti*, also a common ectoparasite of rats in the southeastern U.S., could be experimentally infected with *R. typhi* and transmit rickettsiae from guinea pig to guinea pig. This mite has also been shown to be naturally

Table 2
ECTOPARASITES OF MURINE HOSTS IN THE U.S. SHOWN TO BE NATURALLY INFECTED, EXPERIMENTALLY INFECTED, OR EXPERIMENTAL TRANSMITTERS OF *R. TYPHI*

Order	Genus and species	Natural infection	Experimental Infection	Experimental Transmission	Ref.
Siphonaptera	*Xenopsylla cheopis* (oriental rat flea)[a]	+	+	+	Numerous
	Nosopsyllus fasciatus (northern rat flea)	+	+	+	53, 54
	Leptopsylla segnis (mouse flea)	+	+		54—56
	Echidnophaga gallinacea (sticktight flea)	+	+	+	55—57
Acarina	*Bdellonyssus bacoti* (tropical rat mite)	+	+	+	58—60
Anoplura	*Polyplax spinulosa* (spiny rat louse)		+	+	61

[a] Primary vector.

infected and will readily feed on man. However, *B. bacoti* is at best an inefficient vector, and there is little evidence that it is important in the transmission of typhus either among rats or from rats to man.[56,59]

L. segnis is more commonly found on rats than mice but is less abundant than *X. cheopis*. *L. segnis* can be infected with *R. typhi*, but transmission of infection from rat to rat has not been demonstrated. This flea is most abundant during cooler weather in the spring and is not considered to be an important vector of *R. typhi* among rats. The mouse flea does not bite man.[54]

Nosopsyllus fasciatus is not abundant in the southeastern U.S., preferring more temperate climates; it seldom bites man.[54] *Echidnophaga gallinacea* is an abundant ectoparasite of domestic fowl but is not commonly found on rats. It has been shown to be an experimental vector of *R. typhi*, and it readily bites man.[54] However, neither *N. fasciatus* nor *E. gallinacea* are important in natural transmission of typhus.

Ctenocephalides felis, the common cat flea, is not ordinarily an ectoparasite of rats. However, cat fleas taken from seronegative kittens in Texas were found to be infected with *R. typhi*.[62] Typhus rickettsiae were also recovered from *C. felis* infesting a seropositive opossum that had been trapped in southern California on premises where a typhus case was present.[43]

Arthropods other than *X. cheopis* that are considered to be potential vectors of *R. typhi* outside of the U.S. are not listed here. However, several important observations should be mentioned. Gispen[63] isolated five strains of *R. typhi* from larval trombiculid mites, *Ascoschoengastia indica*, collected from commensal rats in Indonesia. Four of the five rats were seronegative. This mite is parasitic only during larval stages, therefore transovarial transmission of rickettsiae must be considered. *A. indica* does not bite man, but it may be an ancillary vector of *R. typhi* among rats in Indonesia.

Human body lice, *Pediculus humanus humanus*, have been experimentally infected with *R. typhi*.[4,5] Rickettsiae multiply to high titers in gut epithelium and eventually kill the louse. Rickettsiae excreted in feces may remain infectious for several weeks, particularly when temperature and humidity are low.[64] It is theorectically possible that murine typhus occurring in a lousy population may be transmitted from man to man by body lice. This mode of transmission has been reported, but methods used to identify the etiologic agents as *R. typhi* (as distinct from *R. prowazekii*) and difficulty in ruling out flea transmission leave this possibility unsettled.[65,66]

Distribution

Murine typhus has occurred throughout the world in the zone that ranges from about 40° N to 40° S latitudes. Sizeable populations of rats may be present in more temperate foci, but the bionomics of *X. cheopis* require (1) an average environmental midwinter temperature of at least 40°F and (2) an average relative humidity during midsummer of at least 40% in order to sustain flea populations large enough to maintain the disease cycle.[67]

In the Western Hemisphere, murine typhus has been reported from the U.S., Mexico, Central America, and the countries of northern South America. In the Eastern Hemisphere, murine typhus has occurred in central and southern Europe, most of Africa, the Near East, the U.S.S.R., India, China, Japan, the Philippines, Vietnam, Malaya, Indonesia, and Australia. Historically, cases have been most frequent in seaport cities where commensal rat populations are particularly high.

Occurrence of typhus in the U.S. by state and year from 1930 to 1975 is shown in Figures 1 and 2. Of 49,000 cases reported to the U.S. Public Health Service during this 46-year period, 94% occurred in eight southeastern states (Texas, Louisiana, Mississippi, Alabama, Georgia, Florida, and South and North Carolina). The number of cases reported annually increased from about 400 in 1930 to a peak of 5400 in 1944. Results of several surveys indicated that murine typhus was underreported during this 15-year period. After 1944, annual numbers decreased sharply from 5200 cases in 1945 to a low of 18 cases in 1972. The number of reported cases has shown a slight but definite increase in the last 4 years. In 1976, 50 cases were reported provisionally, the highest number recorded since 1967.

Decline in incidence of murine typhus after 1945 paralleled a decline in commensal rat and *X. cheopis* populations. Pertinent factors included better sanitation in endemic areas, rat-proofing of buildings, use of DDT to control rat fleas, pesticides to destroy rats, and a drought in the southeastern states during the early 1950s that reduced rat food supply in rural areas.[68,69] It has also been suggested that early use of broad-spectrum antibiotics has made diagnosis of disease more difficult.[68]

Disease in Animals

Enzootic *R. typhi* infection has little or no effect on rat populations. Widely used experimental animals include guinea pigs, white mice, and white and cotton rats. Established strains of *R. typhi* intraperitoneally inoculated into guinea pigs induced febrile illness after an incubation period of 3 to 7 days. The fever exceeds 40°C for several days and is usually accompanied by swelling and redness of the scrotum in male guinea pigs. *R. typhi* infections of guinea pigs are seldom fatal. Moderate doses of *R. typhi* also induce nonfatal febrile illness in white rats. Rickettsiae can be passed indefinitely from rat to rat by subinoculation of infected tissues, a characteristic that has also been used to differentiate *R. typhi* from *R. prowazekii*.[70] Epidemic typhus rickettsiae cannot be maintained in rats by serial passage.

Large doses of *R. typhi* and *R. prowazekii* are lethal for mice and rats within a few hours after intravenous inoculation.[71,72] This property of viable rickettsiae is ascribed to direct toxic action on endothelial cells of small blood vessels, resulting in permeability of the vascular bed, extravasation of fluid into extravascular tissues, hemoconcentration, and shock.[73,74] Subtoxic doses of *R. typhi* may induce lethal infection in mice 3 to 8 days after inoculation, while subtoxic doses of *R. prowazekii* have no clinical effect.

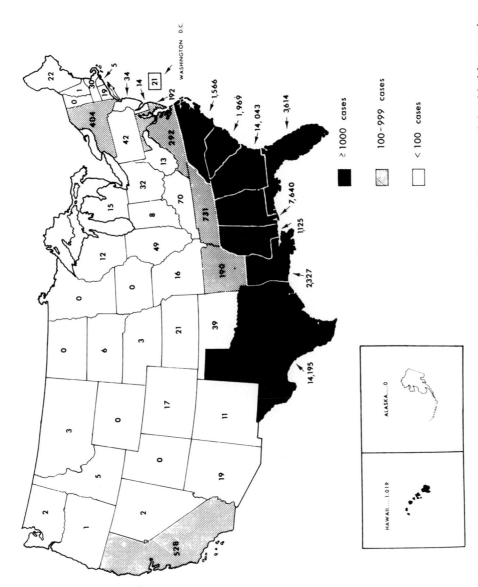

FIGURE 1.   Number of cases of typhus by state, 1930 to 1975. Brill-Zinsser disease was not distinguished from murine typhus.[110]

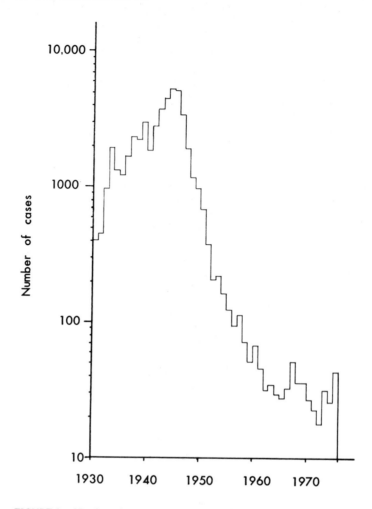

FIGURE 2.   Number of cases of typhus by year, 1930 to 1975. Brill-Zinsser disease was not distinguishable from murine typhus.[111]

Both *R. typhi* and *R. prowazekii* given in large doses cause fatal illness in cotton rats.[39] Cotton rats and guinea pigs are equally susceptible to infection by *R. typhi*.

Viable typhus rickettsiae hemolyze red blood cells of rabbits and sheep, but they have no effect on mouse, guinea pig, and cotton rat erythrocytes.[75] Likewise, large concentrations of rickettsiae will cause in vivo hemolysis and death of rabbits from hyperkaliemia within a few hours.[76] This phenomenon is thought to be another manifestation of the toxic effects of viable rickettsiae on host cells.

A characteristic of all rickettsiae is the ability to persist for long periods in the infected host. Murine typhus rickettsiae have often been recovered from tissues of naturally infected rats with high levels of circulating antibody. *R. typhi* has been shown to persist in blood of experimentally infected white rats for 31 days, in the spleen for 153 days, and in the brain for as long as 370 days.[77] *R. typhi* also has been recovered from the brains of white mice for as long as 150 days and from the brains of guinea pigs for as long as 120 days after infection.

R. typhi is nonlethal for adult *X. cheopis*. The rickettsiae multiply within epithelial cells of the stomach and cells of Malpighian tubules.[53] They are not found in the esophagus, salivary glands, or reproductive organs of infected fleas. The organisms are shed into the feces by way of the Malpighian tubules rather than the gut.

Disease in Man

Murine typhus is clinically indistinguishable from mild epidemic typhus.[78] The incubation period usually ranges from 8 to 12 days and averages 10 days. Onset of illness is sudden in about half of the cases and is characterized by chills, headache, and fever. Mild prodromal complaints may be present along with weakness or prostration, nausea and vomiting, and pains in the chest, back, limbs, and abdomen. A rash appears in about 60% of patients as early as the second day of illness or as late as the eighth day. Usually, it is present by the fifth day. The exanthem is often less pronounced than that seen in epidemic typhus. It usually appears first on the trunk and spreads peripherally to the extremities. The face, palms of the hands, and soles of the feet are seldom affected. The eruption is initially macular and fades on pressure. It may later become maculopapular but is almost never petechial or hemorrhagic. Duration of rash is variable, averaging about 6 days; it terminates during defervescence.

In untreated cases, fever usually reaches a maximum of about 104°F at the end of the first week and falls by lysis during the second week. Headache is often one of the most distressing symptoms, not easily relieved and sometimes persistent throughout the illness. Of all patients 50% have respiratory complaints. A hacking, nonproductive cough is often present, and severe cases may have clinical and roentgenographical evidence of bronchopneumonia. CNS manifestations such as stupor, delirium, coma, and nuchal rigidity may be present in severely ill patients. Signs of myocardial involvement occasionally occur in the elderly. The spleen is palpable in about one third of the patients, and the liver is sometimes enlarged.

Routine clinical laboratory tests are not particularly helpful for diagnosis of murine typhus.[78] A slight leukopenia is usually seen during the first week of disease, and there is often a mild leukocytosis during the second week. The differential white cell count is usually within normal limits, and red blood cell and hemoglobin values are not affected by disease. Abnormalities are seldom detected by urinalysis.

Before specific antibiotic treatment was available, duration of hospitalization from murine typhus averaged about 15 days. In the U.S. between 1930 and 1949, 4.9% of cases reported to the U.S. Public Health Service were fatal. After 1950, broad-spectrum antibiotics were generally used, and case fatality ratios dropped to less than 1%. Fatal illness is most likely to occur in elderly persons.

Histopathology in fatal cases of murine typhus is characterized by generalized proliferative endangiitis, usually involving arterioles, capillaries, and venules.[78] Lesions are ascribed to growth of rickettsiae in vascular endothelial cells. Swelling and proliferation of affected cells may occlude smaller vessels, and thrombosis may result from cellular damage to larger blood vessels. Accumulation of mononuclear cells forming perivascular nodules around smaller vessels is a characteristic feature of murine typhus. Lesions occur in all organs but are particularly noticeable in the brain and skin.

Circulating antibodies may appear as early as 7 days after onset of illness, but effective immunity is usually not evident before the end of the second week.[79] These time relationships are important when considering therapeutic regimens. As in other rickettsial diseases, tetracycline and chloramphenicol are primarily rickettsiastatic, holding the organism in check until the immune mechanism of the host can control infection. If specific therapy is initiated too early and discontinued too soon, relapses may occur 2 to 3 days after cessation of therapy. Once established, immunity is solid—second attacks of disease have not been reported.

Tetracycline given in divided doses of 25 to 50 mg/kg of body weight per day will eliminate the fever within several days. Chloramphenicol given in doses of 3.0 g/day will be similarly effective. However, both antibiotics should be administered until the 14th day after onset even though the patient becomes afebrile much earlier.[79] Doxycycline, a new compound synthetically derived from oxytetracycline, is better absorbed and has longer rickettsistatic activity than other tetracyclines. This antibiotic has had a limited but successful trial in treatment of epidemic typhus.[80] A single dose of 200 mg of doxycycline was as effective as chloramphenicol given in doses of 800 mg four times daily for 15 days. Only 1 of 26 patients relapsed on the single-dose regimen. Doxycycline should also be effective in the treatment of murine typhus.

General Mode of Spread

Murine typhus usually occurs when infected flea feces contaminate the bite wound of *X. cheopis*.[49] Vector fleas will feed intermittently, defecating during blood meals. Rickettsiae are introduced through abraded skin by rubbing or scratching. They are not present in salivary secretions, nor are they regurgitated during feeding.[53,81]

Other modes of spread are less important. Infection occasionally occurs by way of the conjunctivae or respiratory tract. Rickettsiae may be introduced into conjunctival cells by rubbing the eyes with contaminated fingers. Aerosol transmission has occurred in the laboratory and is believed to occur when susceptible hosts are exposed to dust that is heavily contaminated with infected flea feces.[82] In several Australian outbreaks, many patients (some of whom were allergic to fleas) could give no history of flea bite, but they were exposed to aerosols of dust in mouse-and-rat-infested premises. Spread of infection from rat to rat by cannibalism has been demonstrated experimentally.[83] However, excretions from infected rats were not found to be infectious, and attempts to infect rats by feeding on infectious flea feces were unsuccessful.[83,84]

Epidemiology

Intensity of the cycle of *R. typhi* infection in a particular focus is ultimately determined by the presence of rickettsiae, size of the rat population, and degree of flea infestation. The infection cycle is a dynamic process influenced by many complex interacting ecologic and biologic factors. All have to do with the bionomics of the rat host and flea vector as well as the biologic characteristics of the rickettsial agent.

Commensal rats are colonial.[50] They become established in or close to human habitation where environmental temperature is favorable and harborage and food supply are ample. Unless there are intolerable population pressures, individual rats seldom migrate from their home range that is usually 500 yards or less. Life span is about 1 year, and the replacement pool in a particular rat colony comes principally from reproduction rather than immigration. Breeding occurs throughout the year with peaks in the spring and fall. In order to function as a reservoir of infection, a rat population must provide a continual source of rickettsiae for the flea vector. This means that there must also be a continuous and ample supply of susceptible rats. There is little experimental information about the level and duration of rickettsemia in infected rats. Failure of antibody to prevent penetration and replication of *R. typhi* in nonphagocytic host cells suggests that superinfection of commensal rats might occur, similar to that demonstrated for *R. tsutsugamushi* in wild *Rattus*.[26,85]

The size of the vector flea population is dependent upon the number of rats available as a source of blood meals as well as environmental conditions favorable for a vigorous reproduction cycle. Intensity of transmission is dependent upon (1) the number of rats with rickettsemia, (2) the number of rats susceptible to infection, (3) the opportunity for interchange of ectoparasites, and (4) the vector efficiency of the rat flea.   There is no information on the level of rickettsemia necessary to infect *X. cheopis*, but once introduced, rickettsiae multiply to many thousand times the dose ingested.[81] Infected fleas begin to shed rickettsiae after several days and remain infectious for at least 52 days and probably throughout the life of the flea. Temperature and humidity influence the length of the life cycle that may be completed in as few as 4 to 8 weeks.[54] In heated buildings, reproduction may be continuous throughout the year. In rural habitats, adult fleas are most abundant during warmer seasons. Transovarial transmission of rickettsiae does not occur.[81] *R. typhi* may remain viable in infected flea feces for at least 3 days when environmental temperature and humidity are high.[86]

X. cheopis normally prefers rats, but in their absence, this flea will feed readily on man. Murine typhus is a sporadic disease. Clustering of cases is infrequent, and person-to-person spread of rickettsiae does not occur. The disease is present all year in tropical and subtropical regions. In more temperate climates, such as that of the southern U.S., cases are most frequent during late summer and early fall.[32] Murine typhus occurs particularly among persons who are occupationally or otherwise exposed to rats. Thus, morbidity is greater among adults than children, males than females, and those engaged in the food industry than those not so employed. Races are equally susceptible to infection, but disease in the U.S. is less often diagnosed among Blacks than Whites.[87,32] Likewise, all age groups are susceptible, but disease is more severe in elderly than in younger persons.[78]

Diagnosis

Specific diagnosis of murine typhus is based upon isolation of rickettsiae during acute stages of illness or by demonstration of an antibody response to *R. typhi* during convalescence.[88] Isolation of rickettsiae is a specialized procedure that should be attempted only where facilities for containment of infection are adequate.

Rickettsemia occurs during febrile stages of illness. When clotted blood is inoculated intraperitoneally into male guinea pigs, microscopic examination of Gimenez-stained impression smears of the spleen or tunica obtained at the peak of the scrotal reaction reveals numerous intracellular rickettsiae. Isolates are established by subinoculation of blood, brain, or infected tunica into additional guinea pigs or into the yolk sacs of embryonated chicken eggs. Serum from convalescent animals is tested for complement-fixing antibodies 3 to 4 weeks after inoculation of infectious material.

The procedures used most frequently in serologic diagnosis of murine typhus are the Weil-Felix and complement-fixation (CF) tests. Typhus- and many spotted fever-group rickettsiae share an antigen with some strains of *Proteus vulgaris* in O phase. At the end of the first week of illness, agglutinins to Proteus-OX19 and, less frequently, antibodies to Proteus-OX2 begin to increase in patients with typhus. Maximum titers are attained in 3 weeks, and antibodies decline to low levels several months later. Since many persons without rickettsial disease have low levels of agglutinins, the Weil-Felix test is not considered to be positive unless a fourfold increase in titer is demonstrated or a titer of at least 1:160 is attained. Murine typhus cannot be distinguished from epidemic typhus or Rocky Mountain spotted fever on the basis of the Weil-Felix test. Since Weil-Felix antibodies are of the IgM class, a serologic response may not occur in patients who have had previous contact, either by vaccination or illness, with antigens related to the infecting strain.[89] The Weil-Felix test is of little value in serologic surveys of rats.

The CF test became the most widely used serologic procedure following the discovery that typhus rickettsiae could be cultivated in large quantities in the yolk sacs of chicken embryos.[90] CF antibody to typhus appears at the end of the second week of illness, reaches a peak in the third or fourth week, and usually persists in substantial titer for several years.[88] Extraction of aqueous rickettsial suspensions with ethyl ether removes much of the group-reacting antigen, leaving rickettsial cells containing the type-specific component in the aqueous phase.[27,28] Washed antigens can be used to distinguish murine from epidemic typhus on the basis of serologic response except among persons who have had prior contact with the heterologous rickettsia either from vaccination or from infection.[91]

Diagnosis of typhus is based on a fourfold antibody response. Titers equal to or greater than 1:8 are generally considered to be significant. Early CF antibody has a higher antigen requirement than late antibody.[92] Therefore, it is recommended that four times the usual amount of antigen be used in tests of early convalescent sera. Early treatment with specific antibiotics may prevent or delay significant CF antibody responses.[93] The CF test has also proven to be useful and simpler than isolation of rickettsiae in determining prevalence of *R. typhi* infection in surveys of rats.

Other procedures have been used less extensively. An erythrocyte-sensitizing substance obtained by extraction of rickettsiae with sodium hydroxide and adsorbed to sheep or human type O red blood cells has been used to measure hemagglutinating antibody response to infection.[94] The test is sensitive and appears to be specific, but it will not distinguish between murine and epidemic typhus.[94,95]

Rickettsial agglutination techniques have been available for many years, but the requirement for large amounts of antigen has limited their use. A recently developed microagglutination test that requires small amounts of highly purified rickettsial antigen was shown to have advantages over the CF test.[96] Agglutinins appear earlier, and the test is more sensitive in distinguishing between murine and epidemic typhus infections.

Indirect immunofluorescence has also been used in the diagnosis of rickettsial infections.[95,97-100] Indirect immunofluorescence tests are particularly sensitive if suitable conjugates prepared against both IgM and IgG immunoglobulins are used. Using conjugates prepared against a specific immunoglobulin class, immunofluorescence is also helpful in distinguishing primary infection that induces both IgM and IgG antibody responses from recrudescent disease that stimulates only an IgG response.[100]

Neutralizing antibodies appearing during convalescence from typhus will protect white mice against the lethal toxic effects of homologous rickettsiae.[71] The toxin neutralization and protection tests have been used in research laboratories to differentiate *R. typhi* from *R. prowazekii* infections and to evaluate immunogenicity of vaccines.

Prevention and Control

Few diseases in medical annals have yielded as spectacularly to concerted control efforts as murine typhus in the U.S.[45,50,68] Control was directed at the flea vector and the rat host.

Between 1945 and 1968, 10% DDT dust was used to control rat fleas. This insecticide is still effective, but other insecticides are now recommended for controlling *X. cheopis* because of present restrictions on the use of chlorinated hydrocarbon insecticides and the development of DDT resistance in several areas of the world.[54]

Murine typhus control programs should start at the suspected focus of infection and work outward; the following sequence of operations has been effective.[54] The reader is referred to the Center for Disease Control publications 75-8267 and 76-8141 for details.[54,101]

1. Rat and flea surveys to determine the extent and intensity of the problem
2. Application of residual insecticides such as malathion, diazinon, or carbaryl to kill infected fleas
3. Use of anticoagulant rodenticides such as warfarin, Pival®, or Fumarin® against rats
4. Rat trapping and poisoning with "one-dose" rodenticides such as red squill or zinc phosphide, or burrow gassing
5. Improved general sanitation to keep rodent populations at the lowest possible level, with particular attention to refuse storage, collection, and disposal, and harborage elimination

6. Rodent stoppage or rat proofing
7. Continued surveys and maintenance to prevent build-up of disease potentials

Repellents such as dimethylphthalate, benzyl benzoate, and diethyltoluamide should be applied to ankles and clothing to prevent flea attack during control activities. Experimental, inactivated *R. typhi* vaccines were developed, but because of slight demand, they are no longer available.

EPIDEMIC TYPHUS

R. prowazekii is transmitted from person to person by the human body louse, *Pediculus humanus humanus*. Man is the true reservoir of infection, and the louse is the vector. *R. prowazekii* is similar to *R. typhi* in morphology, biochemical composition, metabolic requirements, and interaction with host cells. *R. prowazekii* persists in the host, sometimes giving rise to recrudescent typhus (Brill-Zinsser disease) years after primary infection. Epidemic typhus resembles murine typhus clinically but is usually more severe. Case fatality rates were as high as 20% before broad-spectrum antibiotics were available. Historically, the disease occurred in large epidemics under conditions favorable for louse infestation. Lice became infected while feeding on rickettsemic typhus patients. Rickettsiae multiply in epithelial cells lining the gut of the louse and are shed into the feces. Susceptible individuals are infected by fecal contamination of bite wounds. Procedures for serologic diagnosis and treatment of epidemic typhus are similar to those used for murine typhus. Control measures are directed toward elimination of the louse vector.

The possibility that animals other than man might be natural hosts of *R. prowazekii* has been considered. Reports that ticks and livestock were involved in the infection cycle of epidemic typhus in Ethiopia and Egypt have not been substantiated by further investigation.[102-105] Until recently, there was no conclusive evidence that *R. prowazekii* could be naturally maintained in any host other than man.

Therefore, it was of great interest when rickettsiae indistinguishable from *R. prowazekii* by all immunologic and other biologic methods used to date were isolated from eastern flying squirrels, *Glaucomys volans volans*, trapped in Virginia and Florida.[106] Ten strains from flying squirrels, two from fleas (*Orchopeas howardi*), and one from lice (*Neohaematopinus scuiropteri*) removed from flying squirrels have been recovered.[107] Infection is epizootic in the fall and winter when squirrels aggregate in their tree shelters and is coincident to increased ectoparasite infestation. Evidence obtained thus far indicates that the infection cycle involves only flying squirrels and their ectoparasites.

RICKETTSIA CANADA INFECTION

A rickettsia belonging to the typhus group was isolated from rabbit ticks, *Haemaphysalis leporispalustris*, taken from sentinel rabbits in Ontario in 1963.[108] The organism cross-reacted with *R. typhi* and *R. prowazekii* but not with spotted fever-group rickettsiae in CF tests of guinea pig antisera. However, the rickettsia (strain 2678) was clearly different from other typhus group rickettsiae in CF tests of mouse antisera and in toxin neutralization tests. It was considered to be a distinct species and is designated as *R. canada*.

Additional strains of *R. canada* have not been isolated; however, some serologic evidence indicates that *R. canada* may occasionally be the cause of human infection in the U.S.[109] *R. canada* induces febrile illness but no scrotal reactions in guinea pigs.[108] It grows readily in chick-embryo yolk sac, and high concentrations of rickettsiae are toxic for mice. Subtoxic doses do not cause illness in either suckling or adult mice.

REFERENCES

1. **Moulder, J. W.**, The rickettsias, in *Bergey's Manual of Determinative Bacteriology,* 8th ed., Buchanan, R. E. and Gibbons, N. E., Eds., Williams & Wilkins, Baltimore, 1974, 882.
2. **Tyeryar, F. J., Jr., Weiss, E., Millar, D. B., Bozeman, F. M., and Ormsbee, R. A.**, DNA base composition of rickettsiae, *Science,* 180, 415, 1973.
3. **Ormsbee, R. A. and Peacock, M. G.**, Antigenic structure of rickettsiae of the typhus and spotted fever groups, *Folia Microbiol.* (Prague), 21 (abstr.) 502, 1976.
4. **Balaeva, N. M.**, Study of the properties of *Rickettsia mooseri* cultivated in clothes lice (preliminary communication), *J. Microbiol. Epidemiol. Immunobiol.* (U.S.S.R.), 28, 823, 1957.
5. **Price, W. H., Emerson, H., Nagel, H., Blumberg, R., and Talmadge, S.**, Ecological studies on the interepidemic survival of louse-borne epidemic typhus fever, *Am. J. Hyg.,* 67, 154, 1958.
6. **Dyer, R. E.**, Effect of flea passage on epidemic typhus virus, *Public Health Rep.,* 49, 224, 1934.
7. **Gimenez, D. F.**, Staining rickettsiae in yolk-sac cultures, *Stain Technol.,* 39, 135, 1964.
8. **Wissig, S. L., Caro, L. G., Jackson, E. B., and Smadel, J. E.**, Electron microscopic observations on intracellular rickettsiae, *Am. J. Pathol.,* 32, 1117, 1956.
9. **Anderson, D. R., Hopps, H. E., Barile, M. F., and Bernheim, B. C.**, Comparison of the ultrastructure of several rickettsiae, ornithosis virus, and *Mycoplasma* in tissue culture, *J. Bacteriol.,* 90, 1387, 1965.
10. **Anacker, R. L., Pickens, E. G., and Lackman, D. B.**, Details of the ultrastructure of *Rickettsia prowazekii* grown in the chick yolk sac, *J. Bacteriol.,* 94, 260, 1967.
11. **Wisseman, C. L., Jr.**, Some biological properties of rickettsiae pathogenic for man, *Zentralbl. Bakteriol. Parasitenkd. Infektionskr. Hyg. Orig., Abt. 1:* 206, 299, 1968.
12. **Schaechter, M., Tousimis, A. J., Cohn, Z. A., Rosen, H., Campbell, J., and Hahn, F. E.**, Morphological, chemical, and serological studies of the cell walls of *Rickettsia mooseri, J. Bacteriol.,* 74, 822, 1957.
13. **Wood, W. H., Jr. and Wisseman, C. L., Jr.**, The cell wall of *Rickettsia mooseri.* I. Morphology and chemical composition, *J. Bacteriol.,* 93, 1113, 1967.
14. **Bovarnick, M. R. and Miller, J. C.**, Oxidation and transamination of glutamate by typhus rickettsiae, *J. Biol. Chem.,* 184, 661, 1950.
15. **Wisseman, C. L., Jr., Hahn, F. E., Jackson, E. B., Bozeman, F. M., and Smadel, J. E.**, Metabolic studies of rickettsiae. II. Studies on the pathway of glutamate oxidation by purified suspensions of *Rickettsia mooseri, J. Immunol.,* 68, 251, 1952.
16. **Weiss, E.**, Growth and physiology of rickettsiae, *Bacteriol. Rev.,* 37, 259, 1973.
17. **Bovarnick, M. R., Miller, J. C., and Snyder, J. C.**, The influence of certain salts, amino acids, sugars, and proteins on the stability of rickettsiae, *J. Bacteriol.,* 59, 509, 1950.
18. **Bovarnick, M. R. and Schneider, L.**, The incorporation of glycine-1-C^{14} by typhus rickettsiae, *J. Biol. Chem.,* 235, 1727, 1960.
19. **Cohn, Z. A., Bozeman, F. M., Campbell, J. M., Humphries, J. W., and Sawyer, T. K.**, Study on growth of rickettsiae. V. Penetration of *Rickettsia tsutsugamushi* into mammalian cells in vitro, *J. Exp. Med.,* 109, 271, 1959.
20. **Wisseman, C. L., Jr., Glazier, J., and Grieves, M. J.**, Interaction of rickettsiae and phagocytic host cells. I. *In vitro* studies of phagocytosis and opsonization of typhus rickettsiae, *Arch. Inst. Pasteur Tunis,* 36, 339, 1959.
21. **Beaman, L. and Wisseman, C. L., Jr.**, Mechanisms of immunity in typhus infections. V. Demonstration of *Rickettsia mooseri* — specific antibodies in convalescent mouse and human serum cytophilic for mouse peritoneal macrophages, *Infect. Immun.,* 14, 1065, 1976.
22. **Gambrill, M. R. and Wisseman, C. L., Jr.**, Mechanisms of immunity in typhus infections. II. Multiplication of typhus rickettsiae in human macrophage cell cultures in the nonimmune system: influence of virulence of rickettsial strains and chloramphenicol, *Infect. Immun.,* 8, 519, 1973.
23. **Gambrill, M. R. and Wisseman, C. L., Jr.**, Mechanisms of immunity in typhus infections. III. Influence of human immune serum and complement on the fate of *Rickettsia mooseri* within human macrophages, *Infect. Immun.,* 8, 631, 1973.
24. **Beaman, L. and Wisseman, C. L., Jr.**, Mechanisms of immunity in typhus infections. VI. Differential opsonizing and neutralizing action of human typhus rickettsia-specific cytophilic antibodies in cultures of human macrophages, *Infect. Immun.,* 14, 1071, 1976.
25. **Stork, E. and Wisseman, C. L., Jr.**, Growth of *Rickettsia prowazekii* in enucleated cells, *Infect. Immun.,* 13, 1743, 1976.
26. **Wisseman, C. L., Jr., Waddell, A. D., and Walsh, W. T.**, Mechanisms of immunity in typhus infections. IV. Failure of chicken embryo cells in culture to restrict growth of antibody-sensitized *Rickettsia prowazekii, Infect. Immun.,* 9, 571, 1974.

27. Plotz, H., Bennett, B. L., Wertman, K., Snyder, M. J., and Gauld, R. L., The serological pattern in typhus fever. I. Epidemic, *Am. J. Hyg.*, 47, 150, 1948.
28. Scoville, A. B., Jr., Bennett, B. J., Wertman, K. J., and Gauld, R. L., The serological pattern in typhus fever. II. Murine, *Am. J. Hyg.*, 47, 166, 1948.
29. Wood, W. H., Jr. and Wisseman, C. L., Jr., Studies of *Rickettsia mooseri* cell walls. II. Immunologic properties, *J. Immunol.*, 98, 1224, 1967.
30. Mooser, H., Twenty years of research in typhus fever, *Schweiz. Med. Wochenschr.*, 76, 877, 1946.
31. Neill, M. H., Experimental typhus fever in guinea pigs. A description of a scrotal lesion in guinea pigs infected with Mexican typhus, *Public Health Rep.*, 32, 1105, 1917.
32. Maxcy, K. F., An epidemiological study of endemic typhus (Brill's disease) in the southeastern United States, *Public Health Rep.*, 41, 2967, 1926.
33. Mooser, H., Castaneda, M. R., and Zinsser, H., Rats as carriers of Mexican typhus fever, *JAMA*, 97, 231, 1931.
34. Dyer, R. E., Rumreich, A., and Badger, L. F., A virus of the typhus type derived from fleas collected from wild rats, *Public Health Rep.*, 46, 334, 1931.
35. Keaton, R., Nash, B. J., Murphy, S. N., and Irons, J. V., Complement fixation tests for murine typhus on small mammals, *Public Health Rep.*, 68, 28, 1953.
36. Morlan, H. B., Hill, E. L., and Schubert, J. H., Serological survey for murine typhus infection in southwest Georgia animals, *Public Health Rep.*, 65, 57, 1950.
37. Dyer, R. E., Endemic typhus fever. Susceptibility of woodchucks, house mice, meadow mice, and white-footed mice, *Public Health Rep.*, 49, 723, 1934.
38. Brigham, G. D. and Dyer, R. E., Endemic typhus fever in native rodents, *JAMA*, 110, 180, 1938.
39. Anderson, C. R., Experimental typhus infection in the eastern cotton rat (*Sigmodon hispidus hispidus*), *J. Exp. Med.*, 80, 341, 1944.
40. Rickard, E. R., Postinfection murine typhus antibodies in the sera of rodents, *Am. J. Hyg.*, 53, 207, 1951.
41. Brigham, G. D., Susceptibility of animals to endemic typhus virus, *Public Health Rep.*, 53, 2078, 1938.
42. Beck, M. D. and Allen, A. V., Typhus fever in California, 1916-1945, inclusive. An epidemiologic and field laboratory study, *Am. J. Hyg.*, 45, 335, 1947.
43. Adams, W. H., Emmons, R. W., and Brooks, J. E., The changing ecology of murine (endemic) typhus in southern California, *Am. J. Trop. Med. Hyg.*, 19, 311, 1970.
44. Meleney, H. E., Recent extension of endemic typhus fever in the southern United States, *Am. J. Public Health*, 31, 219, 1941.
45. Love, G. J. and Smith, W. W., Murine typhus investigations in southwestern Georgia, *Public Health Rep.*, 75, 429, 1960.
46. Davis, D. E., Observations on rats and typhus fever in San Antonio, Tex., *Public Health Rep.*, 63, 783, 1948.
47. Heisch, R. B., Grainger, W. E., and Harvey, A.E.C., Feral aspects of rickettsial infections in Kenya, *Trans. R. Soc. Trop. Med. Hyg.*, 56, 272, 1962.
48. Marchette, N. J., Rickettsioses (tick typhus, Q-fever, urban typhus) in Malaya, *J. Med. Entomol.*, 2, 339, 1966.
49. Dyer, R. E., Ceder, E. T., Lillie, R . D., Rumreich, A., and Badger, L. F., Typhus fever. The experimental transmission of endemic typhus fever of the United States by the rat flea *Xenopsylla cheopis*, *Public Health Rep.*, 46, 2481, 1931.
50. Morlan, H. B., Utterback, B. C., Dent, J. E., Wilcomb, M. J., Jr., Griffith, M. E., and Ellis, L. L., Domestic Rats, Rat Ectoparasites and Typhus Control, Public Health Monograph No. 5, Public Health Service Publication No. 209, U.S. Department of Health, Education, and Welfare, Washington, D.C., 1952.
51. Davis, D. E., Observations on rat ectoparasites and typhus fever in San Antonio, Texas, *Public Health Rep.*, 66, 1717, 1951.
52. Smith, W. W., Populations of the most abundant ectoparasites as related to prevalence of typhus antibodies of farm rats in an endemic murine typhus region, *Am. J. Trop. Med. Hyg.*, 6, 581, 1957.
53. Mooser, H. and Castaneda, M. R., The multiplication of the virus of Mexican typhus fever in fleas, *J. Exp. Med.*, 55, 307, 1932.
54. Pratt, H. D. and Stark, H. E., Fleas of Public Health Importance and Their Control, Publication No. 75-8267, U.S. Department of Health, Education, and Welfare, Public Health Service, Center for Disease Control, 1975.
55. Brigham, G. D., Two strains of endemic typhus fever virus isolated from naturally infected chicken fleas (*Echidnophaga gallinacea*), *Public Health Rep.*, 56, 1803, 1941.
56. Standtmann, R. W. and Eben, D. J., A survey of typhus in rats and rat ectoparasites in Galveston, Texas, *Tex. Rep. Biol. Med.*, 11, 144, 1953.

57. **Alicata, J. E.,** Experimental transmission of endemic typhus fever by the sticktight flea, *Echidnophaga gallinacea,* *J. Wash. Acad. Sci.,* 32, 57, 1942.

58. **Dove, W. E. and Shelmire, B.,** Some observations on tropical rat mites and endemic typhus, *J. Parasitol.,* 18, 159, 1932.

59. **Worth, C. B. and Rickard, E. R.,** Evaluation of the efficiency of cotton rat ectoparasites in the transmission of murine typhus, *Am. J. Trop. Med.,* 31, 295, 1951.

60. **Pang, K. H.,** Isolation of typhus rickettsiae from rat mites during epidemic in an orphanage, *Proc. Soc. Exp. Biol. Med.,* 48, 266, 1944.

61. **Mooser, H., Castaneda, M. R., and Zinsser, H.,** The transmission of the virus of Mexican typhus from rat to rat by *Polyplax spinulosus,* *J. Exp. Med.,* 54, 567, 1931.

62. **Irons, J. V., Bohls, S. W., Thurman, D. C., Jr., and McGregor, T.,** Probable role of the cat flea, *Ctenocephalides felis,* in transmission of murine typhus, *Am. J. Trop. Med.,* 24, 359, 1944.

63. **Gispen, R.,** The virus of murine typhus in mites (*Schongastia indica,* fam. Trombiculidae), *Doc. Neer. Indones. Morbis Trop.,* 2, 225, 1950.

64. **Weyer, F.,** Zur Frage der Widerstandsfahigkeit von Rickettsien im Lausekot gegen physikalische Einflusse, insbesondere gegen Warme, *Z. Tropenmed. Parasitol.,* 12, 78, 1961.

65. **Liu, W. T.,** Studies on the murine origin of typhus epidemics in North China. III. Isolation of murine typhus rickettsia from rats, rat-fleas, and body lice of patients during an epidemic in a poorhouse, *Chin. Med. J.,* 62, 119, 1944.

66. **Kalra, S. L. and Rao, K. N. A.,** Typhus fevers in Kashmir State. II. Murine typhus, *Indian J. Med. Res.,* 39, 297, 1951.

67. **Mohr, C. O.,** Entomological background of the distribution of murine typhus and murine plague in the United States, *Am. J. Trop. Med.,* 31, 355, 1951.

68. **Pratt, H. D.,** The changing picture of murine typhus in the United States, *Ann. N.Y. Acad. Sci.,* 70, 516, 1958.

69. **Ecke, D. H.,** Factors influencing the decline in commensal rat infestations in a rural area of southwestern Georgia, *J. Mammal.,* 38, 270, 1957.

70. **Murray, E. S. and Snyder, J. C.,** Brill's disease. II. Etiology, *Am. J. Hyg.,* 53, 22, 1951.

71. **Hamilton, H. L.,** Specificity of the toxic factors associated with the epidemic and the murine strains of typhus rickettsiae, *Am. J. Trop. Med.,* 25, 391, 1945.

72. **Neva, F. A. and Snyder, J. C.,** Studies on the toxicity of typhus rickettsiae. I. Susceptibility of the white rat, with a note on pathological changes, *J. Infect. Dis.,* 91, 72, 1952.

73. **Neva, F. A. and Snyder, J. C.,** Studies on the toxicity of typhus rickettsiae. III. Observations on the mechanism of toxic death in white mice and white rats, *J. Infect. Dis.,* 97, 73, 1955.

74. **Wattenberg, L. W., Elisberg, B. L., Wisseman, C. L., Jr., and Smadel, J. E.,** Studies of rickettsial toxins. II. Altered vascular physiology in rickettsial toxemia of mice. *J. Immunol.,* 74, 147, 1955.

75. **Clarke, D. H. and Fox, J. P.,** The phenomenon of *in vitro* hemolysis produced by the rickettsiae of typhus fever, with a note on the mechanism of rickettsial toxicity in mice, *J. Exp. Med.,* 88, 25, 1948.

76. **Paterson, P. Y., Wisseman, C. L., Jr., and Smadel, J. E.,** Studies of rickettsial toxins. I. Role of hemolysis in fatal toxemia of rabbits and rats, *J. Immunol.,* 72, 12, 1954.

77. **Philip, C. B.,** The persistence of the viruses of endemic (murine) typhus, Rocky Mountain spotted fever, and boutonneuse fever in tissues of experimental animals, *Public Health Rep.,* 53, 1246, 1938.

78. **Stuart, B. M. and Pullen, R. L.,** Endemic (murine) typhus fever: clinical observations of 180 cases, *Am. Intern. Med.,* 23, 520, 1945.

79. **Wisseman, C. L., Jr., Wood, W. H., Jr., Noriega, A. R., Jordan, M. E., and Rill, D. J.,** Antibodies and clinical relapse of murine typhus fever following early chemotherapy, *Ann. Intern. Med.,* 57, 743, 1962.

80. **Huys, J., Freyens, P., Kayihigi, J., and Van den Berghe, G.,** Treatment of epidemic typhus. A comparative study of chloramphenicol, trimethoprim-sulphamethoxazole and doxycycline, *Trans. R. Soc. Trop. Med. Hyg.,* 67, 718, 1973.

81. **Dyer, R. E., Workman, W. G., and Ceder, E. T.,** Typhus fever. The multiplication of the virus of endemic typhus in the rat flea *Xenopsylla cheopis,* *Public Health Rep.,* 47, 987, 1932.

82. **Derrick, E. H. and Pope, J. H.,** Murine typhus, mice, rats and fleas on the Darling Downs, *Med. J. Aust.,* 2, 924, 1960.

83. **Worth, C. B. and Rickard, E. R.,** Transmission of murine typhus in roof rats in the absence of ectoparasites, *Am. J. Trop. Med.,* 31, 301, 1951.

84. **Rickard, E. R.,** Attempted transmission of murine typhus to roof rats by the ingestion of food heavily contaminated with infected flea feces, *Am. J. Trop. Med.,* 31, 311, 1951.

85. **Kuwata, T.,** Analysis of immunity in experimental tsutsugamushi disease, *J. Immunol.,* 68, 115, 1952.

86. Rickard, E. R., The survival of the rickettsias of murine typhus in infected flea feces, Am. J. Trop. Med., 31, 306, 1951.

87. Davis, D. E., Prevalence of typhus complement-fixing antibodies in human serums in San Antonio, Tex., Public Health Rep., 61, 928, 1946.

88. Elisberg, B. L. and Bozeman, F. M., Rickettsiae, in Diagnostic Procedures for Viral and Rickettsial Infections, 4th ed., Lennette, E. H. and Schmidt, N. J., Eds., American Public Health Association, New York, 1969, 826.

89. Elisberg, B. L., Wood, W. H., Jr., and Bellanti, J. A., Serological properties of immune globulins in human murine typhus, Fed. Proc. Fed. Am. Soc. Exp. Biol., 29, 420, 1967.

90. Cox, H. R., Use of yolk sac of developing chick embryo as medium for growing rickettsiae of Rocky Mountain spotted fever and typhus groups, Public Health Rep., 53, 2241, 1938.

91. Plotz, H. and Wertman, K., Modification of serological response to infection with murine typhus by previous immunization with epidemic typhus vaccine, Proc. Soc. Exp. Biol. Med., 59, 248, 1945.

92. Hersey, D. F., Colvin, M. C., and Shepard, C. C., Studies on the serologic diagnosis of murine typhus and Rocky Mountain spotted fever. II. Human infections, J. Immunol., 79, 409, 1957.

93. Stewart, W. H. and Hines, V. D., Murine typhus in southwest Georgia, January 1945-January 1953, Am. J. Trop. Med. Hyg., 3, 883, 1954.

94. Chang, S. M., Snyder, J. C., and Murray, E. S., A serologically active erythrocyte sensitizing substance from typhus rickettsiae, J. Immunol., 70, 215, 1953.

95. Shirai, A., Dietel, J. W., and Osterman, J. V., Indirect hemagglutination test for human antibody to typhus and spotted fever group rickettsiae, J. Clin. Microbiol., 2, 430, 1975.

96. Fiset, P., Ormsbee, R. A., Silberman, R., Peacock, M., and Spielman, S. H., A microagglutination technique for detection and measurement of rickettsial antibodies, Acta Virol., 13, 60, 1969.

97. Bozeman, F. M. and Elisberg, B. L., Serological diagnosis of scrub typhus by indirect immunofluorescence, Proc. Soc. Exp. Biol. Med., 112, 568, 1963.

98. Goldwasser, R. A. and Shepard, C. C., Fluorescent antibody methods in the differentiation of murine and epidemic typhus sera; specificity changes resulting from previous immunization, J. Immunol., 82, 373, 1959.

99. Philip, R. N., Casper, E. A., Ormsbee, R. A., Peacock, M. G., and Burgdorfer, W., Microimmunofluorescence test for the serological study of Rocky Mountain spotted fever and typhus, J. Clin. Microbiol., 3, 51, 1976.

100. Ormsbee, R. A., Peacock, M. G., Philip, R. N., Casper, E. A., Plorde, J., Gabre-Kidan, T., and Wright, L., Serologic diagnosis of epidemic typhus, Am. J. Epidemiol., 105, 261, 1977.

101. Pratt, H. D., Bjornson, B. F., and Littig, K. S., Control of Domestic Rats and Mice, Publication No. 76-8141, U.S. Department of Health, Education, and Welfare, Public Health Service, Center for Disease Control, Atlanta, 1976.

102. Reiss-Gutfreund, R. J., Un nouveau reservoir de virus pour Rickettsia prowazeki: les animaux domestiques et leurs tiques, Bull. Soc. Pathol. Exot., 49, 946, 1956.

103. Imam, I. Z. E. and Labib, A., Evidence of typhus infection in domestic animals in Egypt, Bull. W.H.O., 35, 123, 1966.

104. Ormsbee, R. A., The hypothesis of extra-human reservoirs of Rickettsia prowazeki, in Proc. Int. Symp. on the Control of Lice and Louse-Borne Diseases, Scientific Publication No. 263, Pan American Health Organization, Washington, D.C., 1973, 104.

105. Burgdorfer, W., Ormsbee, R. A., Schmidt, M. L., and Hoogstraal, H., A search for the epidemic typhus agent in Ethiopian ticks, Bull. W.H.O., 48, 563, 1973.

106. Bozeman, F. M., Masiello, S. A., Williams, M. S., and Elisberg, B. L., Epidemic typhus rickettsiae isolated from flying squirrels, Nature (London), 255, 545, 1975.

107. Bozeman, F. M., Williams, M. S., Stocks, N. I., Chadwick, D. P., Elisberg, B. L., Sonenshine, D. E., and Lauer, D. M., Ecologic studies on epidemic typhus infection in the eastern flying squirrel, Folia Microbiol. (Prague), 21 (Abstr.), 507, 1976.

108. McKiel, J. A., Bell, E. J., and Lackman, D. B., Rickettsia canada: a new member of the typhus group of rickettsiae isolated from Haemaphysalis leporispalustris ticks in Canada, Can. J. Microbiol., 13, 503, 1967.

109. Bozeman, F. M., Elisberg, B. L., Humphries, J. W., Runcik, K., and Palmer, D. B., Jr., Serological evidence of Rickettsia canada infection of man, J. Infect. Dis., 121, 367, 1970.

110. Summaries of notifiable diseases submitted by the states to the U.S. Public Health Service, Public Health Rep., 45 to 66, 1930 to 1951.

111. Annual Supplement, Morbidity and Mortality Weekly Report, U.S. Department of Health, Education, and Welfare, Public Health Center, Center for Disease Control, Atlanta, 1952 to 1975.

Q FEVER

H. G. Stoenner

DISEASE

Q fever (abattoir fever, query fever, Balkan grippe) is an acute rickettsial disease generally characterized by abrupt onset with severe headache, chills, remittent fever, malaise, myalgia, and pneumonitis.

ETIOLOGIC AGENT

Coxiella burnetii (Rickettsia diaporica, R. burnetii), the causative agent of Q fever, was isolated and characterized about the same time in Australia and the U.S.[1,2] In Australia, the organism was shown to be the cause of a febrile disease that occurred principally among workers in abattoirs whereas, in the U.S., it was recovered initially from naturally infected *Dermacentor andersoni* ticks. The organism multiplies only in living cells and stains red with Gimenez and Macchiavello stains and purple with Giemsa stain. It grows readily in a variety of arthropod, avian, and mammalian cell cultures. In smears of yolk sac cultures, the organisms are pleomorphic; they may appear as bipolar rods 0.25 μm × 1 μm to 1.25 μm, lanceolate rods 0.25 μm × 0.5 μm, or cocci about 0.25 μm in diameter. In yolk sac preparations examined by electron microscopy, *C. burnetii* has a trilaminar plasma membrane separated from a trilaminar outer membrane by an intermediate dense layer that is comparable to the peptidoglycan layer of Gram-negative bacteria.[3] Also, in some yolk sac preparations, serologically inert forms without limiting membranes are seen.[4,5] These forms may represent infectious particles capable of passing Berkefeld W filters and collodian membranes of mean porosity as low as 65 nm.[2,6] The organism multiplies by binary fission, but the role of atypical subcellular particles in the reproductive cycle has not been clarified.[4-6]

Apparent differences in the serologic reactivity of strains of *C. burnetii* found in early studies were largely explained when phase variation was discovered.[7] The organism exists in animals and ticks in phase I that is reactive only with late convalescent guinea pig serum in the complement-fixation (cf) test. After phase I strains are passed serially in fertile hen eggs, they gradually convert to phase II that reacts with antibodies in both early- and late-convalescent serums of guinea pigs. Apart from serologic differences influenced by phase, only minor antigenic differences among strains have been demonstrated.[8] The major antigens appear to be polysaccharides and are not shared with any of the other rickettsiae.

The resistance of *C. burnetii* to physical and chemical agents is a unique property not shared by other rickettsiae. It survived for at least 586 days in dried tick feces and for 3 months in moist soil of lambing pens.[9,10] It survived in milk at 62°C but not at 63°C for 30 min.[11] Neither 1% phenol nor 1% formalin destroyed the organism within 24 hr.[12] Properties that further distinguish *C. burnetii* from other rickettsiae are its inability to elicit agglutinins against *Proteus* X strains, to cause rash in man, and to induce "toxic" reactions in mice.

TRUE AND ALTERNATE HOSTS

The range of animal hosts involved in the epizootiology of Q fever is extremely broad and extends from ticks to primates. Consequently, it is impossible to distinguish between true and alternate hosts. Nevertheless, the organism is maintained in nature by two cycles that are essentially independent but occasionally overlap. The basic cycle involves many species of wildlife and their ectoparasites, and the second cycle involves domestic animals that serve as the principal source of infection for man.

One may question which cycle is basic, but at least in the U.S., infection of domestic animals, initially detected in the late 1940s, likely originated from wildlife indigenous to this country. At the time Q fever was discovered in California and shown to be widespread among dairy herds in that state, little evidence of infection was found among dairy cattle in the rest of the U.S.[13,14] During the next decade, however, *C. burnetii* became widely disseminated among dairy herds throughout the country.[14] The range of wildlife involved in the basic cycle is shown in Table 1. This list is restricted to species of wildlife in which natural infection has been confirmed by isolation of the organism, and it does not include any species found only to be seropositive.

On a world-wide basis, few studies on Q fever in wildlife have been as comprehensive as those conducted in Utah and California.[17-19] The results of these investigations indicate that widespread epizootics can occur in nature. During the initial year of an 8-year study in Utah, only a single jack rabbit was found to be seropositive; the percentage of infected animals, as based on serology and isolation of *C. burnetii*, increased and reached a peak 6 years later. At that time, 19 of 34 species of wildlife were infected; the finding that 122 of 327 *Dipodomys microps,* 154 of 378 *Lepus californicus,* and 126 of 499 *Peromyscus maniculatus* were seropositive indicates the extent of the epizootic. *C. burnetii* was isolated from ticks, fleas, lice, and mites that parasitized these animals. The California study was initiated while an epizootic was in progress. There the disease affected 4 of 8 species of carnivores and all of 13 species of herbivores, mainly rodents.[17]

A complete listing of hematophagous arthropods found to be naturally infected with *C. burnetii* would require more space than is warranted.[33-35] Ticks, which are principally involved, include 9 species each of *Dermacentor* and *Rhipicephalus,* 10 each of *Haemaphysalis* and *Ixodes,* 15 of *Hyalomma,* 4 of *Amblyomma,* 7 of *Ornithodoros,* and 2 each of *Argas, Boophilus,* and *Octobius megnini.* In addition, *C. burnetii* has been demonstrated in 12 species of mites and at least 3 species of fleas.

The role of these arthropods in the epizootiology of Q fever among wildlife populations has not been clarified. Some may be regarded as "sentinels" that merely ingest an infectious blood meal and transiently retain the organism. Others support growth of the organism in the gut and hemolymph without being able to transmit the agent, whereas some are able to do so directly by bite or indirectly through the medium of infectious feces.[36]

Among domestic animals, cattle, sheep, and goats are the chief sources of infection for man.[13,35,37-41] Other domestic animals, such as horses, camels, and water buffalo, have been found to be seropositive, but their role in the epidemiology of the disease has not been established.[34] Natural infections have been shown to occur in sheep dogs that ingested placentas of infected farm animals.[42]

DISTRIBUTION

Q fever is essentially world-wide in distribution and occurs chiefly in countries where substantial numbers of cattle, sheep, and goats are raised. In 1955, the agent was found in every country surveyed except the Netherlands, Poland, Denmark, Ireland, Sweden, Finland, and Norway.[43] More recent global surveys have not been conducted, but the current distribution of this rickettsia is not likely to differ significantly from that pre-

Table 1
NATURALLY INFECTED WILD VERTEBRATES FROM WHICH
COXIELLA BURNETII HAS BEEN ISOLATED

Host	Country	Ref.
Short-nosed bandicoot (*Isodon macrourus*)	Australia	15
Red kangaroo (*Macropus rufus*)o	Australia	16
Columbian black-tailed deer (*Odocoileus hemionus columbianus*)	U.S. (California)	17
Coyote (*Canis latrans*)	U.S. (California, Utah)	17, 18
Gray fox (*Urocyon cinereoargenteus*)	U.S. (California)	17
Desert woodrat (*Neotoma lepida*)	U.S. (Utah)	17
Bushy-tailed woodrat (*Neotoma cinerea cinerea*)	U.S. (Montana)	20
Spotted skunk (*Spilogale gracilis*)	U.S. (California)	17
Striped skunk (*Mephitis mephitis*)	U.S. (California)	17
Black-tailed jack rabbit (*Lepus californicus*)	U.S. (California, Utah)	17, 18
Brush rabbit (*Sylvilagus bachmani*)	U.S. (California)	17
California ground squirrel (*Spermophilus beecheyi*)	U.S. (California)	17
Golden-mantled ground squirrel (*Spermophilus lateralis tescorum*)	U.S. (Montana)	20
White-tailed antelope squirrel (*Ammospermophilus leucurus*)	U.S. (Utah)	18, 19
Cliff chipmunk (*Eutamias dorsalis*)	U.S. (Utah)	18
Least chipmunk (*Eutamias minimus*)	U.S. (Utah)	18
Yellow-pine chipmunk (*Eutamias amoenus*)	U.S. (Montana)	20
Ord kangaroo rat (*Dipodomys ordii*)	U.S. (Utah)	18, 19
Chisel-toothed kangaroo rat (*Dipodomys microps*)	U.S. (Utah)	18
Botta's pocket gopher (*Thomomys bottae*)o	U.S. (Utah)	18
Deer mouse (*Peromyscus maniculatus*)	U.S. (California, Utah)	17-19
Pinon mouse (*Peromyscus truei*)	U.S. (Utah)	18
Long-tailed pocket mouse (*Perognathus formosus*)	U.S. (Utah)	18
Little pocket mouse (*Perognathus longimembris*)	U.S. (Utah)	18
Western harvest mouse (*Reithrodontomys megalotis*)	U.S. (Utah)	18
Jird (*Meriones shawi*)	Morocco	21
European rabbit (*Orycotolagus cuniculus*)	Morocco	22
Field mouse (*Apodemus sylvaticus*)	Morocco	23
Striped grass mouse (*Lemniscomys barberus*)	Morocco	23
Striped grass rat (*Lemniscomys* sp.)	Africa (Kenya)	24
Redstart (*Phoenicurus phoenicurus*)	Czechoslovakia	25
White wagtail (*Motacilla alba*)	Czechoslovakia	25
Norway rat (*Rattus norvegicus*)	Czechoslovakia	26
House mouse (*Mus musculus*)	Czechoslovakia	26
Red bank vole (*Clethrionomys glareolus*)	Czechoslovakia	26
Least weasel (*Mustela nivalis*)	Czechoslovakia	26
Lesser shrew (*Sorex minimus*)	Czechoslovakia	27
Pigeon (*Columba livia*)	Italy	28
Garden dormouse (*Eliomys quercinus*)	Spain	29
European rabbit (*Oryctolagus cuniculus*)	Spain	29
Talass suslik (*Citellus relictus*)	U.S.S.R.	30
Eurasian grey hamster (*Cricetulus migratorius*)	U.S.S.R.	30
Small jerboa (*Allactaga elater*)	U.S.S.R.	30

Table 1 (continued)
NATURALLY INFECTED WILD VERTEBRATES FROM WHICH COXIELLA BURNETII HAS BEEN ISOLATED

Host	Country	Ref.
Long-eared hedgehog (*Hemiechinus auritus*)	U.S.S.R.	30
Great gerbil (*Rhombomys opimus*)	U.S.S.R.	31, 32
Long-clawed ground squirrel (*Spermophilopsis leptodactylus*)	U.S.S.R.	31
Field sparrow (*Passer montanus pallidus*)	U.S.S.R.	31

viously found. However, prevalence of the disease in man has declined markedly in some countries. In the U.S., infection among dairy herds is widespread throughout the country. Nearly all strains recovered from cattle in recent years are weakly virulent for laboratory animals. Infections among rural populations exposed to these cattle are common, but most are inapparent.[44] During 1975, only 32 clinical cases from five states were reported in the U.S.[45]

DISEASE IN ANIMALS

Observations on naturally occurring infections in cattle suggest that *C. burnetii* does not cause overt disease. Cattle in California that were infected with strains highly virulent for man and guinea pigs did not abort or show any other signs of illness, and the infection did not affect milk production.[13] Furthermore, the leukocyte content of milk from infected quarters of the mammary gland did not differ from that of uninfected quarters.[46] However, considering the heavy population of *C. burnetii* in the placentas of infected cattle, one wonders why abortion does not occur.[47] Pregnant dairy cattle inoculated with a large dose of *C. burnetii* develop fever and abort, but the challenge dose used in these experiments grossly exceeds a natural exposure.[48,49] One must conclude that Q fever rickettsiae do not naturally cause a significant disease in cattle.

Generally, investigators have not noted any evidence of disease in infected flocks of sheep and goats in the U.S.[10,50] A few abortions were seen in infected flocks of sheep in Idaho, but they did not exceed normally expected losses. Furthermore, it was known that many of these flocks were affected to some extent by vibriosis. Abortions have been reported to occur among flocks of sheep and goats in Cyprus and among goats in Switzerland.[51,52] The former were shown to be free of *Chlamydia, Brucella,* and *Vibrio.*

The disease in small laboratory animals used for experimental purposes depends upon the virulence of the strain and dose inoculated.[53] Some highly virulent strains, such as Nine Mile and Idaho J.A., cause a high fever, severe splenomegaly with extensive fibrinous exudate, emaciation, and significant mortality in guinea pigs.[53] Those isolated from wildlife in Utah and California did not cause any fever or other signs of disease. These strains were more infective for hamsters than for mice or guinea pigs.[54,55] Most European, Australian, Balkan, and British strains are moderate in virulence for laboratory animals.

DISEASE IN MAN

The incubation period ranges from 2 to 4 weeks, but in most cases, it is about 18 to 20 days. Onset is usually sudden and characterized initially by fever, chills, severe frontal headache, myalgia, and general malaise. The disease rarely occurs in children under 10 years of age and is more severe in persons 40 years of age and older.

Symptoms and physical findings noted in 180 patients in northern California are

Table 2
SYMPTOMS NOTED IN 180 PATIENTS
WITH Q FEVER, NORTHERN
CALIFORNIA, 1948 TO 1949

Symptom	Number of patients	Percentage of patients
Onset		
Sudden	130	72
Gradual	50	28
Constitutional		
Fever	180	100
Chills	133	74
Chilliness	56	31
Sweating	67	37
Malaise	180	100
General weakness	155	86
Neuromuscular		
Headache	117	65
Muscle pain	85	47
Joint pain	20	11
Retrobulbar pain	23	13
Respiratory		
Cough	43	24
Chest pain	18	10
Sore throat	9	5
Coryza	7	4
G.I.		
Anorexia	77	43
Nausea	40	22
Vomiting	23	13
Diarrhea	9	5

From Clark, W. H., Lennette, E. H., Railsback, O. C., and Romer, M. S., *Arch. Intern. Med.*, 88, 155, 1951. With permission. Copyright 1951, American Medical Association.

summarized in Tables 2 and 3.[56] Maximum temperature elevations range from 104 to 106°F, and daily remissions toward normal usually occur. Temperatures above 102°F are uncommon after the third week of illness, but a few patients may experience daily febrile periods for as long as 3 months. Nearly all patients have chills, especially during the first week of illness; most experience one or more true shaking rigors. Drenching sweats nearly always accompany febrile remissions, and some patients require fluid replacement given parenterally. Severe headache, usually frontal in origin, is a prominent symptom in most cases, often persisting throughout the course of the illness.

Because atypical pneumonia and Q fever share many clinical features, Q fever is often considered to be a primary infection of the respiratory tract. However, only about one half of the patients present signs or symptoms referable to the respiratory tract. These may include chest pain that is usually pleuritic, a dry nonproductive cough, and crepitant rales that bear no constant relationship to pulmonary lesions seen roentgenographically. The occurrence of pulmonary lesions demonstrable by roentgen-ray varies considerably. They are rarely seen in Australian patients but are commonly associated with the disease in Europe and the U.S.[57] In well-documented studies, 28 to 90% of patients had demonstrable lung lesions.[56,58] Lesions most commonly consist of irregular patches of increased density (resembling ground glass) in the peribronchial and alveolar regions of the middle and lower zones of the lungs.[58,59]

Nearly half of the patients complain of anorexia, and vomiting may be so severe that parenteral administration of fluids and medication becomes necessary. Hepatic involvement is common; in the California studies, 5% had jaundice, 11% hepatomegaly, and 7% liver tenderness.[56] When hepatic damage was specifically evaluated, 84% of Australian patients had impaired liver function.[60] Most patients with extensive liver involvement had a protracted course and slow convalescence.[56]

The absence of a skin rash in Q fever generally distinguishes it from other rickettsial diseases. However, transient rashes, variously described as maculopapular erythematous, pruritic red papular, or faint pink macular, have been described.[56,59]

Because of the low mortality of Q fever in man, observations on the pathologic changes seen in this disease are extremely limited.[61-63] Changes attributable to *C. burnetii* are limited essentially to the pleural cavity. Grossly, consolidated lobes resemble those seen in pneumococcal pneumonia, but histologically, they resemble those seen in psittacosis and viral pneumonia.[63] Where the pneumonic process is confluent, alveoli are filled with fibrinocellular exudate consisting chiefly of large mononuclear cells, plasma cells, lymphocytes, and a few neutrophils. Interalveolar septa are thickened and congested, and some capillaries contain hyaline thrombi. Bronchi and bronchioles are filled with a similar exudate. The remarkable feature, consistently described, is the mononuclear nature of the cellular response in the lungs.[61-63]

Complications, chiefly related to damage to the cardiovascular system, are not uncommon in severely affected patients. These include subacute endocarditis, phlebothrombosis, pleurisy, pleural effusions, arthritis, orchitis, epididymitis, esophagitis, massive intestinal hemorrhage, and decubitus ulcers.[59,64] The first is the most serious and is usually fatal unless treated. The latent period between acute disease and appearance of signs of subacute endocarditis may be brief or last more than 1 year. Many patients had rheumatic fever before experiencing Q fever.[65] Subacute endocarditis was characterized by fever, weight loss, clubbing of fingers, joint pains, progressively pronounced heart-valve murmurs, dyspnea, and elevated sedimentation rate and gammaglobulin levels.[65,66] Q fever endocarditis should be suspected when repeated blood cultures do not yield bacterial pathogens.

EPIDEMIOLOGY

As related earlier in this chapter, Q fever rickettsiae are maintained in nature by two independent cycles — one in wildlife and the other in domestic animals. The wildlife cycle involves many species of animals, both herbivores and carnivores. Conceivably, the organism could be spread by the airborne route among these animals. Because most animals consume the placenta after parturition, their feces would be infectious for a brief period, and rickettsiae in the fecal material would contaminate the environment shared by species of wildlife. Some arthropods are capable of transmitting the agent by bite or through the medium of infectious feces.[36] Carnivores could acquire the disease by ingesting infected herbivores.

Among domestic animals, female cattle, sheep, and goats are principally involved in the cycle of infection. Q fever rickettsiae are eliminated from the bodies of female animals in the placentas, ammiotic fluid, and milk. Because of the high concentration of organisms in placentas of parturient animals, they are chiefly responsible for contamination of the environment.

Results of epizootiologic investigations strongly suggest that the agent is disseminated among domestic animals by the airborne route. It has been repeatedly isolated from air samples taken from the environment of infected livestock.[67,68] The salient features of the disease have been reproduced experimentally in pregnant cows exposed to aerosols, some of which contained about 100 minimal infectious guinea pig doses

Table 3
PHYSICAL FINDINGS IN 180 PATIENTS
WITH Q FEVER, NORTHERN
CALIFORNIA, 1948 TO 1949.

Physical findings	Number of patients	Percentage of patients
Respiratory		
Rales	38	21
Altered breath sounds	4	2
Dullness	5	3
"Positive"[a] roentgenograms (65 patients)	(22)	(34)
Abdominal		
Hepatomegaly	20	11
Hepatic tenderness	13	7
Splenomegaly	7	4
Splenic tenderness	4	2
General tenderness	5	3
Neurological		
Nuchal stiffness	9	5
Apathy	4	2
Confusion	9	5
Altered reflexes	2	1
Cardiac		
Irregular rhythm	4	2
Murmur	1	< 1
Cutaneous		
Rash	7	4
Jaundice	9	5

[a]   Includes all abnormalities observed in chest roentgenograms.

From Clark, W. H., Lennette, E. H., Railsback, O. C., and Romer, M. S., *Arch. Intern. Med.*, 88, 155, 1951. With permission. Copyright 1951, American Medical Association.

per milliliter. Cows so exposed had infected placentas and shed the organism in their milk.[69] Although cattle naturally shed *C. burnetii* in their milk for prolonged periods, the agent is not spread by contamination of the teats during the milking process as is the case in bacterial mastitis.[70]

Man most commonly contracts the disease by inhaling organisms released into the environment by infected sheep, cattle, and goats. In southern California, three factors were identified as predisposing to infection: (1) the use of raw milk in the household, (2) residence near a dairy or livestock yard, and (3) employment in industries handling live or recently killed local dairy cows and young calves.[71] Q fever also affected many persons engaged in diverse occupations not directly related to the livestock industry. These people contract Q fever when traveling through a contaminated rural environment or by contact with mobile fomites of various types.[10,72]

Whether or not man can acquire the disease by ingesting raw infected milk has been debated. In England, raw milk was considered to be the source of infection for 41% of the cases studied, and in southern California, the prevalence of antibodies among raw milk users was 12-fold greater than that among persons not using raw milk.[71,73] However, persons who drank raw infective milk during controlled experimental studies experienced seroconversions without any evidence of disease.[74]

Although the disease occurs in the general population of both rural and urban communities, a large proportion of cases occurs among persons engaged in occupations related to the livestock industry. These include animal husbandrymen, dairymen, slaughterhouse workers, creamery workers, and workers in the hide, fat rendering, fertilizer, and animal transportation industries.[71,72] The age and sex distribution of cases varies in different epidemiologic situations. Although the disease occurs chiefly among males of working age (20 to 59), there is no evidence that males are more susceptible. In areas where the disease was associated principally with infected sheep, Q fever had a definite seasonal distribution with a peak incidence during the lambing season and immediately thereafter.[10,50] In contrast, a seasonal distribution was not evident when the disease was associated with dairy cattle herds in which parturition occurs throughout the year.[71,75]

Although the urine, saliva, and excretions of the respiratory tract of Q fever patients are infective, man-to-man transmission of the agent rarely occurs*. In two reported incidents, 38 persons in a hospital in Frankfurt, Germany, contracted the disease from a single patient who had chronic Q fever, and 87% of the patients and 29% of the staff of a mental hospital contracted Q fever from human sources.[34]

DIAGNOSIS

The diagnosis of Q fever in man should be confirmed by isolating *C. burnetii* from tissues or body fluids or by demonstrating a serologic or immunologic response to infection with the organism. For isolating the organism, citrated blood specimens should be obtained during the initial febrile phase before any broad-spectrum antibiotics have been administered. Presence of *C. burnetii* in the blood of a patient is most readily demonstrated by inoculating each of two weanling guinea pigs or hamsters intraperitoneally with 0.5 mℓ whole blood and then testing their sera for antibodies 21 to 30 days later. Suspensions of spleens of seropositive animals then may be inoculated into 5-day-old embryonated hen eggs if yolk sac cultures are desired for further characterization of the strain. Because of the time needed to complete these procedures and the cost of animals, this method is impractical except in special situations when isolating the organism is critical. The hazard of contracting Q fever by working with live organisms should be emphasized, and these procedures should not be attempted without adequate containment facilities needed for the protection of workers.

Demonstration of a humoral response to infection with *C. burnetii* is the most practical means of confirming a diagnosis of Q fever. Acute-phase and one or more convalescent-phase blood samples should be taken so that a significant rise in specific antibody titer can be shown. The CF test and a variety of agglutination tests have been used for detecting antibodies. Of these, the CF test, in which phase II organisms are used for antigen, is the most commonly employed.[76] CF antibodies appear in the blood of 65% of patients during the second week of illness and in about 90% during the fourth week.[77] If chronic Q fever (cardiovascular disease) is considered in the clinical diagnosis, the serums should also be tested against phase I antigen.

A microagglutination technique and a capillary tube test are also widely used for the diagnosis of Q fever in man.[78,79] Agglutinins appear in the serums of about 50% of patients within the first week; during the second week, 92% are seropositive, and by the fourth week, all patients are positive.[77] A radioistope-precipitation test developed about 1962 is extremely sensitive and specific, but its application has been restricted because of the requirement for complex equipment.[80]

---

*Blood taken from exposed donors late in the incubation period may cause Q fever in the recipients. Center for Disease Control, Q fever, California, Morbidity and Mortality Weekly Rep. No. 26, 86, 91, 1977.

A skin test has been used in epidemiological studies on the premise that past infection induces dermal sensitivity to *C. burnetii*.[81] The antigen consists of whole-cell phase I vaccine diluted to contain 0.02 CF units of antigen per milliliter. The results of skin tests correlated with the degree of exposure in various population groups, but the correlation between the results of skin tests and those of CF and CA, tests was not outstanding; the immune population detected by skin test generally exceeded that detected by serologic procedures.[44,81]

Essentially the same isolation procedures used for isolating *C. burnetii* from man are applicable for detecting infection in livestock. However, attempts to isolate the organism should be made from milk and suspensions of placentas rather than blood of seropositive animals.

Sera of livestock are examined by the same serologic procedures used for testing human sera. The regularity of the antibody response of cattle to infection is considered to be comparable to that of man; most infected animals develop detectable levels of antibody. However, a large proportion of seronegative sheep in infected bands have *C. burnetii* in their placentas at parturition.[10,39]

Large populations of dairy cattle can be surveyed for Q fever by testing pooled-herd milk samples with the capillary-tube test.[82] In this test, antibodies in the milk agglutinate the stained rickettsiae and rise with the fat globules to form a bluish layer of cream. Nearly all seropositive cows have detectable levels of antibody in their milk, and the test is sufficiently sensitive to identify most infected herds.

TREATMENT

Chloramphenicol and several tetracycline-group antibiotics used for treating patients are rickettsiostatic rather than rickettsiacidal. Hence, it is sometimes possible to recover *C. burnetti* from patients after several days of treatment.[83] When the rickettsiostatic activity of these antibiotics was measured in infected chick embryos, Terramycin®, Aureomycin®, and Carbomycin® were highly active and erythromycin, chloramphenicol, and streptomycin were only slightly active.[84] However, their efficacy for treating patients affected with Q fever is controversial. Tetracycline, given orally in a dose of 500 mg every 6 hours, had no apparent effect on the course of disease in 78 patientts (British soldiers) in Cyprus.[51] When Aureomycin® was compared with penicillin in treating a series of 45 patients, three types of responses to the former were observed. 71% responding favorably became afebrile within 5 days whereas only 28% of 25 treated with penicillin, which is known to be ineffective, became afebrile within 5 days. A second group of nine patients showed subjective improvement but remained febrile, and a third group of four patients did not show any improvement.[83]
improvement.[83]

PREVENTION AND CONTROL

Q fever in man could be controlled by reducing the amount of environmental contamination originating from infected livestock. This reduction could be achieved by collection and destruction of infected placentas and vaccination of livestock.[86] However, such a program could not be justified (at least in the U.S.) because of the low prevalence of the disease. Furthermore, agencies responsible for the control of animal diseases would not likely support such control programs because livestock are not adversely affected by infection with *C. burnetii*. In areas where the disease is a significant health problem, these control measures could be justified.

Because the results of epidemiological studies have strongly implicated raw milk as a source of infection for man, all raw milk should be pasteurized and all dairy products should be produced from pasteurized milk. Milk must be pasteurized at 161°F for 15 sec to destroy *C. burnetii*.[87]

Laboratory workers handling live organisms often contract the disease, even when exposed to strains that do not cause a significant amount of disease under natural conditions. These workers should be immunized with ten complement-fixing units of antigen given intramuscularly.[88] Before vaccination, each recipient should be skin-tested with a 1:50 dilution of vaccine to detect prior sensitization to *C. burnetii*. Vaccination of sensitized persons is contraindicated because of the hazard of inducing a sterile abscess at the site of vaccination.[88,89] Although Q fever vaccine is not produced commercially, it has been prepared and used in major laboratories where research on the organism is conducted.

REFERENCES

1. **Derrick, E. N.**, *Rickettsia burneti*: the cause of "Q" fever, *Med. J. Aust.*, 1, 14, 1939.
2. **Davis, G. E., Cox, H. R., Parker, R. R., and Dyer, R. E.**, A filter-passing agent isolated from ticks, *Public Health Rep.*, 53, 1, 1938.
3. **Burton, P. R., Stuekemann, J., and Paretsky, D.**, Electron microscopy studies of the limiting layers of the rickettsia, *Coxiella burneti*, *J. Bacteriol.*, 122, 316, 1975.
4. **Anacker, R. L., Fukushi, K., Pickens, E. G., and Lackman, D. B.**, Electron microscopic observations of the development of *Coxiella burnetii* in the chick yolk sac, *J. Bacteriol.*, 88, 1130, 1964.
5. **Rosenberg, M. and Kordova, N.**, Study of intracellular forms of *Coxiella burneti* in the electron microscope, *Acta Virol.*, 4, 52, 1960.
6. **Kordova, N.**, Filterable particles of *Coxiella burneti*, *Acta Virol.*, 3, 25, 1959.
7. **Stoker, M. G. P. and Fiset, P.**, Phase variation of the Nine Mile and other strains of *Rickettsia burneti*, *Can. J. Microbiol.*, 2, 310, 1956.
8. **Fiset, P., Wike, D. A., Pickens, E. G., and Ormsbee, R. A.**, An antigenic comparison of strains of *Coxiella burneti*, *Acta Virol.*, 15, 161, 1971.
9. **Philip, C. B.**, Observations on experimental Q fever, *J. Parasitol.*, 34, 457, 1948.
10. **Stoenner, H. G., Jellison, W. L., Lackman, D. B., Brock, D., and Casey, M.**, Q fever in Idaho, *Am. J. Hyg.*, 69, 202, 1959.
11. **Enright, J. B., Sadler, W. W., and Thomas, R. C.**, Pasteurization of milk containing the organism of Q fever, *Am. J. Public Health*, 47, 695, 1957.
12. **Ransom, S. E. and Huebner, R. J.**, Studies on the resistance of *Coxiella burneti* to physical agents, *Am. J. Hyg.*, 53, 110, 1951.
13. **Huebner, R. J., Jellison, W. L., Beck, M. D., Parker, R. R., and Shepard, C. C.**, Q fever studies in southern California. Recovery of *Rickettsia burneti* from raw milk, *Public Health Rep.*, 63, 214, 1948.
14. **Luoto, L.**, Report on the nationwide occurrence of Q fever infections in cattle, *Public Health Rep.*, 75, 135, 1960.
15. **Derrick, E. H. and Smith, D. J. W.**, Studies on the epidemiology of Q fever. II. The isolation of three strains of *Rickettsia burneti* from the bandicoot *Isoodon torosus*, *Aust. J. Exp. Biol. Med. Sci.*, 18, 99, 1940.
16. **Pope, J. H., Scott, W., and Dwyer, R.**, *Coxiella burneti* in kangaroos and kangaroo ticks in western Queensland, *Aust. J. Exp. Biol. Med. Sci.*, 38, 17, 1960.
17. **Enright, J. B., Frank, C. E., Behymer, D. E., Longhurst, W. M., Dutson, V. J., and Wright, M. E.**, *Coxiella burneti* in a wildlife-livestock environment: distribution of Q fever in wild mammals, *Am. J. Epidemiol.*, 94, 79, 1971.
18. **Sidwell, R. W., Lundgren, D. L., Bushman, J. B., and Thorpe, B. D.**, The occurrence of a possible epizootic of Q fever in fauna of the Great Salt Lake Desert of Utah, *Am. J. Trop. Med.*, 13, 754, 1964.
19. **Stoenner, H. G., Holdenreid, R., Lackman, D., and Orsborn, J. S., Jr.**, The occurrence of *Coxiella burnetii*, *Brucella*, and other pathogens among fauna of the Great Salt Lake in Utah, *Am. J. Trop. Med. Hyg.*, 8, 590, 1959.

20. **Burgdorfer, W., Pickens, E. G., Newhouse, V., and Lackman, D. B.**, Isolation of *Coxiella burnetii* from rodents in western Montana, *J. Infect. Dis.*, 112, 181, 1963.

21. **Blanc, G., Martin, L. A., and Maurice, A.**, Le Merion (*Meriones shawi*) de la region de Goulimine est un reservoir de virus de la Q fever marocaine, *C. R. Acad. Sci.*, 224, 1673, 1947.

22. **Blanc, G. and Bruneau, J.**, Entreitien dans la nature de *Coxiella burnetii* par l'association du lapin de garenne *Oryctolagus cuniculus* (L.) et de la tique *Hyalomma excavatum* C. L. K., *C. R. Acad. Sci.*, 237, 582, 1953.

23. **Blanc, G. and Bruneau, J.**, Isolement du virus de Q fever de deux rongeurs sauvages provenant de la foret de Nefifik (Maroc), *Bull. Soc. Pathol. Exot.*, 49, 431, 1956.

24. **Heisch, R. B.**, The isolation of *Rickettsia burneti* from *Lemniscomys* sp. in Kenya, *East Afr. Med. J.*, 37, 104, 1960.

25. **Syrucek, L., Raska, K., Lim, D., and Harlik, O.**, Q rickettsiosis in birds, *J. Hyg. Epidemiol. Microbiol. Immunol. Czech.*, 4, 22, 1955.

26. **Raska, K. and Syrucek, L.**, Ein Beitrag zur Epidemiologie der Q-Rickettsiose, *Zentralbl. Bakteriol. Parasitenkd. Infektionskr. Hyg. Abt. 1: Orig.*, 167, 267, 1956.

27. **Syrucek, L., Sobeslavsky, O., and Havlik, O.**, Isolation of *Rickettsia burneti* from the pigmy shrew *Sorex minimus* in a focus of Q-rickettsiosis in north-western Bohemia, *Cesk. Epidemiol. Mikrobiol. Immunol.*, 6, 392, 1957.

28. **Babudieri, B. and Moscovici, C.**, Experimental and natural infection of birds by *Coxiella burneti*, *Nature* (London), 169, 195, 1952.

29. **Perez-Gallardo, F., Clavero, G., and Hernandez, F. S.**, Investigaciones sobre la epidemiologia de la fiebre "Q" en Espana, *Rev. Sanid. Hig. Publica*, 26, 81, 1952.

30. **Proreshnaya, T. L., Rapaport, L. P., Evdoshenko, V. G., and Kichatov, E. A.**, A study of natural foci of Q fever in Kirgizia, *J. Microbiol. Epidemiol. Immunobiol.* (U.S.S.R.), 31, 1613, 1960.

31. **Zhmaeva, Z. M., Pchelkina, A. A., Mishchenko, N. K., and Karulin, B. E.**, The epidemiological importance of ectoparasites of birds in a natural focus of Q fever in the south of Central Asia, *Dokl. Vses. Akad. Skh. Nauk.* (in Russian), 101, 387, 1955.

32. **Sterkhova, N. N. and Akhundov, M. G.**, The role of wild rodents in the epidemiology of Q fever, *J. Microbiol. Epidemiol. Immunobiol.* (U.S.S.R.), 30, 153, 1959.

33. **Cracea, E. and Popovici, V.**, *Febra Q La Om Si Animale*, Editura "Ceres," Bucharest, 1975, 111.

34. **Babudieri, B.**, Q fever: a zoonosis, in *Advances in Veterinary Science*, Brandly, C. A. and Jungherr, E. L., Eds., Academic Press, New York, 1959, 106

35. **Berge, T. O. and Lennette, E. H.**, World distribution of Q fever: human, animal, and arthropod infection, *Am. J. Hyg.*, 57, 125, 1953.

36. **Parker, R. R., Bell, E. J., and Stoenner, H. G.**, Q fever — a brief survey of the problem, *J. Am. Vet. Med. Assoc.*, 104, 55; 124, 1949.

37. **Burgdorfer, W., Geigy, R., Gsell, O., and Wiesmann, E.**, Parasitologiische und Klinische Beobactungen an Q-Fieber-Fallen in der Schweiz, *Schweiz. Med. Wochenschr.*, 81, 162, 1951.

38. **Caminopetros, J. P.**, La "Q" fever en Grece. Le lait, source de l'infection pour l'homme et les animaux, *Ann. Parasitol. Hum. Comp.*, 23, 107, 1948.

39. **Welsh, H. H., Lennette, E. H., Abinanti, F. R., and Winn, J. F.**, Q fever in California. IV. Occurrence of *Coxiella burnetii* in the placenta of naturally infected sheep, *Public Health Rep.*, 66, 1473, 1951.

40. **Caporale, G. and Mantovani, A.**, Q fever in Central Italy, *J. Am. Vet. Med. Assoc.*, 119, 438, 1951.

41. **Marmion, B. P. and Stoker, M. G. P.**, Q fever in Great Britain. Epidemiology of an outbreak, *Lancet*, 259, 611, 1950.

42. **Mantovani, A. and Benazzi, P.**, The isolation of *Coxiella burneti* from *Rhipicephalus sanguineus* on naturally infected dogs, *J. Am. Vet. Med. Assoc.*, 122, 117, 1953.

43. **Kaplan, M. M. and Bertagna, P.**, The geographical distribution of Q fever, *Bull. W.H.O.*, 13, 826, 1955.

44. **Stoenner, H. G., Lackman, D. B., Benson, W. W., Mather, J., Casey, M., and Harvey, K. A.**, The role of dairy cattle in the epidemiology of Q fever in Idaho, *J. Infect. Dis.*, 109, 90, 1961.

45. **Center for Disease Control**, Morbidity and Mortality Weekly Reports, Annual Supplement 1975, U.S. Department of Health, Education, and Welfare, Public Health Service, Atlanta, 24, 34, 1976.

46. **Luoto, L., Huebner, R. J., and Stoenner, H. G.**, Q fever studies in southern California. XII. Aureomycin treatment of dairy cattle naturally infected with *Coxiella burnetii*, *Public Health Rep.*, 66, 199, 1951.

47. **Luoto, L.**, Q fever studies in southern California. IX. Isolation of Q fever organisms from parturient placentas of naturally infected dairy cows, *Public Health Rep.*, 65, 541, 1950.

48. **Stoenner, H. G.**, Experimental Q fever in cattle — epizootiologic aspects, *J. Am. Vet. Med. Assoc.*, 118, 170, 1951.

49. **Behymer, D. E., Biberstein, E. L., Reiman, H. P., Franti, C. E., Sawyer, M., Ruppanner, R., and Crenshaw, G. L.,** Q fever (*Coxiella burnetii*) investigations in dairy cattle: challenge of immunity after vaccination, *Am. J. Vet. Res.,* 37, 631, 1976.

50. **Lennette, E. H., Clark, W. H., and Dean, B. H.,** Sheep and goats in the epidemiology of Q fever in northern California, *Am. J. Trop. Med.,* 29, 527, 1949.

51. **Spicer, A. J., Crowther, R. W., Vella, E. E., Bengtsson, E., Miles, R., and Pitzolis, G.,** Q fever and animal abortion in Cyprus, *Trans. R. Soc. Trop. Med. Hyg.,* 71, 16, 1977.

52. **Kilchsperger, G. and Wiesman, E.,** Abortus-Epidemie bei Ziegen, bedingt durch *Rickettsia burneti, Schweiz. Arch. Tierheilkd.,* 91, 553, 1949.

53. **Ormsbee, R. A.,** Q fever rickettsiae, in *Viral and Rickettsial Infections of Man,* 4th ed., Horsfall, F. L., Jr. and Tamm, I., Eds., Lippincott, Philadelphia, 1965, 1144.

54. **Stoenner, H. G. and Lackman, D. B.,** The biologic properties of *Coxiella burnetii* isolated from rodents in Utah, *Am. J. Hyg.,* 71, 45, 1960.

55. **Enright, J. B., Behymer, D. E., Franti, C. E., Dutson, V. J., Longhurst, W. M., Wright, M. E., and Goggin, J. E.,** The behavior of Q fever rickettsiae isolated from wild animals in northern California, *J. Wildl. Dis.,* 7, 83, 1971.

56. **Clark, W. H., Lennette, E. H., Railsback, O. C., and Romer, M. S.,** Q fever in California. VII. Clinical features in one hundred eighty cases, *Arch. Intern. Med.,* 88, 155, 1951.

57. **Powell, O.,** Q fever: clinical features in 72 cases, *Australas. Ann. Med.,* 10, 52, 1961.

58. **Feinstein, M., Yesner, R., and Marks, J.,** Epidemics of Q fever among troops returning from Italy in the spring of 1945. I. Clinical aspects of the epidemic at Camp Patrick Henry, Virginia, *Am. J. Hyg.,* 44, 72, 1946.

59. **Huebner, R. J., Jellison, W. L., and Beck, M. D.,** Q fever — a review of current knowledge, *Ann. Intern. Med.,* 30, 495, 1949.

60. **Powell, O. W.,** Liver involvement in Q fever, *Australas. Ann. Med.,* 10, 52, 1961.

61. **Lillie, R. D., Perrin, T. L., and Armstrong, C.,** An institutional outbreak of pneumonitis. III. Histopathology in man and rhesus monkeys in the pneumonitis due to the virus of "Q" fever, *Public Health Rep.,* 56, 149, 1941.

62. **Perrin, T. L.,** Histopathologic observations in a fatal case of Q fever, *Arch. Pathol.,* 47, 361, 1949.

63. **Whittick, J. W.,** Necropsy findings in a case of Q fever in Britain, *Br. Med. J.,* 1, 979, 1950.

64. **Evans, A. D., Powell, D. E. B., and Burrell, C. D.,** Fatal endocarditis associated with Q fever, *Lancet,* 1, 864, 1959.

65. **Marmion, B. P.,** Subacute rickettsial endocarditis: an unusual complication of Q fever, *J. Hyg. Epidemiol. Microbiol. Immunol.,* 6, 79, 1962.

66. **Kristinsson, A. and Bentall, H. H.,** Medical and surgical treatment of Q fever endocarditis, *Lancet,* 2, 693, 1967.

67. **DeLay, P. D., Lennette, E. H., and DeOme, K. B.,** Q fever in California. II. Recovery of *Coxiella burneti* from naturally-infected air-borne dust, *J. Immunol.,* 65, 211, 1950.

68. **Lennette, E. H. and Welsh, H. H.,** Q fever in California. X. Recovery of *Coxiella burneti* from the air of premises harboring goats, *Am. J. Hyg.,* 54, 44, 1951.

69. **Stoenner, H. G.,** Observations on the epizootiology of bovine Q fever, in *Proc. XV Int. Congr. Vet. Med.,* 1953, 291.

70. **Stoenner, H. G.,** The role of the milking process in the intraherd transmission of Q fever among dairy cattle, *Am. J. Vet. Res.,* 13, 458, 1952.

71. **Bell, J. A., Beck, M. D., and Huebner, R. J.,** Epidemiologic studies of Q fever in southern California, *JAMA,* 142, 808, 1950.

72. **Clark, W. H., Romer, M. S., Holmes, M. A., Welsh, H., Lennette, E. H., and Abinanti, F.,** Q fever in California. VIII. An epidemic of Q fever in a small rural community in northern California, *Am. J. Hyg.,* 54, 25, 1951.

73. **Marmion, B. P., Stoker, M. G. P., McCoy, J. H., Malloch, R. A., and Moore, B.,** Q fever in Great Britain. An analysis of 69 sporadic cases, with a study of the prevalence of infections in humans and cows, *Lancet,* 1, 503, 1953.

74. **Bensen, W. W., Brock, D., and Mather, J.,** Serologic analysis of a penitentiary group using raw milk from a Q fever infected herd, *Public Health Rep.,* 78, 707, 1963.

75. **Beck, M. D., Bell, J. A., Shaw, E. W., and Huebner, R. J.,** Q fever studies in southern California. II. An epidemiological study of 300 cases, *Public Health Rep.,* 64, 41, 1959.

76. **Communicable Diseases Center,** A Guide to the Performance of the Standardized Diagnostic Complement Fixation Method and Adaptation to Micro Test, 1st ed., U.S. Department of Health, Education, and Welfare, Public Health Service, Atlanta, July 1969.

77. Lennette, E. H., Clark, W. H., Jensen, F. W., and Toomb, C. J., Q fever studies. XV. Development and persistence of complement-fixing and agglutinating antibodies to *Coxiella burnetii, J. Immunol.*, 68, 591, 1952.

78. Fiset, P., Ormsbee, R. A., Silverman, R., Peacock, M., and Spielman, S. H., A microagglutination technique for detection and measurement of rickettsial antibodies, *Acta Virol.*, 13, 60, 1969.

79. Luoto, L., A capillary-tube test for antibody against *Coxiella burnetii* in human, guinea pig, and sheep sera, *J. Immunol.*, 77, 294, 1956.

80. Tabert, G. G. and Lackman, D. B., The radioistope precipitation test for study of Q fever antibodies in human and animal sera, *J. Immunol.*, 94, 959, 1965.

81. Lackman, D. B., Bell, J. F., Larson, C. L., Casey, M. L., and Benson, W. W., An intradermal sensitivity test for Q fever in man, *Arch. Inst. Pasteur Tunis*, 36, 557, 1959.

82. Luoto, L. and Mason, D. M., An agglutination test for bovine Q fever performed on milk samples, *J. Immunol.*, 74, 222, 1955.

83. Clark, W. H., Lennette, E. H., and Meiklejohn, G., Q fever in California. III. Aureomycin, in the therapy of Q fever, *Arch. Intern. Med.*, 87, 204, 1951.

84. Ormsbee, R. A., Parker, H., and Pickens, E. G., The comparative effectiveness of aureomycin, terramycin, chloramphenicol, erythromycin, and thiocymetin in suppressing experimental rickettsial infections in chick embryos, *J. Infect. Dis.*, 96, 162, 1955.

85. Luoto, L., Winn, J. F., and Huebner, R. T., Q fever studies in southern California. XIII. Vaccination of dairy cattle against Q fever, *Am. J. Hyg.*, 55, 190, 1952.

86. Biberstein, E. L., Reimann, H. P., Franti, C. E., Behymer, D. E., Rippanner, R., Bushness, R., and Crenshaw, G., Vaccination of dairy cattle against Q fever *(Coxiella burnetti)*: results of field trials, *Am. J. Vet. Res.*, 38(2), 189, 1977.

87. Enright, J. B., Sadler, W. W., and Thomas, R. C., Thermal inactivation of *Coxiella burnetii* and its relation to pasteurization of milk, Public Health Service Monograph 47, U.S. Government Printing Office, Washington, D.C., 1957.

88. Luoto, L., Bell, J. F., Casey, M., and Lackman, D. B., Q fever vaccination of human volunteers. I. The serologic and skin-test response following subcutaneous injections, *Am. J. Hyg.*, 78, 1, 1963.

89. Meiklejohn, G. and Lennette, E. H., Q fever in California. I. Observations on vaccinations of human beings, *Am. J. Hyg.*, 52, 54, 1960.

ADDENDUM

After this chapter was prepared, an outbreak of abortion in a herd of dairy goats in Idaho was tentatively shown to be due to *Coxiella burnetii*. Of 33 mature does, 20 aborted during February and March 1976. Masses of organisms, comparable to the number seen in yolk sac cultures, were observed in placenta smears stained by Stamp's modified Ziehl-Neelsen method. The organism was subsequently isolated and identified as *C. burnetii*. *Leptospira, Toxoplasma gondii, Campylobacter (Vibrio) fetus, Brucella* spp., and other bacteria associated with abortion in livestock were excluded as the cause of these abortions on the basis of appropriate microbiologic cultures and/ or serologic tests.*

In the spring of 1979, four cases of Q fever (one fatality) were diagnosed among staff, students, and employees of a western U.S. medical school in which sheep in late pregnancy were used in experimental surgery, pharmacology, and physiology programs. Epidemiologic studies revealed a surprising number of additional cases among persons occupying the same building, but not involved in the work. The hazards of introducing pregnant sheep into such a setting are obvious. Many of these sheep parturated or aborted within several weeks after surgery and released large numbers of *C. burnetti* into the air circulated throughout the buildings. Ideally, Q fever-free sheep should be used for this work, and it should be possible to protect sheep by vaccination; however, the methodology for developing and maintaing Q fever-free flocks has not been established. Until Q fever-free sources of sheep are available, research personnel should be advised of the hazard, and such research should be conducted in containment facilities that will restrict the agent to the immediate work area.

EDITORIAL COMMENT**

It was only during World War II and the years following that Q fever showed its vast and unsuspected diffusion and was revealed as a health problem of the first order, for both human and veterinary medicine.

In 1941 and *de novo* in 1943 and 1944, numerous epidemics of a febrile disease characterized by pulmonary localization appeared among German occupation forces stationed in southern Italy, Corsica, Yugoslavia, Greece, the Ukraine, Crimea, and Bulgaria. The German military doctors reported the sickness (that they called *balkangrippe* without realizing its etiology. A strange feature was that, in Athens, a high percentage of the German troops contracted the disease, while not only the Greek civilians but also the Italian occupation troops remained relatively unaffected. During this last epidemic, an Athenian doctor, Caminopetros, succeeded in transmitting the disease from man to guinea pig and then successively from animal to animal without isolating the actual agent. The infection was maintained by serial passage until, at the end of the war, Caminopetros, in collaboration with American bacteriologists, was able to identify the infection as Q fever. At the same time in Germany, Herzberg, in collaboration with Imhaeuser, isolated and identified the agent of *balkangrippe* from both a Greek patient and a sample of blood from Italy. It must be noted that by 1942

---

*   Waldhalm, D. G., Stoenner, H. G., Simmons, R. E., and Thomas, L. A., Abortion associated with *Coxiella burnetii* infection in dairy goats, *J. Am. Vet. Med. Assoc.*, 173, 1580, 1978.

** For an excellent review of Q fever beginning with its history, geographical distribution, and appearance as a war-time disease, see Babudieri, B., Q fever: a zoonoses, in *Advances in Veterinary Sciences*, Vol. 5, Brandly, C. A. and Jungherr, E. L., Eds., Academic Press, New York, 1959, 81. Material used with permission of the publisher.

Haemig and Heyden had reported an epidemic of atypical pneumonia, that was most likely due to *C. burnetii* among a battalion of troops in Switzerland.

Another epidemic outbreak of Q fever appeared during the years 1944 and 1945 among American and British soldiers stationed in Italy, Corsica, and Greece. Moreover, there were outbreaks among troops who had left southern Italy and were traveling to the U.S. and, eventually, at Fort Bragg and Camp Patrick Henry among the personnel of laboratories in which the disease had been studied. A special commission of American doctors — the Commission on Acute Respiratory Diseases — was, therefore, set up. They identified the nature of the disease, isolated strains of *C. burnetii*, and pursued a series of interesting epidemiologic and serologic studies. This provided a clear picture of the clinical characteristics of the disease and its epidemiologic behavior.

In southern Europe, the disease raged among the troops of both Germany and the Allies, but most likely some civilians were also attacked although only in sporadic cases. In fact, Robbins and his colleagues confirmed the presence of antibodies to *C. burnetii* in the blood of civilians tested at Pagliana (central Italy) where the disease had appeared in epidemic form among American soldiers. In 1945, Bazzicalupo described a case of Q fever in an Italian civilian who had contact with Americans. Caminopetros again reported cases of the disease among the civilian population in Greece.

With the end of the war and repatriation of the majority of the Allied troops from southern Europe, the disease seemed to disappear from the continent. Therefore, the legend spread in Italy and the Balkans that Q fever must have been imported by the Americans or Australians and, hence, was linked with their presence. For 2 years before the end of 1947, there was no report of Q fever in Europe. The new epidemic cycle began almost at the same time in Italy and southern Germany in the winter of 1947. In contrast to what had been observed before, the disease spread not only in the Italian rural regions but also attacked the population of a major city, Florence. At this time there were two epidemic waves: the first from December 1947 to March 1948 and the second during May 1948. The disease was usually diagnosed as "atypical pneumonia." It was only 2 years later that Babudieri, by testing the sera of 15 individuals who had been ill, demonstrated that Q fever was involved. There were also three more epidemic waves of Q fever in Palermo.

In Germany, the epidemic struck the region of Tubingen, Wurttemberg. From November 1947 until May 1948, there were 2000 confirmed cases of the disease although the number of persons attacked must certainly have been much greater. Numerous other foci appeared in 1949; in 1950 and 1951, they appeared in central Italy, Germany, Eifel, Baden, and southern Bavaria. It was calculated that in Italy about 20,000 cases of the disease occurred within 2 years.

In addition to Italy and Germany, the Balkans, Switzerland, and Israel were attacked. In Switzerland, Wiesmann alone confirmed more than 1000 cases serologically. On the other hand, only a few cases were found in France, England, and Turkey.

Southern Europe, however, did become safe again. The European epidemic wave stopped at almost the same time throughout all of the countries considered during the summer of 1951. In the following years, only small, limited outbreaks were reported, and of these, perhaps one of the most important was that at Sanguinetto in northern Italy. Here, more than 100 persons became ill. In the winter of 1954-1955, there were some clearly defined outbreaks in both Italy and Switzerland.

A new outburst of the disease occurred during the spring of 1958. Many epidemic foci reapeared, particularly in central Italy, and especially in the same places that had suffered from the 1949-1951 epidemic.

During the 1950s, the disease was reported in numerous countries in Africa, but probably the largest outbreaks were among the French troops in North and West Africa. After reorganization of African governments, the disease seemed to disappear.

The most interesting outbreak of recent years was the appearance of Q fever in Cyprus. There had been reports of positive serology as early as 1955. At that time, it was estimated that 68% of the cattle, 40% of the sheep, and 35% of the goats were positive. In 1976, during the displacement of large numbers of persons and introduction of English and Swedish troops to preserve the peace, the disease appeared in epidemic form among the soldiers. A detailed report of this was recently prepared by Alan Spicer and colleagues.

It appears that Q fever is an opportunistic disease that occurs when there is an upheaval in a stable population.

RICKETTSIOSES OF DOMESTIC ANIMALS NOT TRANSMISSIBLE TO MAN

H. G. Stoenner

Most of the rickettsial agents considered in this volume are typically zoonotic be-cause they are maintained naturally in a variety of complex ecosystems, and man be-comes an accidental host when he intrudes into the cycle. In many cases, the animals involved in maintaining cycles of infections are not adversely affected, probably be-cause of the delicate host-parasite relationships that have existed for centuries. How-ever, a number of rickettsial agents cause disease in domestic animals and are not known to affect or even infect man. Brief descriptions of seven of these diseases — heartwater, tick-borne fever, benign ovine and bovine rickettsiosis, canine ehrlichiosis, equine ehrlichiosis, contagious ophthalmia, and salmon poisoning — are provided for comparative purposes. The causative agents of these diseases are immunologically dis-tinct, have a limited host range, do not multiply in fertile hen eggs, and with the excep-tion of *Cowdria ruminatium* and *Ehrlichia phagocytophila* do not cause disease or infection in small laboratory animals. *C. ruminantium*, like *Rickettsia rickettsii*, causes extensive endothelial damage. The agents of tick-borne fever, benign rickettsiosis of sheep and cattle, ehrlichiosis of dogs, and ehrlichiosis of horses invade circulating leu-kocytes. In tick-borne fever and ehrlichiosis of horses, granulocytes are affected, whereas in the other two diseases, lymphocytes and monocytes are affected. *Neorick-ettsia helminthoeca*, the cause of salmon poisoning of dogs, principally invades lymph-oid tissue, and *Colesiota conjunctivae* is limited to the conjunctival epithelium of af-fected animals. The classification of some of these organisms (*C. conjunctivae, E. bovis,* and *E. ovina*) as rickettsiae is tenuous because they have not been thoroughly characterized by modern methods of microbiology and immunology.

HEARTWATER

Heartwater, a tick-transmitted infectious disease of cattle, sheep, and goats, occurs in East and South Africa and the Sudan. Many species of wild ungulates also are susceptible, but most infections are clinically mild or silent. *Cowdria ruminantium,* the causative agent, is chiefly transmitted by *Amblyomma hebraeum* and other *Am-blyomma* species. The organism grows so profusely in vascular endothelium that the lumena of capillaries may be occluded by swollen cells. The severity of disease varies from a mild abortive form to a peracute type characterized by high fever, progressive signs of encephalitis, and sudden death. The organism is most readily demonstrated in "squash smears" of cerebral grey matter stained with Giemsa stain. The dark blue rickettsiae (0.3 μm diameter) are found in the cytoplasm of endothelial cells lining small capillaries.

TICK-BORNE FEVER

Tick-borne fever of sheep and cattle occurs in Great Britain, Norway, Finland, the Netherlands, and India. The disease is characterized by protracted fever with relapses, extensive weight loss, reduced milk production, and abortion. Strains naturally affect-ing sheep differ from those found in cattle. Cross-infections occur, but the disease is milder than that in the natural host. The etiologic agent, *Ehrlichia phagocytophila*, is transmitted by *Ixodes ricinus*. The organism parasitizes granulocytes, of which 50% may be infected during the peak rickettsemia. In Giemsa-stained blood smears, three types of organisms are seen. The smallest (0.5 μm diameter) is a deep purple coccoid- or rod-shaped body near the periphery of the cell. The second type is a larger (1.3 × 2 μm), homogeneously stained body situated more centrally in the cell. The third type appears as a morula containing a number of more deeply stained, distinct bodies.

BENIGN BOVINE AND OVINE RICKETTSIOSIS

This disease occurs in North and South Africa. *Ehrlichia bovis,* the agent causing the disease in cattle, is transmitted by *Hyalomma* species, whereas that affecting sheep, *E. ovina,* is transmitted by *Rhipicephalus bursa.* Available reports mention little information about the clinical disease other than irregular fever of several weeks duration and low mortality. The rickettsiae are found chiefly in circulating monocytes and in cells (monocytes?) of the lung, liver, and spleen, especially the lung. Organisms are usually assembled in round colonies 2 to 10 μm in diameter and may contain closely packed granules 0.5 to 1.0 μm in diameter. Tinctorially, the agent is similar to *E. phagocytophila,* but the percentage of monocytes that contain rickettsiae is much lower.

CANINE EHRLICHIOSIS (TROPICAL CANINE PANCYTOPENIA)

Ehrlichia canis that is transmitted by *Rhipicephalus sanguineus* occurs in India, many countries of Southeast Asia and Africa, and the U.S. Ehrlichiosis that is uncomplicated by concurrent infection with *Babesia* or *Hepatozoon* is a relatively mild disease except in young puppies, in which the disease may be fatal. It is characterized by recurrent fever, a subclinical phase, and a terminal phase marked by profound anemia, emaciation, pancytopenia, thrombocytopenia, and epistaxis. Disease resulting from concurrent infection with *Babesia* or *Hepatozoon* is more severe because of the destruction of erythrocytes by these agents. The organisms parasitize monocytes and lymphocytes; those in monocytes are usually small, acidophilic, single-unit inclusions, whereas most basophilic morulae, consisting of aggregates of small bodies, are found in lymphocytes.

EQUINE EHRLICHIOSIS

This recently discovered disease has been recognized only in California. Although the taxonomic position of the agent has not been established, it is tentatively identified as *Ehrlichia equi. Dermacentor occidentalis* and *D. albipictus* parasitize horses in California, but neither has been shown to be the vector. The disease in horses is characterized by fever, anorexia, depression, edema of the legs, ataxia, leukopenia, and thrombocytopenia. Like *E. phagocytophila,* the agent principally parasitizes neutrophils, and it is morphologically and tinctorially similar to this organism.

CONTAGIOUS OPHTHALMIA

This disease, caused by *Colesiota conjunctivae,* occurs principally among sheep in Africa, Australia, New Zealand, Europe, and North and South America. This organism or similar ones have been associated with conjunctivitis in goats, cattle, swine, and chickens. Flies transmit the organism mechanically. During the initial acute phase, photophobia, purulent discharge, and inflammation and congestion of the conjunctiva are prominent signs. Most animals recover within 1 or 2 weeks, but severe cases may be complicated by keratitis and vascularization and ulceration of the cornea. In smears prepared from conjunctival scrapings of affected animals and stained with Giemsa stain, inclusions resembling those of the psittacosis group are found in the cytoplasm of epithelial cells. The organisms are small, ovoid or short, rod-shaped (0.3 × 0.5 μm) and stain a uniform purplish-red color.

SALMON POISONING

This highly fatal, febrile disease of dogs and other canines occurs in the northwestern U.S. within the geographic distribution of *Goniobasis plicifera silicula*, a snail that is the intermediate host of the vector fluke, *Nanophyetes salmincola*. Dogs contract the disease by ingesting trout or salmon containing encysted metacercariae of the fluke. Initial signs of the disease in dogs are high fever, depression, and inappetence. As the disease progresses, it is characterized by edematous eyelids, rapid weight loss, vomiting, and diarrhea with blood-tinged feces. As death approaches, the temperature becomes subnormal. Diagnosis is most readily confirmed by demonstrating the organism in a lymph node biopsy made during the febrile period. In smears treated with Giemsa stain, purple-stained coccoid bodies (0.3 μm) are scattered or arranged in compact plaques in the cytoplasm of reticular cells and macrophages.

REFERENCES

1. **Henning, M. W.**, *Animal Diseases in South Africa*, 3rd ed., Central News Agency, South Africa, 1956.
2. **Neitz, W. O.**, A consolidation of our knowledge of the transmission of tick-borne diseases, *Onderstepoort J. Vet. Res.*, 27, 115, 1956.
3. **Tuomi, J.**, Studies in epidemiology of bovine tick-borne fever in Finland and a clinical description of field cases, *Ann. Med. Exp. Biol. Fenn.*, 44 (Suppl. 6), 62, 1966.
4. **Tuomi, J.**, Experimental studies on bovine tick-borne fever. IV. Immunofluorescent staining of the agent and demonstration of antigenic relationship between strains, *Acta Pathol. Microbiol. Scand.*, 71, 101, 1967.
5. **Donatien, A. and Lestoquard, F.**, Etat actuel des connaissances sur les rickettsioses animales, *Arch. Inst. Pasteur Alger.*, 15, 142, 1937.
6. **Ewing, S. A.**, Canine ehrlichiosis, in *Advances in Veterinary Science and Comparative Medicine*, Vol. 13, Brandly, C. A. and Cornelius, C. E., Eds., Academic Press, New York, 1969, 331.
7. **Huxsall, D. L., Hildebrandt, P. K., Nims, R. M., and Walker, J. S.**, Tropical canine pancytopenia, *J. Am. Vet. Med. Assoc.*, 157, 1627, 1970.
8. **Gribble, D. H.**, Equine ehrlichiosis, *J. Am. Vet. Med. Assoc.*, 155, 462, 1969.
9. **Beveridge, W. I. B.**, Investigations of contagious ophthalmia of sheep with special attention to the epidemiology of infection by *Rickettsiae conjunctivae*, *Aust. Vet. J.*, 18, 155, 1942.
10. **Dickinson, L. and Cooper, B. S.**, Contagious conjunctivo-keratitis of sheep, *J. Pathol. Bacteriol.*, 78, 257, 1959.
11. **Cordy, D. R. and Gorham, J. R.**, The pathology and etiology of salmon disease in the dog and fox, *Am. J. Pathol.*, 26, 617, 1950.
12. **Philip, C. B., Hadlow, W. J., and Hughes, L. E.**, Studies on salmon poisoning disease of canines. I. The rickettsial relationships and pathogenicity of *Neorickettsia helmintheca*, *Exp. Parasitol.*, 3, 336, 1954.

CHLAMYDIOSIS

A. K. Eugster

INTRODUCTION

Chlamydiae are a group of unique infectious agents; being neither viruses nor bacteria, they represent an intermediate link between the two. Moulder,[1] analyzing the basic biology of chlamydial agents, concluded: "There is an unbridgable gap between viruses and other infectious agents, and this discontinuity is reflected not only in fundamental differences in the biology and chemistry of the agents (chlamydiae) themselves but also in the epidemiology, pathogenesis, and therapy of the disease they produce." This concept, a logical one from an evolutionary standpoint, has led and will continue to lead to unique discoveries of host-parasite interactions in chlamydial infections.

Chlamydiae successfully parasitize a wide variety of hosts including at least 17 mammalian[2] and 130 avian species[3] in many different geographic locations. Diversity is seen, too, in the types of transmission that occur, including inhalation, ingestion, sexual contact, and arthropods. Besides their obvious high adaptability, chlamydiae are also capable of inducing clinically inapparent infections in normal hosts, thus ensuring a large number of carriers. When in such a situation, the delicate host-parasite balance shifts in favor of the parasite due to stress of the host, inapparent infection changes to overt symptoms. The wide host range, high adaptability, and carrier state of chlamydiae are important parameters to be considered in transmission studies and in establishing control measures for these infections.

TAXONOMY

The word "chlamydia" is of Greek origin (chlamys — χλαμυσ) meaning mantle or cloak. It is derived from the term chlamydozoa, originally used in 1912 by Halberstädter[4] to describe intracytoplasmic bodies in conjunctival cells of trachoma patients. Since these organisms are obviously not protozoa, the term chlamydozoa (ζωα — animal) was changed to chlamydia. The genus name *Chlamydia*, under the family name of Chlamydaceae, was first proposed by Jones et al.[5] Taxonomic classification of these organisms has been in a state of scientific controversy until recently. The underlying cause that has plagued microbiologists is the fact that chlamydiae represent a unique infectious entity not readily identified as either viruses or bacteria.

The main differences separating viruses from chlamydiae are that the latter contain both RNA and DNA, are susceptible to sulfonamides and certain antibiotics that inhibit prokaryotic multiplication, and contain their own 70S ribosomes. Chlamydiae differ from common bacteria principally in that they are obligate intracellular parasites and undergo a noninfectious phase during the developmental cycle.

On the infinite scale of life forms, chlamydiae occupy a space somewhere between bacteria and viruses and are at least somewhat morphologically and tinctorially similar to rickettsia. However, the inability of chlamydiae to synthesize ATP and the noninfectiousness of their dividing daughter cells are distinctive characteristics not found in rickettsia.

Page[6] argued for unification of all different human, animal, and avian chlamydial strains into the single genus *Chlamydia*. This concept was supported by the Subcommittee on Chlamydiaceae of the Taxonomy Committee of the American Society for

Table 1
TAXONOMY OF
CHLAMYDIA[7]

Order I
  Rickettsiales
Order II
  Chlamydiales
    Family I
      Chlamydiaceae
        Genus I
          Chlamydia
            Species I
              C. trachomatis
            Species II
              C. psittaci

Microbiology and resulted in its acceptance and inclusion in the recent seventh and eighth editions of *Bergey's Manual of Determinative Bacteriology.*[7] Chlamydiae are placed into Order II that is considered a coordinate with Order I, the Rickettsiales (Table 1).

The principal difference between the two species is that *C. trachomatis,* unlike *C. psittaci,* induces compact cytoplasmic inclusions containing glycogen that can be stained with iodine solutions.[8] Lin and Moulder[9] observed another major difference between the two species — replication of *C. trachomatis* is inhibited by sodium sulfadiazine and that of *C. psittaci* is not.

Those attempting a literature survey should be aware that chlamydia can be listed under the following names, synonyms, or colloquial terms even in recent literature: psittacosis, ornithosis, Levinthal-Coles-Lillie (L.C.L.) bodies, miyagawanella, rickettsiaformis, prowazekia, bedsonia, rakeia, chlamydozoaceae, colesiota, ricolesia, and the psittacosis-trachoma-lymphogranuloma-venereum group of agents.

MORPHOLOGY AND MULTIPLICATION OF CHLAMYDIA

The infectious form of chlamydia, called elementary body, has a diameter of 200 to 300 nm. Viewed under the electron microscope, these particles are spherical (Figures 1 and 2) and on thin sections they reveal an electron-dense homogeneous nucleoid. Ribosome-like structures can be seen in the less dense peripheral material. The particle is surrounded by a trilaminar outer membrane (Figure 3). Jenkins[10] in studying isolated and purified chlamydial-limiting membranes found them to be relatively rigid, morphologically complex, and similar in appearance to bacterial cell walls.

During the developmental cycle, the following forms appear (in chronological order): dispersing forms (also called initial bodies), reticulate bodies, and condensing forms (also known as intermediate forms). Dispersing forms are round or ovoid and measure from 400 to 500 nm in diameter. Reticulate bodies arising from dispersing forms are dividing, pleomorphic, noninfectious forms with a diameter of 500 to 1200 nm (Figures 4 and 5). They are bound by a distinct outer and poorly defined inner trilaminar membrane.[11] Reticulate bodies reorganize through condensing forms into the infectious elementary bodies. Condensing forms have a diameter of 300 to 500 nm, a central nucleoid mass surrounded by a granulo-fibrillar matrix, and are bound by a trilaminar membrane.[12]

The developmental cycle of chlamydiae has long been one of their most interesting aspects and has been studied extensively. Recent electron microscopic and biochemical

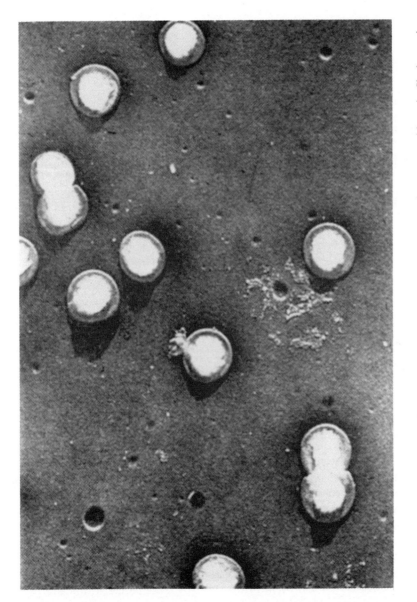

FIGURE 1.   Dense-centered chlamydial forms (elementary bodies) of the mouse meningopneumonitis strain. Shadowcasting. Diameter: 250 nm. (From Tamura, A. and Higashi, N., *Virology*, 20, 596, 1963. With permission.)

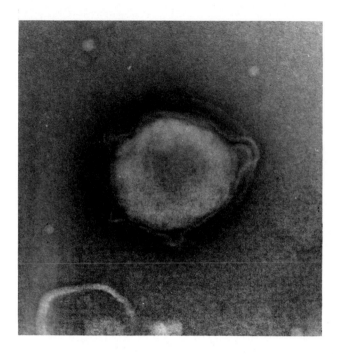

FIGURE 2. Chlamydial elementary body negatively stained; unstained nucleoid, distinct (trilaminar) outer membrane with protrusions. Diameter: 280 nm.

investigations by several researchers have led to a better understanding of the sequence of events in the growth cycle. The small infectious form, commonly called an elementary body, attaches to the cell membrane. Recent work implies that the attachment may be dependent upon specific receptors and certain surface functions of the host-cell membrane. Adsorbtion can be prevented by pretreatment of the host cells with neuraminidase and trypsin.[13,14] At the attachment site, the elementary body is engulfed in an invagination formed by the cell membrane through a process of endocytosis. In susceptible cells, elementary bodies become adsorbed to the host cell within 2 hr after inoculation. At 5 hr, they may be seen at various depths in the cytoplasm, still enclosed in the vacuole that was formed during the host-cell membrane invagination process.[15,16] The invading elementary body then undergoes an internal reorganization within this vacuole. The resulting particle (dispersing form) is larger and has an electron-dense filamentous matrix with ribosome-like particles. Transition of dispersing forms to reticulate bodies concurs with the first division. These large reticulate bodies are pleomorphic and noninfectious; they divide by binary fission without septation, and 20 hr after inoculation the vacuole contains almost exclusively reticulate bodies. At this time, host-cell DNA synthesis and, subsequently, RNA and protein synthesis cease.[17,18] The exact mechanism by which this is accomplished is unknown. Lin,[19] using protein synthesis inhibitors, concluded that a protein synthesized by chlamydiae within the first 10 hr after inoculation is responsible for inhibition of host-cell macromolecular synthesis. Furthermore, he postulated that this was accomplished by preventing the host cell from initiating a new cycle. This apparently occurs during the G-1 phase of the host-cell cycle, obviously an opportune time for a parasite to exploit the host since during the end of the G-1 phase many precursors for host-cell macromolecular synthesis are present.[18] Therefore, arresting the host cell in the G-1 phase gives the chlamydial agent immediate access to material for its own biosynthesis.

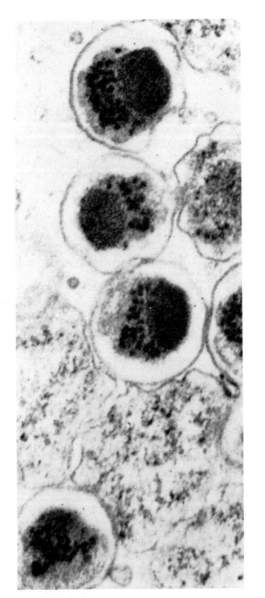

FIGURE 3.   Cross-section of chlamydial elementary bodies. Electron-dense eccentric nucleoid and ribosomes in the cytoplasmic tag. Diameter: 250 nm. (From Anderson, D. R., Hopps, H. E., Barile, M. F., and Bernheim, B. C., *J. Bacteriol.*, 90, 1387, 1965. With permission.)

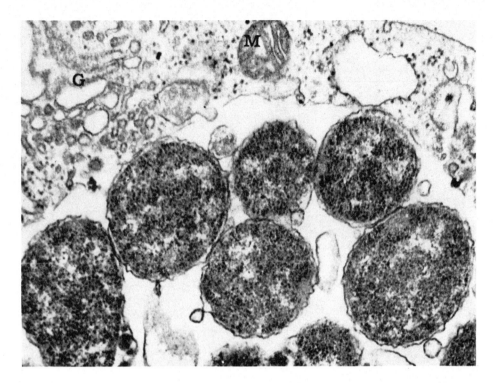

FIGURE 4.   Dispersing chlamydial forms ("initial bodies") within a membrane-bound vacuole of the host cell. Diameter: 600 nm. (From Anderson, D. R., Hopps, H. E., Barile, M. F., and Bernheim, B. C., *J. Bacteriol.*, 90, 1387, 1965. With permission.)

In the second phase of reorganization of chlamydial forms, division of the large reticulate bodies ceases and they become smaller and more spherical. Transition to condensing forms is marked by condensing of the fibrillar matrix and formation of a centrally located nucleoid. This process is asynchronous—some large reticulate bodies are still dividing as emerging elementary bodies are released from the cytoplasmic inclusions into the extracellular environment, capable and ready to infect other cells. The time lapse from inoculation to release of infectious elementary bodies is about 35 to 40 min. A schematic drawing by Storz[2] of the chlamydial developmental growth cycle is presented in Figure 6.

INACTIVATION AND EFFECT OF ANTIMICROBIAL DRUGS ON CHLAMYDIAE

Chlamydiae become easily inactivated at higher temperatures, but they retain their infectivity for years at low temperatures. The rate of heat inactivation differs between different chlamydial isolates. Page,[20] for example, found a pigeon chlamydial isolate that retained its infectivity during a 24-hr incubation at 43°C while a turkey isolate lost its infectivity during this time. Exact heat-inactivation temperatures for all chlamydial isolates is unknown. The old claim that heating at 70°C for 10 min destroys infectivity still holds true; however, some isolates can be destroyed at lower temperatures. Chlamydial agents can be preserved by freezing. Gradual loss of infectivity of a turkey isolate occurred over a span of 400 days at −20°C, and diseased turkeys frozen

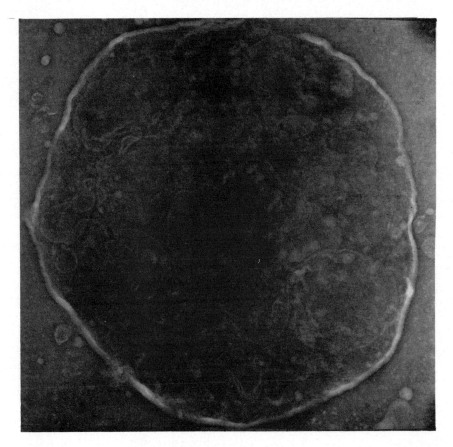

FIGURE 5.   Noninfectious chlamydial reticulate body; negatively stained. Diameter: 1200 nm.

in processing plants retained viable chlamydial agents after 1 year of storage at −20°C.[21] Infectivity is best preserved by suspending the agents in a buffer containing 0.4 M sucrose and 0.02 M sodium phosphate at a pH of 7.0 to 7.4.[22]

At −70°C or in the lyophilized state, chlamydial agents retain their infectivity almost indefinitely. A 0.1% formalin solution or a 0.5% phenol solution inactivates chlamydial agents within 24 to 36 hr. Ether or ethanol at room temperature destroys infectivity within 30 min. The pH range wherein chlamydiae can survive is narrow (7 to 8), and alterations to either side result in gradual destruction of viability.

Proper concentration of disinfectants, such as quartenary ammonium salts, chlorine, iodine, and permanganate solutions, has been shown to inactivate certain chlamydial isolates within 1 to 30 min.[23] However, chlamydial infectivity was preserved for several days in tap and swimming pool water.

The effect of antimicrobial drugs on multiplication of chlamydial agents is quite varied. One of the characteristics used to differentiate between the two chlamydial species is their susceptibility to sulfonamides. *C. trachomatis*, which synthesizes folic acid from para-aminobenzoic acid, is sensitive to sulfadiazine. On the other hand, members of the species *C. psittaci* utilize host-cell folic acid precursors and are, therefore, sulfonamide resistant.[8,9]

Members of both chlamydial species are sensitive to penicillin (avian isolates to a lesser degree than mammalian agents). Penicillin is thought to inhibit bacterial growth by preventing transpeptidation of peptides linking *N*-acetylglucosamine and *N*-acetylmuramic acid in the bacterial cell wall. Bacteria multiplying in the presence of penicillin

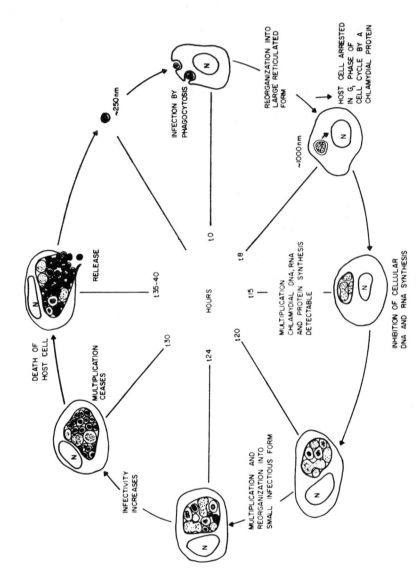

FIGURE 6.   Schematic representation of the developmental cycle of chlamydial agents. (From Storz, J., *Chlamydia and Chlamydia-Induced Diseases*, courtesy of Charles C Thomas, Springfield, Ill., 1971. With permission.)

produce defective cell walls and spheroblasts may be formed. A similar phenomena was noted with chlamydiae grown in the presence of penicillin in developing chick embryos.[24,25] Large aberrant chlamydial forms that resumed normal shape and multiplication after removal of penicillin were produced. Similar to common bacteria, chlamydiae have also been shown to become penicillin resistant.[26] Whether these observations indicate that chlamydial walls do or do not contain muramic acid has not been settled.

Tetracyclines are the most effective inhibitors of chlamydial multiplication and are the drugs of choice in treatment of almost all chlamydial infections, especially psittacosis. They inhibit protein synthesis by preventing attachment of transfer RNA to 30S ribosomes. One of the first chlamydial proteins synthesized is the one that arrests the host-cell cycle in the G-1 phase;[19] it is most likely at this point when tetracyclines act first in inhibiting chlamydial multiplication. Resistant strains have been recovered in the laboratory from tetracycline-treated chick embryos.[27] However, to date, this has not been a problem in the field despite extensive use of prophylactic tetracyclines in avian species. Chlamydiae are also sensitive to tylosin, erythromycin, actinomycin D, and antimetabolites such as halogenated uridines.[28,29]

Many antimicrobial drugs, however, do not interfere with chlamydial multiplication. In the laboratory, these are of great advantage in controlling contamination of various bacteria and fungi in clinical specimens and rendering them suitable for isolation procedures. The most commonly used drugs in this regard are streptomycin, Vancomycin®, and Mycostatin®. These are not known to affect the multiplication of any chlamydial agents.[29]

ZOONOTIC HUMAN CHLAMYDIAL INFECTION (PSITTACOSIS)

Psittacosis is the term commonly used to describe generalized chlamydial infections of man and psittacine birds. Ornithosis is the term applied to the same infection in avian species other than psittacines.

Etiological Agent
The etiological agent is *Chlamydia psittaci.*

Host Spectrum
The primary hosts for these chlamydial strains are numerous avian species. In a literature survey, Meyer[3] found chlamydial infection described in 130 avian species belonging to ten different orders. Of the 130 species, 57 belonged to the parrot family. In fact, from 1874 — when Juergensen[30] was said to have first described the disease as a clinical entity in Europe — til 1938, parrots were the only avian family incriminated as a chlamydial reservoir responsible for outbreaks in humans. Large birds were the source of the pandemics of psittacosis in 1929 and 1930.

A new dimension was added in 1939 when Rasmussen[31] and Haagen and Mauer[32] described 174 human pneumonia cases in the Faroe Islands as psittacosis. This epidemic represented the first recorded example of a chlamydiosis as an occupational disease; it was contracted by persons processing young fulmar petrels for food.

Other investigators[33-36] subsequently found evidence of chlamydial infections by either isolation or presence of antibodies in 13 other species of seashore birds (sea gull, laughing gull, herring gull, lesser black gull, willet, snowy egret, skimmer, sauderling, least tern, common tern, royal tern, gull-billed tern, and glossy ibis).

In 1940, Coles[37] first reported the occurence of chlamydial infections in pigeons in South Africa. This infection was soon incriminated as a public health hazard by Meyer et al.[38] who isolated the chlamydial agent from a flock of racing pigeons and the lung of a woman who died of pneumonia after exposure to these same birds.

The first chlamydial isolation from poultry was made in 1939[39] when the agent was isolated from a flock of white leghorn chickens. A serological diagnosis of chlamydiosis was made in a patient with atypical pneumonia who tended this flock. Chlamydial infections in ducks and their human contacts were first recorded in the U.S. in 1952,[40] and serious economic losses due to chlamydial infections on duck farms were reported from eastern Europe,[41] Austria,[42] and Germany.[43] Clinical case descriptions of psittacosis in humans who had contact with turkeys were recorded in Texas as early as 1937.[44] However, the first report of isolation of the agent from diseased turkeys was made fairly recently. Five outbreaks of psittacosis with 96 cases and seven fatalities occurred in two Texas poultry-dressing establishments between 1948 and 1953.[44] An interesting facet of turkey chlamydial isolates is that there appear to be two different types in terms of mouse pathogenicity. One group of isolates of low pathogenicity for mice produces some visceral lesions in turkeys but rarely clinical illness and mortality. Other isolates are highly fatal in the indicator host (mouse) and also produce unusually high mortalities in turkeys as well as in their human contacts.[44,45] The low pathogenicity of some turkey isolates might explain the large reservoir of chlamydiae in certain turkey flocks. Of flocks tested in Minnesota and Wisconsin, 40% showed serological evidence of exposure to chlamydiae. Human infections in poultry workers tending these flocks were only sporadically of a clinical nature and mainly assumed a subclinical form as evidenced by serological screens. Up to 29% of 200 workers examined had significant titers.[46,47]

The continuing source of turkeys for human chlamydial infections is evident from very recent cases in turkey-processing personnel in the U.S. A total of 154 human cases associated with four turkey processing establishments in three states was recorded in 1974.[48]

Pheasants,[49] geese,[42,50] and mutton birds[51] also should be mentioned since chlamydial infections have been reported in these species. However, of the 130 species parasitized by chlamydia, pleasure and show birds, ducks, geese, and turkeys are the most common source of chlamydial infection of man according to Meyer.[3] Ducks and geese appear to play the same public health role in central and eastern Europe[41-43,50,52,53] as turkeys do in the U.S.

A new epidemiological dimension was added when chlamydiae were isolated from arthropods associated with poultry.[54] Isolations were made from Glycyphagidae, Cheyletidae, and Neoparasitidae as well as from shaft lice of poultry (*Menopon gallinae*) and free-living cheyletid mites. Isolations from these arthropods were made on turkey farms where chlamydiosis was enzootic, whereas no isolations were made on turkey farms free of chlamydial infections. There is no evidence that these arthropods are biological vectors; rather, it is thought that they are only mechanical vectors. Nevertheless, their role in transmission of the agent, especially between rodents and other mammals and avian species, has to be considered. The importance of arthropods as vectors and their role in perpetuating chlamydial inter- and intraspecies endemicity requires further investigation.[55]

It is generally agreed that man is an incidental host for *C. psittaci* and avian species are the primary hosts. However, through the years there have been reports of clinical cases in humans who had no obvious contact with sick birds. An example is the 1943 Louisiana outbreak[56] with a total of 19 cases and eight recognized fatalities (to be discussed in greater detail in a later section). The disease spread among contacts, mainly to nurses of patients who had already contracted the disease. The initial fatal case resulted in 18 additional cases. Secondary spread of the disease from person to person, although usually not as extensive as in this outbreak, has always been known. The question here is the source of the initial infection in persons who supposedly had no contact with any cage or barnyard birds. Retrospective studies have implicated the wild American and snowy egrets as possible sources of infection. Risk of exposure existed in these areas — chlamydial agents with characteristics similar to the ones isolated from the human cases were isolated from these birds in 1950.[56]

Distribution

From 1874, when the disease was first recognized as a separate clinical entity by Juergensen,[30] until 1928, illnesses associated with parrots were reported in Switzerland, Germany, France, England, and the U.S.[57] Outbreaks started after arrival of exotic birds from South America. Mortality in the birds during the long transatlantic shipment was high, and survivors were obviously stressed. These factors, together with overcrowding, probably caused increased excretion of chlamydial agents. The Paris epidemic of 1892 started when two French bird dealers imported 500 parrots from Buenos Aires. The dealers became infected, as did the birds' new owners, their friends and relatives, and a physician tending one of the ill persons. All together, 51 persons fell ill during this epidemic and 16 succumbed to the infection.

The pandemic of 1929 and 1930 renewed interest in the etiology of this disease.[57] It may have started in Argentina where more than 100 human cases were reported in a 3-month period. Eventually, about 1000 cases — with 200 to 300 deaths — occurred in various countries. Until 1930, the cause of psittacosis was thought to be *Salmonella typhimurium* ("Nocard's paracolon bacillus"). Almost simultaneously, Levinthal in Germany,[59] Coles in England,[60] and Lillie in the U.S.[61] observed the characteristic elementary bodies in reticuloendothelial cells of affected humans and birds. However, it was Bedson and co-workers in London,[62] using Berkefeld filtrates of infected tissues, who conclusively established the etiology of psittacosis by transmitting the agent from man to parrots and mice.

Prior to 1934, outbreaks of psittacosis were associated with exotic birds imported from various countries in South America. However, in 1934 chlamydial agents were isolated for the first time from parakeets exported from Australia to California.[63] Subsequently, chlamydiae were also isolated from humans in Australia.[64] With better understanding of the etiology, pathogenesis, and diagnosis of the disease, public health laws regulating the importation of psittacine birds became effective in 1930 in many countries. These measures proved quite effective as human cases traceable to psittacine birds almost disappeared in these countries.

However, sporadic cases in humans continued in the face of import restrictions, and this led to a search for and eventual recovery of chlamydial agents from various barnyard poultry species, wild fowl, and parakeets from local breeding establishments. The significance of these avian species as a source of human infection becomes evident upon examination of a tabulation by Meyer.[65] Statistics derived from world literature and his own records (maintained at the George Williams Hooper Foundation, California) revealed that approximately 5390 human cases of psittacosis occurred between 1931 and 1963, including 89 deaths in 28 countries. The sources of the infection in these cases were psittacines, pigeons, ducks, turkeys, chickens ("poultry"), and seashore birds. In recent years, a relatively high level of endemicity of avian chlamydiosis has been reported in Czechoslovakia, East Germany, and Hungary in duck-raising and -processing establishments and in U.S. turkey industries.[65]

The Disease in Avian Species

Avian chlamydiosis is principally an inapparent or latent infection. However, peracute, acute, subacute, and chronic infections do occur in most species. There are no pathognomonic signs or lesions; the signs are those of a systemic disease. In an outbreak of an avian chlamydiosis, mortality is usually highest in young birds. In the adult bird, a subacute or chronic form occurs with intermittent overt signs followed by asymptomatic periods. The incubation period is quite variable and depends upon virulence of the agent, susceptibility and stress of the host, and route of exposure. In psittacine birds, the incubation period is reported to range from 5 to 98 days,[66] while in experimentally exposed turkeys symptoms can be noticed as early as 2 to 4 days and mortalities 8 to 15 days after infection.[67]

Peracute forms or sudden deaths were noted in parakeets.[66] Australian king parrots may also die suddenly due to chlamydiosis; Burnet[68] reported observing them falling from trees and dying within minutes. Rice birds, finches, and canaries also usually die within a short time and without marked ante-mortem signs.[66]

In the acute form, the first signs noted are usually a bilateral conjunctivitis with serous to purulent exudation, nasal discharge, anorexia, weakness, and reluctance to move. Diarrhea is frequently present, and the feces may be yellowish, rust colored, or blood-tinged. As the infection progresses, eyes may become dull and sunken in, corneas may become cloudy, egg production may decrease drastically, and feathers may be lost by some birds. The birds tend to remain in a fixed position and, when forcefully moved, may stagger and show signs of paralysis.[65]

In the subacute form, similar signs are observed although they are not as severe as in the acute form. However, the course of the disease is protracted, and clinical signs may disappear and then reappear within a few days. These birds usually show retardation in growth and cachexia.[65]

While the above-mentioned clinical forms are useful for a description of the course of the disease, they overlap considerably in nature. Many or all of the different forms can usually be seen at the same time in a given chlamydial epornitic, and it is well to remember that the most prevalent form in the majority of cases is asymptomatic or latent infection. These birds are carriers and shedders of chlamydiae, and the perpetuation of the disease depends upon them.

Carrier and shedding states are the principal factors contributing to transmission. Since avian chlamydiosis has persisted for at least one century (and probably many more), is world-wide in distribution, and has a broad host spectrum, one can assume that transmission does not involve many ecological systems and probably occurs by relatively simple means. Nesting habits of many wild birds are conducive to perpetuation of the infection, as are the artificial, crowded confinements of our domesticated poultry.

The principal routes of excretion of chlamydiae are nasal secretions and feces. Transmission, therefore, occurs most frequently by inhalation and ingestion. Additionally, a bird can be artificially infected by intravenous, intracerebral, intra-air sac, intratracheal, intramuscular, and intraperitoneal inoculation.

Eddie and co-workers[55] isolated chlamydiae from nest mites and avian lice. These ectoparasites may play an important role in transmission of the agent from bird to bird as well as from bird to mammal. Congenital transmission of chlamydiae has been suspected, and if it does occur in nature, it is probably a rarity. Further field and laboratory work is needed to ascertain if chlamydiae localize in the ovaries and pass through the egg.[69]

The oral route of transmission may lead to the shedding state more so than does inhalation. Turkeys infected orally showed few and mild clinical signs but excreted chlamydiae in their feces while inhalation produced a higher infectivity rate and mortality.[67]

The pathogenesis of chlamydiosis that occurs after oral administration of the agent has been studied in turkeys.[67] Events in this experiment simulated those that would most likely occur in an epornitic caused by a virulent strain in a crowded aviary or poultry confinement. Turkeys were fed chlamydiae-containing capsules designed to release their content into the gizzard. The organisms were then reisolated only from the jejunum of one bird on the fifth day after inoculation. The birds did not develop significant clinical signs or humoral antibody titers. Chlamydiae were also isolated from droppings on the runway floor. Two weeks after oral exposure, the birds started to develop chlamydemia and signs and lesions identical to those observed in aerosol-exposed birds. It was concluded that chlamydiae-laden droppings from the oral inoculation had dried, become dust, and were subsequently inhaled, thereby causing respiratory and systemic infections.

After aerosol infection occurred, chlamydiae multiplied primarily in the lungs, air sac, and pericardial sac within 24 hr after exposure. At 48 hr after infection, chlamydemia was detected and the agents were present in various somatic organs such as the liver, spleen, and kidney. Chlamydiae were also found in the nasal turbinates and cloacal contents, important portals in terms of further transmission of the organism.[67]

At necropsy, lesions observed are quite similar in all avian species. Variations are caused by factors such as route of exposure, length of illness, and virulence of the agent and/or susceptibility of the host. The respiratory system, especially the air sacs, is frequently involved. Air sacs are thickened with a fibrinous or fibrinopurulent exudate. The same type of exudate is also frequently deposited on other serous membranes such as those of the pericardium, liver, and intestines. Pronounced congestion of the liver and spleen is common. The liver may also be mottled, saffron colored, and occasionally contain small necrotic foci. Splenomegaly with subcapsular hemorrhages is a common lesion, especially in psittacine birds. This is mainly due to congestion and also occasionally to lymphoid hyperplasia. Spleen enlargement can result in a rupture and consequent sudden death. A catarrhal enteritis with yellowish-green feces caused by biliary stasis (as indicated by the enlarged gall bladder) may be noted. The ingesta has a gelatinous or watery consistency.[65,70]

On microscopic examination of tissues, there are principally two changes that are evident. One is a proliferative response seen mostly in birds that are more resistant to the infection or that harbor chlamydiae of low virulence; the second is a necrotizing lesion seen in acutely ill birds. Carrier animals show a proliferative cell response.

Large amounts of hemosiderin are present in the liver and spleen as a result of extensive cell destruction. Proliferation of lymphoid tissue in the periportal region is an early lesion. Interstitial nephritis and enteritis with hyperplasia of lymphoid tissue are sometimes observed. In natural infections of birds, pneumonia is a rarity.[71]

None of the lesions are sufficiently characteristic to allow a firm diagnosis. *Mycoplasma*, *Salmonella*, and other infectious agents may cause similar lesions. However, fibrinous exudates on various serosal surfaces and enlarged and congested somatic organs should certainly arouse enough suspicion to initiate staining of impression smears for elementary bodies and isolation attempts.

It should also be stressed that turkeys, in particular, may show only minimal or no ante-mortem signs, yet they have typical lesions at necropsy or at the slaughter plant.[72]

Disease in Man

Psittacosis (human chlamydiosis contracted from avian species) should always be suspected in a patient with pneumonia who had recent contact with a diseased or dead bird. However, unfortunately for the epidemiologist and diagnostician, clinically normal birds can also shed the organism and be the source of infection, and occasionally there may be no obvious avian source.

The incubation period varies from 1 to 4 weeks. Onset of symptoms may be sudden or produce low-grade fever of 100 to 102°F that gradually increases as the disease progresses and that may remain high in severe cases. Anorexia, sore throat, photophobia, and severe headache are frequently observed signs. In mild cases, the symptoms noted are those of a flu-like syndrome; body temperature is usually back to normal within 1 week.

Physical examination of the thorax may reveal presence of moist rales or nothing abnormal. Radiographs reveal a patchy infiltration in one or both lungs, usually in the lower part of the lobes. In later stages, extensive consolidation may occur. Patterns observed are usually those of a bronchopneumonia; pleuritis is a rare sequela. Cough may be present, but it is not even a consistent sign in patients with extensive lung involvement. Respiration rates are not increased except in fatal cases when they may go as high as 60/min.

Clinical symptomology varies greatly in severe cases. Nausea, vomiting, signs of hepatitis and myocarditis, and diarrhea or constipation may be present. The liver and spleen may become temporarily enlarged, but in most cases the spleen is not palpable. Hemograms vary considerably and are of little diagnostic value. Generally, the hemogram is either normal or, in the early stages of the disease, a leukopenia with an eosinopenia followed by a leukocytosis is noted. In terminal cases, encephalitis and meningitis — and even delirium — can be present. Death usually results from a pulmonary collapse and toxemia.[73]

Psittacosis is generally more severe in older persons. Infections are rare but do occur in children since they are good candidates for coming into close contact with infected feathers or droppings of their pet birds. Chlamydiae were isolated from children of below 2½ years of age who had respiratory symptoms. In one outbreak, there were two fatalities, two cases of severe respiratory involvement, and two cases with a mild respiratory infection.[74,75]

Relapses do occur, especially if the antibiotic therapy is inadequate. Patients have also been found to shed chlamydiae in their sputum during and after convalescence.[76] Recurrence of psittacosis in the same person years after the first attack more likely represents reinfection rather than relapse.[73]

On necropsy, a bronchopneumonia and lesions associated with a generalized toxemia are observed. Areas of consolidation in the lung vary in extent and are sharply demarcated from the normal lung. Fibrin tags may or may not adhere to the pleural surface, and the predominant microscopic lesion in the lungs is a proliferation of alveolar epithelial cells. In the early phase of the disease, there may be exudate, containing polymorphonuclear cells, present in the alveoli and bronchioles. The exudate disappears unless the disease process becomes complicated by a secondary bacterial infection. In the fully developed lesion, the alveolar lumen contains fibrin, epithelial cells, macrophages, and other mononuclear cells. Some of these cells may contain elementary bodies in their cytoplasm. Absence of major lesions in the larger bronchioles and bronchi and the scarcity of polymorphonuclear cells in the alveolar exudate is quite characteristic although by no means pathognomonic. In uncomplicated psittacosis, no areas of necrosis are found in the lungs. The lesion is entirely due to cell proliferation with some exudation. Absence of necrosis is the reason that lungs return to a normal state during convalescence.[71,73]

Congestion, fatty metamorphosis, and in some cases focal necrosis are the lesions seen in the liver. Kupfer cells may be swollen and contain elementary bodies. The spleen gives the typical picture of a reacting organ and may or may not be enlarged.

Cloudy swelling may be noted in the kidneys and heart, and various lymph nodes and lymphoid tissues invariably show a hyperplasia. Edema and congestion in the brain, spinal cord, and meninges are frequently seen. These and vascular lesions in other organs are thought to be caused by a toxemia that results in proliferative degeneration of the capillary endothelium.[71,73] The problem of the origin of this toxemia — being either the primary effect of toxins produced by the organism or secondarily due to somatic lesions — has yet to be resolved.

Unfortunately for the diagnostician, quite a few systemic febrile illnesses can be confused with psittacosis and need to be differentiated. Typhoid fever, influenza, brucellosis, meningitis, infectious mononucleosis, Legionnaires' disease, Q fever, and viral and mycoplasmal pneumonias need to be excluded, mainly on the basis of laboratory tests. Thorough knowledge of the disease, from its mild, influenza-like form to acute fulminating pneumonia, and a history of contact with birds should lead the physician to at least suspect psittacosis and initiate necessary laboratory tests.

General Mode of Spread

Three modes of transmission of chlamydial agents from bird to man are known. In order of importance, they are (1) inhalation of contaminated air, (2) direct contact with latently infected, sick, or dead birds, their feathers, feces, or nasal secretions, and (3) bite wounds.[65] The human respiratory tract is the principle route of entry, and inhalation of chlamydia-laden aerosols is a fully proven pathway of infection.[77,78] Chlamydiae were observed among the bronchioles in experimentally inoculated non-human primates. It was speculated that the organisms spread from the initial focal site of multiplication via the lymphatics. The main lesion was a pneumonia, but the systemic nature of this disease was also evident in these animals because of isolation of chlamydiae from the blood, liver, and spleen.[78]

Ingestion of chlamydiae is a proven route of entry in birds.[67] In certain mammals (e.g., bovine and ovine animals), chlamydiae have also been shown to localize in the G.I. tract, as well as being excreted in feces. Chlamydial diseases are induced after oral inoculation of calves or lambs.[2,79] Although it has been shown that the G.I. tract is the most important site of the disease and excretion of chlamydia in the feces the most important means of spread in birds and ruminants, little is known in this regard concerning humans. It seems possible that the organisms might be swallowed after contamination of hands by an infected bird. Avian chlamydial agents have been shown to retain their infectivity in mammalian G.I. tracts. Mice that were orally exposed to a turkey chlamydial isolate contracted a generalized infection including pneumonia.[67]

Humans have never been known to contract chlamydial infection by eating infected poultry meat or organs; chlamydiae are relatively easily destroyed by heat.

As noted before, man is considered an incidental host in psittacosis. Nevertheless, person-to-person spread does occur, as evidenced by the 1943 Louisiana epidemic mentioned earlier.[56] A single fatal case gave rise to 18 additional cases among nursing attendants, of which 8 were fatal. In this outbreak, the disease appeared to have spread only to those in attendance at some point during the 48 hr prior to death. A high concentration of highly virulent chlamydiae was present in the sputum of these patients, and the aerosol created by their cough presumably was the source of infection.[56]

Multiple cases in a single-family household have been frequently reported, but these were mainly the result of exposure to the same source (an infected bird) rather than to man-to-man transmission.[73] The general mode of spread of chlamydiae from bird to bird is by ingestion or inhalation. The infective aerosol is created when organism-containing feces and nasal secretions are dry enough to become dust.

Chlamydiae were isolated from certain arthropods that may play a role in spreading the disease.[54] However, the infectious chain certainly does not depend upon an arthropod-vector state. The organism spreads directly from bird to bird and has survived for centuries because of the presence of the carrier state in birds and the low mortality of the disease for them.

Epidemiology

Psittacosis in man is a reportable disease; however, many cases (especially the mild influenza-like respiratory infections) undoubtedly go undiagnosed and hence unreported. Even if the disease is diagnosed as a chlamydial respiratory infection, epidemiological investigation is not always instigated or possible. Andrews reported that the source of the infection and patient's occupation was determined in only 57% of the 333 cases reported in the U.S. in 1950.[80] Therefore, the actual number or even a good estimate of the number of human cases is unavailable.

Sources of the infection in man have changed drastically since the 1929 to 1930 pandemic. Prior to 1930, members of the parrot family were thought to be the only source of infection and, in fact, most of the outbreaks were caused by these birds. Exposure occurred in the home, pet shops, dealing and breeding establishments, and occasionally in zoological gardens. Imposition of important restrictions, establishment of quarantine stations, and use of effective antibiotics after the 1930 outbreaks drastically reduced this source of human infection.

Seabirds, such as petrels, storm birds, and occasionally sea gulls and mutton birds, have been a source of human outbreaks. A major epizootic occurred among adult women in the Faroe Islands who prepared young fulmars for food.[32] These outbreaks ceased when the use of fulmars for food was discontinued. In retrospect, egrets are suspected of having been the source for the Louisiana outbreak of 1943.[56]

Reports from many parts of the world indicate a relatively high incidence and widespread occurrence of mostly asymptomatic chlamydiosis in pigeons.[81] Yet, there was never a major epidemic of pigeon origin even though ample opportunity for exposure existed in most parts of the world. Human chlamydial infections have been traced to pigeon lofts and roving pigeon flocks, nevertheless.[39] Fatalities in human infants[74] and frequent sporadic infections in pigeon dealers and fanciers attest to the public health hazard these birds may present.[82] Contagiousness of the disease for persons in contact with acutely sick pigeons becomes evident from the following two case reports. In one incident, two biochemists and two animal caretakers removing and using pigeon organs for enzyme studies became infected. In the other case, students making psychological evaluations on overtly sick pigeons acquired confirmed clinical and subclinical chlamydiosis.[65]

Psittacosis outbreaks traceable to infected chickens have been few. Chickens rarely show clinical signs although there may be extensive serological evidence for the infection. Of 464 chicken sera tested in several states in the U.S., 18% had positive complement-fixation (CF) titers.[83] A single human case occurred in a chicken-processing plant; however, 25% of the employees, especially those involved in evisceration, had significant antibody titers.[84]

The most extensive epizootic in recent years has been in the form of occupational diseases caused by turkeys in the U.S. and ducks and geese in Europe (especially eastern Europe). This is a direct reflection of different culinary preferences. Outbreaks are seasonal with the highest incidence in the fall months at the height of slaughtering and processing activities. Czechoslovakian epidemiologists made a thorough investigation of the source and nature of human chlamydial infections between 1953 and 1963.[85] They found 478 human cases to be the result of exposure to ducks, 31 cases due to geese, 16 cases due to chickens, 1 case due to turkeys, 5 cases due to pigeons,

Table 2

PLACES OF INFECTION AND OCCUPATION
OF PATIENTS WITH PSITTACOSIS IN
CZECHOSLOVAKIA FROM 1953 TO 1963[85]

Place of infection	Occupation of patient	Number of cases
Poultry industry	Employees	855
	Visitors	8
	Veterinarians	3
	Epidemiologists	1
Small poultry farm	Members of family	179
	Visitors	2
Poultry shops	Merchants	4
Kitchen	Cooks	2
Laboratories	Laboratory workers	6
Unknown	Different occupations	32
Total		1072

and 1 case due to exposure to an imported pheasant. These investigatiors also studied locations where infections occurred and occupations of 1072 infected persons (Table 2).

Another important observation made in these studies was the relatively high frequency of recrudescense of the disease. Of the 1072 human cases, 94 patients had relapses within about 1 month after the first exposure. Within 6 to 60 months, 91 persons had a second attack, that was probably the result of reinfection rather than relapse.[85]

As noted before, turkeys are the main source of infection in the U.S. Meyer[65] lists 510 officially reported human cases and an additional 68 suspected cases that occurred in various parts of the U.S. between 1948 and 1961. The deaths of 11 or possibly 12 persons were associated with these cases. In 1974, 154 human cases originating from turkeys were reported in the U.S.[48] Most of these occurred in employees of turkey-processing plants, but cases were also reported in turkey husbandrymen, caretakers on turkey farms, and a person employed at a turkey-rendering plant. It was shown that chlamydiae-laden aerosols were produced during rendering, i.e., converting turkey carcasses into fertilizer.[77] While domestic poultry accounted for the larger outbreaks of chlamydiosis in man in recent years, individual cases caused by pet birds still occur. Between 1971 and 1973, parakeets were the source of 24 such human cases, pigeons of 22, parrots of 11, canaries of 2, and doves of 1 in the U.S.[86]

No account of psittacosis outbreaks would be complete without mentioning laboratory infections. A total of 108 laboratory-acquired infections with 12 deaths occurred in the U.S. between 1929 and 1956.[65] This fact should serve as a reminder for persons involved in diagnosis of and experimentation with chlamydial agents to use utmost care and proper facilities in carrying out diagnostic procedures and handling contaminated specimens.

An epidemiologist investigating a human outbreak must perform carefully and thoroughly and should not stop the investigation if one source of infection is found. Older reports generally concern household epidemics, and the investigation is usually discontinued after finding one source, such as a diseased parakeet, duck, goose, turkey, etc. The homogeneous-heterogeneous infection chain illustrated by Ortel[87] should always be taken into consideration (Table 3).

This infection chain was well demonstrated in the U.S.S.R. by Terskich.[88] A chla-

Table 3
INFECTION CHAIN OF AVIAN CHLAMYDIOSIS[87]

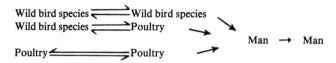

mydial epornitic occurred in wild waterfowl along the coast of the Caspian Sea. The migratory route takes these birds north along the Volga River. Chlamydial infections occurred in two large duck farms located in the vicinity of the nesting sites of these waterfowl, and outbreaks of psittacosis were reported in personnel on these duck farms as well as in those employed in the processing and slaughtering of these ducks.

In studying the ecology of psittacosis, migratory routes, behavior patterns, nesting habits and habitats, and feeding habits of wild birds need to be considered. Birds, such as fulmars, petrels, mutton birds, and pigeons, congregate and nest together and, therefore, produce an environment conducive to the perpetuation of chlamydiosis. On the other hand, bird species of solitary habits rarely become infected and then probably only incidentally.

Intermingling of infected with noninfected birds is the primary means by which the disease is spread and perpetuated. Also, the organism is frequently transferred vertically from the parent bird to the offspring during nesting while they are closely associated. Some young birds may die, but most recover. However, if stress conditions such as crowding, traveling, poor nutrition, and unsatisfactory housing conditions exist, the delicate host-parasite balance shifts in favor of the parasite, and the mortality rate increases drastically. The spread and frequency of transmission between birds and, therefore, the reservoir for human infections — also increases.

During the last 20 years, two important epidemiological factors relative to the transmission of the disease have come to light, although they require further investigative work to attain their true significance. One is the transovarian and the other vector-mediated transmission. Chlamydiae have been isolated from (1) incubator-hatched chickens,[89,90] (2) eggs laid by serologically positive ducks,[91] (3) sea gull eggs,[92] and (4) one egg of a psittacine bird with chlamydiosis.[93] Attempts to isolate chlamydiae from turkey eggs have not been successful.[94] Contamination of the exterior of the eggshell by chlamydiae-containing feces is a possibility and vertical transmission by this route could be suspected. However, this does not appear to be true, at least not for mechanically incubated eggs. Under egg-incubator conditions, a turkey chlamydial agent failed to retain its infectivity for longer than 3 days on turkey eggshells.[94]

While transovarian transmission of chlamydiae does exist in certain avian species, ecology and epidemiology of the disease does not indicate that this route of transmission plays an important role in perpetuation of chlamydiosis. The other factor of epidemiological interest is the role of vectors in the infection chain. Eddie and co-workers[55] have isolated chlamydiae from turkey feather mites, lice collected from chickens, and recently from ticks and fleas.[95] None of these arthropods has yet been shown to be a biological vector for chlamydiae; rather, they appear to be mechanical vectors. A blood-sucking ectoparasite certainly could become infected while parasitizing an animal in a chlamydemic state. Ingestion of chlamydiae-containing ectoparasites is a possible link in the infection chain within the same species and, perhaps more importantly, between different avian species such as wild birds and domesticated fowl.

Interspecies transfer of chlamydiae between birds does occur and is documented in some cases such as between sea gulls and ducks[92] and sparrows, or pigeons and turkeys.[96]

An intriguing epidemiological aspect is the possible interchange of chlamydiae between avian and mammalian species although little is known in this regard. In 1954, an Italian investigator induced lesions of pneumonia in lambs by inoculating them with a chlamydial agent of psittacine origin.[97] In a subsequent study by Pierce and co-workers,[98] ewes were inoculated with a virulent turkey chlamydial isolate. Two died and had pneumonitis and splenomegaly; seven aborted within 27 to 37 days postinoculation and had a severe necrotizing placentitis.

These investigators also studied another interesting parameter — the transfer of the organism back from the infected ewes to turkeys. They placed 20 uninoculated, chlamydiae-free turkeys as contact controls in the same isolation rooms as experimentally infected ewes. Clinical signs and lesions, such as fibrinopurulent pericarditis, aerosaculitis, perihepatitis, and splenomegaly, were noted in 75% of the turkeys. First signs in the turkeys were usually noted 2 weeks after inoculation of the sheep and 1 week after the first signs occurred in the ewes. This corresponds well with the average incubation period of 7 days in turkey chlamydiosis. Chlamydiae were isolated from 11 turkeys that died or were euthanized in *articulo mortis*. The mode of transmission was not established in this study other than that it did not appear to be through contact of the turkeys with infected placentas and aborted fetuses; most turkeys already showed signs at the time the ewes aborted. Chlamydiae isolated from bovine abortions are pathogenic for parakeets.[95]

Does a chlamydial reservoir exist in rodents and wild mammals, and if so, what role do these animals play in the infection chain that leads to man either directly or via birds? The answer has not yet been elucidated. Chlamydiae have been recovered from muskrats and snowshoe hares dying of systemic infection.[99] Mice, guinea pigs, and hamsters have long been used as invaluable experimental indicator hosts. However, we now also know that all three of these species can be naturally infected with chlamydiae (mouse [100], guinea pig [101], hamster [102]). The organisms have also been recovered from opossums.[103] It is unknown at the present if these mammals transmit the disease to other species. Additionally, the level of endemicity and the mode of perpetuation of disease in these species has not been established.

A theory put forward by Schachter[104] relating to the 1943 Louisiana epidemic implicates such an interchange of chlamydiae between wild mammals, birds, and ultimately man. As mentioned earlier, retrospective studies showed that egrets may have been the source for the human outbreaks, and perhaps it was not just coincidental that a cataclysmic die-off of muskrats closely preceded the epidemic.[104] Even though this infection chain is basically speculative, it bears mention because it may well serve the astute epidemiologist as a working hypothesis.

The level of endemicity of avian chlamydial infections (psittacosis) in man is difficult to establish even though numerous serological surveys have been reported. The majority of these surveys were based on the CF test using a group-specific antigen. This heat-stable antigen is shared by all avian and mammalian chlamydial agents. Therefore, the CF test only indicates that a particular host contains group-specific antibodies. It is of no value in differentiating whether man or other species have been infected with an avian chlamydial isolate of the *C. psittaci* species or an agent of the *C. trachomatis* species.

In view of the recent increased incidence of human nongonoccal urethritis and its etiological association with *C. trachomatis*,[105] it becomes obvious that serological test results based on the group-specific CF test need to be interpreted cautiously. Epidemiologists trying to analyze occupational chlamydiosis found it difficult to interpret positive CF antibody titers in employees before they became involved in outbreaks. In retrospect, it can be theorized that these positive titers were perhaps not caused by infection with an avian chlamydial agent but rather by nonzoonotic human chlamydiosis.

Diagnosis

A separate section will be devoted to this subject since diagnostic methods are similar for all chlamydial infections.

Prevention and Control

Since the advent of effective antibiotic treatment (mainly tetracyclines), human chlamydiosis of avian origin has been drastically reduced and is no longer considered a major public health problem. Enough is known in the case of exotic psittacine birds to suppress or interrupt the infection chain. The severe import restrictions or total embargos imposed by many countries after the 1929 to 1930 pandemic have been retracted. These have been largely replaced by prophylactic treatment of imported birds in special treatment centers or quarantine stations or by a licensed veterinarian either at the point of shipment or destination. This change came about largely through the extensive work of Meyer and co-workers[106] who first implemented an effective method of eradicating the infection from birds by using tetracycline-medicated feed. Arnstein et al.[107,108] evaluated several treatment schedules and found 0.44% chlorotetracycline in cooked mash or 0.5% chlorotetracycline in dry pelleted feed effectively eliminates the infection in parrots. The level of antibiotic in the feed had to be maintained for 45 consecutive days since chlamydiae could still be recovered from the feces after only 30 days of treatment.

In parakeets, hulled millet seed impregnated with 5 mg chlorotetracycline per gram and administered for 14 consecutive days was effective.[106] Medicated cooked mash for parrots and hulled millet seeds for parakeets are the treatments accepted by the U.S. Food Drug Administration for chlamydiosis in psittacine birds. Measures used to prevent the infection in them cannot be applied to domesticated poultry, mainly because routine use of antibiotic-treated feed is economically unfeasible. In such a massive program, resistance of chlamydiae to tetracyclines could also become a reality. To date, tetracycline-resistant strains have been induced only in the laboratory.[27]

Success in treating chlamydiosis in turkeys appears to depend upon the virulence of the strain. Flocks infected with a strain of low virulence (i.e., causing few mortalities) were given feed containing 400 g of chlorotetracycline per ton for 7 to 14 days, and this was quite successful in eliminating the infection.[69] The same or even higher levels of treatment, however, did not control the infection of a highly virulent chlamydial turkey strain.[69,96] As in turkeys, antibiotic treatment of ducks and geese is also only partially effective in the prevention and control of chlamydiosis.[109]

The U.S. Department of Agriculture prohibits movement in inter- and intrastate commerce of poultry carcasses and offal in which chlamydiosis has been confirmed. Avian and human chlamydiosis (psittacosis) are reportable diseases. The observant poultry owner and his veterinarian should bring any diseased birds in which clinical signs and/or necropsy lesions even remotely resemble chlamydiosis to a competent diagnostic laboratory. It is important to isolate sick birds and establish a diagnosis early in the disease course. Clinically sick birds shed high numbers of chlamydiae and, if not detected early, contaminate the environment to such a degree that control measures within a flock become useless. In outbreaks with a high mortality, depopulation of the entire flock may be the only alternative. In other outbreaks, a treatment schedule usually consisting of 200 g of chlorotetracycline per ton of dry mash for 21 consecutive days may be initiated under veterinary supervision. Proper withholding times prior to slaughter need to be observed.

In breeding establishments, birds to be introduced into an existing flock should be checked clinically, serologically, and possibly even by culturing their excreta; the health status of the flock or origin should also be ascertained.

In the absence of an effective vaccine — which does not appear to be forthcoming in the near future without extensive research into the basic and peculiar immunological aspects of chlamydial infections — eradication of chlamydiosis in poultry does not seem likely. Basically, the reasons for this are ubiquitousness of the chlamydial reservoir and lack of knowledge about the ecology of the disease. The interchange of organisms between wild birds (especially pigeons, waterfowl, sparrows, and migratory birds) and domesticated poultry, the role of rodents as a reservoir, the role of arthropods as vectors of the organism between avian species and possibly even between rodents and birds, and the role of our domesticated mammals as a source of avian chlamydiosis or vice versa are all problems that must await complete answers that will come via extensive experimentation and field research.

Prevention of the disease and measures that can be taken to protect poultry farmers, workers in poultry-processing plants, and consumers must be discussed. As pointed out above, the most important and essential aspect in this regard is the early recognition of chlamydiosis on the poultry farm. Unfortunately, initial recognition of the disease frequently occurs at the poultry-processing plant. Ideally, an infected flock should never reach the plant.

It is obvious that complete protection of man is impossible as long as avian chlamydiosis exists. However, total eradication is probably not obtainable for reasons listed above. For poultry and pet owners, awareness of the disease must be continuously stimulated through distribution of information and educational material by proper agencies. Some measures the owners should consider are (1) proper hygiene and feeding, (2) avoidance of crowding, (3) elimination of stagnant, contaminated water, (4) installation of running water and concrete drainage channels, and possibly (5) repeated serological testing of an entire flock or part of a large flock. Production of aerosol and the intimate contact that frequently occurs between pet birds should be prevented.

Unfortunately, in the processing plant most workers have already been exposed once a positive diagnosis of chlamydiosis in carcasses has been made. Therefore, it is important to use all possible means to prevent infected flocks from entering the plant. One safeguard would be thorough ante-mortem inspection of the flock (on the farm) by the poultry meat inspector.

Prolonged transportation with little or no food and water in overcrowded cages should be avoided. Under such stress conditions, latent infections easily convert to active infections and result in increased shedding of chlamydiae. Frequent disinfection of the entire plant, increased scalding time (at temperaures higher than 56°C), mechanical defeathering, and evisceration are all measures that minimize the creation of aerosol and should be applied where feasible. Ventilation systems, if not installed properly, can do more harm than good.

The consumer-at-large has never been at risk. As stated before, man is not known to contract the disease by ingestion. Chlamydiae are sensitive to heat, and even temperatures of 60°C for 5 min will render them noninfectious. Thus, properly cooked poultry is not a source of infection.

Perhaps the most important method of protecting persons in contact with birds is to stimulate awareness of the disease through distributing educational and informative material. Physicians near poultry-processing plants should be cognizant and informed. The worst outbreaks occurred when the infection was not recognized until several persons died from chlamydial pneumonitis.

Now, with the availability of effective treatment most human deaths can be prevented if chemotherapy is initiated early in the course of the disease. Optimally, prevention should involve serological monitoring of high-risk personnel.

NONZOONOTIC HUMAN CHLAMYDIAL INFECTONS AND THEIR POSSIBLE COUNTERPARTS IN ANIMALS

Genital Chlamydial Infections
Diseases

A sexually transmitted chlamydial disease that John Hunter delineated as a clinical entity in 1786 is lymphogranuloma venereum (LGV). The following synonyms have been used to describe this disease: climatic bubo, tropical bubo, venereal bubo, sixth venereal disease, lymphogranuloma inguinale, granulomatous lymphomatosis, poradenitis, lymphopathia venereum, esthiomene, and *maladie de Nicolas et Favre.*[73]

Recently, chlamydiae have been shown to be a major cause of venereally transmitted nongonococcal urethritis and cervicitis. The organism has also been found in the genital tract of clinically normal individuals,[105] leading to the false conclusion that chlamydiae might be part of the normal genital flora. Abundant epidemiological and biochemical evidence clearly shows that these organisms are true parasites and are always pathogenic at the cellular level. Therefore, chlamydiae in the genital tract of clinically normal persons indicates a latent infection, a common feature of chlamydiosis in almost all affected species.

Etiological Agent

The organism involved in these infections belongs to the species *C. trachomatis.*

Host Spectrum

LGV appears to be a disease peculiar to man; a similar disease has not been reported in animals. Monkeys are susceptible to experimental injection and develop meningitis after intracerebral inoculation with human LGV isolates.[110] After injection of monkeys by various parenteral routes, local inflammation develops at the site of inoculation with enlargement of regional lymph nodes.[73] The exact symptoms and lesions seen in man have not been reproduced in monkeys, however. Mice and chick embryos are susceptible and are widely and successfully used in isolation attempts. Only erratic experimental inoculation success has been obtained in less susceptible animals such as guinea pigs, rabbits, squirrels, marmots, harvest mice, rats, cats, dogs, sheep, fowl, pigeons, rice birds, and parakeets.[73] Urethral infection was produced in baboons that were inoculated with a chlamydial isolate recovered from a man with nonspecific urethritis.[111]

Distribution

Since LGV is not a reportable disease in most places, its actual prevalence is unknown. An almost world-wide distribution is likely, judging from case reports.[112] Poor hygiene probably contributes more to its prevalence than other factors such as climate. The disease is especially prevalent in tropical countries, the Mediterranean, and the southern and eastern U.S. The incidence of LGV was reported as eight cases per 10,000 admissions in a New York hospital and 1.9% of 34,766 patients admitted to a venereal disease clinic in San Francisco in 1940.[73] It has rarely been diagnosed in recent years, perhaps due to higher socioeconomic standards and consequent improved hygienic conditions.

Chlamydiae associated with nongonococcal or postgonococcal urethritis, cervicitis, or vaginitis have been found to be highly prevalent in countries, such as England and the U.S., where an extensive search for these organisms has been made in recent years. Chlamydiae have been isolated from 30 to 40% of patients with nongonococcal urethritis as opposed to 10 to 30% of those with gonococcal or postgonococcal urethritis and 0 to 7% of those with no symptoms. The organisms have also been frequently recovered from the cervices of women. Isolation rates reported from various venereal disease clinics in the U.S. and England range from 18 to 36% in patients with cervicitis to 4.0% in persons with vaginitis only and 0 to 3.5% in asymptomatic women.[105,113]

Disease in Animals

Symptoms and lesions of LGV in man are not known to occur naturally in animals nor have they been reproduced in their entirety in experimentally inoculated animals. Laboratory animals, such as mice and chick embryos, are susceptible. These are the most useful indicator hosts for chlamydiae in general, and the lesions induced by inoculation with the LGV agent are not different from those induced by most other chlamydial agents. Mice inoculated intracerebrally develop meningitis while intranasal instillation incites pneumonia. Monkeys inoculated by various routes develop a local reaction at the site of injection with subsequent enlargement of regional lymph nodes.

Chlamydiae isolated from the human genital tract — other than those recovered from persons affected with LGV — are infective in the usual chlamydial indicator hosts as well as in monkeys, in which experimental urethritis was recently induced.[111]

Few studies have been reported on the natural occurrence of venereal chlamydiosis in animals. Chlamydial elementary bodies have been demonstrated in vaginal discharges of cows with infertility problems.[114] Storz and co-workers[115] isolated chlamydiae from the semen of bulls affected with seminal vesiculitis syndrome. These chlamydial isolates did induce microscopic lesions of orchitis, epididymitis, and ampullitis when inoculated intravenously or intramuscularly into susceptible bulls and rams, and chlamydiae were reisolated from the semen.[116] Histological changes seen in the sex and accessory sex organs were of a granulomatous nature typical of chlamydiae-induced lesions (Figure 7). Little is known about chlamydial infections of the female genital tract of animals. Omori and co-workers[117] were able to induce endometritis by experimental inoculation of the uterus. It is conceivable, therefore, that venereally transmitted chlamydial diseases can occur in some animals. However, clinical consequences in the sexual partner are unknown, and these limited observations must await further investigation before conclusions can be made.

Disease in Man

LGV manifests itself in either an acute or chronic form. The incubation period varies but may be as short as a few days. The first lesion after venereal exposure is usually a vesicule on the prepuce, glans penis, or in the vaginal mucosa, cervix, urethra, or anal region. The vesicules rupture, leaving shallow erosions that may become ulcerous. These lesions may heal and a complete recovery can occur, or the disease may progress to involve the regional and usually the inguinal lymph nodes. Deep pelvic and perianal lymph nodes may also become enlarged, especially in case of vaginitis and proctitis.

In the male, buboes form in inguinal nodes. The lymphadenitis may resolve spontaneously or lead to suppuration of the nodes. At this stage, the patient may also show signs such as anorexia, nausea, vomiting, sweats, chills, generalized muscle pains, headaches, epistaxis, and bronchitis. If the chlamydiae surpass the regional lymph nodes, a generalized lymphadenitis, leukocytosis, hypergammaglobulinemia with a reversed A/G ratio, and a hepato-splenomegaly usually occur.

Occasionally, a well-defined syndrome that may manifest itself early or late in the

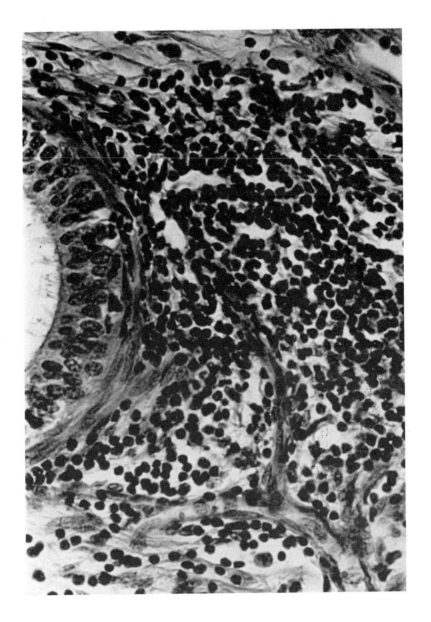

FIGURE 7.   Inflammatory reaction adjacent to an efferent duct of the epididymis of a ram inoculated parenterally with chlamydiae from the semen. (Hematoxylin-eosin stain.)

infection is seen. It is characterized by signs of esthiomene and elephantiasis of the penis, scrotum, and rectal stenosis. Proctitis and vaginorectal and perianal fistulas are reported sequelae of LGV.[118] A person recovering from LGV does have a certain immunity; if injected intra- or subcutaneously with material containing the agent, no clinical signs are produced except a hypersensitivity reaction at the site of inoculation, similar to the reaction produced with inactivated chlamydiae in the Frei test. However, relapses, can occur in LGV.[119] The disease must be differentiated from malignancy of lymph nodes and rectum, tuberculosis, buboes due to supperative lesions in the lower extremities, gonorrhea, syphilis, tularemia, and plague.

Nongonococcal urethritis is diagnosed after exclusion of gonorrhea in patients who have scanty to moderate urethral discharge and variable dysuria. While not all nongonococcal urethral infections are caused by chlamydiae, the symptoms and lesions are the same. Subclinical urethritis is common, and these cases are usually detected because a sex partner has a clinical visible infection and therefore enters a clinic for examination. In the minority of cases, the condition is severe with purulent discharges. Only laboratory tests can differentiate this condition from gonorrhea.

The true incubation period of nongonococcal urethritis is unknown but is considered to be about 8 to 14 days (or longer) after exposure during sexual intercourse. Symptoms in females are frequently absent or minor; acute or recurrent cystitis usually brings the patient to a physician. Vaginal discharge caused by erosive cervicitis, urethritis, or proctitis (rarely) may be encountered.[120]

These genital infections in males and females can only be associated with chlamydiae through isolation. Organisms such as *Trichomonas vaginalis, Mycoplasma, Candida albicans, Corynebacteria,* Neisseria gonococcus, and *Trepanoma pallidum* must be excluded by proper laboratory tests. Multiple infections may exist.

Chlamydiae have also been incriminated in a disease of man known as Reiter's syndrome. Symptomology in this disease includes a nongonococcal urethritis, in addition to polyarthritis and conjunctivitis or iritis. It will be discussed in more detail under "Chlamydial Joint Infections."

General Mode of Spread

The usual mode of transmission is venereal in LGV and nongonococcal urethritis. However, on rare occasions, LGV has been contracted from contaminated clothing. Surgeons and hospital personnel have become infected in the process of removing affected lymph nodes and tending and bathing patients, respectively.[73]

Epidemiology

Genital chlamydial infections are found in persons who are in the sexually active period of life. Few cases have been observed in children; LGV is not thought to be a congenital infection. However, a urogenital chlamydial infection of the mother may cause infection in the newborn. Chlamydial agents of the same species are responsible for conjunctivitis in human neonates. The genital origin of this infection has been established, and transmission is thought to occur during passage of the fetus through the infected birth canal. This disease is discussed in more detail under "Ocular and Conjunctival Chlamydial Infections."

While classical LGV has become a rare disease in many western countries, chlamydial genital infections leading to urethritis, cervicitis, and vaginitis are increasing (or at least their recognition is). In a recent study, Schachter and co-workers[105] found chlamydial infections to be the most common venereal disease. Of approximately 70 patients with cervicitis, 36.6% were infected with chlamydiae, 20.5% with *Candida* sp., 13.7% with *Trichomonas vaginalis*, 6.8% with Neisseria gonococcus, and 5.7%

with herpesvirus. Multiple etiology is probably more common than is generally realized. Of 18 patients with gonorrhea, 2 also had chlamydial infection and 1 of 17 also harbored a herpesvirus.[105] Other investigators found an even higher incidence of dual chlamydial-gonococcal infection.[113] The highest chlamydial isolation rate was found in patients with nongonococcal genital infections. In one study, 57% of those with nongonococcal urethritis harbored chlamydial agents.[105] Nongonococcal urethritis has become more common than gonococcal urethritis in England[113] and the U.S.[121]

The increased frequency of isolation and successful experimental infection in monkeys[111] seem to establish chlamydiae as a major cause of genital infection, either symptomatic or asymptomatic. However, many questions remain to be answered. What is the incubation period? Why is the chlamydial isolation rate higher in persons with "altered" endocrine functions, as occurs during pregnancy or through use of oral contraceptives? Why are chlamydiae isolated more frequently when symptoms have persisted for a greater length of time? Why does not the increased number of sexual partners and promiscuity prior to examination lead to an increased chlamydial isolation rate as it does in the case of gonorrhea? Why do patients already have chlamydial antibodies in their blood when they have shown symptoms for only 2 to 7 days?[113,122]

Many of these problems can probably be explained on the basis of the known tendency of chlamydiae to cause persistent and latent infections. However, more expanded research efforts into the pathogenesis and epidemiology of chlamydiosis and the establishment of animal models are needed in order to fulfill Koch's postulates or at least revisions thereof.

Diagnosis

Methods for isolation and serological procedures will be covered under the separate heading "Diagnostic Procedures." One test, however, bears special mention in regard to diagnosing LGV. The Frei test[123] is based upon a delayed-type hypersensitivity reaction and is extensively used in diagnosing the disease. To a limited extent, it has also been tried in various other chlamydioses of man and animals. The original antigen made by Frei in 1925 consisted of pus from a bubo of an LGV patient. Today, the Frei antigen consists of a phenol-treated suspension of infected chick-embryo yolk sacs. The test is performed by injecting 0.1 mℓ of the antigen intradermally into one forearm and 0.1 mℓ of a control antigen consisting of normal yolk into the other. The test is read 48 and 72 hr later. A raised red papule, surrounded by erythema and measuring 6 × 6 mm, is considered positive if the control antigen response is 5 × 5 mm or less or is absent, as is usually the case. The Frei test usually becomes positive 1 week to 6 months (generally 2 to 3 weeks) after onset of symptoms.[120] A positive patient may retain this reactivity for many years, perhaps throughout life. It should be remembered that the Frei test, as the CF test, is a group-specific test for chlamydiae. Antigens prepared from various chlamydial organisms such as avian, mouse, or feline isolates elicited the same response in LGV patients as antigens prepared with an isolate from a LGV patient.[124] Patients affected with chlamydial infections other than LGV, such as pneumonia (psittacosis), may also be positive to the Frei test.

Prevention and Control

Perhaps the most important control measures in human genital infection at this stage are (1) distribution of informative literature to physicians and (2) establishment of new public health or venereal disease laboratories (or expansion of existing ones) capable of isolating and identifying chlamydiae. Diagnosis of genital chlamydial infections other than classical LGV is presently in the research stage, and only a few specialized laboratories are gathering information needed for expansion in this area. Unfortunately, while useful as a screening procedure, the relatively simple CF test is not reliable for diagnosis since rising titers are rarely demonstrated. This is because of the difficulty of obtaining an acute sample.

Isolation and identification of chlamydiae is, at present, the only absolute diagnostic means. Finding the asymptomatic carrier is important in controlling genital chlamydial infection. Our modern plans for combating syphilis and gonorrhea should be applied to chlamydial genital infections as well.

Early treatment with tetracyclines and oxytetracyclines given orally at 1 to 2 g daily for 5 to 7 consecutive days or even longer appears to be the remedy of choice.[120] Without treatment, symptoms may gradually disappear in some cases. However, treatment is always indicated since it will relieve discomfort and prevent later complications.

Chlamydial genital infections including LGV do not respond to penicillin. It is unfortunate that penicillin is sometimes administered without initiation of a laboratory diagnosis.

Ocular and Conjunctival Chlamydial Infections
Diseases

A disease of man probably recognized at the time of the Egyptian dynasties is trachoma, also known as granular conjunctivitis. In 1912, Halberstadter[4] first observed the characteristic intracytoplasmic inclusion bodies in Giemsa-stained conjunctival epithelial cells of trachoma patients. However, it was not until 1957 that the agent was isolated for the first time and propagated in chick embryos.[125] Trachoma is often acquired during childhood and takes a very slow progressive course with frequent periods of quiescence followed by acute exacerbations. Occasionally, the disease may start acutely in adults. Trachoma lesions are limited to the eye and conjunctiva.

Another chlamydial disease of man is inclusion conjunctivitis. Jones and co-workers[126] isolated chlamydiae from this condition in 1959. The disease is basically a genital infection of adults, and the fetal conjunctivae become exposed during passage through the infected birth canal. The neonate usually starts showing symptoms of a follicular conjunctivitis with purulent discharge at 1 week of age. Adults may contract the disease in swimming pools polluted with chlamydiae-containing genital excretions.[127] Agents that produce trachoma and inclusion conjunctivitis are indistinguishable in laboratory tests, but the absence of pannus formations and conjunctival scars (characteristic lesions in trachoma) in inclusion conjunctivitis of neonates is one argument used to advance the idea that these agents are different. However, Jones and Collier[128] were able to induce pannus formation in adult human volunteers inoculated with a chlamydial isolate from an infant with inclusion conjunctivitis. Genital infections other than LGV are commonly called TRIC agents (TR = trachoma, IC = inclusion conjunctivitis). Most recent evidence indicates that trachoma and inclusion conjunctivitis are caused by the same chlamydial organism and that different manifestations are the result of age, route of infection, immune status, and possibly other physiological factors of the host.

While eye lesions in conjunction with a systemic chlamydiosis have long been recognized in avian species, lesions restricted to the eye were, until 1960, thought to be a peculiar chlamydial manifestation seen only in man. In 1960, Yerasimides[129] isolated a chlamydial agent from the ocular discharge of a cat with acute conjunctivitis. The organisms were also incriminated as the cause of conjunctivitis in dogs,[130] guinea pigs,[131] sheep,[132] piglets,[133] and cattle in the early stages of the disease.[134] Conjunctivitis is also frequently seen in sheep affected with chlamydial polyarthritis (see "Chlamydial Joint Infections").

Etiological Agents

The human agents responsible for trachoma and inclusion conjunctivitis belong to the species *C. trachomatis*. All animal strains isolated from eye lesions belong to the species *C. psittaci*.

Host Spectrum

Besides the above mentioned species, in which chlamydial eye infections occurred naturally, conjunctivitis was also experimentally induced with TRIC agents in monkeys.[135]

Distribution

Trachoma and inclusion conjunctivitis have a world-wide distribution. The greatest number of cases today are found in Egypt and the Middle East. In certain villages in North Africa, nearly the entire population may be affected with trachoma. Algeria had more than one million cases in 1953, and Morocco had approximately 250,000. An equally large percentage of the population is infected in other North African nations (e.g., Tunisia, Egypt, and Libya). Trachoma is endemic in most African countries, although it is not as extensive outside of North Africa.[136]

The disease is also endemic in many countries in Asia, especially Southwest Asia. In 1953, Jordan reported 80,000 occurrences; Iraq reported 500,000. The prevalence of trachoma has declined in countries bordering the Mediterranean Sea and in the Balkan States. There are foci in many South American countries where trachoma is endemic. In 1963, Argentina reported 369 cases; Paraguay reported 10. Only minor foci still exist in the U.S. and Canada.[136] The distribution of inclusion conjunctivitis is unknown, except for isolated case reports all originating in Europe or North America.

Disease in Animals

The main lesion in all species (guinea pig, cat, dog, sheep, cattle, and piglets) in which chlamydial eye infections have been reported is a follicular conjunctivitis. The animals are photophobic; conjunctivae are hyperemic, and the enlarged submucosal lymphoid follicles may become singly visible or confluent. Chemosis, keratitis, and pannus formation can also occur. Some animals such as piglets become anorectic, depressed, and feverish.[133] The disease in sheep is usually bilateral while in cats it is frequently unilateral, at least initially. However, the opposite eye usually develops similar lesions within 5 to 7 days if not treated. A large percentage of cats may develop conjunctivitis in catteries in which the disease is endemic. Kittens of affected queens frequently develop a severe conjunctivitis. Chlamydial organisms, however, have not been demonstrated in the birth canal of the queens.[137]

In sheep, the incidence may reach 90% in a given flock, especially if they are held in close confinement (such as feedlots). In an extensive outbreak in Colorado, 10 to 25% of the sheep also had polyarthritis.[132] Intracytoplasmic inclusions identical to those seen in human patients may be seen in Giemsa-stained conjunctival epithelial cells of affected animals (Figure 8). Untreated cases may become superinfected with other microbes such as various bacteria (including *Mycoplasma*), that may result in severe corneal ulceration and eventual loss of the eye.

The disease in animals has been experimentally reproduced. The response in cats that were inoculated 4 months after the original exposure varied from a very mild to a severe infection.[137] Experimental work suggests an incubation period ranging from 3 to 7 days. Low antibody titers are usually present during convalescence, and it is dif-

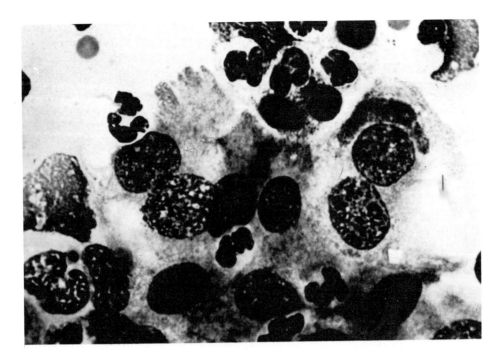

FIGURE 8.   Conjunctival scraping from a natural case of ovine chlamydial conjunctivitis. Helmet-shaped chlamydial inclusion in one epithelial cell. (Giemsa stain.)

ficult to demonstrate a rising titer. This is not surprising in view of the localized nature of the infection.

Disease in Man

The onset of trachoma in children is insidious. Follicular conjunctivitis is the first sign; in later stages, pannus formation, that always starts in the upper quadrants (unlike in other diseases), corneal ulcerations, and scar formations are observed. In adults, the disease may start acutely with considerable irritation, lacrimation, and exudation. In the acute stage, trachoma is highly communicable. The disease progresses slowly over months or years, regardless of whether the onset was acute or insidious. In later stages, cicatrization resulting in deformities of the eye lid, corneal opacification, and cornification of the conjunctival and corneal epithelium occur. Chronic trachoma patients may experience occasional exacerbations of the symptoms, that result in shedding of the infectious agents.

Inclusion conjunctivitis is usually seen between the 5th and 14th day of life. It is characterized by an acute purulent conjunctivitis. The infection is usually self-limiting, and symptoms gradually begin to disappear 14 days after onset. Inclusion conjunctivitis in adults is a follicular conjunctivitis with little discharge. Symptoms may persist for weeks or even months (rarely) and then disappear without treatment. Unlike in trachoma, pannus formation and corneal opacification never occur in children and only very seldomly in adults with inclusion conjunctivitis.[127]

General Mode of Spread

The TRIC organism is spread by direct contact with ocular secretions of infected persons or material soiled therewith. Flies, such as *Musca sorbens*, may act as mechanical carriers but are not a necessary link in the infection chain.

Conjunctivitis is acquired by the infant in the infected birth canal of its mother. In adults, the disease may be contracted by direct contact with infected infants or in improperly chlorinated swimming pools contaminated with infected genital secretions.

The period of highest communicability is when active lesions are present. In the late stages of trachoma, when cicatrization is extensive, communicability is very low. However, during relapses, resulting in exacerbation of lesions, the concentration of organisms in the ocular discharge increases.[127] Chlamydial conjunctivitis in animals is also transmitted by direct contact, and no vector is known to be involved.

Epidemiology

The principal reservoir of the infection is the species in which the disease occurs. Sporadic or accidental interspecies transfer can occur, however. The eyes of a laboratory technician became infected while he was working with an avian (parakeet) chlamydial isolate.[138] The patient developed ptosis, follicular conjunctivitis, papillary hypertropy, and in the later stages corneal epithelial erosions and keratitis. An avian chlamydial agent was isolated before tetracycline treatment was started, and a rising antibody titer was noted; however, no signs of a systemic infection were present. The patient was placed on 1 g/day of tetracycline taken orally for 2 months. The course was protracted, and it was not until about 5 months after onset that the lesions completely disappeared.

In another case, the conjunctiva of an investigator working with a chlamydial isolate from an aborted lamb became infected. The source of infection was an aerosol produced during sonication. This particular ovine chlamydial strain hadbeen passed 94 times in mouse L-cells at the time of the human exposure. Treatment was initiated with 1 hr of exposure and consisted of a 1% chloromycetin® ophthalmic ointment. Despite the early treatment, the patient developed an acute conjunctivitis 1 to 2 days after infection. Conjunctival scrapings taken the fourth day contained epithelial cells with typical inclusion when stained with Giemsa and specific fluorescein-labeled antiserum.[139]

An interesting observation in this study was that this ovine chlamydial isolate did not appear attenuated after 94 passages in cell cultures. It was obviously pathogenic to the human eye and caused the same placental and fetal lesions in pregnant ewes as prior to tissue-culture passaging.[139] A chlamydial agent was also isolated from a man and his pet cat; both suffered from a follicular-type conjunctivitis.[140]

The extent of transmission from animals to man is unknown. An interesting but unconfirmed field observation is that employees of sheep feedlots, where extensive outbreaks of conjunctivitis and polyarthritis occur, also frequently show photophobia and conjunctivitis.[141]

These case reports on laboratory infections certainly indicate that members of the species *C. psittaci* can replicate in the human conjunctiva and cause lesions. Therefore, one should consider these diseases at least as potential zoonoses.

In man, infection with TRIC agents has long been thought to be restricted to the eye and genital tract. However, it is now clearly established that TRIC agents can also invade the throat, causing follicles and granulation on the posterior pharyngeal wall. Occasional accompanyment of a middle ear infection in trachoma could possibly be explained by the presence of an infection in the throat and extension via the Eustachian tube.[142]

Route of entry and exit of chlamydiae from the host is an important epidemiological parameter. In human TRIC infections, a systemic chlamydiosis and chlamydemia have not yet been reported. Entry and exit routes are limited to ocular, nasopharyngeal, and urogenital mucosal surfaces. TRIC agents inoculated parenterally into susceptible baboons do disseminate via lymph and blood and replicate mainly in the regional lymph nodes and spleen. However, no lesions in the eyes were noted after parenteral inoculation.[143] On the other hand, animal eye infections may be part of a systemic infection as is frequently seen in avian chlamydiosis. In sheep flocks, 10 to 25% of animals with conjunctivitis also have polyarthritis. Experimental inoculation of lambs by the intravenous, intramuscular, or intraarticular route invariably results not only in polyarthritis but also in follicular conjunctivitis.[132] Of course, it should be realized that chlamydiae isolated from ovine and bovine conjunctivitis and polyarthritis as well as the agent of bovine encephalomyelitis all belong to one major serotype and are closely related antigenically.[144]   A chlamydial agent of the species *C. psittaci* that was originally isolated from muskrats in Canada also induces eye lesions in intravenously inoculated rabbits.[145] The first lesion is a bilateral uveitis followed by an iritis indicating a hematogenous route of entry into the eye. Keratoconjunctivitis was frequently observed in these animals. Factors perpetuating endemicity are lack of personal hygiene and basic sanitation, towels and toilet articles used in common, fly controls, etc.

Diagnosis

Diagnosis of TRIC in hyperendemic areas is usually made on the basis of clinical symptoms alone. In areas where TRIC infections are uncommon (and in animals), diagnosis should be aided by laboratory tests (discussed under a separate heading).

Prevention and Control

Trachoma might be considered a family disease and is most prevalent in poor families. As socioeconomic conditions and resultant sanitation improve, prevalence levels decline proportionately. There is no vaccine available for humans or animals, and vaccine research with chlamydiae has been generally disappointing. In many vaccine trials, a significant antibody response (as measured by the CF test) was elicited. However, it has been shown repeatedly that these circulating antibody titers bear no relation to the state of resistance to conjunctival challenge. In fact, frequently the conjunctival responses are enhanced in postvaccination challenges and pannus formation may be more pronounced. Some think pannus formation, seen mainly in severe cases or repeated reinfections, occurs more as a result of a hypersensitivity reaction of the host than as a direct consequence of the infection.[146,147]

Treatments of choice today are tetracyclines or erythromycin given systemically. The standard course of treatment is oral administration of these antibiotics for 3 weeks.[127] Ophthalmic ointment containing these drugs has to be given at least four times daily to be effective. In countries with a high prevalence of human trachoma, treatment with topical tetracycline or erythromycin is often used. Sulfonamides such as sulfadiazine, given systemically or topically, are also effective. However, occasional side effects such as erythema multiforme, associated with cicatrizing conjunctivitis, have been noted with sulfonamides.[127]

Preventive measures in human TRIC infections should include educating the public about the disease. Treatment should be emphasized in preschool children in hyperendemic areas. Personal hygiene, basic sanitation, and nutrition are important parameters that, if improved, help reduce the prevalence of the disease.

Proper chlorination of water in swimming pools probably helps prevent transmission of the TRIC agent. In animals such as sheep, conjunctivitis is especially prevalent in overcrowded, artificial confinements such as feedlots. Individual systemic treatment of animals with tetracyclines is effective if given early in the disease course. Inclusion of high levels of chlorotetracyclines in feed aids in controlling the disease but does not prevent it.

Chlamydial Joint Infections

Diseases

Polyarthritis is a well-established and well-recognized chlamydial disease in sheep and calves. The organism was first isolated in 1960 from sheep[148] and 4 years later was isolated from calves.[149] The disease in lambs has also been referred to as "stiff lamb disease." Chlamydiae have been recovered recently from two foals with a naturally occurring polyarthritis.[150] Schachter and co-workers[151] added a new human pathogenetic potential for these organisms when they isolated a chlamydial agent from the synovia of a patient affected with Reiter's syndrome. The classical triad of symptoms in Reiter's syndrome consists of a nonspecific urethritis, conjunctivitis, and arthritis, but it may also be accompanied by other symptoms or only two features of the triad, usually urethritis and arthritis.

In comparison, it is interesting to note that similar organ systems are frequently involved in animals. For example, sheep affected with polyarthritis also frequently have conjunctivitis.[132] Arthritis in man is also a rare complication in systemic human chlamydioses such as psittacosis and LGV.

Etiological Agent

Organisms causing polyarthritis in lambs and calves belong to the same serotype of the species *C. psittaci*. They are antigenically closely related or perhaps identical.[144] The agent isolated from patients with Reiter's syndrome belongs to the species *C. trachomatis*.

Host Spectrum

To date, chlamydiae have only been recovered from synovial tissues of the following species with naturally occuring polyarthritis: ovine, bovine, equine, and human (mostly patients with Reiter's syndrome). In general, animals used for isolation, such as chick embryos, mice, and guinea pigs, are also susceptible to infection with these agents. Dogs inoculated parenterally with an ovine polyarthritis strain developed a systemic chlamydiosis, evidenced by reisolation of the agent from various organ systems and development of signs such as pneumonia, diarrhea, fever, and arthritis.[152]

A chlamydial agent isolated from synovial tissues of a patient with Reiter's syndrome produced only a local reaction in monkeys after repeated intraarticular inoculation.[153] However, inoculation of these human isolates into rabbits induced a polyarthritis in all 28 principles and also uveitis in 2 of them.[154]

Distribution

To date, chlamydial polyarthritis in sheep has only been described in the U.S. in various states of the intermountain region and Texas.[2] In view of the cosmopolitan range of chlamydiae in general, it would not be surprising to confirm this disease in sheep in other parts of the world as well.

Chlamydial polyarthritis in calves has been confirmed in the U.S.[149] Austria,[155] and possibly Australia.[156] In the U.S. chlamydiae have only been isolated from a polyarthritic foal.[150] However, they have also been recovered from horses with bronchopneumonia in Rumania[157] and horses with an hepato-encephalopathy in Spain.[158]

Reiter's syndrome in man is probably distributed world-wide. However, chlamydial isolates from synovial tissues of these patients have only recently been obtained in laboratories in France, England, Denmark, the U.S.S.R., and the U.S. where an extensive search for these organisms is underway.

Disease in Animals

Chlamydial polyarthritis in lambs has been observed on ranges as well as in feedlots. The morbidity varies but may reach 75%, especially in feedlots. Prevalence of the disease is higher in older lambs (weighing 25 to 50 kg) than in smaller, younger ones. Clinical features consist of varying degrees of stiffness, lameness, reluctance to move, anorexia, and a fever that ranges from 39 to 42°C in the acute stage. No signs of diarrhea are usually observed, but the agents are frequently recovered from the feces, spleen, and kidney, indicating systemic involvement. Mortality is low, and most lambs start improving 2 weeks after onset of symptoms; however, a few lambs remain permanently crippled. Affected joints are rarely enlarged. Lambs may "warm out" of stiffness and lameness following forced exercise.[159,160]

Polyarthritis in calves is a close counterpart to the disease in lambs. However, the mortality rate in calves is higher (almost 100%) and the morbidity rate is lower. Usually, only young calves less than 3 weeks of age are affected. Calves are frequently born weak but do show a normal desire to suck the dam's colostrum. They become stiff, are reluctant to move, and may show fever and diarrhea; they usually die 2 to 10 days after onset of symptoms.[149]

Koch's postulates have been fulfilled to the full extent in regard to chlamydial polyarthritis in lambs and calves. The disease has been reproduced by inoculation via various parenteral routes. Unlike man, in whom the G.I. tract has not been shown to be of prime importance in the pathogenesis of chlamydial infections, the G.I. tract in animals is considered to be one of the most important sites of entry, initial multiplication, and dissemination of chlamydiae. This holds true not only for chlamydial polyarthritis in lambs and calves but also for chlamydial abortion, encephalomyelitis, and avian chlamydiosis.

Polyarthritis in calves can invariably be induced by oral inoculation. The pathogenetic events that occur subsequent to oral exposure and lead to chlamydial polyarthritis are depicted in Figure 9. These events were traced by reisolation of chlamydiae and fluorescent antibody (FA) tests on various organs at different intervals postinoculation.[161]

Isolation of chlamydiae from the bile points toward an interesting cycle between the intestines, portal vascular system, liver, bile, and small intestines. Intestinal infections in orally inoculated calves persist after initiation of systemic infection and polyarthritis. Although both lamb and calf chlamydial polyarthritis agents induce a systemic infection under experimental and natural conditions, they do have a specific propensity for synovial tissues since the most extensive multiplication occurred in joints and major symptoms and lesions are those of polyarthritis.

Similar macro- and microscopic lesions are seen in the affected joints of calves and lambs. Weight-bearing joints and also atlantooccipital joints are most severely affected. Synovial cavities contain excessive, turbid, grayish-yellow fluid and fibrin plaques. The synovial membrane is usually swollen and petechiated. Erosions on the articular surfaces are not present. Periarthritis, tendovaginitis, and tendofasciitis are commonly seen. Various somatic organs including the small intestine may reveal petechiation, edema, and hyperemia. Conjunctivitis is frequently seen together with polyarthritis in lambs. Unlike in man, the genital tract has not been proven to be of importance in the pathogenesis of polyarthritis in calves and lambs. More studies are needed to elucidate its role in animal chlamydiosis.[2,79,149,159,160]

Chlamydial polyarthritis in lambs must be differentiated from osteomalacia, mineral deficiences, erysipelas, bluetongue, and *Mycoplasma* infections. Differential diagnosis in chlamydial polyarthritis of calves must include mineral deficiences, especially selenium, abnormal osteogenesis, naval infections, and possibly *Mycoplasma* infections.

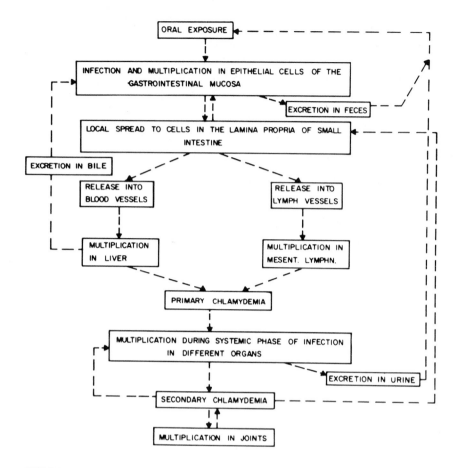

FIGURE 9.   Pathogenetic events following oral chlamydial exposure of calves as traced
by reisolation of the agent and immunofluorescence.

Disease in Man

The typical disease course of Reiter's syndrome starts with a nonspecific urethritis
7 to 14 days after a sexual episode, followed by conjunctivitis and arthritis. Besides
the classical triad of symptoms, other signs and lesions, such as balanitis, anterior
uveitis, tendonitis, stomatitis, pericarditis, myocarditis, thrombophlebitis, ankylosis of
the spine, and encephalopathy, are occasionally seen.[162] Microscopic lesions in the synovial membrane in Reiter's syndrome are characterized by the presence of mononuclear cells containing polymorphonuclear inclusions and by the plugging of small blood
vessels with platelets and polymorphonuclear cells.[163] Polymorphonuclear inclusions
within mononuclear cells can rarely be seen in chlamydial polyarthritis of lambs and
calves (Figure 10).

Recurrences of the disease, that may take place within weeks, months, or years of
each other occur in about 70% of the patients. In these patients, genital infections are
usually not detected while other signs such as uveitis, sarcoileitis, and cardiac involvement are more prominent. It has been estimated that about 0.5 to 2% of patients with
nonspecific urethritis develop Reiter's syndrome.[162] This disease is generally considered
a relatively rare sequela to a venereally acquired urethritis. However, it has also been
known for centuries that about 1% of patients develop arthritis and conjunctivitis
following dysentery. The etiology of dysentery was established as shigellosis in many
but not all cases. The dysenteric form of Reiter's syndrome is identical to the venereal

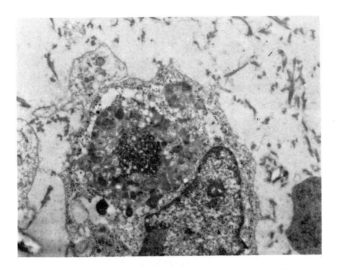

FIGURE 10.   Polymorphonuclear inclusion within the cytoplasm of a mononuclear cell in synovial tissues of calves with experimentally induced chlamydial polyarthritis.

form apart from the original site of the infection. Indeed, cases described originally by Reiter are retrospectively thought to be due to dysentery and not to a venereally transmitted infection.[162] This poses an interesting problem in terms of etiology and pathogenesis of the disease. It is generally agreed that chlamydiae are not the sole cause of Reiter's syndrome. What evidence, then, incriminates chlamydiae as at least partially responsible for the syndrome?

1.   Chlamydiae are known to cause polyarthritis, conjunctivitis, and genital infections in some animals.
2.   Chlamydiae are known to cause urethritis and genital infections in man. In several laboratories throughout the world, chlamydiae have been recovered from 20 to 40% of patients with urethritis or cervicitis/vaginitis. In most cases, no other pathogens were present. Experimental urethritis has been produced in monkeys with these isolates.
3.   Chlamydiae have been recovered from the synovial membrane and fluid, urethra, and conjunctivae of patients with Reiter's syndrome. The isolation rate from synovial tissues is generally low, but in a recent study it was reported to be as high as 17.2% of 29 patients.[164] The low isolation rate can to some degree be attributed to the frequent prior antibiotic treatment regime of these patients; this is known to interfere with isolation attempts. However, the fact that in some competent laboratories chlamydiae could not be recovered from patients with Reiter's syndrome[165] and that an identical syndrome can be seen following a shigella dysentery point toward a more complex etiology. It is difficult to conceive that widely different infectious agents by themselves would lead to a common pathological expression.

An attractive hypothesis has been put forward recently in view of the finding of a histocompatability antigen (HL-A27) in patients with Reiter's syndrome.[166,167] Therefore, arthritis (especially rheumatoid) may be defined as a reaction in joints that is associated with infection elsewhere in the body with the inciting organism absent from the joint itself. The stipulation that a host genetic factor is responsible for the mediation of common lesions following multiple initial etiological stimuli

— be they shigella dysentery, salmonellosis, yersinia, or a chlamydial urethritis — is an enlightening concept. It would also explain why only approximately 1% of patients with dysentery or chlamydial urethritis subsequently develop Reiter's syndrome. This concept received impetus from recent research with the histocompatability antigen HL-A27. This antigen has been found in (1) 70 to 90% of patients with Reiter's syndrome, (2) 87% of those with yersinia arthritis, (3) 10% of those with nonspecific urethritis, and (4) 6 to 14% of normal humans.[166,167]

The exact function of HL-A27 has not been determined. Several theories regarding the pathogenesis of Reiter's syndrome can be put forward. HL-A27 antigen may be so closely related to antigenic determinants of the invading microbe that (1) the host is unable to mount an effective immune response or, alternatively, (2) the host immune system becomes hypersensitive because of this "molecular mimicry," and the disease is perpetuated as a hypersensitivity reaction in the absence of the original inciting agent. On the other hand, the HL-A27 antigen may have nothing to do with the disease process. It may only serve as a marker—albeit a valuable one because of its close association with the locus of immune-response genes.

That susceptibility to Reiter's syndrome may be inherited receives support from reports describing the disease in brothers and several members of the same family.[162] First-degree relatives have been shown to have a higher incidence of forms of arthritis known to be associated with the HL-A27 antigen.[166]

The role of chlamydiae and other microbes in Reiter's syndrome may be one of inducing the initial insult, but the ultimate determination of whether Reiter's syndrome succeeds this insult may be governed by the genetic make-up of the host.

General Mode of Spread

Chlamydiae causing polyarthritis in calves and lambs are spread by direct contact within the species. The agent is excreted in the feces, urine, and ocular discharges if a conjunctivitis is concurrently present.[2] A vector has not been shown to be involved. Transmission between calves and lambs has not been reported although it seems conceivable in view of the relatedness of these agents.

Reiter's syndrome is mainly a venereally transmitted disease although post-shigella dysentery cases also occur. There has never been a case of human polyarthritis or Reiter's syndrome associated with polyarthritis outbreaks in calves and lambs.

Epidemiology

There is no evidence linking chlamydial polyarthritis in ruminants with other animals such as rodents or avian species. Avian chlamydiae do multiply and cause disease in ruminants when experimentally inoculated. They induce similar lesions in sheep as they do in man, such as bronchopneumonia and splenomegaly. However, none of the inoculated sheep showed polyarthritis.[98]

Perpetuation of the disease most likely depends upon the presence of latent carriers, and evidence points to the intestinal tract as the main organ system responsible for dissemination of the organism.[161] Outbreaks of polyarthritis in feedlots usually occur 2 to 4 weeks after transport from different points of origin to the lot.[168] The infection is acquired by inhalation of chlamydiae-laden dust and by ingestion.

In the western world, Reiter's syndrome is commonly considered to follow a venereal infection, while in the eastern world, it often succeeds shigella dysentery. As discussed above, present thinking is that patients with Reiter's syndrome appear to have an inherited characteristic that renders them susceptible if the proper inciting agent is encountered.

Presence of the histocompatability antigen HL-A27 in more than 70% of patients with Reiter's syndrome is an important finding. Its possible use as a diagnostic marker is, at present, only an intriguing prospect.

In 1818, Sir Benjamin Brodie first described what is now known as Reiter's syndrome and thought that it was caused by a venereally transmitted infectious agent. Progress in uncovering the etiology, epidemiology, and pathogenesis of this disease has been slow.

Diagnosis

Methods used in the diagnosis of polyarthritis in ruminants are discussed under "Diagnostic Procedures." Diagnosis of Reiter's syndrome is mainly clinical, based upon the triad of symptoms (arthritis, conjunctivitis, and urethritis) and history of a preceding venereal infection or dysentery. The laboratory can aid diagnosis by determining the presence of HL-A27 antigens or existence of chlamydiae with immunofluorescent techniques or isolation from any or all of the three lesion sites. Testing for chlamydial antibodies is of little value since rising titers are seldom observed.

ANIMAL CHLAMYDIAL INFECTIONS WITHOUT RECOGNIZED COUNTERPARTS IN HUMANS

Intestinal Infections

Chlamydiae have been recovered from the feces and intestinal tract of many apparently health (as well as diseased) species, except perhaps man. In 1951, York and Baker[169] isolated chlamydiae from the feces of about 60% of clinically normal calves. These naturally infected calves excreted chlamydiae for periods of 6 months, providing a rich source of organisms for contamination of the environment. Chlamydiae have since been recovered from the feces of cattle in various states of the U.S., Europe, Australia, and Japan. A similar intestinal chlamydial infection is also common in goats and sheep and has been reported from Japan, Europe, and the U.S.[2] Chlamydiae have also been isolated recently from the feces of dogs in England[170] and pigs in Austria.[171]

This inapparent intestinal infection in mammals is clearly comparable to the one that occurs in birds; here, chlamydiae are also excreted in the feces over long periods, sometimes without clinical symptoms and sometimes with symptoms of severe diarrhea in the course of a systemic chlamydiosis.[65]

While the majority of infected animals show no symptoms, diarrhea is occasionally associated with the infection. An interesting point is that many animals, even after clinical recovery, remain infected and continue to excrete the agent in the feces. In one case, for example, chlamydiae were recovered from the feces of a cow for 1 year.[172] Therefore, it is not surprising to find that the majority of animals with a localized intestinal infection have no or only low levels of humoral chlamydial antibodies.[173]

Pregnant ewes experiencing chlamydiae-induced abortions also frequently harbor the agent in the intestinal tract. In this regard, it is important to remember that the ovine and bovine chlamydial abortion strain and those isolated from intestinal tracts of clinically normal sheep and cattle are antigenically closely related and belong to the same serotype.[144,173]

Calves experimentally inoculated by the oral route with an enteric chlamydial isolate develop diarrhea.[161] Infection usually remains localized in the intestines but may reach the mesenteric lymph nodes; it has been traced by reisolation,[174] immunofluorescence,[174] and electron microscopy.[175] Fluorescing chlamydial inclusions were consistently observed in the cytoplasm of mucosal epithelial cells on the tips of the jejunal and ileal villi (Figure 11). Electron microscopic studies revealed that chlamydiae en-

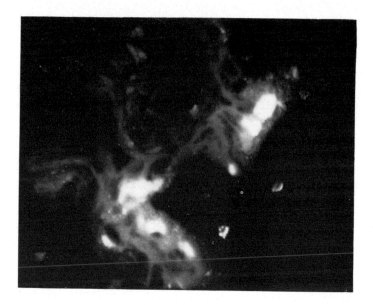

FIGURE 11.   Frozen section of the ileal mucosa of a calf that was orally inoculated with a chlamydial agent and stained with fluorescein-labeled specific chlamydial antiserum. Fluorescing intracytoplasmic inclusions in intestinal epithelial cells.

tered through the brush border of epithelial cells via endocytosis (Figure 12). Chlamydial polyarthritis strains traversed the epithelial mucosal cells and entered the lamina propria mucosae. After further multiplication in the lamina propria, they eventually entered endothelial cells and were subsequently liberated into lymphatic channels. Chlamydiae were also shown to multiply in macrophages, which, because of their mobility, certainly aided the spread of these organisms. In addition to the quiescent intestinal chlamydial infection, G.I. tract infections are also of major importance in the pathogenesis and epidemiology of other chlamydial infections. Lambs and ewes suffering from chlamydial polyarthritis have an intestinal infection simultaneously, and the disease can be reproduced by oral inoculation.[2,159,160] A fecal chlamydial isolate from "normal" sheep induced typical pneumonia after intratracheal inoculation.[176] Pregnant ewes superinfected parenterally with their own chlamydial fecal isolate aborted.[177]

Absence of clinical signs in many chlamydial intestinal infections is probably based on a balanced host-parasite relationship. Any alteration of this balance in favor of chlamydiae may result in the various aforementioned clinical manifestations. Storz and co-workers[178] observed marked shifts in the bacterial ecology of the intestinal tract in calves with experimentally induced chlamydial enteritis. High numbers of *Escherichia coli* were observed in the abomasum and small and large intestines in the principals while in control calves *E. coli* inhabited mainly the large intestine.

Little is known about the involvement of the intestinal tract in various human chlamydial infections. Rectal strictures and rectovaginal fistulas have long been recognized as sequelae in patients with LGV. Dunlop and co-workers[179] isolated chlamydiae from the rectum of a woman who gave birth to an infant with symptoms of inclusion conjunctivitis and also from two adults with chlamydial conjunctivitis.

It is surprising, in view of the ample evidence of latent chlamydial intestinal infections in animals, that no thorough study of chlamydial flora in "normal" humans has been undertaken. The challenging statement by K. F. Meyer[3] still awaits scientific eval-

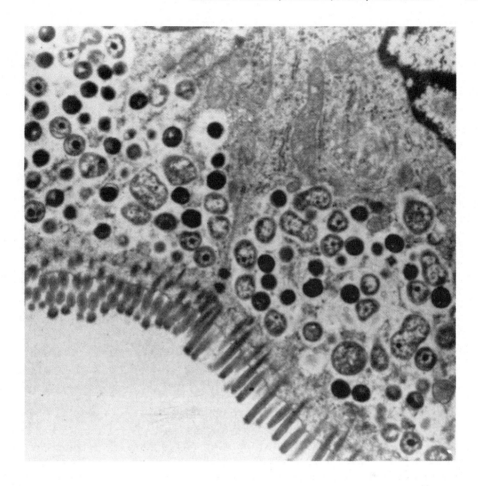

FIGURE 12.   Intestinal absorptive epithelial cells infected with chlamydiae. Various developmental chlamydial forms located between the nuclei and brush border (uranyl acetate-lead citrate stain). (From Doughri, A. M., Altera, K. P., Storz, J., and Eugster, A. K., *Exp. Mol. Pathol.*, 18, 10, 1973. With permission.)

uation: "Today it is imperative that the search for psittacosis-lymphogranuloma venereum-chlamydia agents in the excretions and secretions of man be systematically pursued . . . ."

Abortions

Chlamydial agents have been identified as the cause of spontaneous abortions in ewes,[180] cattle,[181] domestic rabbits,[182] pigs,[183] and goats.[184] Ovine chlamydial abortions were first recognized in 1950 in Scotland.[180] Since then, the disease has also been reported from Sardinia, Germany, France, the Balkan States, Cyprus, North Africa, Spain, and throughout the western U.S.[2] The distribution of bovine chlamydial abortions is similar.

Chlamydial infection of pregnant ewes and cows may result in abortions (usually during the last trimester of gestation), stillbirths, or weak calves. The incidence of abortion is generally low (1 to 5%) in a given flock or herd in which the disease is enzootic, but it may reach 30% in a flock of ewes exposed for the first time. There are no clinical signs in ewes or cows that indicate abortion is imminent. Following abortion, ewes usually recover without complications except occasional retainment of the placenta. In cows, on the other hand, retained placentas are a common sequela.

All of the various epidemiological aspects of this disease in cows and ewes have not been explored. Evidence collected to date implicates the ewe itself as the key in perpetuating the infection. Aborting ewes also frequently have an intestinal infection.[173] Chlamydial agents isolated from the feces of cattle induced abortion when inoculated parenterally into pregnant cows. Also, fecal isolates reinoculated parenterally into the same heifer caused abortion.[185] The same results were obtained with sheep.[177] Chlamydial isolates obtained from feces and aborted fetuses of cows and ewes are antigenically closely related or identical.[144]

The possibility of the highly contaminated aborted fetuses and placentas serving as a source of infection, and its spread via birds, scavengers, rodents, flies, and other vectors remain to be explored. Chlamydiae have been isolated from poultry arthropods,[54] ticks (*Dermacentor occidentalis*), and fleas.[95] These isolates have not been typed, and no experimental forced feeding studies have been reported. There is no evidence that these arthropods are biological vectors for chlamydiae; rather, they are thought to be mechanical carriers. The concept of vector transmission received impetus from studies in California where most chlamydial abortions in cattle occur after their return in the fall from foothill pastures.[181] While vectors may be involved occasionally, transmission of chlamydiae does not appear to depend upon them. Chlamydial abortions, for example, have occurred in stabled dairy herds in cold climate zones during winter months.[186]

Transmission of the agent between cattle and sheep seems possible in view of the positive experimental cross-infection results; however, it has not been reported to occur under natural conditions, nor is it necessary for maintaining the infection. In certain areas, chlamydial infections in cattle appear regional. For example, chlamydial abortions and encephalomyelitis in cattle were found only in western Texas.[187,188] This is also the major sheep-raising area in that state, and chlamydiae have been isolated from polyarthritic sheep there.[189] However, in most instances management practices preclude a direct interchange of the infection between sheep and cattle. Ecological and epidemiological factors, natural modes of transmission, and detection of reservoirs of the infection need to be further explored in regard to chlamydial abortion in ruminants.

Using antibiotics to prevent abortion in cows and ewes would be difficult since no signs of impending abortion are noted. Starting by at least the end of the first trimester of pregnancy, 2.5 to 5 mg of crude tetracycline in pelleted alfalfa hay would have to be given daily to all animals. In most cases, this is economically unfeasible.

Prevention and control of the disease through vaccination would certainly aid in conquering these diseases. In view of consistent failure to induce resistance in animals and man to various chlamydiosis, recent work by McKercher and associates[190] is encouraging. Multiple intradermal injections with an inactivated chlamydial bovine abortion strain induced resistance in cattle that withstood experimental challenge by the same route. The same vaccine given intramuscularly or subcutaneously was not effective. Further work is needed to expand this research effort.

Chlamydiae were also isolated from 4 of 22 human aborted conceptuses. Preliminary studies indicated that at least two of the isolates were — unlike trachoma, inclusion conjunctivitis, and human genital chlamydial isolates — sulfonamide resistant. The report did not indicate whether any of the four women, whose abortion specimens yielded chlamydiae with characteristics of the *C. psittaci* species, had any contact with livestock during or prior to pregnancy.[191] Giroud and co-workers[182,192] isolated agents with chlamydial properties from the cerebrospinal fluid of a febrile child and from an aborted human fetus and its placenta in the Congo. These patients had definite contact with sheep, goats, or cattle suffering from pneumonia or abortions. A case was reported from Britain, wherein a woman exposed to sheep developed a high chlamydial titer after aborting a 6-month-old fetus.[193] In neither of these case reports were chlamydial isolation attempts from animals on the farm undertaken.

Storz[2] reported an interesting case of a man who became ill while tending ewes that were aborting due to experimental chlamydial infection. The patient developed an acute febrile illness with headache, conjunctivitis, and nausea within a few days after cleaning the premises where the ewes had aborted. Chlorotetracycline therapy was initiated and the man made an uneventful recovery. He did develop high chlamydial antibody levels in his serum. A case of fatal pneumonitis with an alveolar-capillary block was reported in a California rancher[194] from whom a chlamydial agent was isolated from cardiac blood at autopsy. This man was the owner of cattle that experienced abortions, subsequently diagnosed as a result of chlamydial infection. A laboratory infection was reported by Barwell,[195] wherein the agent causing chlamydial abortion in ewes was isolated from the sputum of a laboratory worker.

These isolated cases, while too few from which to draw any conclusions, nevertheless should alert one to the possibility that the pathogenetic potential of chlamydia to cause abortions may also exist in man and that chlamydial abortion strains of animals may multiply and cause human disease.

Encephalomyelitis

Sporadic cases of chlamydial encephalomyelitis were first recognized in cattle in 1940.[196,197] The disease has since been observed in cattle in various parts of the U.S., Japan, Czechoslovakia, Australia, Canada, and Hungary.[2]

Animals of all ages can become infected, but the disease is especially prevalent in calves between 2 and 12 months of age. Affected calves become markedly depressed, anorectic, and sometime exhibit an intermittent diarrhea. The main symptoms are fever in the early stages of the disease and general inactivity evidenced by stiffness and lameness. These symptoms may be seen in a large percentage of calves in a given herd or may go unnoted depending upon the severity. Only a few of the affected calves eventually show CNS signs. Such calves exhibit an ataxic gait, staggering, and signs of paralysis that eventually prevent them from rising. Occasionally, calves also show opisthotonus, fall over small objects, and exhibit other CNS signs that might be confused with those seen in rabies.

A generalized, systemic chlamydial infection occurs concurrently or precedes involvement of the brain. This is evidenced by isolation of the organism from various somatic organs and the necropsy findings of a fibrinous peritonitis, pleuritis, and pericarditis.[188,196] Chlamydial encephalomyelitis in cattle is, therefore, basically a systemic disease with occasional involvement of the CNS.

Chlamydiae were also isolated from opossums in Columbia affected with a severe meningitis that resulted in convulsive seizures and paralysis of the hind extremities.[198] Agents with chlamydial properties were also isolated from dogs affected with encephalitis.[199]

An acute generalized encephalitis was also noted in an aborted bovine fetus from which chlamydiae were isolated.[187] Meningitis and encephalitis may also accompany a systemic chlamydiosis in avian species.[65]

Involvement of the central and peripheral nervous systems, resulting in various encephalitic symptoms, insomnia, disorientation, apathy, and even delirium, occurs sometimes in human chlamydioses contracted from avian sources (psittacosis). Human cases of encephalomyelitis attributable to contact with affected cattle have not been reported under natural conditions. One accidental laboratory infection, in which the agent causing bovine chlamydial encephalomyelitis was recovered from the blood of the patient, has been reported.[200]

Pneumonias Other than Zoonotic Avian Chlamydiosis

Pneumonia has been recognized as the main symptom of human chlamydiosis contracted from avian species (psittacosis) since the disease in man was first described almost a century ago.[57] Chlamydia-induced pneumonias have since been described in many other animals. In 1942, chlamydiae were isolated from pneumonic lesions of cats.[201] Affected cats start sneezing and coughing and subsequently exhibit a mucopurulent nasal discharge, conjunctivitis, rhinitis, and dyspnea. Cats usually recover within 2 to 4 weeks but may remain asymptomatic carriers. The disease is transmitted horizontally by contact with the highly contagious ocular and nasal secretions and aerosol. The disease may spread rapidly through a susceptible cattery. In cats, this chlamydia-induced disease can only be differentiated from herpesvirus- or picornavirus-induced respiratory infections with the aid of laboratory tests. A modified live chlamydial vaccine against feline chlamydial pneumonitis prepared from infected yolk sacs is available commercially in the U.S. There is some controversy about its effectiveness; however, it has been shown by at least one source that vaccinated cats are resistant to challenge with the virulent chlamydial cat pneumonitis strain.[202] Cats, by the nature of their habitat, could conceivably contract chlamydiae from infected mice, birds, and domesticated or wild mammals. This infection chain has not yet been proven, and what danger, if any, infected cats represent as man's companions has not been elucidated.

In one case, a chlamydial agent was isolated from a man with an acute follicular keratoconjunctivitis. This isolate did not have the biological characteristics of chlamydiae that cause trachoma and inclusion conjunctivitis. Rather, it appeared to belong to the species *C. psittaci*, that causes various animal chlamydial infections including feline pneumonitis. The patient owned a cat that had rhinitis and conjunctivitis. A chlamydial agent was subsequently isolated from this cat as well as another in the same household.[140]

Chlamydia-induced pneumonias have also been reported in sheep,[203] goats,[204] cattle,[117,205] pigs,[206] and foals;[157] in ruminants, the disease has been reported from many areas of the world. Distribution is probably more a reflection of concentrated diagnostic efforts in certain areas than an actual indication of the incidence of the disease.

Clinical signs and lesions in cattle, sheep, and goats are similar, consisting of fever, nasal discharge, cough, symptoms of a bronchopneumonia, and occasionally diarrhea. If uncomplicated, the disease is usually benign. Several authors emphasize the importance of predisposing factors, such as stress or concurrent infections with other microbial agents (e.g., *Pasteurella* sp., *Hemophilus*, and *Mycoplasma*), in the pathogenesis of chlamydial pneumonia.[207,208] As evidence, they cite the increased occurrence of pneumonias during movement of animals and in periods of highly variable fall and winter weather.

The ability of chlamydial agents isolated from the feces of clinically normal ruminants to experimentally induce pneumonia and the simultaneous isolation of chlamydiae from feces of animals naturally affected with pneumonia certainly point toward a causative involvement of the G.I. tract in the disease.[117,176,207,209] It is also interesting to note that the world-wide distribution of chlamydial pneumonia corresponds well with the epidemiology of clinically inapparent intestinal infections in cattle, sheep, and goats.

The occurrence of pneumonia may indeed be based upon existence of a latent intestinal infection. Changes in microbiological, immunological, and physiological factors and/or a combination thereof may lead to activation of the intestinal infection, resulting in a systemic chlamydiosis and bronchopneumonia.

Chlamydiosis in Laboratory and Wild Mammals

Mice and guinea pigs are common indicator hosts for chlamydiae and have been used extensively in the past for isolation and propagation of both species (*C. trachomatis* and *C. psittaci*). The important epidemiological questions are (1) Do wild mammals become infected with chlamydiae, (2) If so, do they represent a reservoir, and (3) Can the agent be transmitted to man and his domesticated animals?

The first question can be answered affirmatively. Many colonies and strains of clinically normal laboratory mice have been found to be latently infected with chlamydiae.[210] The infection can be activated by serial blind passages in mice, and treatment of affected colonies with tetracyclines is effective in eliminating the infection. This murine chlamydial isolate is reported to be sulfadiazine sensitive — a characteristic of *C. trachomatis* spp. — and represents the only *C. trachomatis* isolate from mammals other than man. Evidence indicates that it is of mouse origin; however, the possibility that it represents a human chlamydial agent introduced into the mouse colony cannot be excluded. Chlamydial agents belonging to the *C. psittaci* species have recently been recovered from mouse colonies.[211]

Storz[101] reported a systemic chlamydiosis with a high mortality rate in a laboratory herd of guinea pigs. The realization of natural chlamydial infections (especially latent ones) in mice and guinea pigs is of obvious diagnostic importance. These animals should be used for isolation purposes only after careful screening for the presence of chlamydiae.

Serological evidence suggests that chlamydial infections exist in several species of wildlife although at different prevalence levels. Debbie[212] found significant titers in about 200 of 500 deer tested in the state of New York and in Canada. Only eight serological reactors were found in more than 2000 sera of different wildlife species in Utah. These included deer, mice (*Peromyscus maniculatus*), jack rabbits (*Lepus californicus*), pocket mice (*Perognathus parvus*), and cottontail rabbits (*Sylvilagus sp.*).[213] In a later survey in the same area, 50 reactors (CF test) were found among 2305 wild animals tested. Animals with significant CF titers were found among rodents, lagomorphs, felids, and deer.[214] Serological evidence as well as isolation results showed that chlamydial infections also exist at a high prevalence rate in fur seals (*Calirhinus ursinus*) of the Pribilof Islands.[215]

From organ pools of 170 wild mammals in California, Eddie et al.[95] recovered chlamydiae from one wood rat (*Neotoma fuscipes*) and two pinon mice (*Peromyscus truci*). The organisms were also recovered in Columbia from common and wooly opossums captured in the wild and then housed in captivity for 45 days.[198]

A chlamydial agent identified as *C. psittaci* was isolated during an epizootic in muskrats and snowshoe hares (*L. americanus*) in Canada.[99] Entire populations of these two species died in the stricken areas. This epidemiological picture does not correspond with the one typically seen in almost all chlamydiosis, i.e., high prevalence of latent infections with occasional overt signs.

Then how is infection in these lagomorphs maintained? In experimental studies, it was learned that snowshoe hares are extremely susceptible and invariably die when inoculated by various parenteral and oral routes. However, only a mild disease with complete recovery could be induced in muskrats and rabbits by experimental inoculation.[216] The reason for the cataclysmic die-off between 1959 and 1961 may well have been confirmed using plaque reduction tests.[144] Two major serotypes were established: Starved, cachectic, and diseased animals were a common sight, and an existing parasite-host balance must certainly have shifted in favor of the parasite. An existing latent chlamydial infection in muskrats could very well have become activated and spread rapidly in those stressed and starved animals. Highly susceptible snowshoe hares live in close association with muskrats, and an interspecies transmission of chlamydiae is conceivable. This is a plausible example of a chlamydial infection possibly acting as a successful population control method in a particular ecosystem.

These few reports point to the potential importance of wildlife as a reservoir for chlamydial infection. Numerous theoretical infection chains, patterned by our knowledge of animal ecosystems, come to mind; however, lack of investigative work in this area prevents the drawing of any affirmative conclusions at this time.

CONCLUSION

The reader may have become bewildered by the multitude of symptoms and lesions chlamydiae are capable of inducing in such a broad host spectrum. Are all these diseases and syndromes caused by different chlamydial agents, or does the distribution of lesions merely present a tissue tropism? At present, there are two biochemically, biologically, and antigenically differentiable *Chlamydia* species (*C. trachomatis* and *C. psittaci*) recognized. *C. trachomatis* has been isolated only from man with the possible exception of the "Nigg" isolate from mice.[210] It causes trachoma, inclusion conjunctivitis, genital infection, and probably plays a role in the pathogenesis of Reiter's syndrome in man. Agents isolated from these different lesions and sites are antigenically related. However, there are some antigenic differences, and 12 subgroups have been proposed within this species.[217] Until proven otherwise, man will be considered the only host for this chlamydial species. Maintenance and perpetuation of the infection in man is dependent upon presence of latent infections and venereal as well as horizontal transmission.

All remaining chlamydial isolates — including all those from domesticated and wild animals (except perhaps the mouse pneumonitis isolate), avian species, and arthropods — belong to the species *C. psittaci*. How many different serotypes and subgroups exist within this species is not known precisely. Avian chlamydial isolates responsible for latent and systemic diseases in birds and pneumonitis in man (psittacosis) are antigenically unrelated to mammalian isolates.[144] Strain differences do exist within avian isolates. In turkeys, for example, one isolated chlamydial strain is of very low virulence, mainly causing latent infections, while another strain is of high virulence, causing severe epornitics with high mortality rates.

Latency is also a dominant feature in avian chlamydiosis and is responsible for its endemicity. Man is not required in this infection chain; rather, he is an incidental host.

Earlier work by Storz[2] on establishing serotypes within ruminant isolates has recently been confirmed using plague reduction tests.[144] Two major serotypes were established: type 1 includes isolates obtained from ovine and bovine abortion and enteric infections, and type 2 is comprised of isolates from ovine and bovine chlamydial polyarthritis, conjunctivitis, and bovine encephalomyelitis. These two serotypes are distinct, and it is interesting to note that diseases induced by serotypes 1 and 2 have not been observed to occur simultaneously under natural conditions. Evidence is accumulating that indicates that the intestinal tract frequently serves as the primary as well as continuing site of multiplication for both of these serotypes in ruminants. This important pathogenetic finding has obvious epidemiological implications.

Judging from world literature, mammalian chlamydial types are certainly not as infectious for humans as avian chlamydiae. There has never been a major zoonosis attributed to the mammalian type. However, there are enough reported cases to substantiate the fact that chlamydiae of nonhuman mammalian origin can multiply in man and produce disease.

DIAGNOSTIC PROCEDURES

The same diagnostic techniques can generally be applied to all chlamydial infection. Laboratory diagnosis of chlamydiosis is based upon: (1) isolation of the agent, (2) demonstration of the agent directly, either morphologically or immunologically, (3) demonstration of rising antibody levels between the acute stage of the disease and convalescence, and (4) histological examination of tissue changes as an aid in differential diagnosis. There are, however, no pathognomonic changes recognizable in chlamydiae-infected tissues.

Isolation of Chlamydiae

Chances for recovering chlamydiae are best early in the disease course. In selecting tissue sites for isolation, it is important to recall pathogenetic events leading to the particular disease. Isolation attempts obviously should be made from diseased tissues but should not be limited to them. For example, in bovine chlamydial encephalitis the organisms may no longer be recoverable from CNS tissues at the time of death, but they may still be present in the pericardial fluid, lung, liver, spleen, or intestinal tract. Feces in live animals or small intestinal mucosa and somatic organs in dead animals should always be cultured in addition to synovial tissue and fluid in chlamydial polyarthritis of ruminants. In chlamydial abortions of ewes and cows, feces of the dams should also be cultured along with placentas and a composite of fetal organs and fluids.

In cases of human chlamydial pneumonitis, sputum, tracheal swabs or washings, blood, and vomitus may yield chlamydiae while the patient is alive. On autopsy, a complete set of tissues and exudates — not only lung tissues — should be cultured. In this case, of course, investigation of the source of infection should be initiated even when only suspicions of the disease exist. In poultry-slaughtering establishments, any tissues with suspicious lesions uncovered by the post-mortem inspector should be examined; however, more importantly, a careful ante-mortem inspection should be undertaken and representative organ samples of diseased or even clinically normal birds should be cultured. Air sacs, exudates, spleen, liver, lung, and intestines are tissues of choice for chlamydial isolation attempts in birds. The astute epidemiologist should not stop if no avian source is obvious but should direct the search for a source toward wild or domesticated mammals or more obscure avian sources.

In localized infections such as conjunctivitis, urethritis, or cervicitis, scrapings of epithelial cells are obtained with Prince ring forceps, curettes, spatulas, or other suitable instruments. Cells are suspended in media for isolation and are also smeared onto slides for direct staining. In the early stages of trachoma, the upper tarsus and fornix appear to be the best sites for demonstrating the organism, while in conjunctivitis in neonates the lower tarsal conjunctiva and fornix are reported to be the best.[217] Handling and preparation of specimens for inoculation should be done under a safety hood whenever possible. Most laboratory infections are caused by inhalation of infected aerosol or accidental inoculation. *C. psittaci* of avian origin has been responsible for most laboratory infections, but all chlamydial organisms should be considered hazardous to human health and treated as such in laboratories. Even serologists using plugged pipettes may create an aerosol by pipetting sera from chlamydemic animals.

Best isolation results are obtained if specimens are inoculated into the proper indicator host as soon as possible. If an overnight delay is anticipated, specimens should be placed and processed in a buffer that contains protein or sucrose as a stabilizing component. This may be simply a nutrient broth, serum-containing tissue culture medium, or, as frequently used, a phosphate buffer containing sucrose and streptomycin (known as Bovarnick's buffer).[22] For overnight storage, specimens should be kept at 4°C. For long-term storage, chlamydiae may be preserved for years at −70°C or in a lyophilized state.

Feces or tissues heavily contaminated with extraneous bacteria are homogenized in a medium (such as Bovarnick's buffer[22]) containing 1 to 10 mg/mℓ streptomycin, 1 mg/mℓ Vancomycin®, and 1 mg/mℓ kanamycin. Bacitracin at 1000 units/mℓ or nystatin at 50 units/mℓ may also be used. The recent observation that gentamicin at concentrations of up to 100 μl/mℓ did not interfere with multiplication of *C. trachomatis* should aid in decontaminating specimens.[219] In the author's laboratory, gentamicin at a concentration of 50 μl/mℓ is routinely used, and various *C. psittaci* species of mammalian origin have been isolated in its presence.[220] Tetracyclines, Chloromycetin®, and penicillin cannot be used, since these antibiotics interfere with multiplication of chlamydiae.

Generally, a 20 to 40% suspension of tissues, feces, or exudates to be examined is prepared and centrifuged at 1000 × g for 30 min. The middle layer of the supernatant serves as inoculum. In the case of feces or other heavily contaminated specimens, the centifugation step may be repeated twice. Specimens, such as blood, joint fluid, and ascitic fluid, that are drawn aseptically, may be used directly as inoculum.

When inoculating tissue cultures or chicken embryos, it is advisable to make serial dilutions of tissues suspensions or fluids since this not only serves as a means of quantifying the number of organisms present but, perhaps more importantly, as a means of diluting out toxic effects and extraneous contaminants. The most widely used indicator hosts for isolation of chlamydiae are 7-day-old chicken embryos, tissue cultures, mice, and guinea pigs.

Chicken Embryos

Intra-yolk sac inoculation of 6- to 8-day-old developing chicken embryos is now the most widely used method for isolation of chlamydiae. All known chlamydial strains can infect and multiply in cells of the yolk sac membrane.[2] It is important to obtain fertile eggs from flocks free of *Mycoplasma* infections that are being fed a ration free of antibiotics. The most commonly used incubation temperature for inoculated chicken embryos is 37°C. With chlamydiae isolated from the human conjunctivae, incubation temperatures of 34 to 35°C reportedly yield better results.[221] Death of chick embryos within 2 to 3 days after inoculation is considered to be caused by bacterial contamination or nonspecific reasons and these embryos are discarded. Yolk sac membranes of embryos that die 3 to 4 days after inoculation and thereafter are harvested. There is an inverse relationship between time of death and concentration of the organism in the inoculum. Generally, embryos start dying about 5 days postinoculation; this is somewhat dependent upon the chlamydial strain and, of course, concentration. Yolk of infected embryos is usually thinner than normal, and the trophoblastic villi of yolk sac membranes may be partially absent or reduced in size. A prominent lesion in infected embryos is a severe congestion of yolk sac blood vessels, and the embryo itself, especially the legs and toes, is frequently hyperemic (Figure 13).

After stripping off excess yolk, an impression smear of the yolk sac membrane yields typical elementary bodies. The stain usually used is the one originally described by Giménez.[222] Elementary bodies stain bright red and are perfectly spherical (Figure 14) while reticulate bodies are much larger and appear blue. Isolation attempts from clinical material frequently do not result in chicken embryo deaths in the first passage.

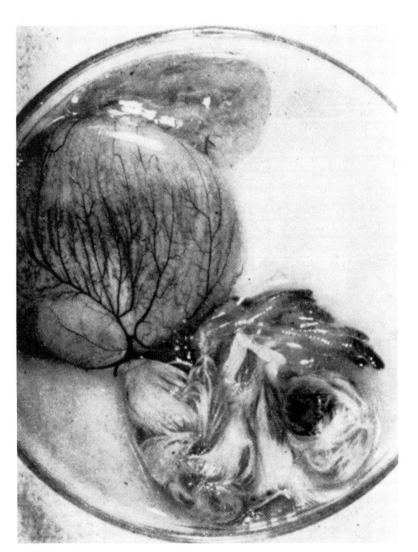

FIGURE 13. Chicken embryo and yolk sac 10 days after inoculation with a chlamdial agent. Note congestion of yolk sac blood vessels and hyperemia and congestion of toes. (From Storz, J., *Chlamydia and Chlamydia-Induced Diseases*, courtesy of Charles C Thomas, Springfield, Ill., 1971. With permission.)

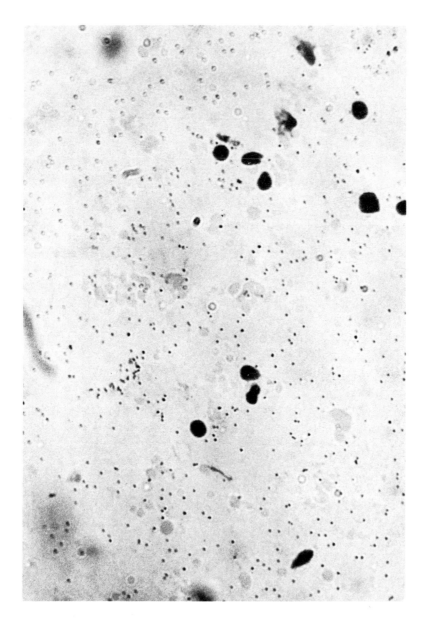

FIGURE 14.   Yolk sac smear of a chick embryo 7 days after inoculation with a chlamydial agent.   Numerous dark dots are elementary bodies. (Gimenez stain.)

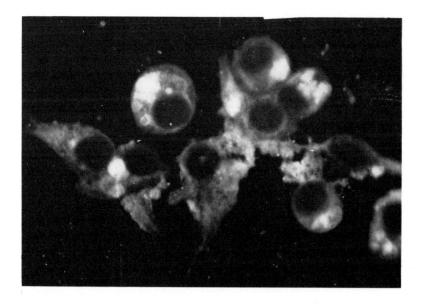

FIGURE 15.   Fluorescing chlamydial inclusions in mouse L-cells inoculated with chlamydial agents (stained with fluorescein-labeled chlamydial antibodies).

Yolk sac membranes are then harvested between 10 to 19 days postinoculation and passed "blindly" three to six times before a sample is called negative. Characteristic death patterns may become obvious only after several passages in chicken embryos. A typical incubation period (3 to 6 days), the linear inverse relationship between concentration and time of death of the embryos, and tinctorial properties of chlamydiae in stained yolk sac smears offer presumptive evidence for the presence of chlamydiae. This may be confirmed by preparing a 20 to 50% infected yolk sac suspension, heating it for 30 min at 100°C, then testing it against known antisera in the CF test.

Cell Cultures

Cell cultures have not yet been widely used for chlamydial isolation. However, they have been extensively employed in studies of chlamydial infection at the cellular level. The host spectrum of chlamydiae in cell cultures is unknown. Chick embryo fibroblasts, mouse cell lines such as L-cells and McCoy cells, or human cell lines such as Chang liver and various diploid cells support the growth of certain chlamydial strains. Most strains do multiply in various cell cultures to some extent; however, in many cases it is difficult to make serial passages.

While cell cultures are not the indicator host of choice for isolation of *C. psittaci*, Gordon and associates[223] reported equal or better isolation rates from human patients with *C. trachomatis* infections when they used irradiated cell cultures rather than chicken embryos. The McCoy cell line was subjected to 5000 rad of gamma- or X-irradition 5 days prior to inoculation with human conjunctival, urethral, or genital specimens. Presence of chlamydiae was detected by recognition of glycogen-containing inclusions — characteristic of the *C. trachomatis* species — after staining with iodine solutions or Giemsa. Evidence that chlamydiae are present in infected cultures can also be obtained by reacting them with known chlamydial antisera in the CF test or by demonstrating specific intracytoplasmic fluorescence when stained with a fluorescein-labeled chlamydial antiserum (Figure 15).

Many chlamydial strains produce varying degrees of cell destruction after some adaptive period. Partial purification of the inoculum by centrifuging clarified infected yolk suspension through a 25% sucrose solution improved the initiation of infection in cell cultures.[129] Addition of 10% calf serum to the crude inoculum also provided a more favorable condition for infection and replication of chlamydiae.

Mice

Before using mice, guinea pigs, or other laboratory animals, two parameters need to be clarified: (1) the animals should not be on antibiotic-containing feed and (2) they themselves should be free of any natural chlamydial infection. The latter may be checked by serially passing tissue suspensions in the given species and/or by serological testing for chlamydial antibodies.

Mice have been extensively used for isolation of *C. psittaci* of avian origin and from humans affected with psittacosis. Some human *C. trachomatis* isolates as well as some *C. psittaci* isolates of mammalian origin have been shown to be nonpathogenic to mice on primary isolation attempts. Therefore, it may be prudent to perform isolation attempts in both mice and chicken embryos.

Young laboratory mice can be inoculated with a 10 to 20% suspension intraperitoneally, intranasally, or intracerebrally. Death may occur as soon as 2 days or as late as 30 days after inoculation, depending upon the virulence and concentration of the organism. Some mice may recover, and in some cases one to three blind passages at 7 to 14 days are required. Mice dying 2 to 3 days postinoculation show few, if any, grossly visible abnormalities such as a bloated duodenum after intraperitoneal administration or congestion of lungs after intranasal instillation. When death occurs 5 to 15 days post-intraperitoneal inoculation, splenomegaly, liver necrosis, and peritonitis are usually visible. Stained-impression smears from those organs with lesions reveal numerous cells containing chlamydial elementary bodies in their cytoplasm. Lobules or entire lungs may become consolidated after intranasal inoculation, and elementary bodies are found in lung impression smears or sections.

Intracerebral inoculation frequently results in a more rapid diagnosis. However, the purity of the inoculum (in terms of being free from extraneous microbial agents and toxins) is perhaps more critical when using this route than when the intraperitoneal or intranasal route is employed. Mice often develop paralysis and somnolescence within 1 or 2 days and usually die within 3 to 5 days. Chlamydiae are demonstrated in meningeal impression smears; histologically, the lesions consist of a meningoencephalitis with pronounced perivascular cuffing.

Guinea Pigs

It is not uncommon to find natural chlamydial infections in herds of guinea pigs.[101] Testing for chlamydiae prior to use of these animals is, therefore, mandatory. It should be remembered that, when using guinea pig serum as a source of complement, false-positive results may be obtained in chlamydial CF tests if the serum originated from an infected herd and, therefore, contains chlamydial antibodies.

Guinea pigs have frequently been used in the past to isolate *C. psittaci* strains of mammalian origin. Avian isolates, except those from turkeys and egrets, appear to be less pathogenic for guinea pigs than for mice or chicken embryos. Intraperitoneal inoculation of guinea pigs elicits a febrile illness that terminates fatally within 5 to 10 days. Prominent lesions are a fibrinous peritonitis, splenomegaly, and liver necrosis. Demonstration of elementary bodies in lesion material or rising antibody titers serve as evidence of the infection.[224]

Direct Morphological and Immunological Demonstration of Chlamydiae

Impression smears or frozen sections from lesion material always offer a good diagnostic tool, not only for detecting the presence of chlamydiae, but also for detecting other microbes and differentiating inflammatory cells. For example, the presence of high numbers of eosinophils in conjunctival smears may also lead the diagnostician to consider an allergenic problem.

Generally, the chances of demonstrating chlamydiae in direct impression smears are enhanced if the smears are made early in the acute stage of the disease. Therefore, chlamydial inclusions can frequently be seen in impression smears of acute cases of human and animal conjunctivitis; unfortunately, they are rarely observed in more chronic diseases such as trachoma. Inclusions consisting of purplish-colored elementary bodies (when stained with Giemsa) can be seen in the cytoplasm of conjunctival epithelial cells (Figure 8), free in the exudate, or phagocytosed in neutrophils. Chlamydial inclusions are also occasionally found in impression smears made from epithelial scrapings of the cervix and urethra. Direct demonstration of chlamydiae in synovial tissues of polyarthritic animals or persons with Reiter's syndrome is rarely successful. In any event, absence of chlamydial inclusions in direct impression smears by no means rules out chlamydial infection. It is a useful first step in chlamydial diagnosis but should always be followed by isolation attempts.

Staining of smears or frozen sections with fluorescein-labeled chlamydial antibodies adds specificity and sensitivity if the test procedure is properly standardized. Apart from its diagnostic value, this technique has greatly aided in elucidating the pathogenesis of various chlamydial infections.[174] It serves as a rapid and specific method of establishing the presence of a chlamydial infection in cell cultures, especially since the problem of nonspecific staining in this system is minor compared to staining problems that arise with direct tissue smears or sections.

Serological Tests

CF Test

All chlamydiae share a heat-stable antigen that fixes complement in the presence of chlamydial antibodies. The CF test (and variations thereof) has been and still is the most widely used serological test for chlamydial infections. However, like other serological tests, it has limitations that need to be recognized. Very few humoral antibodies may be present in strictly localized superficial chlamydial infections such as trachoma or urogenital infections. Only about 50% of humans with eye and genital infections have chlamydial CF titers of 1:16 or higher, and only 15% of men with chlamydial urethritis have significant CF titers.[225] The CF test is a group-specific test, and the recently recognized high prevalence of urogenital chlamydial infections in man has to be considered when evaluating serological surveys for psittacosis or other chlamydial infections.

Thus, a positive serological result on a single serum sample supports a diagnosis of chlamydiosis but by no means proves it. Height of titers might be of some aid when all parameters of the disease are considered together. The only way a serological diagnosis of chlamydiosis can be made is by demonstrating a rising titer (at least a fourfold increase) between the time samples are taken during the acute stage of the disease and convalescence. Chlamydial antibodies may not be present in measurable amounts if the infection is aborted early with antibiotic therapy. It should also be pointed out that presence of complement-fixing chlamydial antibodies is by no means in itself an indication of host resistance. Chlamydiae have been repeatedly isolated from blood in the presence of high levels of humoral antibodies.[226]

Group-specific chlamydial antigens are commercially available; however, their quality varies. These antigens may be prepared from any one chlamydial strain by boiling chlamydial suspensions and extracting them with deoxycholate, acid, alkali, diethyl ether, phenol, or water. A detailed method that uses heat and phenol is described by Meyer et al.[224]

Guinea pig complement should always be checked for chlamydial antibodies before use. The CF test may be performed in standard test tubes or micro titer plates. If the microsystem is used, it is still advisable to standardize the complement and hemolytic system in tubes prior to their use in the micro CF test.

Most avian species other than pigeons do not fix guinea pig complement. In these species, an indirect CF test[227] or a direct CF test that is modified by the addition of unheated normal chlamydiae antibody-free rooster serum needs to be employed.[228]

Agglutination Test

Slide and tube agglutination tests have been used occasionally in determining chlamydial antibodies, especially in avian species. The reaction is also group-specific, as in the CF test. Nonspecific clumping of the antigen has presented a problem. If the purity of the antigen is improved, this may serve as a valuable and rapid serological tool for laboratories unequipped to use the more sophisticated CF test. A capillary-tube agglutination test was devised by Mason,[229] wherein Giemsa-stained chlamydial suspensions were drawn halfway into 0.4 mm capillary tubes, followed by antiserum. The tubes were then inverted and allowed to stand at room temperature for 4 to 24 hr. As the stained chlamydiae traveled down through the antiserum, agglutination became visible. Agglutinating antibodies appear earlier after experimental inoculation of turkeys but disappear more rapidly than CF antibodies.

Agar Gel Diffusion (AGP) Test

The AGP test is also a simple and rapid serological test. It is slightly less sensitive than the CF test in detecting chlamydial antibodies and was originally applied to human sera from trachoma patients.[230] Page found it a reliable test in detecting antibodies in turkeys and parakeets but, for unknown reasons, not in pigeon and sparrow sera.[231] The antigen used is a partially purified, chlamydiae-containing yolk sac suspension extracted with 1% sodium deoxycholate; the method is described in detail by Page.[231] This same antigen may also be used in the CF test. The main advantage of the AGP test when compared to the CF test is simplicity. However, CF tests are generally considered more sensitive than AGP tests, and this probably also holds true in the case of chlamydial serology.

Immunofluorescence

An indirect microimmunofluorescence (IFA) test is reportedly more sensitive than the CF test.[232] The IFA test measures specific antibodies to a particular chlamydial serotype. This test has been applied mainly to detect *C. trachomatis* antibodies in serum and conjunctival exudates; however, it should be equally applicable to *C. psittaci* serology.

Chlamydial elementary bodies of yolk-sac origin are placed on a glass slide in concentrations determined by pretitrations. After fixation in acetone, these slides may be stored frozen for months and probably years. After the thawed slide is dry, serial dilutions of the serum to be tested are placed on the slide in dots, incubated, and then washed. This is followed by addition of the second antibody, i.e., a fluorescein-labeled antispecies serum. Any antibody in the original serum adhering to the chlamydial elementary body after washing then becomes labeled by the fluorescein-tagged antispecies antibody.[232] It certainly would also seem possible to use infected cell cultures instead of yolk sac smears as substrates in the IFA test.

Serum Neutralization and Plaque Reduction Test

Multiplication of chlamydiae and their infectivity can be neutralized with high-titered antisera. The test may be performed in chicken embryos, mice, or preferably tissue cultures. The plaque reduction test using mouse L-cells has been successfully employed in serotyping chlamydial agents.[144] These tests are quite valuable in the reference laboratory but are presently not applicable to any large scale epidemiological investigation.

EDITORIAL COMMENT

A review of general chlamydia infections that caused eye problems appeared in *Clinical Trends*, January 1977. The article stated that *C. trachomatis* now causes more ophthalmia neonatorum in the U.S. than does gonococcus. Statistics from England indicate that it causes eye problems five to six times more frequently there. Although silver nitrate prophylaxis at birth is still standard in both countries, it is ineffective against this organism. This statement was made by Dr. John W. Chandler at the American Academy of Ophthalmology and Otolaryngology meetings in Las Vegas. Dr. Chandler's full report was published in the journal *Transactions of the American Academy of Ophthalmology and Otolaryngology, 83, 302, 1977.*

REFERENCES

1. **Moulder, J. W.**, *The Psittacosis Group as Bacteria,* John Wiley & Sons, New York, 1964.
2. **Storz, J.**, *Chlamydia and Chlamydia-induced Diseases,* Charles C Thomas, Springfield, Ill., 1971.
3. **Meyer, K. F.**, The host spectrum of psittacosis-lymphogranuloma venereum (PL) agents, *Am. J. Ophthalmol.*, 63, 1225; 199, 1967.
4. **Halberstädter, L.**, Trachom und Chlamydozoenerkrankungen der Schleimhaute, in *Handbuch der Pathogenen Protozoen,* von Prowazek, S., Ed., Barth, Leipzig, 1912, 172.
5. **Jones, H., Rake, G., and Stearns, B.**, Studies on lymphogranuloma venereum. III. The action of the sulfonamides on the agent of lymphogranuloma venereum, *J. Infect. Dis.*, 76, 55, 1945.
6. **Page, L. A.**, Revision of the family Chlamydiaceae Rake (rickettsiales): unification of the psittacosis-lymphogranuloma-venereum-trachoma group of organisms in the genus *Chlamydia*, Jones, Rake and Stearns, 1945, *Int. J. Syst. Bacteriol.*, 16, 223, 1966.
7. **Buchanan, R. and Gibbons, N.**, Eds., *Bergey's Manual of Determinative Bacteriology,* 8th ed., Waverly Press, Baltimore, 1974, 914.
8. **Gordon, F. B. and Quan, A. L.**, Occurrence of glycogen in inclusions of the psittacosis-lymphogranuloma venereum-trachoma agents, *J. Infect. Dis.*, 115, 186, 1965.
9. **Lin, H. S. and Moulder, J. W.**, Patterns of response to sulfadiazine, D-cycloserine and D-alanine in members of the psittacosis group, *J. Infect. Dis.*, 116, 372, 1966.
10. **Jenkin, H. M.**, Preparation and properties of cell walls of the agent of meningopneumonitis, *J. Bacteriol.*, 80, 639, 1960.
11. **Mitsui, Y., Fujimoto, M., and Kajima, M.**, Development and morphology of trachoma agent in the yolk sac cell as revealed by electron microscopy, *Virology*, 23, 30, 1964.
12. **Costerton, J. W., Poffenroth, L., Wilt, J. C., and Kordova, N.**, Ultrastructural studies of *Chlamydia psittaci* 6BC *in situ* in yolk sac explants and L-cells: comparison with Gram-negative bacteria, *Can. J. Microbiol,* 21, 1433, 1975.
13. **Kuo, C. C., Wang, S. P., and Grayston, J. T.**, Effect of polycations, polyanions and neuraminidase on the infectivity of trachoma-inclusion conjunctivitis and lymphogranuloma venereum organisms in HeLa Cells: sialic acid residues as possible receptors for trachoma-inclusion conjunctivitis, *Infect. Immun.*, 8, 74, 1973.

14. **Moulder, J. W., Hatch, T. P., Byrne, G. I., and Kellog, K. R.,** Immediate toxicity of high multiplicities of *Chlamydia psittaci* for mouse fibroblasts (L-cells), *Infect. Immun.,* 14, 277, 1976.

15. **Armstrong, J. A. and Reed, S.,** Nature and origin of initial bodies in lymphogranuloma venereum, *Nature* (London), 201, 371, 1964.

16. **Friis, R. R.,** Interaction of L-cells and *Chlamydia psittaci:* entry of the parasite and host responses to its development, *J. Bacteriol.,* 110, 706, 1972.

17. **Schechter, E. M.,** Synthesis of nucleic acid and protein in L cells infected with the agent of meningopneumonitis, *J. Bacteriol.,* 91, 2069, 1966.

18. **Crocker, T. T., Pelc, S. R., Nielsen, B. I., Eastwood, J. M., and Banks, J.,** Population dynamics and deoxyribonucleic acid synthesis in HeLa cells infected with an ornithosis agent, *J. Infect. Dis.,* 115, 105, 1965.

19. **Lin, H. S.,** Stability of the nucleic acids of L-cells after infection with the meningopneumonitis agent, *J. Bacteriol.,* 96, 2049, 1968.

20. **Page, L. A.,** High body temperature of pigeons and sparrows as a factor in their resistance to an agent of the psittacosis group, *Bull. Wildl. Dis. Assoc.,* 1, 49, 1965.

21. **Page, L. A.,** Thermal inactivation studies on a turkey ornithosis virus, *Avian Dis.,* 3, 67, 1959.

22. **Bovarnick, M. E., Miller, J. C., and Snyder, J. C.,** The influence of certain salts, amino acids, sugars and proteins on the stability of rickettsiae, *J. Bacteriol.,* 59, 509, 1950.

23. **Nabli, B. and Tarizzo, M. L.,** The effect of antiseptics and other substances on TRIC agents, *Am. J. Ophthalmol.,* 63, 1541/515, 1967.

24. **Weiss, E.,** The effect of antibiotics on agents of the psittacosis-lymphogranuloma group. I. The effect of penicillin, *J. Infect. Dis.,* 87, 249, 1950.

25. **Walz, A.,** Morphologische Studien an einem Psittakosestamm und seine Veränderungen unter dem Einfluss von Penicillin, *Zentralbl. Bakteriol. Parasitenkd. Infektionskr. Hyg. Abt. 1: Orig.,* 188, 29; 174, 1963.

26. **Gordon, F. B., Andrew, V. W., and Wagner, J. C.,** Development of resistance to penicillin and to chlortetracycline in psittacosis virus, *Virology,* 4, 156, 1957.

27. **Gordon, F. B., Mamay, H. K., and Trimmer, R. W.,** Studies with drug-resistant strains of psittacosis virus. II. Derivation of strains with dual drug resistance from mixed culture of singly resistant strains, *Virology,* 11, 486, 1960.

28. **Pollard, M. and Starr, T. J.,** Study of intracellular virus with acridine orange fluorochrome, *Prog. Med. Virol.,* 4, 54, 1962.

29. **Gordon, F. B. and Quan, A. L.,** Drug susceptibilities of the psittacosis and trachoma agents, *Ann. N.Y. Acad. Sci.,* 98, 261, 1962.

30. **Juergensen, T.,** *Ziemssen's Handbuch der speziellen Pathologie und Therapie. Handbuch der Krankheiten des Respirations-Apparatus,* Vol. 2, Vogel, Leipzig, 1894, 3.

31. **Rasmussen, R. K.,** Über eine durch Sturmvögel übertragbare Lungenerkrankung auf den Faröern, *Zentralbl. Bakteriol. Parasitenkd. Infektionskr. Hyg. Abt. 1: Orig.,* 132, 240, 1939.

32. **Haagen, E. and Mauser, G.,** Über eine auf den Menschen übertragbare Virus-Krankheit bei Sturmvogeln und ihre Beziehungen zur Psittakose, *Zentrabl. Bakterial. Parasitenkd. Infektionskr. Hyg. Abt. 1: Orig.,* 132, 238, 1939.

33. **Pollard, M.,** Ornithosis in sea-shore birds, *Proc. Soc. Exp. Biol. Med.,* 64, 200, 1947.

34. **Miles, J. A. R. and Shrivaston, J. B.,** Ornithosis in certain sea-birds, *J. Anim. Ecol.,* 20, 195, 1951.

35. **Rubin, H., Kissling, R. E., Chamberlain, R. W., and Edison, M. E.,** Isolation of a psittacosis-like agent from the blood of snowy egrets, *Proc. Soc. Exp. Biol. Med.,* 78, 696, 1951.

36. **Pollard, M.,** Psittacosis in seashore birds, in *Psittacosis, Diagnosis, Epidemiology and Control,* Beaudette, F. R., Ed., Rutgers University Press, New Brunswick, N.J., 1955, 99.

37. **Coles, J. D. W. A.,** Psittacosis in domestic pigeons, *Onderstepoort J. Vet. Sci. Anim. Ind.,* 15, 141, 1940.

38. **Meyer, K. F., Eddie, B., and Yanamura, H. Y.,** Ornithosis (psittacosis) in pigeons and its relation to human pneumonitis, *Proc. Soc. Exp. Biol. Med.,* 49, 609, 1942.

39. **Meyer, K. F. and Eddie, B.,** Spontaneous ornithosis (psittacosis) in chickens — the cause of a human infection, *Proc. Soc. Exp. Biol. Med.,* 49, 522, 1942.

40. **Meyer, K. F. and Eddie, B.,** Reservoirs of the psittacosis agent, *Acta Trop.,* 9, 204, 1952.

41. **Strauss, J.,** Ornithosis in Czechoslovakia, *Acta Virol.* (Engl. ed.), 1, 132, 1957.

42. **Fürst, W., Kovac, W., and Moritzsch, H.,** Enten als Virusreservoir für Ornithoseerkrankungen des Menschen, *Wien. Klin. Wochenschr.,* 69, 223, 1957.

43. **Oretel, S.,** Serologische und epidemiologische Untersuchungen während einer Ornithose-Epidemie bei Angestellten eins Geflügelschlachthofes, *Zentralbl. Bakterial. Parasitenkd. Infektionskr. Hyg. Abt. 1: Orig.,* 180, 441, 1960.

44. Irons, J. V., Denley, M. L., and Sullivan, T. D., Psittacosis in turkeys and fowls as a source of human infection, in *Psittacosis: Diagnosis, Epidemiology and Control*, Beaudette, F. R., Ed., Rutgers University Press, New Brunswick, N.J., 1955, 44.

45. Page, L. A., Ecologic considerations in turkey ornithosis, *Am. J. Vet. Res.*, 21, 618, 1960.

46. Graber, R. E., Ornithosis-psittacocis in Wisconsin, a preliminary report of a human outbreak transmitted from turkeys, *Wis. Med. J.*, 56, 341, 1957.

47. Graber, R. E. and Pomeroy, B. S., Ornithosis (psittacosis): an epidemiological study of a Wisconsin human outbreak transmitted from turkeys, *Am. J. Public Health*, 48, 1469, 1958.

48. Center for Disease Control, Morbidity and Mortality, Weekly Report, U.S. Department of Health, Education and Welfare, Public Health Service, Atlanta, 23(36), 309, 1974.

49. Ward, C. G. and Birge, J. P., Psittacosis (ornithosis) following contact with pheasants: report of a case, *JAMA*, 150, 217, 1952.

50. Strauss, J., Ornithosis in men and ducks microbiologically identified, *Cesk. Epidemiol. Mikrobiol. Imunol.*, 5, 281, 1956.

51. Mykytowycz, R., Dane, D. A., and Beech, M., Ornithosis in the petrel, *Puffinus tenuirostris* (Temminck), *Aust. J. Exp. Biol. Med. Sci.*, 33, 629, 1955.

52. Dömök, I., Ornithosis epidemics of the last two years in Hungary, *Arch. Gesamte Virusforsch.*, 13, 323, 1963.

53. Parnas, J. and Szmuness, W., Untersuchungen über Ornithose, *Zentralbl. Bakteriol. Parasitenkd. Infektionskr. Hyg. Abt. 1: Orig.*, 183, 141, 1961.

54. Meyer, K. F. and Eddie, B., Feather mites and ornithosis, *Science*, 132, 300, 1960.

55. Eddie, B., Meyer, K. F., Lambrecht, F. L., and Furman, D. P., Isolation of ornithosis bedsoniae from mites collected in turkey quarters and from chicken lice, *J. Infect. Dis.*, 110, 231, 1962.

56. Treuting, W., Epidemiology of Louisiana pneumonitis, in *Psittacosis, Diagnosis, Epidemiology and Control*, Beaudette, F. R., Ed., Rutgers University Press, New Brunswick, N.J., 1955, 111.

57. van Rooyen, C. E., The early history of psittacosis, in *Psittacosis, Diagnosis, Epidemiology and Control*, Beaudette, F. R., Ed., Rutgers University Press, New Brunswick, N.J., 1955, 3.

58. Nocard, E., Rapport General sur les Travaux du Conseil d'Hygiène Publique et de Salubrité du Département de la Seine, 1890-1894, 1893, 278.

59. Levinthal, W., Die Ätiologie der Psittakosis, *Klin. Wochenschr.*, 9, 654, 1930.

60. Coles, A. C., Microorganisms in psittacosis, *Lancet*, 1, 1011, 1930.

61. Lillie, R. D., Psittacosis: rickettsia-like inclusions in man and in experimental animals, *Public Health Rep.*, 45, 773, 1930.

62. Bedson, S. P., Western, G. T., and Simpson, S. L., Observations on the etiology of psittacosis, *Lancet*, 1, 235, 1930.

63. Meyer, K. F. and Eddie, B., Psittacosis in importations of psittacine birds from the South American and Australian continent, *J. Infect. Dis.*, 65, 234, 1939.

64. Burnet, E. M. and MacNamara, J., Human psittacosis in Australia, *Med. J. Aust.*, 2, 84, 1936.

65. Meyer, K. F., Ornithosis, in *Diseases of Poultry*, 5th ed., Biester, H. E. and Schwarte, L. H., Eds., Iowa State University Press, Ames, 1965, 675.

66. Meyer, K. F., The ecology of psittacosis and ornithosis, *Medicine* (Baltimore), 21, 175, 1942.

67. Page, L. A., Experimental ornithosis in turkeys, *Avian Dis.*, 3, 51, 1959.

68. Burnet, F. M., A note on occurrence of fatal psittacosis in parrots living in the wild state, *Med. J. Aust.*, 1, 545, 1939.

69. Page, L. A. and Bankowski, R. A., Investigation of a recent ornithosis epornitic in California turkeys, *Am. J. Vet. Res.*, 20, 941, 1959.

70. Burkhart, R. L. and Page, L. A., Chlamydiosis (ornithosis-psittacosis), in *Infectious and Parasitic Diseases of Wild Birds*, Davis, J., Anderson, R., Karstad, L., and Trainer, D., Eds., Iowa State University Press, Ames, 1971, 118.

71. Sprunt, D. H., The pathology of psittacosis, in *Psittacosis, Diagnosis, Epidemiology and Control*, Beaudette, F. R., Ed., Rutgers University Press, New Brunswick, N.J., 1955, 33.

72. Carlson, H. C., Whenhahm, G. R., and Bigland, C. H., Ornithosis in turkeys in Alberta, *Avian Dis.*, 5, 31, 1961.

73. Meyer, K. F., Psittacosis-lymphogranuloma venereum agents, in *Viral and Rickettsial Infections of Man*, 4th ed., Horsfall, F. L. and Tamm, J., Eds., Lippincott, Philadelphia, 1965, 1006.

74. Berman, S., Freundlich, E., Glaser, K., Abrahamov, A., Ephrati-Elizur, E., and Bernkopf, H., Ornithosis in infancy, *Pediatrics*, 15, 752, 1955.

75. Ephrati-Elizur, E. and Bernkopf, H., Isolation of six strains of ornithosis virus from children with infections of the respiratory tract, *J. Infect. Dis.*, 98, 45, 1956.

76. Meyer, K. F. and Eddie, B., Immunity against some bedsonia in man resulting from infection and in animals from infection or vaccination, *Ann. N.Y. Acad. Sci.*, 98, 288, 1962.

77. **Spendlove, I. C.,** Production of bacterial aerosols in a rendering plant process, *Public Health Rep.,* 72, 176, 1957.

78. **McGavran, M. H., Beard, C. W., Berendt, R. F., and Nakamura, R. M.,** The pathogenesis of psittacosis. Serial studies on rhesus monkeys exposed to a small-particle aerosol of the Borg strain, *Am. J. Pathol.,* 40, 653, 1962.

79. **Eugster, A. K.,** Pathogenetic Studies on Intestinal Chlamydial Infection of Calves, Ph.D. thesis, Colorado State University, Fort Collins, 1970.

80. **Andrews, J. M.,** The importance of psittacosis in the United States, *J. Am. Vet. Med. Assoc.,* 130, 109, 1957.

81. **Mohr, W.,** Untersuchungen und Beobachtungen zur Verbreitung und Klinik der Ornithose (Psittakose) in Deutschland, *Z. Gesamte Inn. Med. Ihre Grenzgeb.,* 9, 1005, 1954.

82. **Dekking, F.,** Epidemiology of ornithosis and psittacosis, *Arch. Gesammte Virusforsch.,* 13, 316, 1963.

82. **Karrer, H., Meyer, K. F., and Eddie, B.,** The complement-fixation inhibition test and its application to the diagnosis of ornithosis in chickens and in ducks. II. Confirmation of the specificity and epidemiological application of the test, *J. Infect. Dis.,* 87, 24, 1950.

84. **Rindge, M. E., Jungherr, E. L., and Scruggs, I. H.,** Serological evidence of occupational psittacosis in poultry-plant workers, *N. Engl. J. Med.,* 260, 1214, 1959.

85. **Strauss, J. and Sery, W.,** Ornithose in der CSSR. Epidemiologisch-virologische Aspekte, *Arch. Exp. Veterinaermed.,* 18, 61, 1964.

86. **Center for Disease Control,** Human psittacosis in he United States, 1971-1973, *J. Infect. Dis.,* 131, 193, 1975.

87. **Ortel, S.,** Die Ornithose-Situation in der DDR auf Grund epidemiologischer und serologischer Untersuchungen, *Arch. Exp. Veterinaermed.,* 18, 89, 1964.

88. **Terskich, I. I.,** Epidemiologie der Ornithose in der USSR, *Arch. Exp. Veterinaermed.,* 18, 19, 1964.

89. **Davis, D. J. and Vogel, J. S.,** Recovery of psittacosis virus from chicks hatched from inoculated eggs, *Proc. Soc. Exp. Biol. Med.,* 70, 585, 1949.

90. **Storz, J., Call, J. W., and Miner, M. L.,** Meningo-encephalitis in young chickens resulting from infection with an ornithosis agent, *Avian Dis.,* 7, 480, 1963.

91. **Lehnert, C.,** Zur Frage der Übertragung des Ornithosevirus über das Brutei bei Enten, *Berl. Muench. Tieraerztl. Wochenschr.,* 75, 151, 1962.

92. **Illner, F.,** Zur Frage der Übertragung des Ornithosevirus durch das Ei, *Monatsh. Veterinaermed.,* 17, 116, 1962.

93. **Meyer, K. F. and Eddie, B.,** Ecology of avian psittacosis, particularly in parakeets, in *Progress in Psittacosis Research and Control,* Beaudette, F. R., Ed., Rutgers University Press, New Brunswick, N.J., 1958, 52.

94. **Davis, D. E., Delaplane, J. P., and Watkins, J. R.,** The role of turkey eggs in the transmission of ornithosis, *Am. J. Vet. Res.,* 18, 409, 1957.

95. **Eddie, B., Radovsky, F. J., Stiller, D., and Kumada, N.,** Psittacosis-lymphogranuloma venereum (PL) agents (*Bedsonia, Chlamydia*) in ticks, fleas and native mammals in California, *Am. J. Epidemiol.,* 90, 449, 1969.

96. **Bankowski, R. A. and Page, L. A.,** Studies of two epornitics of ornithosis caused by agents of low virulence, *Am. J. Vet. Res.,* 20, 935, 1959.

97. **DiDominizio, G.,** Contributo allo studio delle lesioni anatomistopatologiche de virus del gruppo psittacosi ornithosi in animali: Pappagalli, Cocorite, Agnelli, *Atti Soc. Ital. Sci. Vet.,* 8, 499, 1954.

98. **Pierce, K. R., Carroll, L. H., and Moore, R. W.,** Experimental transmission of ornithosis from sheep to turkeys, *Am. J. Vet. Res.,* 25, 977, 1964.

99. **Spalatin, J., Fraser, C. E. Q., Connel, R., Hanson, R. P., and Berman, D. T.,** Agents of psittacosis-lymphogranuloma venereum group isolated from muskrats and snowshoe hares in Saskatchewan, *Can. J. Comp. Med. Vet. Sci.,* 30, 260, 1966.

100. **Gonnert, R.,** Die Bronchopneumonie, eine neue Viruskrankheit der Maus, *Zentralbl. Bakteriol. Parasitenkd. Infektionskd. Hyg. Abt. 1: Orig.,* 147, 161, 1941.

101. **Storz, J.,** Über eine natürliche Infektion eines Meerschweinchenbestandes mit einem Erreger aus der Psittakose-Lymphogranuloma Gruppe, *Zentralbl. Bakteriol. Parasitenkd. Infektionskr. Hyg. Abt. 1: Orig.,* 193, 432, 1964.

102. **Kempf, A. H., Wheeler, A. H., and Nungster, W. J.,** Isolation of an agent belonging to the psittacosis-lymphogranuloma group of viruses, *J. Infect. Dis.,* 76, 135, 1945.

103. **Rocca-Garcia, M.,** Viruses of the lymphogranuloma-psittacosis group isolated from opossums: opossum virus B, *Nature* (London), 211, 502, 1967.

104. **Schachter, J.,** Psittacosis, in *Diseases Transmitted from Animals to Man,* Hubbert, W. T., McCulloch, W. F., and Schnurrenberger, P. R., Eds., Charles C Thomas, Springfield, Ill., 1975, 369.

105. **Schachter, J., Hanna, L., Hill, E., Massad, S., Sheppard, C. W., Conte, J., Cohen, S., and Meyer, K. F.,** Are chlamydial infections the most prevalent venereal disease?, *JAMA*, 231(12), 1252, 1975.

106. **Meyer, K. F., Eddie, B., Richardson, J. H., Schipkowitz, N. L., and Muir, R. J.,** Chemotherapie in the control of psittacosis in parakeets, in *Progress in Psittacosis Research and Control*, Beaudette, F. R., Ed., Rutgers University Press, New Brunswick, N.J., 1958, 163.

107. **Arnstein, P. and Meyer, K. F.,** Psittacosis-ornithosis, in *Current Veterinary Therapy*, Kirk, R. W., Ed., W. B. Saunders, Philadelphia, 1966, 543.

108. **Arnstein, P., Eddie, B., and Meyer, K. F.,** Control of psittacosis by group chemotherapy of infected parrots, *Am. J. Vet. Res.,* 29, 2213, 1968.

109. **Strauss, J., Smejkal, F., Vondracek, V., and Kuzusnik, Z.,** Feeding of chlortetracycline (aureomycin) to ducks with latent ornithosis, *Vet. Med.* (Prague), 6, 807, 1961.

110. **Hellerström, S. and Wassen, E.,** Meningo-enzephalitische Veränderungen bei Affen nach intracerebraler Impfung mit Lymphogranuloma inguinale, *C. R. Int. Dermatol. Syphol.* (Paris), 1147, 1930.

111. **Digiacomo, R. G., Gale, J. L., and Wang, S. P.,** Chlamydial Infection of the male baboon urethra, *Br. J. Vener. Dis.,* 51, 310, 1975.

112. **Favre, M. and Hellerström, S.,** The epidemiology, etiology and prophylaxis of lymphogranuloma inguinale, *Acta Derm. Venereol.,* 34(30), 1, 1954.

113. **Richmond, S. J. and Sparling, F.,** Genital chlamydial infections, *Am. J. Epidemiol.,* 103, 428, 1976.

114. **Hidiroglov, M. and Prevost, R.,** Quelques observations sur la sterilité des bovins occasionnée par un virus du groupe psittacose, *Rec. Med. Vet.,* 135, 259, 1959.

115. **Storz, J., Carroll, E. J., Ball, L., and Faulkner, L. C.,** Isolation of a psittacosis agent (chlamydia) from semen and epididymis of bulls with seminal vesiculitis syndrome, *Am. J. Vet. Res.,* 29, 549, 1968.

116. **Eugster, A. K., Ball, L., Carroll, E. J., and Storz, J.,** Experimental genital infection of bulls and rams with chlamydial (psittacosis) agents, *Proc. Sixth Int. Conf. Cattle Diseases,* Heritage Press, Stillwater, Okla., 1970, 327.

117. **Omori, T., Ishii, S., and Matumoto, M.,** Miyagawanellosis of cattle in Japan, *Am. J. Vet. Res.,* 21, 564, 1960.

118. **Greenblatt, R. B., Dienet, R. B., and Baldwin, K. R.,** Lymphogranuloma venereum and granuloma inguinale, *Med. Clin. North Am.,* 43, 1493, 1959.

119. **Koteen, H.,** Lymphogranuloma venereum. II. Historical background, *Medicine* (Baltimore), 24, 3, 1945.

120. **King, A. and Nicol, C., Eds.,** Nonspecific urogenital infections, in *Venereal Diseases,* Baillière Tindall, London; Williams & Wilkins, Baltimore, 1975, 257.

121. **Volk, J. and Kraus, S. J.,** Nongonococcal urethritis: a venereal disease as prevalent as epidemic gonorrhea, *Arch. Intern. Med.,* 134, 511, 1974.

122. **Hilton, A. L., Richmond, S. J., and Milne, J. D.,** Chlamydia A in the female genital tract, *Br. J. Vener. Dis.,* 50, 1, 1974.

123. **Frei, W.,** Eine neue Hautreaktion bei "Lymphogranuloma inguinale," *Klin. Wochenschr.,* 4, 2148, 1925.

124. **Barwell, C. F.,** Some observations on the antigenic structure of psittacosis and lymphogranuloma venereum viruses, *Br. J. Exp. Pathol.,* 33, 258, 1952.

125. **T'ang, F. F., Chang, H. L., Huang, Y. T., and Wang, K. C.,** Studies on the etiology of trachoma with special reference to isolation of the virus in chick embryo, *Chin. Med. J.,* 75, 429, 1957.

126. **Jones, B. R., Collier, L. H., and Smith, C. H.,** Isolation of virus from inclusion blennorrhoea, *Lancet,* 1, 902, 1959.

127. **Thygeson, P.,** Trachoma, inclusion conjunctivitis, lymphogranuloma venereum, in *Tropical Medicine,* Hunter, G., Swartzwelder, J., and Clyde, D., Eds., W. B. Saunders, Philadelphia, 1976, 249.

128. **Jones, B. R. and Collier, L. H.,** Inoculation of man with inclusion blennorrhea virus, *Ann. N.Y. Acad. Sci.,* 98, 212, 1962.

129. **Yerasimides, T. G.,** Isolation of a new strain of feline pneumonitis virus from a domestic cat, *J. Infect. Dis.,* 106, 290, 1960.

130. **Voigt, A., Dietz, O., and Schmidt, W.,** Klinische und experimentelle Untersuchungen zur Ätiologie der Keratitis superficialis chronica (Überreiter), *Arch. Exp. Veterinaermed.,* 20, 259, 1966.

131. **Murray, E. S.,** Guinea pig inclusion conjunctivitis virus. I. Isolation and identification as a member of the psittacosis-lymphogranuloma-trachoma group, *J. Infect. Dis.,* 114, 1, 1964.

132. **Storz, J., Pierson, R. E., Marriott, M. E., and Chow, T. L.,** Isolation of psittacosis agents from follicular conjunctivitis of sheep, *Proc. Soc. Exp. Biol. Med.,* 125, 857, 1967.

133. **Pavlov, N., Milanov, M., and Tschilev, D.,** Recherches sur la rickettsiose kerato-conjunctivale du porc en Bulgarie, *Ann. Inst. Pasteur Paris,* 105, 450, 1963.

134. **Dyml, B.,** Isolation of a virus of the psittacosis-lymphogranuloma group from cattle with infectious kerato-conjunctivitis, *Vet. Med.* (Prague), 7, 358, 1965.

135. **Alexander, E. R. and Chiang, W. T.,** Infection of pregnant monkeys and their offspring with TRIC agents, *Am. J. Ophthalmol.,* 63, 1145, 1967.

136. **Gelman, A. C.,** Distribution of selected communicable diseases in tropical and subtropical areas of the world, in *Tropical Medicine,* Hunter, G., Swartzwelder, J., and Clyde, D., Eds., W. B. Saunders, Philadelphia, 1976, 843.

137. **Cello, R. M.,** Ocular infections in animals with PLT (Bedsonia) group agents, *Am. J. Ophthalmol.,* 63, 1270; 244, 1967.

138. **Schachter, J., Arnstein, P., Dawson, C. R., Hanna, L., Thygeson, P., and Meyer, K. F.,** Human follicular conjunctivitis caused by infection with a psittacosis agent, *Proc. Soc. Exp. Biol. Med.,* 127, 292, 1968.

139. **Becerra, V. and Storz, J.,** Tissue culture adaption and pathogenic properties of an ovine chlamydial abortion strain, *Zentralbl. Veterinaermed. Reihe B,* 21, 290, 1974.

140. **Schachter, J., Ostler, H. B., and Meyer, K. F.,** Human infection with the agent of feline pneumonitis, *Lancet,* 1, 1063, 1969.

141. **Storz, J.,** personal communication, 1976.

142. **Scott, G.,** TRIC infection of the ocular, ENT and urogenital systems in whites, *S. Afr. Med. J.,* 42, 928, 1968.

143. **Collier, L. H. and Smith, A.,** Dissemination and immunogenicity of live TRIC agent in baboons after parenteral injection, *Am. J. Ophthalmol.,* 63, 1589; 563, 1967.

144. **Schachter, J., Banks, J., Sugg, N., Sung, M., Storz, J., and Meyer, K. F.,** Serotyping of chlamydia: isolates of bovine origin, *Infect. Immun.,* 11, 904, 1975.

145. **Iverson, J. O., Spalatin, J., Fraser, C. E., and Hanson, R.,** Ocular involvement with chlamydia psittaci (strain M56) in rabbits inoculated intravenously, *Can. J. Comp. Med.,* 38, 298, 1974.

146. **Collier, L. and Blyth, W.,** Immunogenicity of experimental trachoma vaccines in baboons, *J. Hyg.* (Cambridge), 64, 529, 1966.

147. **Wang, S. and Grayston, J. T.,** Pannus with experimental trachoma and inclusion conjunctivitis agent infection of Taiwan monkeys, *Am. J. Ophthalmol.,* 63, 1133; 107, 1967.

148. **Mendlowski, B. and Segre, D.,** Polyarthritis in sheep. I. Description of the disease and experimental transmission, *Am. J. Vet. Res.,* 21, 68, 1960.

149. **Storz, J., Smart, R. A., and Shupe, J. L.,** Virusbededingte Polyarthritis bei Kälbern, *Nord. Veterinaermed.,* 16, 109, 1964.

150. **McChesney, A., Becerra, V., and England, J.,** Chlamydial polyarthritis in a foal, *J. Am. Vet. Med. Assoc.,* 165(3), 259, 1974.

151. **Schachter, J., Barnes, M. G., Jones, J. P., Engleman, E. P., and Meyer, K. F.,** Isolation of bedsoniae from the joints of patients with Reiter's syndrome, *Proc. Soc. Exp. Biol. Med.,* 122, 283, 1966.

152. **Maierhofer, C. A. and Storz, J.,** Clinical and serologic response of dogs to infection with the chlamydial agent of ovine polyarthritis, *Am. J. Vet. Res.,* 30, 1961, 1969.

153. **Schachter, J., Barnes, M., Jones, J., Engleman, E., Meyer, K. F., and Weber, H.,** The Role of *Bedsonia* Infection in Human and Experimental Arthritis, in 4th Panam. Congr. of Rheumat., Mexico City, 1962.

154. **Smith, D., James, P., Schachter, J., Engleman, E., and Meyer, K. F.,** Experimental *Bedsonia* Arthritis in Rabbits, in Annu. Meet. Am. Rheumatism Assoc., Seattle, 1968.

155. **Kölbl, O. and Psota, A.,** Miyagawanellen-Isolierungen bei Polyarthritis, Pneumonie, Encephalomyelitis and interstitieller Herdnephritis (Fleckniere) der Kalber, *Wien. Tieraerztl. Monatsschr.,* 55, 443, 1968.

156. **Littlejohns, I. R., Harris, A. N. A., and Harding, W. B.,** Sporadic bovine encephalomyelitis, *Aust. Vet. J.,* 37, 53, 1961.

157. **Popovici, V. and Hiastru, F.,** Izolarea microorganismelor din grupul *Bedsonia* de la cabaline, *Rev. Med. Vet.* (Bucharest), 11, 56, 1968.

158. **Blanco, A. L.,** Estudios sobre les pneumoenteritis de los bovinos, *Rev. Patronato Biol. Anim.,* 10, 5, 1966.

159. **Storz, J., Shupe, J. L., James, L. F., and Smart, R. A.,** Polyarthritis of sheep in the intermountain region caused by a psittacosis-lymphogranuloma agent, *Am. J. Vet. Res.,* 24, 1201, 1963.

160. **Storz, J., Shupe, J. L., Marriott, M. E., and Thornley, W. R.,** Polyarthritis of lambs induced experimentally with a psittacosis agent, *J. Infect. Dis.,* 115, 9, 1965.

161. **Eugster, A. K. and Storz, J.,** Pathogenetic events in intestinal chlamydial infections leading to polyarthritis in calves, *J. Infect. Dis.,* 123, 41, 1971.

162. **Csonka, G. W.,** Reiter's disease, *Br. J. Hosp. Med.,* 7, 8, 1972.

163. **Norton, W. L. and Storz, J.,** Observations on the polyarthritis of sheep produced by an agent of the psittacosis-lymphogranuloma venereum-trachoma group, *Arthritis Rheum.,* 10, 1, 1967.

164. Schachter, J., Can chlamydial infections cause rheumatoid arthritis?, in *Infection and Immunology in the Rheumatic Diseases*, Dumonde, D. C. and Path, M. R., Eds., Blackwell Scientific, Oxford, 1976, 151.

165. Ford, D. K., Non-gonococcal urethritis and Reiter's syndrome: personal experience with etiological studies during 15 years, *Can. Med. Assoc. J.*, 99, 900, 1968.

166. Brewerton, D. A., Caffrey, M., Nicholls, A., Walters, D., Oates, J. K., and James, D. C. O., Reiter's disease and HL-A27, *Lancet*, 2, 996, 1973.

167. Aho, K., Ahvonen, P., Lassus, A., Sievers, K., and Tiilikainen, A., HL-A27 in reactive arthritis, *Arthritis Rheum.*, 17(5), 521, 1974.

168. Pierson, R. E., Polyarthritis in Colorado feedlot lambs, *J. Am. Vet. Med. Assoc.*, 150, 1487, 1967.

169. York, C. J. and Baker, J. A., A new member of the psittacosis-lymphogranuloma group of viruses that causes infection in calves, *J. Exp. Med.*, 93, 587, 1951.

170. Frazer, G., Norwall, J., Withers, A. R., and Gregor, W. W., A case history of psittacosis in the dog, *Vet. Rec.*, 85, 54, 1969.

171. Kölbl, O., Untersuchungen über das Vorkommen von Miyagawanellen beim Schwein, *Wien. Tieraerztl. Monatsschr.*, 56, 332, 1969.

172. Matumoto, M., Omori, T., Morimoto, T., Harada, K., Inaba, Y., and Ishii, S., Studies on the disease of cattle caused by a psittacosis-lymphogranuloma group virus. VIII. Sites for the virus to leave the infected host, *Jpn. J. Exp. Med.*, 25, 223, 1955.

173. Storz, J. and Thornley, W. R., Serologische und aetiologische Studien über die intestinale Psittakose-Lymphogranuloma-Infektion der Schafe, *Zentralbl. Veterinaermed.*, 13, 14, 1966.

174. Eugster, A. K., Joyce, B. K., and Storz, J., Immunofluorescence studies on the pathogenesis of intestinal chlamydial infections in calves, *Infect. Immun.*, 2(4), 351, 1970.

175. Doughri, A. M., Altera, K. P., Storz, J., and Eugster, A. K., Electron microscopic tracing of pathogenetic events in intestinal chlamydial infections of newborn calves, *Exp. Mol. Pathol.*, 18, 10, 1973.

176. Dungworth, D. L. and Cordy, D. R., The pathogenesis of ovine pneumonia. II. Isolation of virus from faeces; comparison of pneumonia caused be faecal, enzootic abortion and pneumonitis viruses, *J. Comp. Pathol. Ther.*, 72, 71, 1962.

177. Storz, J., Superinfection of pregnant ewes latently infected with a psittacosis-lymphogranuloma agent, *Cornell Vet.*, 53, 469, 1963.

178. Storz, J., Collier, J. R., Eugster, A. K., and Altera, K. P., Intestinal bacterial changes in chlamydia-induced primary enteritis of newborn calves, *Ann. N.Y. Acad. Sci.*, 176, 162, 1971.

179. Dunlop, E. M., Hare, M. J., Darougar, S., Jones, B. R., and Rice, N. S., Detection of chlamydiae (*Bedsonia*) in certain infections of man. II. Clinical study of genital tract, eye, rectum, and other sites of recovery of chlamydiae, *J. Infect. Dis.*, 120(4) 463, 1969.

180. Stamp, J. T., McEwen, A. D., Watt, J. A. A., and Nisbet, D. J., Enzootic abortion in ewes. I. Transmission of the disease, *Vet. Rec.*, 62, 251, 1950.

181. Storz, J., McKercher, D. G., Howarth, J. A., and Straub, O. C., The isolation of a viral agent from epizootic bovine abortion, *J. Am. Vet. Med. Assoc.*, 137, 509, 1960.

182. Giroud, P., Observations et donnés expérimentales concernant les avortements chez l'homme et l'animal (rickettsioses, toxoplasmoses, néo-rickettsioses ou group psittacose), *Arch. Inst. Pasteur Tunis*, 34, 187, 1957.

183. Bohac, J. and Mensik, J., Bedsonia Group Agents as a Cause of Enzootic Abortions of Pigs, paper presented at the Conference on Diseases of Pigs, College of Veterinary Medicine, Brno, Czechoslovakia, 1965.

184. McCauley, E. H. and Tieken, E. L., Psittacosis-lymphogranuloma venereum agent isolated during an abortion epizootic in goats, *J. Am. Vet. Med. Assoc.*, 152(12), 1758, 1968.

185. Lincoln, S., Kwapien, R. P., Reed, D. E., Whiteman, C. E., and Chow, T. L., Epizootic bovine abortion: clinical and serologic responses and pathologic changes in extragenital organs of pregnant heifers, *Am. J. Vet. Res.*, 31, 2105, 1969.

186. Storz, J., Call, J. W., Jones, R. W., and Miner, M. L., Epizootic bovine abortion in the intermountain region: some recent clinical, epidemiologic and pathologic findings, *Cornell Vet.*, 57, 21, 1967.

187. Eugster, A. K. and Jones, L. P., Isolation of chlamydia from an aborted bovine fetus, *Southwest. Vet.*, 27, 143, 1974.

188. Eugster, A. K. and Herrmann, W. W., Chlamydial infections in young calves, *Southwest. Vet.*, 25, 283, 1972.

189. Eugster, A. K. and Jones, L. P., Polyarthritis in sheep caused by chlamydial agents, *Southwest. Vet.*, 24, 283, 1971.

190. McKercher, D. G., Crenshaw, G. L., Wada, E. M., Mauris, C. M., and Franti, C. E., Vaccination against epizootic bovine (chlamydial) abortions, *J. Am. Vet. Med. Assoc.*, 163(7), 889, 1973.

191. **Schachter, J.,** Isolation of bedsoniae from human arthritis and abortion tissues, *Am. J. Ophthalmol.,* 63, 1082/56, 1967.

192. **Giroud P., Roger, F., and Dumas, N.,** Résultats concernant l'avortement de la femme dû à un agent dû groupe de la psittacose, *C. R. Acad. Sci.* (Paris), 242, 697, 1956.

193. **Roberts, W., Grist, N. R., and Giroud, P.,** Human abortion associated with infection by ovine abortion agent, *Br. Med. J.,* 4, 37, 1967.

194. **Barnes, M. G. and Brainerd, H.,** Pneumonitis with alveolar-capillary block in a cattle rancher exposed to epizootic bovine abortion, *N. Engl. J. Med.,* 271, 981, 1964.

195. **Barwell, C. F.,** Laboratory infection of man with virus of enzootic abortion of ewes, *Lancet,* 2, 1369, 1955.

196. **McNutt, S. H. and Waller, E. F.,** Sporadic bovine encephalomyelitis, *Cornell Vet.,* 30, 437, 1940.

197. **Boughton, I. B.,** Sporadic bovine encephalomyelitis, *Tex. Vet. Bull.,* 3, 1, 1941.

198. **Rocca-Garcia, M.,** Viruses of the lymphogranuloma-psittacosis group isolated from opossums in Columbia, opossum virus A, *J. Infect. Dis.,* 85, 275, 1949.

199. **Giroud, P., Groulade, P., Roger, F., and Dortois, N.,** Réactions positives vis-à-vis d'un antigène du groupe de la psittacose chez le chien, au cours de divers syndrome infectieux, *Bull. Acad. Vet. Fr.,* 27, 309, 1954.

200. **Meyer, K. F. and Eddie, B.,** Psittacosis, in *Diagnostic Procedures for Virus and Rickettsial Diseases,* Lennette, E. H. and Schmidt, N. J., Eds., American Public Health Association, New York, 1964, 603.

201. **Baker, J. A.,** Virus obtained from pneumonia of cats and its possible relation to cause of atypical pneumonia in man, *Science,* 96, 475, 1942.

202. **Bittle, T. L.,** Feline pneumonitis, *J. Am. Vet. Med. Assoc.,* 158, 942, 1971.

203. **McKercher, D. G.,** A virus possibly related to the psittacosis-lymphogranulmaneumonitis group causing a pneumonia in sheep, *Science,* 115, 543, 1952.

204. **Omori, T., Ishii, S., Harada, K., Ischikawa, O., Murase, N., Katada, M., and Araumi, W.,** Study on an infectious pneumonia of goats caused by a virus. I. Isolation of the causative agent and characteristics, *Exp. Rep. Gov. Exp. Stn. Anim. Hyg. Tokyo,* 27, 101, 1953.

205. **Kiuchi, M. and Inaba, Y.,** Study on so-called "bovine influenza," *Exp. Rep. Gov. Exp. Stn. Anim. Hyg. Tokyo,* 25, 37, 1952.

206. **Sorodoc, C., Surdan, C., and Sarateanu, D.,** Investigation on the identification of the virus of enzootic pneumonia in swine, *Stud. Cercet. Inframicrobiol.,* 12, 355, 1961.

207. **Palotay, J. L. and Christensen, N. R.,** Bovine respiratory infections. I. Psittacosis-lymphogranuloma venereum group of viruses as etiological agents, *J. Am. Vet. Med. Assoc.,* 134, 222, 1959.

208. **Romvary, J.,** Respiratory disease caused in suckling calves by a PLV virus, *Acta Vet. Acad. Sci. Hung.,* 14, 469, 1964.

209. **Omori, T., Morimoto, T., Harada, K., Inaba, Y., Ishii, S., and Matumoto, M.,** Miyagawanella: psittacosis-lymphogranuloma group of viruses. I. Excretion of goat pneumonia virus in feces, *Jpn. J. Exp. Med.,* 27, 131, 1957.

210. **Nigg., C.,** Unidentified virus which produces pneumonia and systemic infection in mice, *Science,* 95, 49, 1942.

211. **Gerloff, R. K. Watson, R. O.,** A chlamydia from the peritoneal cavity of mice *Infect. Immun.,* 1, 64, 1970.

212. **Debbie, J. G.,** Chlamydia (psittacosis) antibody study in white-tailed deer, *Bull. Wild. Dis. Assoc.,* 3, 152, 1967.

213. **Stoenner, H. G., Holdenried, R., Lackman, D., and Osborn, J. S.,** The occurence of *Coxiella burnetii, Brucella* and other pathogens among the fauna of the Great Salt Lake desert in Utah, *Am. J. Trop. Med. Hyg.,* 8, 590, 1959.

214. **Sidewell, R. W., Lundgren, D. L., and Thorpe, B. D.,** Psittacosis complement-fixing antibodies in sera from fauna of the Great Salt Lake Desert in Utah, *Am. J. Trop. Med. Hyg.,* 13, 591, 1964.

215. **Eddie, B., Sladen, W. J., Sladen, B. K., and Meyer, K. F.,** Serological studies and isolation of *Bedsonia* agents from northern fur seals on the Pribilof Islands, *Am. J. Epidemiol.,* 84, 405, 1966.

216. **Iversen, J. O., Spalatin, J., and Hanson, R. P.,** Experimental chlamydiosis in wild and domestic lagomorphs, *J. Wildl. Dis.,* 12, 215, 1976.

217. **Fraser, C. E. O.,** Analytical serology of the chlamydiaceae, *Analytical Serology of Microorganisms,* Kwapinski, J. B. G., Ed., John Wiley & Sons, New York, 1969, 257.

218. **Braley, A. E.,** Intracellular bodies of conjunctival epithelial cells, *Arch. Ophthalml.,* 24, 681, 1940.

219. **Wentworth, B. B.,** Use of gentamycin in the isolation of subgroup A chlamydia, *Antimicrob. Agents Chemother.,* 3, 698, 1973.

220. **Eugster, A. K.,** unpublished data.

221. **Thygeson, P. and Hauna, L.,** TRIC agents, in *Diagnostic Procedures for Viral and Rickettsial Infections,* Lennette, E. H. and Schmidt, N. J., Eds., American Public Health Association, New York, 1969, 904.
222. **Giménez, D. F.,** Staining rickettsiae in yolk-sac cultures, *Stain Technol.,* 39, 135, 1964.
223. **Gordon, F. B., Harper, I. A., Quan, A. L., Treharne, J. D., Dwyer, R. S. C., and Garland, I. A.,** Detection of chlamydia (bedsonia) in certain infections of man. I. Laboratory procedures: comparison of yolk sac and cell culture for detection and isolation, *J. Infect. Dis.,* 120, 451, 1969.
224. **Meyer, K. F., Eddie, B., and Schachter J.,** Psittacosis-lymphogranuloma venereum agents, in *Diagnostic procedures for Viral and Rickettsial Infections,* Lennette, E. H. and Schmidt, N. J., Eds., American Public Health Association, New York, 1969, 869.
225. **Schachter, J.,** Chlamydiae, in *Manual of Clinical Immunology,* Rose, N. and Friedman, N., Eds., American Society for Microbiology, Washington, D.C., 1976, 494.
226. **Ata, F. A.,** Factors Influencing Clearance of Chlamydial Agents in Sheep, Ph.D. thesis, Colorado State University, Fort Collins, 1970.
227. **Karrer, H., Meyer, K. F., and Eddie, B.,** The complement-fixation inhibition test and its application to the diagnosis of ornithosis in chickens and ducks. I. Principles and techniques of the test, *J. Infect. Dis.,* 87, 13, 1950.
228. **Brumfield, H. P. and Pomeroy, B. S.,** Direct complement fixation by turkey and chicken serum in viral systems, *Proc. Soc. Exp. Biol. Med.,* 94, 146, 1957.
229. **Mason, D. M.,** A capillary tube agglutination test for detecting antibodies against ornithosis in turkey serum, *J. Imunol.,* 83, 661, 1959.
230. **Barron, A. L. and Collins A. R.,** Studies on trachoma agent by double diffusion gel precipitation, *Am. J. Ophthalmol.,* 63, 1487, 1967.
231. **Page, A.,** Application of an agar gel precipitin test to the serodiagnosis of avian chlamydiosis, in *Proc. 17th Annu. Meet. American Association Veterinary Laboratory Diagnosticians,* American Asociation of Veterinary Laboratory Diagnosticians, Madison, Wis., 1974, 51.
232. **Wang, S. P. and Grayston, J. T.,** Human serology in *Chlamydia trachomatis* infection with immunofluorescence, *J. Infect. Dis.,* 130, 388, 1974.
233. **Tamura, A. and Higashi, N.,** Purification and chemical composition of meningopneumonitis virus, *Virology,* 20, 596, 1963.
234. **Anderson, D. R., Hopps, H. E., Barile, M. F., and Bernheim, B. C.,** Comparison of the ultrastructure of several rickettsiae, ornithosis virus, and Mycoplasma in tissue culture, *J. Bacteriol.,* 90, 1387, 1965.

EDITORIAL COMMENT — CHLAMYDIA

In *Science,* February 24, 1978, Katz and Nash report on the agent of Legionnaires' Disease. In their abstract, they state: "The Legionnaires' disease organism was isolated from lung tissue taken from two fatalities of the Legionnaires' disease epidemic that occurred in Philadelphia during 1976. In yolk sac tissue the agent grew as a small coccobacillary microorganism, which was Gram variable and Gimenez positive. Intracellular coccoid and bacillary forms, detected by electron microscopy, within and without vacuoles, underwent multiplication by septate binary fission. Some of the intracellular forms resembled obligate intracellular pathogens. On defined bacteriologic media, the organisms were predominantly bacillary. The organism conforms to the morphologic criteria of a prokaryocyte."

They go on to state that the extracellular and intracellular growth exhibited by the microorganism are compatible with transmission to humans from a form that is native to the environment, possibly involving an animal reservoir. Moreover, their spore-like structures suggest resistance to the environment. Some of the intracellular cytoplasmic coccoid and bacillary structures are morphologically similar to obligate intracellular pathogens of the order Chlamydiales, the order Rickettsiales, and small bacilli.

It is possible that the organism of Legionnaires' disease is related to an environmental microbe from which the larger obligate intracellular pathogens have evolved.

APPENDIX

CURRENT DEVELOPMENTS IN *C. TRACHOMATIS* INFECTIONS IN MAN

J. Schachter

With the exception of a few strains recovered from rodents, *Chlamydia trachomatis* organisms have been isolated only from man. It would appear that as *C. psittaci* has become extremely well adapted to its natural hosts, *C. trachomatis* has become equally well adapted to man. The organisms depend upon contact transmission and are highly successful parasites. Although they were first demonstrated in 1907 in the conjunctiva of patients with trachoma,[1] it is only recently that we have begun to understand how widespread parasitism is in man. Indeed, we are now beginning to discover that the diversity of diseases associated with *C. trachomatis* infection in humans may be similar to the spectrum of diseases seen in animals infected with *C. psittaci*. Undoubtedly, the *C. psittaci* strains are more invasive than *C. trachomatis* that (except for the lymphogranuloma venereum strains) seems to be restricted to mucous membranes and, specifically, columnar epithelial cells in these membranes. However, these epithelial cells are present in large contiguous areas of the body and the organisms have been recovered from the eye, eustachian tube, throat, and lung as well as from a number of sites within the male and female genital tract.

As *C. psittaci* is an extraordinarily common parasite of animals, *C. trachomatis* seems to be equally common in man. The disease distribution appears to differ according to socioeconomic class and geographic locale. Trachoma, still the leading preventable cause of blindness, is primarily a disease of children and is spread by direct contact. It is found in emerging nations and is associated with poor sanitation and living conditions.[2,3] Agents virtually identical to the trachoma organisms are commonly found in the industrialized world, but here rather than infecting the eyes of children, they more often infect the genital tracts of adults.[3-5] *C. trachomatis* is currently recognized as being among the most common, if not the most common, of the sexually transmitted pathogens.[6] Chlamydiae are major identifiable causes of nongonococcal and postgonococcal urethritis.[3-5] They probably cause a significant proportion of cervicitis and may be involved in pelvic inflammatory disease and epididymitis.[7,8] Because they are found in the genital tract of the female, chlamydiae also may be transmitted to the neonate where they can cause superficial ocular infection as well as more serious systemic diseases.

The high prevalence rate of infection with these organisms makes chlamydial infections one of the more significant public health problems currently being identified. It is clear that the next few years will greatly increase our understanding of human chlamydial infections. Recent research findings, based largely on improved diagnostic methods, promise significant advances in the near future. The following comments are drawn from an editorial on the expanding clinical spectrum of *C. trachomatis* infections.[9]

Beem and Saxon have recently reported the recovery of *C. trachomatis* from nasopharyngeal and tracheobronchial aspirates collected from infants with a distinctive pneumonic syndrome.[10] The disease was characterized by an afebrile course, chronic diffuse pulmonary involvement, tachypnea, a distinctive cough, and elevated levels of serum IgG and IgM. Of 20 infants with this syndrome who were studied, 18 (90%)

were found to have chlamydial infection of the respiratory tract. Of these 20, 11 (55%) had conjunctivitis either by history or examination. It is obvious that respiratory tract colonization by *C. trachomatis* is a common outcome of natally acquired infection, as 10 of 12 (93%) infants with inclusion conjunctivitis but with no respiratory disease yielded chlamydiae from the nasopharynx. Infants with respiratory disease and chlamydial infection had significantly higher antichlamydial antibody titers than were found in the infants with ocular disease only. Only 2 of 15 infants (13%) with various other illnesses had chlamydiae in the respiratory tract. Because of the high recovery rate and extremely high antibody levels to *C. trachomatis* in the case of pneumonia, Beem and Saxon have suggested that chlamydiae are etiologically associated with the disease and may be a significant cause of respiratory disease in infants.

A chlamydial etiology for this syndrome has not yet been proven. Support for an etiologic role has come from the recovery of *C. trachomatis* from a lung biopsy taken from an infant with pneumonia.[11] This finding has been repeated in my laboratory.* Establishment of an etiologic relationship will also involve demonstration of clinical response to antichlamydial chemotherapy or development of an appropriate animal model to fulfill Koch's postulates. However, the preliminary findings are so compelling that for purposes of this discussion an etiologic association between chlamydiae and neonatal pneumonia will be assumed.

In a personal communication, Beem reports that the number of infants studied has now been expanded to approximately 50 with the distinctive syndrome of pneumonia and 50 in the other diseases category. Results of the expanded series confirm the initial findings. In addition, Beem has stated his belief that some of the infants with chlamydial respiratory infection may also have secretory otitis media and obstructive nasopharyngeal problems.

Since their data were first presented at a series of meetings in the spring of 1976, the findings of Beem and Saxon have provoked considerable interest in a number of clinical specialties. *C. trachomatis* is a pathogen commonly found in the gential tract,[3-5] and it is considered to be one of the major causes of nongonococcal urethritis in men. Although the organism may cause cervicitis, its pathogenic potential in women is unclear. Transmission of chlamydiae from the infected cervix to the neonate has been recognized since the first decade of this century.[12]

Until the report of Beem and Saxon, however, the only disease attributed to chlamydiae in neonates was inclusion conjunctivitis of the newborn (inclusion blennorrhea). Early circumstantial findings have also suggested that chlamydiae may be associated with vaginitis in infants.[13,14]

In retrospect, there is considerable evidence in the literature which suggests that *Chlamydia* might be involved in neonatal respiratory disease. For example, Freedman and co-workers[15] observed rhinitis in a series of infants with inclusion blennorrhea, and Scott[16] reported recovery of the agent from throat swabs collected from infants in a trachoma-endemic area. However, these children all had conjunctivitis. The possibility that the inclusion conjunctivitis agent could persist in the respiratory tract after the ocular disease had been treated was shown in one infant with pneumonia whose throat cultures were positive in the absence of ocular disease or infection.[17] This infant probably had a clinical condition identical to that elucidated by Beem and Saxon. However, the published data of Beem and Saxon, involving 20 infants with such infection, prove that the earlier observations were neither unique nor uncommon.

The possibility that *C. trachomatis* may be involved in otitis media is another logical extension of previous anecdotal reports. Otitis is a common problem in children in

---

* The George Williams Hooper Foundation, Karl Friedrich Meyer Laboratories, San Francisco.

areas that are endemic for trachoma, but etiology is generally ascribed to the usual bacterial pathogens. However, otitis has been observed in adult volunteers infected with *C. trachomatis* by the ocular route.[18] Hearing loss has been associated with inclusion conjunctivitis and in one case the chlamydiae were recovered from fluid obtained by myringotomy.[19,20] It is obvious that for purposes of this discussion the auditory canal can be considered an extension of the respiratory tract exposed to *C. trachomatis*.

Serologic surveys for chlamydial antibody have found that as many as 10% of some pediatric populations have specific microimmunofluorescence antibodies to *Chlamydia*.[21] Review of the histories of seropositive patients did not reveal any clear-cut clinical association between a specific disease and antichlamydial antibodies. Since Alexander and Chiang have presented evidence that newborn subhuman primates passing through an infected cervix may become sensitized to *Chlamydia* without developing disease,[22] it was thought that some of the antibodies found in human infants resulted from subclinical infections.

The results of Beem and Saxon now raise the possibility that chlamydiae may be significant pathogens in respiratory disease of infants less than 3 months of age. As is typical of most initial reports with great potential, the report of Beem and Saxon raises more questions than it answers. The most important question, perhaps, is how should the disease be treated? Their patients were highly selected. Prospective studies are needed to define the incidence and clinical spectrum of the infection. Prevalence studies in appropriate clinics would also be useful to determine the significance of the respiratory tract infections. Approximately one half of Beem and Saxon's patients had inclusion blennorrhea, which usually has an incubation period of 7 to 14 days and apparently precedes the onset of respiratory tract disease by 2 weeks to 2 months. What percentage of infants with inclusion blennorrhea develop respiratory tract infections? Conversely, what percentage of patients with respiratory tract infections have antecedent conjunctivitis? The infants in Beem and Saxon's series with inclusion conjunctivitis received topical tetracycline, yet when seen for respiratory tract infection, most (10/12) still had infection of the conjunctiva. It is obviously important to determine whether this represents failure of topical tetracycline treatment, inadequate administration of the drug, or persistent infection of the upper respiratory tract that allowsseeding of the conjunctiva. Many of Beem and Saxon's patients had no history of conjunctivitis. It would be important to determine whether this reflects ocular infections so mild that they were overlooked, or whether the respiratory tract may be infected in the absence of ocular infection.

A logical assumption would be that the ocular infection results in infection of the respiratory tract through drainage of the ocular discharges. If, however, the respiratory tract may be directly infected by contamination at birth, pneumonia may occur in the absence of antecedent infection of the eye.

The reservoir of these infections is clearly the cervix of the mother. Since a number of studies have shown that chlamydial carriage in pregnant women may range from 3 to 13%, it is obvious that the number of exposed infants must be quite high. If the risk of developing pneumonia is sufficiently high and the spectrum of the neonatal disease sufficiently broad to include severe respiratory tract disease, a number of questions arise. Should routine screening of pregnant women include tests for chlamydial infection of the cervix? Should pregnant women with chlamydial infection be treated? Should efforts be made to develop a Crede-like prophylaxis for chlamydial infection? Is the eye the only primary site of infection with *C. trachomatis*? Should systemic therapy replace topical therapy in the treatment of inclusion conjunctivitis?

In addition, one must consider the possibility that the report of Beem and Saxon represents just the beginning of an expansion of the clinical spectrum of neonatal chlamydial infections. If ocular infection or exposure at birth results in an infected respiratory tract, is it not likely that infective material reaches the G.I. tract and may cause disease there? Presently available information suggests that the chlamydial agent responsible for inclusion conjunctivitis grows only in columnar epithelial cells. Thus, the agents are known to infect the conjunctiva, the urethra, the quamo-columnar junction of the cervix, and the rectal mucosa, as well as the respiratory tract. It would seem reasonable, in appropriate epidemiologic circumstances, to look for infection with *C. trachomatis* in any anatomic site containing cells capable of supporting this infection. Undoubtedly, a number of research projects are currently aimed at answering some of the questions presented above, and the results will be eagerly awaited.

Some preliminary results from prospective studies are available. The most ambitious study has been performed by Alexander, Chandler, and associates at the University of Washington, Seattle.[23,24] They studied 142 unselected pregnant women and found 18 (12.7%) to have chlamydial infection of the cervix. Of the 18 infants born to these women, 9 (50%) developed conjunctivitis, and 12 (67%) developed serum antibodies against genital chlamydiae. Although the baseline infection rate in pregnant women in this clinic seems to be relatively high in comparison to other similar populations studied, the percentage of infants developing conjunctivitis was quite similar in another prospective study. This study (made in San Francisco) was based on an infection rate of 5% in pregnant women.[25] Results, as yet unpublished, showed that of the 25 infants at risk, 10 (40%) developed laboratory-confirmed inclusion conjunctivitis. The results from these two studies suggest that approximately 40 to 50% of those infants exposed at birth developed conjunctivitis. The incidence of respiratory tract infection is unknown. Beem and Saxon's report suggested that respiratory tract colonization may be a better indicator of exposure at birth than conjunctival infection. However, accepting the range of cervical infections and neonatal infections found in these prospective studies leads to minimum estimates of between 2 and 6% of all newborns acquiring chlamydial infection at birth. The potential public health significance of these infections is obvious.

REFERENCES

1. **Halberstaedter, L. and von Prowazek, S.**, Zur Atiologie des Trachoms, *Dtsch. Med. Wochenschr.*, 33, 1285, 1907b.
2. **Jones, B. R.**, Prevention of blindness from trachoma, *Trans. Ophthalmol. Soc. U.K.*, 95, 16, 1975.
3. **Grayston, J. T. and Wang, S. P.**, New knowledge of chlamydiae and the diseases they cause, *J. Infect. Dis.*, 132, 87, 1975.
4. **Richmond, S. J. and Sparling, P. F.**, Genital chlamydial infections, *Am. J. Epidemiol.*, 103, 428, 1976.
5. **Schachter, J., Causse, G., and Tarizzo, M. L.**, Chlamydiae as agents of sexually transmitted diseases, *Bull. W.H.O.*, 54, 245, 1976.
6. **Schachter, J., Hanna, L., Hill, E. C., Massad, S., Sheppard, C. W., Conte, J. R., Jr., Cohen, S. N., and Meyer, K. F.**, Are chlamydial infections the most prevalent venereal disease?, *JAMA*, 231, 1252, 1975.
7. **Mardh, P. A., Ripa, T., Svensson L., and Westrom, L.**, *Chlamydia trachomatis* infection in patients with acute salpingitis, *N. Engl. J. Med.*, 296, 1377, 1977.
8. **Harnisch, J. P., Alexander, E. R., Berger, R. E., Monda, G., and Holmes, K. K.**, Aetiology of acute epididymitis, *Lancet*, 1, 819, 1977.
9. **Schachter, J.**, The expanding clinical spectrum of infections with *Chlamydia trachomatis*, *Sex. Transmit. Dis.*, 4, 116, 1977.

10. **Beem, M. O. and Saxon, E. M.**, Respiratory tract colonization and a distinctive pneumonia syndrome in infants infected with *Chlamydia trachomatis, N. Engl. J. Med.,* 296, 306, 1977.

11. **Frommell, G. T., Brush, F. W., and Schwartzman, J. D.**, Isolation of *Chlamydia trachomatis* from infant lung tissue, *N. Engl. J. Med.,* 296, 1150, 1977.

12. **Lindner, K.**, Gonoblennorrhoe, Einschlussblennorrhoe, und Trachoma, *Graefe's Arch. Ophthalmol.,* 78, 345, 1911.

13. **Thygeson, P. and Stone, W., Jr.**, Epidemiology of inclusion conjunctivitis, *Arch. Ophthalmol.,* 27, 91, 1942.

14. **Mordhorst, C. H.**, Studies on oculogenital TRIC agents isolated in Denmark, *Am. J. Ophthalmol.,* 63, 1282, 1967.

15. **Freedman, A., Al-Hussaini, M. K., Dunlop, E. M., et al.**, Infection by TRIC agent and other members of the bedsonia group; with a note on Reiter's Disease, *Trans. Ophthalmol. Soc.,* 86, 313, 1966.

16. **Scott, J. G.**, TRIC infections (Bedsoniae), *Med. Proc.,* 14, 410, 1968.

17. **Schachter, J., Lum, L., Gooding, C. A., et al.**, Pneumonitis following inclusion blennorrhea, *J. Pediatr.,* 87, 779, 1975.

18. **Dawson, C. R., Wood, T. R., and Rose, L.**, Experimental inclusion conjunctivitis. III. Keratitis and other complications, *Arch. Ophthalmol.,* 78, 341, 1967.

19. **Gow, J. A., Ostler, H. B., and Schachter, J.**, Inclusion conjunctivitis with hearing loss, *JAMA,* 229, 519, 1974.

20. **Dawson, C. R. and Schachter, J.**, TRIC agent infections of the eye and genital tract, *Am. J. Ophthalmol.,* 63, 1288, 1967.

21. **Schachter, J.**, Chlamydiae, in *Manual of Clinical Immunology,* Rose, N. R. and Friedman, H., Eds., American Society for Microbiology, Washington, D.C., 1976, 494.

22. **Alexander, E. R. and Chiang, W. T.**, Infection of pregnant monkeys and their offspring with TRIC agents, *Am. J. Ophthalmol.,* 63, 1145, 1967.

23. **Alexander, E. R., Chandler, J., Pheiffer, T. A., Wang, S-P., Holmes, K. K., and English, M.**, Chlamydial maternal-neonatal infection: a pilot study, in *Nongonococcal Urethritis and Related Oculogenital Infections,* Holmes, K. K. and Hobson, D., Eds., American Society for Microbiology, Washington, D.C., 1977.

24. **Chandler, J. W., Alexander, E. R., Pheiffer, T. A., et al.**, Ophthalmia neonatorum associated with maternal chlamydial infections, *Trans. Am. Acad. Ophthalmol. Otolaryngol.,* 83, 302, 1977.

25. **Schachter, J., Hill, E. C., King, E. B., Coleman, V. R., Jones, P., and Meyer, K. F.**, Chlamydial infection in women with cervical dysplasia, *Am. J. Obstet. Gynecol.,* 123, 753, 1975.

EDITORIAL COMMENT — CHLAMYDIOSIS IN WILD BIRDS

The occurrence of chlamydiosis in turkeys in Texas with its economic and public health implications has been known since the 1949—1950 turkey processing season. There was about a 10- to 11-year period from 1963 to April 1974 when no known outbreaks occurred. There were severe outbreaks in the spring and again in the fall of 1974. Spread continued in 1975 and one flock was found infected in 1976. Since then no known outbreaks have occurred.

To determine the source of the infection, J. E. Grimes, College of Veterinary Medicine, Texas A & M University, has studied the incidence of chlamydia in wild birds and has experimentally infected doves, cowbirds, and grackles. He has found doves and cowbirds refractory to disease. Only 1 of 16 doves challenged shed chlamydia. The grackles, on the other hand, were readily infected and shed large numbers of the chlamydia. When known infected grackles were placed in cages with healthy turkeys, the latter show signs of disease 21 days later, including depression and sulfur-yellow droppings on day 23. Cloacal swabs taken from the turkeys at this time yielded chlamydiae. At day 28 postexposure, the turkeys were sacrificed and necropsied. Spleens were enlarged and mottled, and pericardits, perihepatitis, or air sacculitics was observed. Chlamydiae were isolated from the tissues. The turkeys had a CF titer of 1.32 at termination of the experiment.

From this experiment, it is apparent that transmission of chlamydiae from grackles to turkeys can be done experimentally and probably occurs in nature. Grackles are dirty, messy birds that excrete watery cloacal droppings that would readily contaminate ranges and feeding grounds. Grimes plans to continue the chlamydiae studies in wild birds to determine which may be important in transmitting disease to turkeys as well as other birds and possibly man.

CAT SCRATCH DISEASE

S. S. Kalter

INTRODUCTION

Cat scratch disease (synonyms: cat scratch fever, benign lymphoreticulosis, benign inoculation lymphoreticulosis, regional lymphadenitis, *la maladie des griffes de chat*) is a self-limiting, generally nonfatal, extremely protean disease characterized by malaise, headache, low-grade fever, lymphadenopathy (regional or generalized), and development of a papule at the scratch site. Cat scratches, however, may not be necessary for development of the disease, or they may go unnoticed; other vectors have been reported.

HISTORY

The first description of cat scratch disease (1931) was attributed to Dr. R. Debre of the University of Paris. A 10-year-old boy was observed with a suppurating lymphadenitis in the epitrochlear area. Numerous cat scratches were apparent, but they were much more severe on the hand located on the side of the body with adenitis than on the opposing hand. A diagnosis of tuberculosis (that was quite common in France at the time was suggested—with the bacterium supposedly entering through the scratches. Further testing, including tuberculin skin tests and a variety of bacteriologic examinations, failed to support a diagnosis of tuberculosis or that of any other human infectious disease. The adenitis regressed within a few weeks, and the patient recovered uneventfully with minimal therapy. During the next few years, additional cases were observed, and Dr. R. Debre referred to these as "cat scratch disease" in his teaching practice.

In 1946, Dr. F. Hanger at the College of Physicians and Surgeons, New York City, developed an epitrochlear and infraclavicular lymphadenitis that was Frei-test negative. Fluid aspirated from these nodes was prepared as a skin test antigen by Dr. H. Rose, who employed the same procedure used to prepare Frei antigen. For a time, this antigen was referred to as the Hanger-Rose antigen, and the skin test was referred to by the same name. The skin test was positive not only on Dr. Hanger but also on another individual who had previously shown a similar clinical condition. A known lymphogranuloma venereum patient tested negative with the Hanger-Rose antigen but positive with Frei antigen. What this positive skin test represented, however, was not understood.

At this same time, Hanger was intrigued by Dr. L. Foshay's studies in Cincinnati on tularemia. Specifically, it was the atypical cases of tularemia that clinically resembled his own disease that were of interest to Hanger. He supplied Foshay with some of the antigen prepared by Rose, that led Foshay to prepare skin test material. Foshay never reported his findings on this entity. He called the disease "atypical tularemia" and "cat fever" because of the patients' history of cat scratches. Foshay's studies led Debre to prepare skin test antigen and to test a series of similar patients in France.

In France, Debre and collaborators[1] continued their studies with the first case report given in 1950. Another French group, headed by D. P. Mollaret and including J. Reilly, R. Bastin, and P. Tournier, was independently observing this same disease and also reported their findings in 1950.[2] It is intersting to note that experimental attempts to isolate or transmit the disease agent were carried on by Mollaret et al. with transmission from human to human successfully reported. The first report in English was presented by Greer and Keefer[3] in 1951. In Washington, D.C., Daniels and Mac-Murray[4] (1951) were largely responsible for stimulating interest in the disease with their studies on a large series of patients and by making skin test antigen available. A comprehensive review was provided in 1967 when Warwick[5] listed 567 references to this disease. Margileth[6] also provided a good review of available literature.

ETIOLOGIC AGENT

Numerous agents have been suggested as etiologically responsible for cat scratch disease, but thus far none has been unequivocally demonstrated to be the causative organism. Attempts to isolate the responsible agent have generally included inoculating patient suppurative material, lymph node homogenates, or blood into a wide variety of bacteriological media, embryonated eggs, mice of various ages, numerous laboratory animals (including rabbits, guinea pigs, rats, different species of monkeys [very few apes have been used]) human volunteers, and cell cultures derived from many different animal (including human) sources.

Three main groups of organisms have been reported to be responsible for cat scratch disease: atypical mycobacteria, chlamydiae, and herpesviruses. Other organisms with less convincing support have also been reported. An indication that several organisms or at least antigenic variants of a given organism may be responsible for the disease has been suggested by the fact that skin test antigen prepared from pooling the pus of several patients yields more positives than antigen prepared from an individual patient.

Most investigators have given up associating mycobacteria with the disease, principally because many cat scratch patients are tuberculin negative. Infection with mycobacteria does occur, and although the disease resembles cat scratch disease, such patients are cat scratch skin test negative.

A relationship between cat scratch disease and the psittacosis-lymphogranuloma venereum group of agents is based principally upon serologic findings. Large series of serologic studies (many uncontrolled) have demonstrated a high percentage of positives (about 20 to 30%) among cat scratch patients when they are tested by various serologic procedures, usually complement-fixation. However, careful analysis of these studies, while supporting the higher number of positives, fails to show any significant antibody increases among convalescent sera, and titers in the sera are generally lower than those found among cases due to chlamydiae.

Many investigators now feel that the increased number of positives probably reflects either a low-level antigenic crossing or coincidental exposure among cat scratch patients to *Chlamydia*-infected animals or birds. In support of the psittacosis group as the responsible agent, Chervonskii et al.[7] reported the isolation of an agent (HE) that they classified as a member of the genus *Chlamydia* from three patients with clinical cat scratch disease. This organism, isolated by inoculation of albino mice and chick embryos, produced infection in mice, guinea pigs, monkeys, and chickens. Confirmation of these have not appeared.

Another agent suggested by several investigators to be the responsible organism is a herpesvirus. Various feline herpesviruses (rhinotracheitis) have been suggested without any conclusive evidence. Furthermore, studies reported from the Southwest Foundation for Research and Education clearly failed to show any relationship to the Epstein-Barr virus (EBV) despite the fact that 100% of eight patient lymph nodes examined by election microscopy contained characteristic herpesviruses.[8,9]

The need to demonstrate unequivocally the etiologic agent of this disease continues. Several laboratories have gathered preliminary evidence that suggests transmission of an agent to nonhuman primates, unfortunately still without confirmation. Such isolation attempts should be encouraged.

TRUE AND ALTERNATE HOSTS

Apparently, cat scratch disease is found naturally only in humans since no other animal species has thus far been reported to have this or any similar-appearing disease. Even the cat, considered to be the major recognized vector, does not become overtly ill. Dogs have also been reported to carry the agent, but they, like cats, have failed to show evidence of any disease. Since the agent has been transmitted by rose thorns, monkey, rabbit, and dog scratches, dog bites, porcupine quills, fish hooks, and other materials, the contaminating source(s) or host(s) may indeed be extremely varied.

DISTRIBUTION

The prevalence of cat scratch disease is directly related to the interest of the physician. Because of this, the actual distribution may only be surmised. However, since cases have been unquestionably observed and diagnosed in Europe, the U.S., Australia, and Canada, the disease may be assumed to be world-wide in distribution. In addition to the need for an interested physician, clinical judgement requires a suitable laboratory test to support the clinical findings. The only reliable supportive test is the skin test, and appropriate antigen is limited. Thus, a number of suspected cases have gone unconfirmed because of failure to finalize the diagnosis and, conversely, cases have been diagnosed as "cat scratch disease" without supportive data.

The exact number of cases is unknown, and the number per 100,000 persons varies from source to source. Adding to the difficulty in determining the endemicity of this disease is the fact that the skin test is a hypersensitivity reaction, and a patient is skin test positive for life. The testing of adults provides a greater prevalence than does testing of young children. Such groups as veterinarians have a somewhat higher number of skin test positives (30%) than other populations of similar age (3 to 20%).[10] There does not appear to be any increased evidence of clinical disease, however, among veterinarians. The greatest frequency of disease occurs among young children, whereas familial cases are known but infrequent.

DISEASE IN ANIMALS

Cat scratch disease has not been reported to occur naturally in animals. Experimental studies have been extremely limited and may be misleading because of the lack of a specific etiologic agent. Thus far, all reports of experimental disease in animals have been unconfirmed. At the Southwest Foundation for Research and Education, limited transmission studies through two young baboons in series were discontinued because of a lack of additional animals. Regional lymphadenopathy and conversion to skin test positive was observed, however, in both animals. Lymphadenopathy was noted approximately 10 days postinoculation as measured from the time of cat scratch.

DISEASE IN HUMANS

The disease in humans is extremely variable, but it is usually mild. However, severe generalized cases with CNS involvement and death are reported. Again, because diagnosis may not be fully established, some questions regarding the validity of a number of cases may be raised. To fully establish a diagnosis of cat scratch disease, the following criteria have been recommended by a number of investigators:

1. Absence of any laboratory evidence in support of another etiologic agent
2. A histopathologic finding in a lymph node that is compatible with this disease
3. A positive skin test with a reliable skin test antigen
4. Association with a cat scratch, preferably an evident scratch

In patients meeting these criteria, the usual clinical findings are as follows. After an incubation period of 3 to 28 days, the patient, generally a child, will present mild constitutional symptoms. A low-grade fever may or may not be present (approximately 25% in adults, more frequent in children), hence the term "disease" rather than "fever". There may be some evidence of malaise, anorexia, and headache. A flu-like syndrome may be indicated.

These symptoms alone generally do not bring the patient to the attention of a physician. The most alarming symptom and reason for concern to the patient (or parent) is development of a lymphadenopathy in the region of a scratch or other skin injury. A papule or pustule (primary lesion) — but no lymphangitis — develops in most patients at the site of the skin break. Skin lesions may be overlooked or considered as unrelated. The enlarged lymph node varies from pea to grapefruit size. Usually restricted to the region draining the scratched area, bilateral and generalized adenopathy have been reported. The nodes are frequently tender and suppurate in about half of the cases.

Treatment of involved nodes depends upon the individual case. Chemotherapy is not indicated unless concomitant bacterial infection occurs. Small nodes usually regress within 2 to 10 weeks. Larger nodes may need to be aspirated or surgically excised. Drainage, aspiration, or removal of the node results in rapid subsiding of the symptoms. Histopathologic examination of the excised (or biopsied) node is helpful in finalizing the diagnosis but is not in itself pathognomonic. Most patients recover without complications following disappearance of the enlarged node.

Laboratory tests, with the exception of the histopathologic findings, are of little value. The tests are of value, however, for exclusion of other agents. Differential diagnosis is necessary to exclude lymphogranuloma venereum, tularemia, brucellosis, tuberculosis, other mycobacterial lymphadenopathies, infectious mononucleosis, coccidioidomycosis, histoplasmosis, and various lymphoproliferative diseases (Hodgkin's disease, sarcoidosis, etc.).

Atypical forms of the disease have been reported with sufficient frequency to make diagnosis difficult. Parinaud's oculoglandular syndrome is most common, and any ocular lesion with a regional lymphadenopathy should be considered as possibly being cat scratch disease. Neurologic manifestations, usually in the form of an encephalitis, are among the more serious of the clinical complications. In these cases, convulsions and coma occur abruptly 1 to 6 weeks after initial symptoms appear. Most patients develop a pleocytosis in their cerebrospinal fluids, and elevated proteins are noted. Generally, complete recovery occurs following transient sequelae, but deaths have been reported. Other forms of neurologic involvement include encephalomyelitis, encephalomyeloradiculitis, polyneuritis, and paraplegia. Respiratory tract involvement includes pharyngitis and pneumonia. Erythema nodosum is one of the more frequently reported of the skin reactions, but thrombocytopenic purpura also occurs. Osteolytic lesions and arthralgia have been described. Other rare complications and clinical findings have also been reported.[5]

In addition to atypical forms of disease, extreme variations in duration of illness

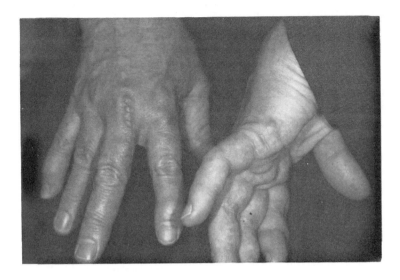

FIGURE 1.   Multiple linear lesions on hands of a patient with cat-scratch disease.
(From Wooldridge, W. E., *Consultant*, 18(4), 77, 1978. With permission.)

may be noted. Two to six weeks is generally reported as the length of illness of most
cases. Some individuals "relapse," with repeated episodes of glandular tenderness and
clinical disease persisting 6 to 12 months. A small number of patients have been observed to manifest symptoms for periods of more than 2 years.

The histopathologic findings on catscratch-diseased lymph nodes are nonspecific,
but they are helpful when collated with clinical and skin test findings. Several characteristic stages may be observed, but they are not pathognomonic. The earliest finding
is one of a reticulum cell hyperplasia that may resemble one of the lymphoproliferative
disorders. An increase in the number of lymphoid follicles and germinal centers containing many reticulum cells is observed at this stage, followed by the appearance of a
tubercle-like granuloma with small abscesses developing. This inflammatory lesion
contains numerous cell types surrounding the microabscesses. In addition to the various inflammatory cells, giant cells (Langhans' type) may be observed.

Microscopically at this stage of the disease, nodes resemble a suppurative lymphadenitis, especially those due to lymphogranuloma venereum, tularemia, brucellosis, etc.
As the microabscesses coalesce, larger abscesses develop with caseous degeneration
resembling tuberculosis being most prominent. These abscesses are surrounded by epithelioid cells that contain infiltrating lymphocytes (giant cells) and may resemble the
Sternberg cells seen in Hodgkin's disease. A fibroblastic invasion connotes the start
of the healing process.

GENERAL MODE OF SPREAD

It is generally agreed that the "healthy" cat is the vector involved in transmitting
the agent or agents. Other mechanisms, as indicated above, have been associated with
transmission. While familial outbreaks are generally not the rule, it has been noted
that several members of a family may develop the disease following sequential cat
scratches. In one family with four children who contracted the disease, the first
youngster that was scratched developed the most severe form of the illness while the
last youngster scratched developed the mildest form. Dilution of virus or coincidence?

Human-to-human transmission has not been observed, so isolation of patients is not required.

EPIDEMIOLOGY

Cat scratch disease occurs throughout the year, but a number of investigators suggest an autumn-winter peaking. These investigators, it should be noted, are reporting from geographic areas where there are relatively cold seasons. In San Antonio, Tex., cat scratch disease occurs without any major seasonal peaking. Association with cats, generally kittens, is nearly always reported. It is almost impossible to find an individual without some form of such contact. Even "cat haters" usually recall contact with a cat at a neighbor's or friend's house or at the market, etc. Since a scratch is not necessary, this type of contact may have some relevance.

It is not known with any certainty whether or not epidemics occur. Epidemics have been reported, but because of several factors, such reports must be considered with the following factors in mind. Because this disease is not reportable and diagnosis is dependent upon physician interest, the exact prevalence in a community is unknown. Furthermore, if a number of cases occur in one area and undiagnosed cases occur in other areas, a misrepresentation of the situation develops. Endemic regions are recorded, but, again, the above factors may contribute toward erroneous interpretations. Family epidemics have been known to occur, but some investigators feel that these represent contact with several cats rather than scratches by an individual cat. We have alluded above to a known familial outbreak involving a single cat.

Because of the overall lack of information, it is almost impossible to provide a true epidemiologic pattern for cat scratch disease. Reservoirs are unknown; transmission other than by cat scratch is not clearly understood; age factors are unclear although children are most often affected. Until an etiologic agent is precisely defined, it appears that many epidemiologic considerations will continue to be unresolved.

DIAGNOSIS

Because cat scratch disease has only been reported in humans, despite its name, the discussion shall be restricted to diagnosis in this species. Lack of a specific etiologic agent adds to the difficulty of specific diagnosis. However, as described in other sections, enough information and diagnostic capabilities are available to provide a reasonably accurate diagnosis of the disease. It is important, therefore, to recognize that no single criterion may be used for a definitive diagnosis. Close correlation of clinical, histopathologic, and laboratory (including skin test) findings is necessary in order to diagnose this disease.

Probably the most reliable test is the skin test; it has a high degree of significance when the clinical findings are compatible with cat scratch disease and all other laboratory findings are negative. Negative features of the skin test are (1) it is a hypersensitivity reaction and (2) a patient is positive for life. The prevalence of second attacks is unknown, and the possible transmission of a human agent contaminating the skin test material must be considered. Fortunately, the antigen may be autoclaved in the course of preparation, providing a reassuring note.

It has been this author's experience to use only pooled materials for skin tests. Sufficient data are available to demonstrate that many cases go unrecognized when a skin test with antigen prepared from a single patient is used. The significance of this finding unfortunately remains obscure. As stressed above, the use of similar diagnostic procedures has failed to disclose any animals with this disease. Little reliance should be placed upon serologic tests since there are no data to support use of any such procedures.

CONCLUSION

Cat scratch disease, in spite of its relative clinical "unimportance," is a most interesting disease. Its ability to simulate other entities is of diagnostic importance and deserves further study. It is difficult to suggest just which studies would be most useful. Most obvious is the need for ascertaining the cause of the disease. Previous experiments regarding transmission of infectious material to nonhuman primates suggests that further investigations should be conducted utilizing this approach.

Immunologic parameters are also worth consideration. Serologic tests require known antigens and are, therefore, dependent upon the isolation of a causative agent. Schulkind and Ayoub[11] have found that cat scratch patients have a transient, depressed, cell-mediated responsiveness, and this observation is of some interest.

It is suggested that a more concerted effort be made to define cat scratch disease. Emmons et al.[12] have recently demonstrated that serologic testing of sera from cat scratch disease patients against suspected etiologic agents is inconclusive. Present-day methodology clearly indicates that this disease could be defined if given the proper interest. For an interesting historical review of the early recognition of this disease, a report by Carithers[13] should be consulted.

REFERENCES

1. Debre, R., Lamy, M., Jammet, M. L., Costil, L., and Mozziconacci, P., La maladie des griffes de chat, *Bull. Soc. Med. Hopitaux Paris*, 66, 76, 1950.
2. Mollaret, P., Reilly, J., Bastin, R., and Tournier, P., Sur une adenopathie regionale subaigue et spontanement curable, avec intradermo-reaction et lesions ganglionnaires particulieres, *Bull Soc. Med. Hop.*, 66, 424, 1950.
3. Greer, W. E. and Keefer, C. S., Cat-scratch disease: a disease entity, *N. Engl. J. Med.*, 244, 545, 1951.
4. Daniels, W. B. and MacMurray, F. G., Cat scratch disease: nonbacterial regional lymphadenitis, *AMA Arch. Intern. Med.*, 88, 736, 1951.
5. Warwick, W. J., The cat-scratch syndrome, many diseases or one disease? *Prog. Med. Virol.*, 9, 256, 1967.
6. Margileth, A. M., Cat scratch disease: nonbacterial regional lymphadenitis. The study of 145 patients and a review of the literature, *Pediatrics*, 42, 803, 1968.
7. Chervonskii, V. I., Terskikh, I. I., and Beklevshova, A. Y., Isolation and study of agent of benign lymphoreticulosis (cat scratch fever) in man, *Vopr. Virusol.*, 8, 264, 1963.
8. Kalter, S. S., Kim, C. S., and Heberling, R. L., Herpes-like virus particles associated with cat scratch disease, *Nature* London), 224, 190, 1969.
9. Kalter, S. S., Heberling, R. L., and Ratner, J. J., Titers of antibody to Epstein-Barr virus in patients with cat scratch disease, *J. Infect. Dis.*, 126, 464, 1972.
10. Kalter, S. S., A survey of cat scratch disease among veterinarians, *J. Am. Vet. Med. Assoc.*, 144, 1281, 1964.
11. Schulkind, M. L. and Ayoub, E. M., Cell-mediated immunity in cat scratch disease, *J. Pediatr.*, 85, 199, 1974.
12. Emmons, R. W., Riggs, J. L., and Schachter, J., Continuing search for the etiology of cat scratch disease, *J. Clin. Microbiol.*, 4, 112, 1976.
13. Carithers, H. A., Cat scratch disease, notes on its history, *Am. J. Dis. Child.*, 119, 200, 1970.

Mycobacterial Diseases

MYCOTIC AND ACTINOMYCOTIC ZOONOSES

L. Ajello, W. Kaplan, and A. Padhye

INTRODUCTION

Almost 150 species of fungi have been recorded as agents of disease in man and animals. Some of these organisms are basically pathogens that can infect normal individuals; others are saprophytes that assume a pathogenic role under certain conditions of reduced host resistance. Factors that can render a host susceptible to such opportunists include the administration of certain broad-spectrum antibiotics, corticosteroids, immunosuppressive therapy, irradiation, hyperalimentation, and the existence of certain underlying diseases. In recent years there has been a remarkable increase in the number of opportunistic fungus infections, and the list of opportunistic fungi is ever increasing. Interestingly, this rise in prevalence has occurred mainly in developed countries where advancements in medical practice have led to use of the very factors that can predispose man to infection by opportunists.

In addition, in developed countries there are more mycological diagnostic laboratories and personnel with the expertise necessary to diagnose fungus diseases. The diseases caused by the basically pathogenic fungi pose important medical problems in many parts of the world. Some of these diseases are cosmopolitan; others have a limited geographic distribution. All present a diagnostic and therapeutic challenge.

Fungi can infect all organs and structures of the body. Any classification of mycotic diseases based on clinical expression or taxonomic position of the agent can be considered as arbitrary. However, for the sake of convenience and better understanding of the diseases, the mycoses may be grouped into four categories: (1) superficial, (2) cutaneous, (3) subcutaneous, and (4) systemic.

Superficial mycoses — The superficial mycoses include disorders that involve the outermost layer of the skin and hair. Diseases included in this category are black piedra, white piedra, tinea nigra palmaris, and tinea versicolor. These diseases are primarily of cosmetic importance, but severe cases can cause discomfort.

Cutaneous mycoses — In this category are placed those disorders that involve the skin and its appendages to a greater extent than do the diseases classified as superficial mycoses. Dermatophytoses and cutaneous forms of candidiasis are the most common cutaneous mycoses.

Subcutaneous mycoses — This group includes those diseases that usually involve the subcutaneous tissues and the skin. Internal organs may also occasionally be affected. The diseases included in this category are chromoblastomycosis, mycetomas, some forms of phaeohyphomycosis, rhinosporidiosis, and sporotrichosis.

Systemic mycoses — These diseases are caused by fungi that infect internal organs of the body. It must be emphasized that the subcutaneous tissues and the skin may also be affected. Infections may be asymptomatic or may manifest varying degrees of severity. In some cases, the systemic mycoses may be fatal. The more common systemic mycoses are aspergillosis, blastomycosis, systemic forms of candidiasis, coccidioidomycosis, cryptococcosis, histoplasmosis, and zygomycosis.

Protothecosis is caused by members of the genus *Prototheca,* that some researchers consider to be achloric algae and others classify as fungi. This disease can also appear in a systemic form. Some of the systemic mycoses, such as blastomycosis, coccidioidomycosis, and histoplasmosis, are caused by well-recognized pathogenic fungi, but many of the systemic mycoses are caused by opportunistic fungi.

Nearly all of the fungus diseases that affect man can also affect lower animals. This common susceptibility, however, does not imply communicability. There is no evidence that systemic mycoses are naturally transmissible from one host to another. Rather, all available evidence indicates that both man and lower animals contract these diseases by exposure to sources in the environment. Most of the causative agents exist in nature in organic wastes or debris or in soil enriched with organic matter. In suitable and often restricted habitats, these fungi grow and successfully compete with other microorganisms present in the substrates. The systemic mycotic agents, therefore, are true saprophytes. However, under favorable conditions, as when inhaled or introduced subcutaneously by trauma, they can cause infection and disease in either an apparently healthy individual or a compromised individual, depending upon the pathogenic potential of the fungus.

The subcutaneous mycoses are also not considered to be communicable diseases, and their etiologic agents also have a saprophytic existence in nature. They occur in soil, decaying organic matter, or on vegetation. Most human or animal infections result from traumatic inoculation of the fungus into subcutaneous tissue or skin.

With the exception of tinea versicolor, the superficial mycoses are not considered to be communicable. The etiologic agents of most of these disorders probably occur as free-living saprophytes in the environment, and infections are contracted by exposure to such sources. The fungus that causes tinea versicolor has not been found to occur in nature as a free-living organism. It is assumed that the infection spreads by direct or indirect exposure to contaminated, desquamated epidermal cells.

In contrast to the other mycoses, dermatophytoses are communicable. More than 30 distinct species of dermatophytes are recognized. Some, termed anthropophilic dermatophytes, are adapted for parasitism of man. Others, termed zoophilic dermatophytes, are basically pathogens of lower animals, but they can also infect humans. Still others, called geophilic dermatophytes, are soil fungi that have the added capacity to infect the skin and its appendages of man and animals. The various forms of ringworm caused by zoophilic dermatophytes are true zoonotic diseases.

Most of the mycoses are exogenous diseases. A few, such as candidiasis, are endogenous. Etiologic agents of the endogenous mycoses occur as commensals in the G.I. tract and on the skin and mucous membranes. They are opportunists, and under certain conditions of reduced systemic or local resistance, these usually innocuous fungi can cause disease.

In the succeeding chapters, the mycoses transmissible from animals to man or man to animals and those common to animals and man are discussed in detail. Mycoses that only affect man or are rarely encountered are summarized briefly. For convenience, individual chapters are organized into superficial, cutaneous, subcutaneous, and systemic mycoses.

In addition to the fungus diseases, medical mycology has traditionally encompassed diseases caused by actinomycetes. These organisms are higher bacteria and include such disease agents as *Dermatophilus congolensis, Actinomyces bovis* and other members of the genus *Actinomyces,* members of related microaerophilic genera, *Nocardia asteroides* and other species of that genus, and members of related aerobic genera. The diseases caused by the actinomycetes are covered in Section A, Volume I.

SUPERFICIAL MYCOSES

W. Kaplan

Superficial mycoses are a group of fungus diseases confined to the outermost layer of the skin and hair. Disorders included in this category are black piedra, white piedra, tinea nigra, and tinea versicolor. Two of these diseases, black piedra and white piedra, affect man and lower animals. They will be covered in detail. Tinea nigra and tinea versicolor are only known to affect man; therefore, they will be briefly summarized.

BLACK PIEDRA

Etiologic Agent

Piedraia hortae is the causative agent of the disease in man and many species of lower primates classified in nearly all major divisions of this order of animals.[1] Recently a second species, *P. quintanilhai,* was described as the agent of black piedra in some lower primates and other mammals in central Africa.[2] However, some investigators question its validity as a distinct species.

P. hortae is an ascomycete. In culture, its colonies are dark brown to black, compact, and conical; they are covered with short, grayish aerial mycelium. Microscopically, they consist of dematiaceous, closely septate hyphae of varying diameter with terminal and intercalary chlamydospores. *P. hortae* has been reported to form asci and ascospores when cultured on special media. On hair, *P. hortae* forms black nodules that are composed of closely septate, dematiaceous hyphae. Within locules, it produces asci that usually contain eight single-celled, curved fusiform ascospores bearing a single polar filament at each end.

True and Alternate Hosts

P. hortae causes disease in man and a great diversity of lower primates. *P. quintanilhai* has caused disease in various primates and other wild mammals including the water mongoose, large spotted genet, two-spotted palm civet, and African giant squirrel.

Distribution

Black piedra is endemic in man and lower primates in humid regions of tropical and subtropical America, Indonesia, Indochina, Malaya, and Thailand. The disease is also endemic in lower primates in India and primates and other wild mammals in Africa. In endemic areas black piedra is a relatively common affliction, affecting large numbers of individuals annually.

Disease in Animals

In all affected animals the disease appears in the form of discrete brown to black hard nodules on the hair shaft. The infection in lower primates commonly causes severe pilar damage, and infected hairs are frequently broken at the site of nodule formation.

Disease in Man

The disease in man, as in lower animals, appears in the form of discrete brown to black hard nodules on the shaft of scalp hairs. However, unlike in animals, human infections are superficial and cause only minimal pilar damage. Black and white piedras may occur in a mixed infection.[3]

General Mode of Spread

There is no evidence that black piedra is a transmissible disease. Rather, all available evidence suggests that the disease is contracted by exposure to sources in nature.

Epidemiology

Our present day knowledge of the epidemiology of black piedra and ecology of the etiologic agent(s) is fragmentary. A number of investigations suggest that the infection is contracted by exposure to sources in the environment. The occurrence of piedra in a diversity of primates indigenous to humid, tropical and subtropical regions of Africa, Asia, and the New World suggests the widespread existence of *P. hortae* in the forests of these continental land masses.

Diagnosis

A diagnosis of black piedra is established by microscopic examination of nodules to detect the presence of dematiaceous, closely septate branched hyphae. Asci and ascospores are often observed but need not be present for a diagnosis to be made. Culture of nodules and isolation of the etiologic agent are readily carried out on Sabouraud's dextrose agar with antibacterial antibiotics.

Prevention and Control

Unknown.

WHITE PIEDRA

Etiologic Agent

Trichosporon cutaneum (T. beigelii) is the etiologic agent of this disease. In culture, this fungus grows rapidly, producing a cream-colored, yeast-like colony that, with age, becomes yellowish-gray and develops a wrinkled surface. Microscopically, the colony consists of hyaline hyphae and numerous arthrospores and some blastospores. In and on hair, the fungus forms hyphae, arthrospores, and blastospores.

True and Alternate Hosts

T. cutaneum is the agent of white piedra in man and horses; one case has been reported in a black spider monkey.[4]

Distribution

White piedra is more sporadic in occurrence and less common than black piedra. It occurs in temperate and tropical regions of Europe, Asia, South America, and the U.S.

Disease in Animals

White piedra is characterized by formation of soft, white to light-brown nodules on and within hair shafts. The extensive intrapilar growth of the fungus causes severe destruction so that hair often breaks or splits. In horses, the disease usually involves the mane, tail, and forelock.

Disease in Man

White piedra in man generally affects hair of the beard and mustache; occasionally other hairy parts of the body are affected. The disease is characterized by formation of soft, white to light-brown nodules on and within hair shafts that are often less discrete than those of black piedra and may appear as a sheath surrounding the shaft.[3]

Frequently the fungus invades the interior of the hair and causes severe damage. Such hairs are often broken or split.

General Mode of Spread
There is no evidence that white piedra is a transmissible disease. All available evidence indicates that the infection is contracted by exposure to sources in the environment.

Epidemiology
Knowledge of the epidemiology of white piedra is fragmentary. The etiologic agent has been isolated from a variety of natural substrates. It has been recovered from wood pulp in Sweden and Italy, sewage of a dairy plant in England, and soil and decaying plant material in Israel. In view of this apparent widespread occurrence in the environment, man and lower animals are undoubtedly often exposed to the fungus. However, cases of this disease are uncommon. Undoubtedly there are many factors that render hairs susceptible to infection by this fungus, but such factors are unknown. There is no evidence, as stated above, that the disease is transmissible from one host to another.

Diagnosis
A diagnosis of white piedra is established by the microscopic examination of nodules to detect the presence of the characteristic hyaline hyphae, arthrospores, and blastospores. Culturing the nodules to isolate the etiologic agent is also useful in making a diagnosis.

Prevention and Control
Unknown.

TINEA VERSICOLOR

Tinea versicolor is a mild, superficial fungus infection of the skin characterized by scaly discolored patches. Infections are chronic, usually noninflammatory and asymptomatic, and most patients seek medical assistance for cosmetic reasons; lesions in some patients are more active and cause pruritus. The disease has been diagnosed only in man — no animal cases have been recognized. Lesions appear most often on the face, neck, shoulders, arms, and trunk. The disease is extremely prevalent in many tropical and subtropical regions of the world and is less common in temperate climates. The causative agent, *Pityrosporum (Malassezia) furfur,* has not been found as a free-living saprophyte in the environment. It is thought that the infection spreads from person to person directly or indirectly by exposure to contaminated desquamated epidermis. Observation of the characteristic clusters of spherical yeast-like cells and short hyphae by direct microscopic examination of scrapings establishes a diagnosis. Tests to isolate the etiologic agent are not usually performed.

TINEA NIGRA

Tinea nigra is a superficial, usually asymptomatic mycotic infection of the epidermis caused by the fungus *Exophiala (Cladosporum) werneckii.* The disease has been recognized only in man — no cases have been reported in animals. Lesions usually occur on the palms of the hands and are flat and brown to black in color; they may have a slightly elevated border and show very little scaling. Generally there is no inflammation, and the lesions are usually asymptomatic.

The disease is most commonly observed in tropical areas although cases are occasionally seen in temperate regions. The etiologic agent occurs as a saprophyte in the environment, and infections apparently are contracted by exposure to such sources. A diagnosis is established by finding branched, septate dematiaceous hyphae and sometimes elongated budding cells upon direct microscopic examination of skin scrapings and isolation of the etiologic agent. Tinea nigra is primarily of cosmetic importance. However, it has been mistaken a number of times for rapidly enlarging nevi. This confusion has led to unnecessary surgery.

REFERENCES

1. **Kaplan, W.,** The occurrence of black piedra in primate pelts, *Trop. Geogr. Med.,* 11, 115, 1959.
2. **Van Uden, N., DeBarros-Machado, A., and Castelo-Branco, R.,** On black piedra in central African mammals caused by the ascomycete *Piedraia quintanilhai* Nov. Spec., *Rev. Biol.* (Lisbon), 3, 271, 1963.
3. **Mackinnon, J. E. and Schouten, G. B.,** Investigaciones sobre las enfermedales de los cabellos denominadas "piedra," *Arch. Soc. Biol. Montevideo,* 10, 227, 1947.
4. **Kaplan, W.,** Piedra in lower animals, a case report of white piedra in a monkey and a review of the literature, *J. Am. Vet. Med. Assoc.,* 134, 113, 1959.
5. **Emmons, C. W., Binford, C. H., Utz, J. P., and Kwon-Chung, K. J.,** *Medical Mycology,* 3rd ed., Lea & Febiger, Philadelphia, 1977, 168.

CUTANEOUS MYCOSES

A. A. Padhye

DERMATOPHYTOSES

Dermatomycoses are infections of human and animal epidermal tissues caused by a homogenous group of fungi known as dermatophytes. Unlike the agents of superficial mycoses, dermatophytes penetrate and parasitize keratinous body tissues (skin, hair, feathers, horns, nails) and cause the disease dermatophytosis (dermatomycosis, ringworm, tinea).

Dermatophytes were considered hyphomycetous fungi until recently, classified exclusively under the subdivision Deuteromycotina (Fungi Imperfectii). Some of these species, however, are now known to reproduce sexually and are classified in the family Gymnoascaceae of the subdivision Ascomycotina. Most dermatophytes have a worldwide distribution although some species are geographically limited.

The more than 35 different species of dermatophytes currently recognized belong to three genera: *Epidermophyton*, *Microsporum*, and *Trichophyton*. Individual species differ significantly with respect to their host preference. Some are basically animal parasites (zoophilic) although most of these are also pathogenic for humans to some degree. Others are essentially soil inhabitants (geophilic) that only rarely infect humans and animals. Still others are primarily parasites of man (anthropophilic), only rarely causing ringworm in lower animals (Table 1). They are not known to live in soil as saprophytes.

MICROSPORUM CANIS

Etiologic Agent — *M. canis (M. felineum, M. lanosum);* Perfect State — *Nannizzia otae*[1]

Colonies of *M. canis* are fast-growing on Sabouraud dextrose agar; they are white, fluffy at first, and then become silky with bright yellow pigment showing through peripheral regions. After 2 to 3 weeks, the aerial mycelium becomes dense and tan-colored with a bright yellow periphery and orangish-brown pigment on the reverse side of the colony.

Macroconidia are usually numerous, large, fusiform, and thick-walled and have verruculose walls with as many as 14 septa. Microconidia are usually scanty, small, clavate, sessile, or borne on short stalks along the sides of hyphae. *M. canis* has no special nutritional requirements. It grows luxuriantly and sporulates abundantly on rice grain medium.

An infected hair fluoresces bright yellowish-green under a Wood's light. By microscopic examination, an infected hair in a 10% KOH mount exhibits a sheath (ectothrix) that surrounds the hair and consists of mosaically patterned spaces of 2 to 3 μm in diameter. Infected skin or nail scrapings show hyphae that are hyaline, septate, and branched. Frequently, hyphal cells break into small chains of arthrospores.

True and Alternate Hosts

M. canis is the principal agent of feline and canine ringworm. It causes more than 98% of feline and more than 70% of canine ringworm cases in the U.S.[2] It is also the causal agent of ringworm in monkeys and horses and has been isolated occasionally

Table 1
CLASSIFICATION OF THE IMPORTANT SPECIES OF
DERMATOPHYTES THAT CAUSE RINGWORM IN ANIMALS

Genus	Zoophilic	Geophilic	Anthropophilic
Microsporum	*M. canis*	*M. gypseum*-complex	*M. audouinii*
	M. distortum		
	M. equinum	*M. nanum*	
Trichophyton	*T. equinum*		*T. rubrum*
	T. gallinae		
	T. mentagrophytes		
	var. *mentagrophytes*		
	var. *erinacei*		
	var. *quinckeanum*		
	T. verrucosum		

from a variety of animals such as the bat, bear, canary, chimpanzee, chinchilla, cow, donkey, fox, guinea pig, jaguar, lion, rabbit, and sheep.[3,4]

Distribution
M. canis infections of cats, dogs, and humans are common throughout the world. Sporadic outbreaks are fairly common, especially in urban areas.

Disease in Animals
The clinical manifestations of ringworm in cats due to *M. canis* are often inconspicuous. At other times, they are mild, noninflammatory, and result in hair loss. In some cases, a more inflammatory reaction accompanied by encrustation is observed. Such lesions frequently appear on the face and paws with whiskers and sometimes claws becoming infected. In more generalized infections lesions may be distributed on several body areas. Lesions in dogs are more obvious than those in cats, with dogs often evidencing circular lesions as large as 2.5 cm in diameter on any part of the body.

Disease in Man
Although *M. canis* is basically a zoophilic dermatophyte, it is frequently transmitted to man by animals. Most of the "animal-type" ringworm cases in urban areas are the result of animal contact, particularly with kittens that have *M. canis* lesions. These infections are most common in children but do occur occasionally in adults. In children, ringworm of the scalp with scaly, dry, diffuse lesions is seen with rare instances of kerion formation. *M. canis* can infect any part of the body, but lesions are most commonly seen on the glabrous skin and scalp. Lesions of the glabrous skin are circular, erythematous, and have sharp margins.

General Mode of Spread
M. canis is spread by direct contact among animals or indirectly by contaminated fomites. Human-to-human transmission also occurs, and in many cases of infection there is no history of any direct contact with animals.

Epidemiology
Since this fungus is the principal cause of ringworm in cats and dogs, these two hosts serve as the reservoir for spreading infection. Young and old animals, whose general resistance is lowered by disease or malnutrition, are most commonly infected. Animal-to-animal spread of infection through direct or indirect contact is well known.

The fungus is frequently transmitted by animals (especially by kittens with lesions) to human contacts. Person-to-person transmission of *M. canis* also occurs although after several human passages the fungus loses its infectivity for man and dies. Therefore, large-scale epidemics caused by *M. canis* are not observed among humans. Ringworm infection due to *M. canis* is transmissible by humans to lower animals, and although the frequency of such transfer is not well known, its existence represents a potential health hazard. Apart from adding to the reservoir of infections in animals, such passage strengthens the survival of the fungus.

Diagnosis

Direct examination of skin scrapings from active lesion borders in 10% KOH shows the presence of branched hyphae and arthrospores. Observations of infected hair — with the help of a Wood's lamp and culture of the infected material on Sabouraud dextrose agar — are necessary for identification of the fungus.

Prevention and Control

Infections in animals (especially cats) can persist at a subclinical level without obvious lesions for months or even years and become generalized in animals that are in poor condition. The first essential step of any control program is to isolate the infected animals. Recommendations for treatment include: (1) painting lesions with tincture of iodine or using sulfur dust or mercuric chloride ointment,[5] (2) washing dogs regularly with detergent, and (3) using griseofulvin therapy on cats,[6,7] dogs, and humans.

MICROSPORUM DISTORTUM

Etiologic Agent — *M. distortum;* Perfect State — Unknown

M. distortum grows moderately rapidly on Sabouraud dextrose agar and forms submerged to velvety or fluffy colonies. The colony is either flat or radially grooved and very pale buff to buff; the reverse side is also pale buff. Macroconidia are distorted, have up to ten septa, and are thick-walled with a verruculose outer wall. Microconidia are often abundant, long, single-celled, and pyriform. *M. distortum* infects hair and produces an ectothrix-type invasion. Under a Wood's lamp, infected hairs fluoresce a bright yellowish-green.

True and Alternate Hosts

M. distortum is a fairly common etiologic agent of feline and canine ringworm in New Zealand.[8-10] A few human cases have been described in the U.S. and traced to contacts with South American pet monkeys or dogs.[11] The natural reservoir of this species is unknown.

Distribution

Most cases of *M. distortum* have been reported in New Zealand and the U.S. In the southern part of New Zealand's South Island (rural areas of central Otago), *M. distortum* has been recorded more frequently than in the northern part.[9,10]

Disease in Animals

In animals, the lesions are similar to those caused by *M. canis*. Lesions in cats are usually on the back of the neck, inconspicuously small, and crusted. Baldness due to loss of infected hair can occur. The infection is uncommon in horses but can infect extensive areas of the animals with scaling and crusting when it does occur.

Disease in Man

Human infections are similar to those caused by *M. canis*. Most patients have scalp lesions that appear as bald, scaling patches containing crusted, broken hairs that fluoresce green under a Wood's lamp. The few lesions observed on the neck, face, trunk, arm, hand, or leg area develop as small, circular, red scaly patches with inconspicuous central healing.

General Mode of Spread

Present data indicates that cats, monkeys, and other such hosts may prove to be the reservoir for *M. distortum*.[9] Little is known regarding the spread of the infection from animal to animal. There is little evidence to suggest that person-to-person transmission of *M. distortum* occurs. Although more than one person in a family has been found to be infected, present data suggest exposure to a common source rather than intrapersonal transfer of infection.

Epidemiology

All epidemiological data indicate that cats and monkeys may be the reservoir of *M. distortum*. *M. distortum* lesions in cats resemble those caused by *M. canis* to such an extent that the two infections cannot be differentiated without isolation of the causal organism. Animal-to-animal spread of infection through direct or indirect contact occurs. Infections are more common in young kittens than older cats, and more common in children than adults. The most common lesion in humans is scaly and appears on the skin although lesions on other areas of the body have also been observed.

Diagnosis

Samples of infected hair in KOH mounts and of skin scrapings show the presence of branching hyphae and arthrospores. As with *M. canis*, an infected hair fluoresces green under a Wood's lamp and exhibits an ectothrix invasion under a microscope. Final identification rests on the isolation and culture of the fungus and the ensuing production of its characteristic distorted macroconidia.

Prevention and Control

Preventive and control measures for infections due to *M. distortum* are the same as those presented previously for *M. canis* infections.

MICROSPORUM EQUINUM

Etiologic Agent — *M. equinum;* Perfect State — Unknown

M. equinum has been confused with *M. canis*. Conant[12] at first recognized it as a distinct species and distinguished it from *M. canis* on the basis of the smaller size of its macroconidia. Dowding and Orr[13] described a strain of *M. canis* with short macroconidia similar to those of *M. equinum* and suggested that *M. equinum* be included in the former species (*M. canis*). Conant[12] accepted this recommendation, and *M. equinum* has since been considered a synonym of *M. canis* by many authors.

Colonies on Sabouraud dextrose agar are velvety, becoming powdery in older cultures. They are radially furrowed and are pale buff to pale salmon colored. Macroconidia are more abundant toward the center of the colony. They are elliptical to broadly fusiform with thick, verruculose walls that have up to eight septa. Macroconidia are borne terminally or on short lateral branches that arise acutely from hyphae. Microconidia are pyriform to clavate, unicellular, smooth, and sessile or borne on short stalks. *M. equinum* forms numerous macroconidia on polished rice grain medium.

The organism infects hair and produces a small-spored ectothrix-type hair invasion. Under a Wood's lamp, infected hair fluoresces bright yellowish-green.

True and Alternate Hosts

M. equinum is primarily a pathogen of the horse but can transmit the infection to humans. Other animals such as cats, dogs, guinea pigs, and rabbits have been experimentally infected.

Distribution

M. equinum is apparently the source of endemic equine ringworm and sometimes causes severe epizootics in large stables. Although most reported outbreaks have been among army horses, outbreaks of ringworm in race horses have been recorded. *M. equinum* is the most common cause of equine ringworm in such countries as France, Algeria, and the U.S.S.R., in contrast with North and South America where it has been isolated only rarely and is superseded by *Trichophyton equinum*.[3] *M. equinum* has been recorded in (1) Africa (Algeria, Zaire, Malagasay, Morocco, Sudan), (2) Asia (Iran, Java, U.S.S.R.), (3) Australasia and Oceania (Fiji), (4) Europe (Belgium, Bulgaria, Denmark, France, Germany, Greece, Italy, the Netherlands, Norway, Romania, U.S.S.R.), (5) North America (New Jersey, New York), and (6) South America (Uruguay).[3]

Disease in Animals

Equine lesions cannot be distinguished clinically from those caused by other species. Usually they are dry, raised, and scaly and lead to circumscribed, balding patches. They may occur on any part of the animal but are most common in the saddle and girth regions. Although adjacent lesions may become confluent, areas of infection are never extensive or heavily crusted.

Disease in Man

Reports of the infection in humans usually describe the lesion as small and erythematous, most often appearing on the glabrous skin of the arms and beard (tinea barbae).

General Mode of Spread

Infection among horses is probably transmitted by direct or indirect contact between healthy and infected animals. Equine infections may be transmitted to humans.

Epidemiology

Since transmission of ringworm among horses probably occurs chiefly as a result of contact between healthy and infected animals, outbreaks[6] commonly occur in large stables. The disease is common among race horses that are constantly being moved from one race track to another. Individuals who attend horses and use the same tools may transfer infections from one animal to another and are themselves vulnerable to the disease.

Diagnosis

A diagnosis of equine or human ringworm due to *M. equinum* is established by direct microscopic examination of skin scrapings and hair in KOH preparations and by growth of the causal fungus in culture. An infected hair fluoresces green under a Wood's lamp.

Prevention and Control

Washing stables with a disinfectant, using a blowtorch on the walls, or applying some other cleaning procedure is essential to ensure that infections do not spread or recur. Infected animals can be treated with a detergent wash and griseofulvin.

TRICHOPHYTON EQUINUM

Etiologic Agent — *T. equinum;* Perfect State — Unknown

Colonies of *T. equinum* are fast-growing, white, and cottony with bright yellow pigment in the peripheral region. The reverse side of the colonies is yellow at first and turns pink to reddish brown with age.

Macroconidia are rare. They are long, narrow, and smooth-walled and are produced by some isolates only on such specialized media as bean pod agar. Microconidia are usually numerous, small, smooth, clavate, and are borne along the sides of hyphae. Most isolates of *T. equinum* have a nutritional requirement for nicotinic acid that is unique among dermatophytes. This requirement is satisfied by the hair of horses, donkeys, and mules but not by the hair of man or other animals. Strains independent of this requirement have been isolated from horses in New Zealand and Australia and are identified as *T. equinum* var. *autotrophicum.*[14]

Infected hairs do not exhibit fluorescence. When observed in KOH mounts, spores (5 to 8 μm) forming a sheath or isolated chains on the hair surface become evident. Scrapings from skin lesions show branched, hyaline, septate hyphae that may have formed arthrospores.

True and Alternate Hosts

This species has a relatively narrow host range. *T. equinum* is a pathogen of donkeys, horses, and mules and only rarely infects other lower animals. Infections among humans are usually confined to persons in contact with infected animals. *T. equinum* var. *autotrophicum* demonstrates the same host range.

Distribution

Infections due to *T. equinum* have been reported from Europe, North America, and Asia and are probably world-wide in distribution. The *autotrophicum* var. has only been reported from New Zealand and Australia to date.

Disease in Animals

Clinical manifestations in horses are similar to those described for *M. equinum* except that infected hairs do not fluoresce under a Wood's lamp.

Disease in Man

In man, infections of the glabrous skin are commonly observed; lesions are usually small and erythematous.

General Mode of Spread

Transmission of infection among horses is by direct or indirect contact through use of contaminated harnesses, grooming equipment, or fomites. Humans contract the infection through contact with infected horses or by handling contaminated grooming equipment.

Epidemiology

The epidemiology of infection caused by *T. equinum* is identical to that discussed earlier for *M. equinum.*

Diagnosis

A diagnosis of equine or human ringworm due to *T. equinum* is established by direct microscopic examination of skin scrapings and infected hair in KOH preparations and by culturing on Sabouraud dextrose agar. The nutritional requirement for nicotinic acid is peculiar to *T. equinum.*

Prevention and Control

The means for controlling and preventing further spread of infection are (1) disinfection of stables and equipment, (2) isolation of the infected animals, (3) treatment with griseofulvin, or (4) the local application of other antifungal agents.

TRICHOPHYTON GALLINAE

Etiologic Agent — *T. gallinae;* Perfect State — Unknown

On Sabouraud dextrose agar, colonies are downy and white (turning pink or buff with age), usually producing a characteristic pigment that is initially yellow but becomes strawberry-red and diffuses into the agar. If the cultures are maintained for a long time, pigment production may not be evident.

When produced by certain strains, macroconidia are blunt-tipped, smooth, and slipper-shaped or clavate with 5 to 10 cells. Microconidia are sparse, small, pyriform to elongate, and are borne along the sides of hyphae or in clusters.[3,15] Branched, septate, hyaline hyphae are present in KOH mounts of skin scrapings from crusty lesions. A sparse ectothrix invasion is present in infected scalp hair.

True and Alternate Hosts

T. gallinae is the principal agent of ringworm in birds, especially chickens. Infections due to *T. gallinae* have also been recorded in the canary,[16] chicken,[17-19] duck,[3] quail,[20] pigeon,[21] turkey,[16] cat,[22] dog,[3] laboratory mouse,[22] monkey,[23] and man.[24]

Distribution

T. gallinae is widely distributed geographically. Sporadic outbreaks of fowl infections have been reported from Australia, Brazil,[18,19] England, France, New Zealand, Puerto Rico, Tasmania, Venezuela, Yugoslavia, and Zaire.[19]

Disease in Animals

Characteristic symptoms in birds include a thick white crusting of the comb and wattles; however, in severe cases the infection may become generalized and involve the base of the feathers and development of circular favic lesions on the underlying skin occurs. In young birds, these lesions sometimes extend to the necks, thighs, and ventral surfaces of the wings and are accompanied by loss of feathers.

Disease in Man

The infection in humans is primarily confined to the scalp and glabrous skin; it is most commonly seen in children.

General Mode of Spread

Among fowl the infection can be transmitted directly or indirectly. The fungus can remain viable at room temperature in infected scales for 12 months. These scales can infect young birds either by direct contact or fomites.

Epidemiology

Though world-wide in distribution, fowl favus occurs sporadically. Among birds it is markedly contagious, and although infections are transmissible to man,[24] this rarely occurs, perhaps due to the low virulence of *T. gallinae* for humans.

Diagnosis

Diagnosis is established by directly examining the infected material in KOH mounts and by growing the causal fungus on Sabouraud dextrose agar. Final identification of *T. gallinae* is based upon its morphological characters, especially the strawberry-red pigment that diffuses into the agar.

Prevention and Control

Isolation of infected birds and attention to general hygiene are factors of major importance in eradicating and preventing outbreaks. Removing crusts with soap and water and using disinfectants are recommended treatments.

TRICHOPHYTON MENTAGROPHYTES

Etiologic Agent — *T. mentagrophytes* var. *mentagrophytes, T. mentagrophytes* var. *erinacei,* and *T. mentagrophytes* var. *quinckeanum;* Perfect State — *Arthroderma benhamiae*[25] and *A. vanbreuseghemii*[26]

On Sabouraud dextrose agar, colonies are finely or coarsely granular, flat or only slightly folded (var. *mentagrophytes*) and velvety to fluffy to powdery, becoming distinctly folded (var. *quinckeanum*). The reverse side of colonies is red, yellow, ochraceous (var. *mentagrophytes*), bright yellow (var. *erinacei*), or colorless (var. *quinckeanum*).

Microconidia are usually globose and occasionally pyriform to short clavate; they are borne along the sides of simple or branched hyphae (occasionally) or on complexly branched hyphae in grapelike clusters often surrounded by antler-like and spiral hyphae. Spiral hyphae are most commonly seen in the var. *mentagrophytes* and are rare in the other two varieties. Macroconidia are produced in greater abundance by some isolates than others. They are smooth, clavate, and composed of 2 to 5 cells or more.

Infected hair does not fluoresce under a Wood's lamp. Hairs infected with *T. mentagrophytes* reveal a sheath of surface (ectothrix) spores (3 to 5 μm in diameter) in isolated chains. Scrapings from skin lesions or nails show hyaline, branched, septate hyphae that break into arthrospores.

True and Alternate Hosts

The granular variety (var. *mentagrophytes*) is a zoophilic dermatophyte that causes ringworm in many lower animal species, both domestic and wild. These include rodents and larger mammals. This fungus is an important cause of ringworm in dogs, horses, rabbits, mice, and rats and commonly in such fur-bearing animals as chinchillas and foxes. *T. mentagrophytes* var. *erinacei* is a natural resident and pathogen of hedgehogs and occasionally mice and rats. The var. *quinckeanum* is the principal agent of mouse favus and has been isolated from cats, cattle, dogs, fowl, horses, man, rabbits, and sheep. The diverse list of host animals from which *T. mentagrophytes* has been isolated is too long to cite here. Readers are urged to refer to textbooks detailing fungal diseases of animals.[3]

Distribution

T. mentagrophytes is a dermatophyte with world-wide distribution. The var. *quinckeanum* is also cosmopolitan, but the var. *erinacei* has so far been reported only in New Zealand and England.

Disease in Animals

Infections due to *T. mentagrophytes* also manifest a diversity of clinical forms. In wild rodents, the disease may be asymptomatic while in laboratory animals it may produce scaly, erythematous lesions with loss of fur or hair. Among dogs, 10% of all ringworm cases are caused by *T. mentagrophytes*.[27] Infections of both cats and dogs by *T. mentagrophytes* are less frequent than those caused by *M. canis*. Diagnostic clinical differences between infections caused by *M. canis* and *T. mentagrophytes* have not been clearly defined, but scutula in both cats and dogs suggest that infection is due to the var. *quinckeanum*.[3]

Disease in Man

Human cases of this fungus are seen mainly in rural areas. In Michigan, nearly half of the cases of suppurative ringworm in rural residents are due to *T. mentagrophytes* var. *mentagrophytes*. This dermatophyte can infect any part of the body, causing boggy, kerion-type lesions. Lesions caused by var. *quinckeanum* can develop scutula.[3]

General Mode of Spread

Although infections among rural residents caused by the different varieties of *T. mentagrophytes* can often be traced to contact with domestic animals, the animal source cannot always be identified. Wild animals, particularly rodents of the type commonly encountered on farm premises, have been found to be carriers of this dermatophyte.[2,28-30]

Epidemiology

In both urban and rural areas, infections are usually contracted through direct or indirect contact with domestic animals; additionally, in rural areas infections are caused by contact with wild rodents that enter barns, feed storage bins, and other similar areas. Such infested sites may serve as indirect sources of human infection by means of infected hair shed by the rodents.

Diagnosis

The diagnosis in animals and man is established by direct microscopic examination in KOH mounts of skin scrapings, nail clippings, or infected hair and by culture of the causal fungus on Sabouraud dextrose agar.

Prevention and Control

Preventive and control measures against the spread of infection include the use of disinfectants, decontamination of tools and barn equipment, and isolation of infected animals, followed by treatment with antifungal agents.

TRICHOPHYTON VERRUCOSUM

Etiologic Agent — *T. verrucosum (T. discoides, T. album, T. ochraceum, T. faviforme*[31]); Perfect State — Unknown

A colony on Sabouraud dextrose agar is glabrous, rarely downy, white to ochraceous, and has abundant chlamydospores that are sometimes solitary but usually occur in chains. The growth rate is slow at 25°C but accelerates at 37°C. Microconidia are produced occasionally in downy cultures, especially in those grown on thiamine-supplemented media.

A nutritional requirement of *T. verrucosum* is thiamine. Many isolates also require inositol.[31] Unlike other dermatophytes, its growth rate usually accelerates at 37°C.

Infected hairs do not fluoresce under a Wood's lamp. In KOH mounts, arthrospores of 8 to 10 μm in diameter forming a sheath or isolated chains are seen on the surface of hair (large-spored ectothrix). Skin scrapings and nail clippings mounted in KOH show hyaline, branching, septate hyphae breaking into arthrospores.

True and Alternate Hosts

T. verrucosum is the principal agent of bovine ringworm in the U.S. and other parts of the world. It is also an occasional cause of ringworm in the buffalo, canary, cat, dog, donkey, goat, horse, mule, pig, and sheep.[3] Most infections in these occasional hosts can be traced to bovine sources.

Distribution

In the U.S., almost all cases of bovine ringworm are caused by *T. verrucosum*. This dermatophyte is widespread and has a world-wide distribution.

Disease in Animals

Cattle are the preferred hosts for *T. verrucosum*, and infections are observed more frequently in calves than older animals. Whether calves are inherently more susceptible to the infection or differences in husbandry practices account for the difference in incidence is unknown.[2] Lesions are discrete and vary in size from 1-cm circular lesions to much larger. Sometimes scaliness and loss of hair are the only symptoms. More commonly, lesions are white at first but then become thick, yellowish-brown, and crusty. They are most frequently observed on the head or neck,[32] but flanks, rump, and limbs may also become involved.

Disease in Man

T. verrucosum is also infectious for man with both adults and children being susceptible. Human cases are encountered mainly in rural areas. In Michigan, according to Georg et al.,[29] nearly half of the cases of suppurative ringworm in humans residing in rural areas were due to this dermatophyte. Lesions are inflammatory, usually located on the face, and frequently appear as a sycosis of the lips and chin. *T. verrucosum* causes kerion-type, boggy lesions in children. The infection is usually contracted from animals. The fungus grows inside the hair shaft and forms an external sheath of spores 8 to 10 μm in diameter.

General Mode of Spread

Bovine ringworm in the U.S. occurs most commonly in the fall and winter months when animals are kept in barns although outbreaks do occur during the warm months of the year. Since calves are commonly kept confined during winter months, there are many opportunities for initial spread of the infection, as well as for constant reinfection within a group of animals and contamination of the environment by an infected group of calves. Contraction of infection by man from infected cattle occurs frequently[32-34] and is an important aspect of the epidemiology of human ringworm.

Epidemiology

The incidence of bovine ringworm is generally higher in winter than summer. During the winter when animals are kept inside barns, *T. verrocosum* apparently spreads from animal to animal by direct contact. McPherson[35] has shown that since *T. verrucosum* retains its viability for as long as 4.5 years in skin scrapings, a building that is unused during the summer months could still contain much infected material the following autumn. Spores in the infected scales are protected from the action of ultraviolet light.

The dermatophyte can also grow temporarily on many substrates and thus may persist for some time as a saprobe on the farm. The contaminated environment surrounding infected cattle suggests that transmission may also occur through fomites. Human infections are generally contracted from infected cattle, but it is unlikely that cattle contract the infection from humans.

Diagnosis

A clinical diagnosis of *T. verrucosum* ringworm is confirmed by examination of infected hair of skin scrapings in KOH mounts. Infected hairs show an endothrix-type invasion. Specific identification of *T. verrucosum* must be made on selective isolation media, such as Sabouraud dextrose agar, that contain chloramphenicol and cyclohex-imide. *T. verrucosum* has specific nutritional requirements — some isolates require thiamine while others require a combination of thiamine and inositol. Growth is more rapid at 37°C than at room temperature.[31]

Prevention and Control

One of the many measures advocated for preventing or controlling this infection is spraying infected and healthy animals with a fungicide such as captan, thus reducing the reservoir of infection. Thorough cleansing of calf sheds breaks up the succession of epidemics among calves kept in a particular shed. This can be done by spraying both the walls and woodwork with Bordeaux mixture or another copper-containing fungicide. Successful griseofulvin therapy has been reported by Lauder and O'Sullivan[36] and Pearson and Rankin.[37]

MICROSPORUM GYPSEUM

Etiologic Agent — *M. gypseum* complex; Perfect State — *Nannizzia incurvata*,[38] *N. gypsea*,[39] and *N. fulva*[39]

A colony on Sabouraud dextrose agar is fast-growing, flat, coarsely or finely granular, and buff to rosy-buff. The reverse side of the colony is rosy-buff to cinnamon and has an irregularly fringed border. Macroconidia are numerous and ellipsoidal to fusiform or predominantly cylindrical. They contain as many as five septa and are rough and moderately thick-walled. Microconidia are sparse clavate, sessile, or on short pedicels.

Until recently, *M. gypseum* was regarded as a single species. Although differences in cultural characteristics had been noted among isolates, they were considered to be within the normal range of species variation. Based upon sexual reproduction, the three perfect species, *N. gypsea*,[39] *N. incurvata*,[38] and *N. fulva*,[39] are now differentiated. Since members of this complex are generally encountered in their imperfect or conidial states and have not been shown to differ in their natural history, the *M. gypseum* complex is treated here as a single species.

The *M. gypseum* complex species form ectothrix chains (spores of 5 to 8 μm) on the hairs of infected animals. In skin scrapings, hyaline, branched, septate hyphae that form arthrospores are observed in KOH mounts.

True and Alternate Hosts

M. gypseum complex is an important cause of ringworm in dogs and other lower animals. It is also a significant agent of ringworm in horses and occasionally causes the disease in cats and other animals such as goats, jaguars, lions, monkeys, pigs, baboons, cattle, chimpanzees, chinchillas, fowl, gerbils, guinea pigs, laboratory mice, leopards, parrots, rabbits, rats, rodents, and tigers.[3,27,40,41] Human infections are infrequent.

Distribution

The *M. gypseum* complex species are cosmopolitan, geophilic dermatophytes.

Disease in Animals

In the U.S., this complex of species is an important cause of ringworm in dogs (close to 24%) and a minor cause of ringworm in cats (about 10%).[27,42] Infections appear to occur mainly during summer and fall. In winter and spring, a few cases are reported in the South but virtually none are noted in the North.

The lesions in dogs are circular, with the development of alopecia, erythema, scaling, and peripheral yellowish-white crusts. In cats, varying degrees of tissue involvement and tissue response to invasion are noted. Lesions are dry and diffuse with erythema and alopecia. There have also been reports of kerion formation in domestic-short-hair cats, with raised, boggy lesions that suppurate at many points on the head area.[40] In horses, circular patches of alopecia on the back, rump, shoulders, or other areas are seen.[41]

Disease in Man

M. gypseum complex species are an occasional cause of ringworm of the scalp, nails, and glabrous skin. Scalp infections may present a clinical picture of kerion with small-spored ectothrix invasion of the hair. Tinea capitis infections may also manifest themselves as dry scaly patches that occasionally simulate alopecia. Infection may spread to the nails and glabrous skin.

General Mode of Spread

Soil often contains members of the *M. gypseum* complex. In the past they were regarded as zoophilic dermatophytes in the belief that animals served as reservoirs of infection for man. Basically, infections spread through the exposure of animals to soil sites where *M. gypseum* complex species are present rather than by direct contact with infected animals.

Epidemiology

Ajello[43] reported recovery of this dermatophyte complex from 37 of 116 soil samples collected from various localities in Tennessee and Georgia. Subsequent analyses of domestic and foreign soils by other workers have yielded similar results. Infections in dogs occur mainly in the summer and fall and are rarely reported in winter and spring in most parts of the U.S. Additional available data also suggest a similar seasonal pattern in other animals. Soil is the ultimate reservoir of this dermatophyte complex for both man and animals.

Diagnosis

M. gypseum complex infections in cats cannot be detected under a Wood's lamp because infected hairs do not fluoresce.[40] Ringworm is confirmed by direct microscopic examination of hairs and skin scales in KOH mounts and by isolation of the causal dermatophyte on Sabouraud dextrose agar.

Prevention and Control

Since *M. gypseum* complex species are soil dermatophytes of widespread occurrence, there are no special preventive or control measures available. Isolation of infected animals, disinfection of the surrounding environment, and treatment of infected animals with antifungal agents are the measures to be followed in controlling the spread of infection.

MICROSPORUM NANUM

Etiologic Agent — *M. nanum*; Perfect State — *Nannizzia obtusa*[44]

A colony on Sabouraud dextrose agar is fast-growing, powdery to granular, and buff-colored; the reverse side is pale brown. Macroconidia are numerous, ovate to clavate, have as many as three septa (majority have one septum), and are rough-walled. Microconidia are sparse, pyriform to cylindric, smooth, and thin-walled.

M. nanum invades hair and causes an ectothrix-type invasion with spores of 5 to 8 μm in chains surrounding the hair surface. Skin scrapings in KOH mounts show hyaline, branched, septate hyphae.

True and Alternate Hosts

M. nanum is primarily a parasite of pigs, only rarely infecting humans.[45,46]

Distribution

M. nanum occurs as a free-living soil saprophyte in areas populated by swine. It is widespread in North America (U.S., Canada), Australasia, and Africa and has also been reported from some Asian countries (India) as well as Europe (Italy).[3a]

Disease in Animals

M. nanum is the principal cause of porcine ringworm, a widespread disease in the U.S. Lesions usually have a reddish background that is frequently obscured by brownish crusts. Some lesions become very extensive and eventually cover a large part of the body surface. Alopecia and pruritis are generally absent.[45] Lesions can be confused with urine scald and mange.

Disease in Man

Human infections due to *M. nanum* are rare and lesions resemble those caused by the *M. gypseum* complex. In tinea capitis, a kerion-type reaction may be produced. Hair invasion has been described as being of the ectothrix type. Some hairs from persons with scalp infections fluoresce under a Wood's lamp.[45]

General Mode of Spread

Most human infections are generally noted in rural areas where swine are raised, but the infection need not be contracted directly from infected animals. Most cases are probably infected by exposure to the organism in soil.

Epidemiology

The fungus occurs as a free-living saprophyte in soil of areas populated by swine. Most porcine infections are contracted either through direct exposure to the fungus in soil or contact with an infected animal. Most human cases are usually found in rural areas where swine are raised. The infection may be contracted on rare occasions through direct contact with infected swine, but most human cases are probably contracted from exposure to the fungus in the environment.

Diagnosis

Microscopic examination of the infected hair reveals ectothrix invasion. Some hairs from persons with scalp infections fluoresce under a Wood's light. Specific identification is based upon morphological characteristics of the isolate.

Prevention and Control
Control methods are similar to those described earlier for the *M. gypseum* complex.

ANTHROPOPHILIC DERMATOPHYTES

Some anthropophilic species of dermatophytes occasionally have been found to infect animals. The anthropophilic species are basically pathogens of man. Animals have not been found to play a role in the epidemiology of these diseases. During the course of a survey of ringworm in animals, Kaplan and Georg[47] diagnosed three cases of ringworm in dogs caused by the anthropophilic species *M. audouinii*. All three dogs were less than 1 year old and had had close contact with children being treated for chronic tinea capitis due to *M. audouinii*. Kaplan and Gump[48] also diagnosed a case of ringworm in a young dog caused by *T. rubrum*, another anthropophilic dermatophyte. The dog's owner had been suffering for many years from a chronic case of athlete's foot due to *T. rubrum* and he had a habit of rubbing the dog with his bare feet.

In a few instances, human-to-animal transmission does occur. Investigators in the U.S. and elsewhere have reported spontaneous anthropophilic dermatophyte infections in lower animals.[42,49] Although few in number, such cases do indicate that close contact between humans suffering from anthropophilic dermatophyte infections and pets, particularly young ones, constitutes a potential health hazard for the animal involved.[2]

CANDIDIASIS (MONILIASIS, THRUSH)

Candidiasis is a general term that covers diseases caused by mycelial yeasts of the genus *Candida* especially *C. albicans*. Although infections in animals are most commonly restricted to the alimentary canal, generalized infections do occur. Candidiasis of poultry, especially turkeys, is an economically important disease. *C. albicans* infections in other animals, such as cattle, cat, dogs, pigs, and sheep, have been described. Systemic *C. albicans* infection in animals is discussed under the heading of systemic mycoses. In this presentation, only cutaneous candidiasis is described. *C. albicans*, although at times a primary pathogen, is frequently found as part of the normal flora of healthy animals.

Etiologic Agent — *Candida albicans*
A colony on Sabouraud dextrose agar is fast-growing, creamy smooth or wrinkled, creamy white, and soft and has globose, short ovoid, 5- to 7-μm blastospores. Terminal thick-walled chlamydospores and mycelium are produced on special media.

The identification of yeasts, a highly specialized branch of mycology, was greatly facilitated by publication of Lodder's scholarly monograph.[50] The identification system is based upon type of sporulation, morphology of spores, development of mycelium on defined media, and fermentation and assimilation reactions with a variety of compounds. Several techniques are used for the specific identification of *C. albicans*.[2-5]

True and Alternate Hosts
C. albicans was first described as the causal agent of thrush in infants. It is a normal inhabitant of the flora of the human alimentary canal.[55] Ainsworth and Austwick[55] found it and other yeasts to be associated with both normal and abnormal animals, and their records suggested that these yeasts were more commonly associated with the lungs and alimentary canal than other sites of the body. Candidiasis has been recog-

nized in lower animals for more than 50 years; however, other than those pertaining to poultry, early data regarding animal infections are scanty.[54] Yeasts are common saprobes, and several species of *Candida* are frequently isolated from the air and soil.[55] Candidiasis has been reported in birds (fowl, turkeys, duck, geese, guinea-fowl, pigeons, partridges), cattle, sheep, dogs, cats, hedgehogs, guinea pigs, monkeys, baboons, mice, various other rodents, and man.[55]

Distribution

C. albicans is an ubiquitous yeast and its occurrence as a disease agent has been reported from all parts of the world.[56]

Disease in Animals

Cutaneous candidiasis in animals is rare. In 1968, it was described in 180 members of a group of 450 garbage-fed swine.[57] No deaths occurred, but packers complained that the hams had to be skinned before they were used. Kral and Uscavage[58] described the case of a dog that had candidiasis lesions over much of the skin area. These had developed following a long period of oral and parenteral antibiotic therapy. Schwartzman and associates[59] induced cutaneous infection in dogs. Lesions resembled those of pyotraumatic dermatitis. Neither equine nor feline cutaneous candidiasis has been documented.

Disease in Man

Candidiasis, especially the human systemic variety, is recognized frequently in patients whose resistance has been compromised by other diseases, who are debilitated from such conditions as diabetes mellitus, or whose normal defense mechanisms have been impaired by immunosuppressive, broad-spectrum antibiotic, and steroid therapy. Clinical manifestations of candidiasis are varied. They can be divided into: (1) mucocutaneous candidiasis (glossitis, stomatitis, chelitis, perleche, vaginitis, and balanitis; bronchial, pulmonary, alimentary (involving esophagus), enteric, or perianal candidiasis), (2) cutaneous candidiasis (intertrigenous, paronychia, and onythomycosis; diaper rash, candidal granuloma), and (3) systemic candidiasis (urinary tract infection, endocarditis, meningitis, septicemia).[60]

Cutaneous candidiasis may directly involve intertrigenous areas of the glabrous skin, or it may be a secondary colonization of preexisting lesions on any part of the body. Intertrigo is most commonly seen in the axillae, groin, intermammary folds, intergluteal folds, interdigital spaces, and the umbilicus. Lesions are well-defined, weeping, scalded skin areas with an erythematous base and a scalloped border. They are surrounded by satellite eruptions of vesicles, pustules, or bullae. Clinical variations do occur, and the lesions may appear dry and scaly. Cutaneous candidiasis is usually associated with two types of patients: (1) those with such metabolic disorders as diabetes, obesity, or chronic alcoholism that predispose them to candidal colonization or (2) those predisposed to infection by various environmental conditions such as moisture, occlusion, maceration, or continual immersion in water.

Paronychia and onychomycosis are the most common forms of cutaneous candidiasis. They are often seen in people whose occupations require that they frequently immerse their hands in water. Diaper rash is commonly seen in newborns as a result of preexisting oral or perianal candidiasis. It also occurs in infants raised under unhygienic conditions, such as wet and irregularly changed diapers. Candidal granuloma of children is very rare. Hauser and Rothman[61] reviewed 13 cases. The lesions were quite distinct and were described as primary vascularized papules that were covered with thick, adherent, yellowish-brown crusts. They sometimes develop into horns or protrusions 2 cm long. The face is most commonly involved, but lesions are also found on the scalp, fingernails, trunk, and legs. Defects of the immune system predispose to this form of disease.

General Mode of Spread

Candida spp. are so commonly present in the G.I. tract of both man and animals and are so infrequently encountered in nature that it seems proper to consider the disease that they cause as being endogenous in origin. The host, who is compromised by other diseases, debilitated from conditions such as diabetes mellitus, or whose defense mechanisms have been impaired by therapy with immunosuppressive drugs, is predisposed to infection by the *Candida* spp. Other factors favorable to candidiasis are vitamin A deficiency, a high-glucose diet, or deficient essential fatty acid nutrition.[62-64]

Epidemiology

The epidemiology of cutaneous candidiasis in animals is not fully understood. In certain circumstances, individual transmission occurs in man and animals. Fecal contamination of meat at the slaughterhouse or of animal feed may account for spread of the disease from animal to man or animal to animal.

Diagnosis

Diagnosis of candidiasis is confirmed by direct examination of scrapings in KOH mounts, isolation of the causal fungus, and histopathological examination of the tissues. *C. albicans* can be differentiated from other *Candida* species by such morphological characteristics as formation of germ tubes or development of chlamydospores on special media. It also has characteristic assimilation and fermentation patterns.

Prevention and Control

The addition of copper sulfate to drinking water is both a control and a prophylactic measure. Addition of nystatin to animal feed is also recommended as an effective measure for controlling and preventing epidemics of candidiasis.[50]

REFERENCES

1. **Hasegawa, A. and Usi, K.,** *Nannizzia otae* sp. nov., the perfect state of *Microsporum canis* Bodin, *Jpn. J. Med. Mycol.,* 16, 148, 1975.
2. **Kaplan, W.,** Epidemiology and public health significance of ringworm in animals, *Arch. Dermatol.,* 96, 404, 1967.
3. **Ainsworth, G. C. and Austwick, P. K. C.,** *Fungal Diseases of Animals,* 2nd ed, Commonwealth Agricultural Bureaux, Slough, England, 1973, 10.
3a. **Morganti, L., Bianchedi, M., Ajello, L., and Padhye, A.,** First european report of swine infection by *Microsporum nanum, Mycopathologia,* 59, 179, 1976.
4. **Jungerman, P. F. and Schwartzman, R. M.,** *Veterinary Medical Mycology,* Lea & Febiger, Philadelphia, 1972, 3.
5. **Kirk, H.,** Organo-mercury compounds in veterinary medicine, *Vet. Rec.,* 58, 299, 1946.
6. **Dawson, C. O. and Noddle, B. M.,** Treatment of *Microsporum canis* ringworm in a cat colony, *J. Small Anim. Pract.,* 9, 613, 1968.
7. **O'Sullivan, J. G.,** Griseofulvin treatment in experimental *Microsporum canis* infection in the cat, *Sabouraudia,* 1, 103, 1961.

8. Smith, J. M. B., Animal mycoses in New Zealand, *Mycopathol. Mycol. Appl.*, 34, 323, 1968.
9. Smith, J. M. B., *Microsporum distortum* ringworm in New Zealand, *Aust. J. Dermatol.*, 11, 131, 1970.
10. Smith, J. M. B., Rush-Munro, F. M., and McCarthy, M., Animals as a reservoir of human ringworm in New Zealand, *Aust. J. Dermatol.*, 10, 169, 1969.
11. Kaplan, W., Georg, L. K., Hendricks, S. L., and Leeper, R. A., Isolation of *Microsporum distortum* from animals in the United States, *J. Invest. Dermatol.*, 28, 449, 1957.
12. Conant, N. F., A statistical analysis of spore size in the genus *Microsporum*, *J. Invest. Dermatol.*, 4, 265, 1941.
13. Dowding, E. S. and Orr, H., The dermatophyte *Microsporum lanosum*, *Mycologia*, 31, 76, 1939.
14. Smith, J. M. B., Jolly, R. D., Georg, L. K., and Connole, M. D., *Trichophyton equinum* var. *autotrophicum*; its characteristics and geographical distribution, *Sabouraudia*, 6, 296, 1968.
15. Georg, L. K., Cultural and nutritional studies of *Trichophyton gallinae* and *Trichophyton megninii*, *Mycologia*, 44, 470, 1952.
16. Kral, F., Skin diseases, *Adv. Vet. Sci.*, 7, 183, 1962.
17. Carnaghan, R. B. A., Gitter, M., and Blaxland, J. D., Favus in poultry: an outbreak of *Trichophyton gallinae* infection, *Vet. Rec.*, 68, 600, 1956.
18. Londero, A. T., Fischman, O., and Ramos, C. D., *Trichophyton gallinae* in Brazil, *Sabouraudia*, 3, 233, 1964.
19. Londero, A. T., Ramos, C. D., and Fischman, O., Four epizooties of *Trichophyton gallinae* infection on chickens in Brasil, *Mykosen*, 12, 31, 1969.
20. Gullion, G. W., Gambel quail disease and parasite investigations in Nevada, *Am. Midl. Nat.*, 57, 414, 1957.
21. Gierloff, B. C. H. and Katic, I., Griseofulvin treatment of ringworm in animals, *Nord. Vet. Med.*, 13, 571, 1961.
22. Dvorak, J. and Otcenasek, M., Geophilic, zoophilic and anthropophilic dermatophytes. A review, *Mycopathol. Mycol. Appl.*, 23, 294, 1964.
23. Gordon, M. A. and Little, G. N., *Trichophyton (Microsporum?) gallinae* ringworm in a monkey, *Sabouraudia*, 6, 207, 1968.
24. Torres, G. and Georg, L. K., A human case of *Trichophyton gallinae* infection. Disease contracted from chickens, *Arch. Dermatol. Syphilol.*, 74, 191, 1956.
25. Ajello, L. and Cheng, S. Y., The perfect state of *Trichophyton mentagrophytes*, *Sabouraudia*, 5, 230, 1967.
26. Takashio, M., Etude des phenomenes de reproduction lies au vieillissement et au rejeunissement des cultures de champignons, *Ann. Soc. Belge Med. Trop.*, 53, 427, 1973.
27. Kaplan, W. and Ivens, M. S., Observations on the seasonal variations in incidence of ringworm in dogs and cats in the United States, *Sabouraudia*, 1, 91, 1961.
28. Georg, L. K., The role of animals as vectors of human fungus diseases, *Trans. N.Y. Acad. Sci.*, 18, 639, 1956.
29. Georg, L. K., Hand, E. A., and Menges, R. A., Observations on rural and urban ringworm, *J. Invest. Dermatol.*, 27, 335, 1956.
30. Kaplan, W., Georg, L. K., and Ajello, L., Recent developments in animal ringworm and their public health implications, *Ann. N.Y. Acad. Sci.*, 70, 636, 1958.
31. Georg, L. K., The relation of nutrition to the growth and morphology of *Trichophyton faviforme*, *Mycologia*, 42, 693, 1950.
32. Gentles, J. C. and O'Sullivan, J. G., Correlation of human and animal ringworm in west of Scotland, *Br. Med. J.*, 2, 678, 1957.
33. Blank, F., Ringworm in cattle due to *Trichophyton discoides* and its transmission to man, *Can. J. Comp. Med.*, 17, 277, 1953.
34. Blank, F. and Craig, G. E., Family epidemics of ringworm contracted from cattle, *Can. Med. Assoc. J.*, 71, 234, 1954.
35. McPherson, E. A., The influence of physical factors on dermatomycosis in domestic animals, *Vet. Rec.*, 69, 674, 1957.
36. Lauder, I. M. and O'Sullivan, J. G., Ringworm in cattle. Prevention and treatment with griseofulvin, *Vet. Rec.*, 70, 949, 1958.
37. Pearson, J. K. L. and Rankin, J. E. F., Griseofulvin in the treatment of bovine ringworm, *Vet. Rec.*, 74, 564, 1962.
38. Stockdale, P. M., *Nannizzia incurvata* gen. nov., sp. nov., a perfect state of *Microsporum gypseum* (Bodin) Guiart et Grigorakis, *Sabouraudia*, 1, 41, 1961.
39. Stockdale, P. M., The *Microsporum gypseum* complex (*Nannizzia incurvata* Stockd., *N. gypsea* (Nann.) comb. nov., *N. fulva* sp. nov.), *Sabouraudia*, 3, 114, 1963.

40. **Kaplan, W., Georg, L. K., and Bromley, C. L.,** Ringworm in cats caused by *Microsporum gypseum,* *Vet. Med.,* 52, 347, 1957.

41. **Kaplan, W., Hopping, J. L., and Georg, L. K.,** Ringworm in horses caused by the dermatophyte, *Microsporum gypseum, J. Am. Vet. Med. Assoc.,* 131, 329, 1957.

42. **Georg, L. K.,** Animal Ringworm in Public Health, Diagnosis and Nature, Publication No. 727, U.S. Department of Health, Education, and Welfare, Public Health Service, Washington D.C., 1960.

43. **Ajello, L.,** The dermatophyte, *Microsporum gypseum* as a saprophyte and parasite, *J. Invest. Dermatol.,* 21, 157, 1953.

44. **Dawson, C. O. and Gentles, J. C.,** The perfect states of *Keratinomyces ajelloi* Vanbreuseghem, *Trichophyton terrestre* Durie and Frey, and *Microsporum nanum* Fuentes, *Sabouraudia,* 1, 49, 1961.

45. **Ajello, L., Varsavsky, E., Ginther, O. J., and Bubash, G.,** The natural history of *Microsporum nanum, Mycologia,* 56, 873, 1964.

46. **Bubash, G. R., Ginther, C. J., and Ajello, L.,** *Microsporum nanum:* first recorded isolations from animals in the United States, *Science,* 143, 366, 1964.

47. **Kaplan, W. and Georg, L. K.,** Isolation of *Microsporum audouinii* from a dog, *J. Invest. Dermatol.,* 28, 313, 1957.

48. **Kaplan, W. and Gump, R. H.,** Ringworm in a dog caused by *Trichophyton rubrum, Vet. Med.,* 53, 139, 1958.

49. **Chakraborty, A. N., Ghosh, S., and Blank, F.,** Isolation of *Trichophyton rubrum* (Castellani) Sabouraud, 1911, from animals, *Can. J. Comp. Med.,* 18, 436, 1954.

50. **Lodder, J., Ed.,** *The Yeasts: A Taxonomic Study,* 2nd ed., North-Holland Amsterdam, 1970.

51. **Kutscher, A. H., Seguin, L., Zegarelli, E. V., Rankow, R. M., Mercandante, J., and Piro, J. D.,** Growth characteristics of *Candida albicans* on Pagano-Levin culture medium, *J. Invest. Dermatol.,* 33, 41, 1959.

52. **Mackenzie, D. W. R.,** Serum tube identification of *Candida albicans, J. Clin. Pathol.,* 15, 563, 1962.

53. **Raubitschek, F.,** Taurocholate agar for chlamydospore production by *Candida albicans, Mycopathol. Mycol. Appl.,* 9, 285, 1958.

54. **Winner, H. I. and Hurley, R.,** *Candida albicans,* J & A Churchill, London, 1964.

55. **Ainsworth, G. C. and Austwick, P. K. C.,** *Fungal Diseases of Animals,* 2nd ed., Commonwealth Agricultural Bureaux, Slough, England, 1973, 63.

56. **Jungerman, P. F. and Schwartzman, R. M.,** *Veterinary Medical Mycology,* Lea & Febiger, Philadelphia, 1972, 61.

57. **Reynolds, I. M., Miner, P. W., and Smith, R. E.,** Cutaneous candidiasis in swine, *J. Am. Vet. Med. Assoc.,* 152, 182, 1968.

58. **Kral, F. and Uscavage, J. P.,** Cutaneous candidiasis in a dog, *J. Am. Vet. Med. Assoc.,* 136, 612, 1960.

59. **Schwartzman, R. M., Deubler, M. J., and Dice, P. F.,** Experimentally induced cutaneous moniliasis (*Candida albicans*) in the dog, *J. Small Anim. Pract.,* 8, 327, 1965.

60. **Rippon, J. W.,** Medical mycology in *The Pathogenic Fungi and the Pathogenic Actinomycetes,* W. B. Saunders, Philadelphia, 1974, 175.

61. **Hauser, F. and Rothman, S.,** Monilial granuloma: report of a case and review of the literature, *Arch. Dermatol.,* 61, 297, 1950.

62. **Jeoffery, S. M. S. and Kenzy, S. G.,** Nutritional factors influencing experimental *Candida albicans* in chickens. I. Effect of vitamin A deficiency, *Avian Dis.,* 4, 138, 1960.

63. **Sayedain, S. M. and Kenzy, S. G.,** Nutritional factors influencing experimental *Candida albicans* infection in chickens. II. Effect of purified glucose diet, *Pak. J. Sci. Res.,* 14, 54, 1962.

64. **Wagstaff, R. K., Jensen, L. S., Tripathy, S. B., and Kenzy, S. G.,** Essential fatty acid deficiency and *Candida albicans* infection in the chick, *Avian Dis.,* 12, 186, 1968.

THE SUBCUTANEOUS MYCOSES

W. Kaplan and L. Ajello

INTRODUCTION

The subcutaneous mycoses are a group of fungus diseases that involve the subcutaneous tissue and skin. Dissemination to the internal organs occurs only on rare occasions. The etiologic agents are classified among several unrelated genera. Most of these fungi have a saprophytic existence in nature, and most human and animal infections result from the traumatic implantation of these agents into the skin or subcutaneous tissue.

Tissue responses to these etiologic agents and the type and severity of lesions depend upon the fungus species involved and the host. In most cases, lesions tend to remain localized. Four subcutaneous mycoses — sporotrichosis, eumycotic mycetomas, phaeohyphomycosis, and rhinosporidiosis — affect both man and lower animals. They will be covered in detail. Another subcutaneous mycosis, chromoblastomycosis, is known only as a human disease and will be briefly summarized.

SPOROTRICHOSIS

Etiologic agent — *Sporothrix (Sporotrichum) schenckii*

S. schenckii is a dimorphic fungus. When cultivated at room temperature, it develops in a mycelial form. When grown at 37°C in vitro or in tissues of a living host, it develops in a yeast form. Characteristically, mycelial-form cultures grow rapidly and have a wrinkled or folded membranous surface that is at first whitish in color but eventually becomes brownish or, in some strains, black. In some isolates, fine, grayish, velvety aerial mycelium may appear at the outer borders. Microscopic examination reveals relatively fine, branched, septate, hyaline mycelium and numerous conidia. Conidia are produced in abundance on delicate sterigmata along the hyphae and terminally on conidiophores. Yeast-form colonies are moist, creamy, and white in color. Microscopic examination reveals single and budding yeast-like cells that vary in size and shape; they may be round, oval, or cigar-shaped. Single and budding cells identical in appearance to those found in yeast-form cultures occur in infected tissues and in exudates. Asteroid bodies are occasionally seen in tissues.[1]

True and Alternate Hosts

The disease occurs in man and a diversity of lower animals, including dogs, cats, horses, mules, cattle, camels, swine, rats, mice, and chimpanzees.[2]

Distribution

Sporotrichosis occurs throughout the world in temperate as well as tropical zones.

Disease in Animals

In horses, mules, and donkeys, the disease is generally limited to skin, subcutaneous tissues, and lymphatics. The classical lesion is a subcutaneous nodule that develops at the primary site of infection. As the disease progresses, a series of subcutaneous nodules develop along the course of the lymphatics that drain the area of the primary lesion. Lymphatic vessels may become corded, and the nodules eventually ulcerate and discharge pus. In addition to this classical lymphangitic form, a subcutaneous form in which nodules develop without involvement of the lymphatics has also been described in horses. In dogs, both cutaneous and disseminated forms of the disease as well as the classical form have been reported. The disease is too infrequent in other animal species to permit its characterization. The incubation period of sporotrichosis in animals is unknown.

Disease in Man

The most common form of this disease in man is a series of chronic subcutaneous nodules. The primary lesion usually occurs on an exposed part of the body, commonly on the hand, arm, or neck and occasionally on the foot or leg; from here, the infection spreads along the course of lymphatic drainage of the area. Lymphatic vessels become corded, and a series of secondary nodules are formed. Eventually the nodules ulcerate and discharge pus. Single lesions of the skin and underlying tissue are not uncommon. Infections of the bones, joints, lungs, and other internal organs are occasionally observed. Skin and subcutaneous tissue lesions usually show areas of ulceration with pus formation and a thickening of the epidermis with infiltrations of lymphocytes and occasional giant cells. Both suppurative and granulomatous tissue reactions occur in systemic lesions. The classical lymphatic form may develop within 1 week to 3 months or longer after injury.

General Mode of Spread

Infections in man and in animals are contracted by exposure to sources in the environment. The disease is not contagious; however, infections can result from contamination of the broken skin with infectious material from persons or animals with sporotrichosis.

Epidemiology

S. schenckii grows as a saprophyte in the environment. It is found in soil and on plants and a variety of plant materials. Infections are usually contracted by accidental inoculation of the fungus into skin or subcutaneous tissue. Pulmonary infections, however, may result from inhalation of the fungus. Human infections occur most commonly among farmers, gardeners, nurserymen, florists, and other individuals who work outdoors or handle plant products. Sporotrichosis has been reported at all ages and in both sexes. Apparent variations in frequency of occurrence according to race and sex are probably due to differences in occupation or exposure. The disease is not transmitted from host to host; however, one may become infected by the accidental inoculation or contamination of broken skin with lesion exudates or other infectious material from persons or animals with sporotrichosis.

Diagnosis

Laboratory studies are essential for the accurate diagnosis of sporotrichosis. Only a few *S. schenckii* cells are generally present in clinical materials from spontaneous cases. As a result, they are usually not detected by direct microscopy unless special fungal stains such as the Gomori methenamine-silver nitrate procedure or the Gridley method are used. The fluorescent-antibody (FA) procedure is very useful for rapid diagnosis of this disease. Cultural examination of clinical material is an excellent method for making a definitive diagnosis. Serologic tests using the latex agglutination and the tube agglutination procedures are also helpful for diagnosis.

Prevention and Control

When practical, treatment of plant materials with an antifungal product or by another method that destroys *S. schenckii* is of value. Care should be taken when infectious material is handled to preclude the possibility of accidental infection.

MYCETOMAS

Etiologic Agents — *Curvularia geniculata* and *Petriellidium boydii*

Synonyms for mycetoma (eumycotic) are Madura foot and maduromycosis. Only the two species of fungi noted above have been found to cause mycetomas in lower animals.[3] A description of each follows.

C. geniculata is a common dematiaceous filamentous fungus that lives in soil as a saprophyte. However, it has pathogenic potentialities when introduced into the body.

On Sabouraud's dextrose agar at 25°C, *C. geniculata* develops colonies that are cottony in texture and brownish on their surface. The reverse side becomes dark as growth progresses. The colony is made up of septate, dark-walled (dematiaceous) mycelium of 3 to 5 μm in diameter. At maturity, large multicellular conidia are borne by septate, filiform conidiophores in an acropleurogenous manner, i.e., the dark-walled conidia are borne at the tip as well as the sides of the conidiophore. There they arise through pores in the wall of the conidiophore. The smooth, curved conidia range in size from 18 to 27 μm in length by 8 to 14 μm in width. Curvature results from increased growth of the penultimate cell of the conidia that are 3 to 5-celled and lack a protuberant hilum.

C. geniculata is the imperfect state of the ascomycete *Cochliobolus geniculata*.

P. boydii (Allescheria boydii) is an ascomycete whose imperfect state is generally referred to as *Monosporium apiospermum*. It is commonly present in soil as a saprophyte.

On Sabouraud's dextrose agar, *P. boydii* forms a rapidly growing colony that is loose in texture; it is white at first but becomes brownish with age. The growth is made up of septate, hyaline mycelium of 2 to 4 μm in diameter. Numerous unicellular spores are produced on simple filamentous conidiophores that vary greatly in length. Smooth conidia are borne singly or in clusters. They vary in form from elliptical to globose to ovate and have a truncate base; their average size is 7.3 × 4.4 μm. Some isolates form bundles of conidiophores that are known as coremia. Conidiophore walls in the coremia tend to be dematiaceous.

Many isolates of *P. boydii*, especially when grown on corn meal agar, undergo sexual reproduction and produce perithecia. Perithecia are dark-colored, spherical structures that range in size from 50 to 200 μm in diameter. The perithecial wall is made up of modified mycelial cells. Asci with eight ascospores are produced within the perithecia. However, ascus walls are evanescent, and the asci are rarely seen. At maturity, elliptical ascospores escape from the perithecia through rupture of the peridial wall. They measure 5.0 to 6.5 × 3.4 μm. Ascospores are distinguished from asexual conidia by the fact that they are pointed at each end and thus lack a truncated base.

True and Alternate Hosts

Both *C. geniculata* and *P. boydii* are known as etiologic agents of disease in humans and lower animals. *C. geniculata* is a rare cause of endocarditis and keratitis in man. *P. boydii* is much more common as a disease agent in humans than is *C. geniculata*. It is the most frequent cause of mycetomas in the U.S., and cases have also been reported in Africa, Asia, Europe, and Latin America. *P. boydii* also causes pulmonary and systemic infections in man. Such infections probably occur more frequently than is currently recognized.[5] Animal infections caused by *C. geniculata* have been diagnosed only in dogs.[6,7] *P. boydii* has been incriminated as an agent of mycetoma in dogs and horses and as a cause of mycotic abortion in cattle and horses.[8-10] Its mycelium was also found to be present in the epidermis of a dog with chronic eczema.[11]

Distribution

As soil saprophytes, both *C. geniculata* and *P. boydii* have a cosmopolitan distribution. Infections by *C. geniculata*, however, have only been reported from Sri Lanka and the U.S. *P. boydii* cases have occurred in Africa, Asia, Canada, Latin America, and the U.S.[12,13]

Disease in Animals

Eumycotic mycetomas are chronic granulomatous infections that manifest themselves in time as tumor-like swellings on various parts of the body. They are caused by fungi that develop in the lesions in the form of granules. Diagnostic granules are composed of tightly interwoven septate (2 to 4 μm in diameter) hyphae that are frequently distorted into grotesque shapes. The mycelium may or may not be embedded in a cement-like substance. The size, color, shape, and texture of the granules is distinctive for most of the etiologic agents.

Mycetoma lesions have a localized inception almost always at the site of a traumatic incident. The etiologic agent is generally introduced into the wound by a contaminated thorn, sliver of wood, soil, or similar material. The infection slowly develops as the fungus multiplies and spreads by contiguity. Lymphatic and blood vessel dissemination is rare. Tissues as well as bone are invaded by some of the fungi. In advanced cases, there is considerable tumefaction and development of draining sinus tracts.

In mycetomas, *C. geniculata* produces black to dark brown granules that are 0.5 to 1.5 μm in diameter. They are soft when first collected but become hard when exposed to the air. The granules vary greatly in form, ranging from spherical to ovoid, or they may be highly irregular in shape. The periphery of the granules is made up of a dense mass of interwoven dark-walled hyphae and chlamydospores. These fungal elements are embedded in a cement-like material. The interior of a granule is vacuolar and contains normal septate hyphae and distorted, bizarre-shaped mycelial elements. They are not embedded in cement.

Granules of *P. boydii* are soft and white to yellowish; they range in size from 0.5 to 2 mm in diameter. They are made up of hyaline septate mycelium (2 to 5 μm in diameter) that becomes swollen and distorted, especially at the periphery of the granules. The granules do not contain a cement.

Disease in Man

Both the symptomatology and pathology of mycetomas in man are similar to that described for the lower animals. In contrast to the limited etiology in animals, eumycotic mycetomas in humans are caused by many more genera and species of fungi. Among the described etiologic agents are (1) *Acremonium (Cephalosporium) falciforme,* (2) *A. kiliense,* (3) *A. recifei,* (4) *Aspergillus nidulans,* (5) *Corynespora cassicola,* (6) *Curvularia lunata,* (7) *Exophiala (Phialophora) jeanselmei,* (8) *Madurella grisea,* (9) *M. mycetomii,* (10) *Neotestudina rosatii,* (11) *Pyrenochaeta romeroi,* (12) *Zopfia (Leptosphaeria) senegalensis,* and (13) *Z. tompkinsii.* Contamination of traumatic wounds is the mode of entry of these fungi. The incubation period is long, involving periods of several months in many instances.

General Mode of Spread

Mycetomas are not contagious and are not transmitted from animals to man or man to man.

Epidemiology

The etiologic agents of the mycetomas occur as saprophytic fungi in soil or parasites of plants. They must be introduced into muscular tissue through some break in the skin to induce infection and cause disease. The geographic distribution of the myceto-mas is influenced by climate. Most mycetomas occur in the tropical areas of Africa, Asia, and Latin America. However, the incidence and prevalence of mycetomas is also governed by the degree of exposure of the body to contaminated soil and plant mate-rials.

Diagnosis

Eumycotic mycetomas are diagnosed by demonstrating the presence of mycotic granules in tissue or in exudate from draining sinus tracts. The granules must be ex-amined to determine whether or not they are composed of septate mycelial filaments that average 3 to 5 μm in diameter. Clinical manifestations such as tumefaction and presence of sinus tracts are not, per se, pathognomonic of mycetomas. The basic ele-ment that defines a mycetoma is the granule. The size, texture, color, and internal make-up of the granules are in most cases species-specific, but definitive identification of the fungus involved depends upon its isolation and study of its morphological char-acteristics.

Prevention and Control

Prevention of wounds that can become contaminated by mycetoma agents would reduce the incidence of this disease. In humans, field workers should wear shoes, long-sleeved shirts, and trousers. In the tropics, economic and climatic conditions often make the wearing of protective clothing impractical. Even more difficult would be the protection of domestic animals from traumatic incidents.

PHAEOHYPHOMYCOSIS

Synonyms are phaeosporotrichosis, chromoblastomycosis (in part), and chromo-mycosis (in part). This is a group of diseases of man and lower animals caused by hyphomycetous fungi that develop in the host's tissues in the form of dark-walled, septate mycelial elements.[14]

Etiologic Agents

Only *Dactylaria gallopava* and *Drechslera spicifera*, two species of fungi, have been incriminated and fully described as agents of phaeohyphomycosis in lower mammals. The etiology of human cases is much more extensive. In addition to the above-men-tioned species, such fungi as the following are also included: (1) *Cercospora apii*, (2) *Cladosporium bantianum (trichoides)*, (3) *Curvularia senegalensis*, (4) *Drechslera ha-waiiensis*, (5) *Exophiala (Phialophora) jeanselmei*, (6) *E. (P.) spinifera*, (7) *Henderson-ula toruloidea*, (8) *P. parasitica*, (9) *P. richardsiae*, (10) *Phoma hibernica*, (11) *Pyren-ochaeta unguis-hominis*, and (12) *Wangiella (Phialophora) dermatitidis*.

Dactylaria gallopava is a thermophilic, dematiaceous fungus found in warm habi-tats. It has been isolated from hot springs, thermal soils, and self-heated coal waste piles.[15] It is a fast-growing mold that develops dark brown, velvety colonies on Sa-bouraud's dextrose agar. On the reverse of the colonies, a reddish-brown diffusable pigment develops. Microscopic examination reveals yellowish-brown septate hyphae that measure 1.5 to 3.5 μm in diameter. Simple, short, hyaline to lightly pigmented condiophores are present and are septate and denticulated. They bear clavate to cunei-form two-celled dark-walled conidia that measure 12 to 16 × 4 to 5 μm. Isolates grow well at temperatures as high as 60°C. At 42°C, good sporulation occurs with most isolates.

Drechslera spicifera is the imperfect or asexual state of the ascomycete *Cochliobolus spicifera*. It is basically a saprophytic fungus that commonly occurs in soil throughout the world. It is most prevalent, however, in tropical countries. *D. spicifera* has been isolated from many different species of plants and is known to be a plant pathogen. *D. spicifera* grows rapidly on Sabouraud's dextrose agar that is free of the antifungal antibiotic cycloheximide (Acti-dione®). It produces a flat, velvety growth that is blackish-brown; the reverse side of the colony is black.

Microscopic examination reveals that the colony is made up of septate, dark-walled mycelium. At maturity, numerous conidia are produced. These are borne on simple, flexuous conidiophores that are 4 to 9 μm wide and as long as 300 μm. They are either solitary or in small groups. Older conidiophores bear numerous scars that mark the attachment point of the conidia. Oblong spores are straight and cylindric with rounded ends. Conidia are smooth-walled and divided into several compartments by development of these pseudosepta. They range from 20 to 40 μm in length and 9 to 14 μm in width. The spores are golden brown.

When appropriate mating strains of *D. spicifera* are paired, the perfect stage — known as *Cochliobolus spicifera* — develops. Sexual reproduction results in the development of black globose to ellipsoidal perithecia. These measure 460 to 710 μm in height and 350 to 650 μm in diameter. Perithecia have an ostiolate beak that ranges from 280 to 670 μm in height and 60 to 150 μm in diameter. At maturity, asci are produced that contain one to eight filiform ascospores. These hyaline ascospores have 6 to 16 septa and measure 135 to 240 × 3.75 to 7.0 μm.

True and Alternate Hosts

Infections caused by *D. gallopava* or *D. spicifera* are not contagious. Human infections caused by *D. gallopava* have yet to be reported. It is known only as a disease agent of chickens and turkeys.[16,17] Until recently, disease caused by *D. spicifera* had been reported only in cats and horses.[18,19] In 1975, however, human cases of keratitis due to this fungus were diagnosed in Argentina and Florida.[20,21]

Distribution

The fungi involved with zoonotic phaeohyphomycosis are cosmopolitan in their distribution. Infections caused by them, however, have been few. *D. gallopava* infections have been diagnosed only in Australia and the U.S. *D. spicifera* cases have been reported from Canada and the U.S.

Disease in Animals

Invasion of the brain by the mycelium of *D. gallopava* causes birds to develop CNS disturbances. Early clinical signs are those of muscular incoordination, leg paralysis, and torticollis. These signs are not pathognomonic for *D. gallopava* infections. The disease must be differentiated from viral diseases that give essentially similar clinical signs. This can be done only by histological examination of brain tissue and isolation and identification of the fungus. Histologically, brain tissue shows necrotic areas with giant cells and dematiaceous, septate mycelial filaments of 1.2 to 2.4 μm in diameter.

D. spicifera infections involve the epidermis, dermis, and subcutaneous tissues of the host. Infections tend to be chronic and are not known to involve the vital organs. Cutaneous plaques, subcutaneous nodules, or granulomatous enlargements of the extremities develop in the host after an unknown period of incubation. Etiology of such pathological developments can only be determined by examining tissue for presence of fungal elements and culturing the tissue. In tissue, *D. spicifera* exists in the form of septate, dark-walled mycelium measuring 2 to 4 μm in diameter. However, bizarre-shaped and enlarged mycelial elements may also abound in the tissue.

The mycelium of the etiologic agents that cause phaeohyphomycosis is never organized in the form of granules. These are only produced by the several fungi that cause mycetomas. This is an important point to remember since many cases of phaeohyphomycosis have been mistakenly classified as mycetomas.

Disease in Man

D. gallopava infections in man have not been reported. *D. spicifera* is now known to cause mycotic keratitis in humans. In the one fully described human case, the patient developed an ulcer in the cornea with an irregular border. Scrapings from the eye, when examined in KOH, revealed the presence of dematiaceous mycelial fragments. The incubation period is unknown.

General Mode of Spread

The fungi of phaeohyphomycosis enter the body at a traumatized site. Infectious elements of the fungi may be blown into the eye by air currents and cause keratitis.

Epidemiology

Both *D. gallopava* and *D. spicifera* are soil fungi, and humans and animals are directly infected from that source. There is no known transmission from one victim to another.

Diagnosis

Direct examination or histological study of tissue is the basis for determining the mycotic nature of an infection suspected of being phaeohyphomycosis. Fresh tissue smears in scrapings can be examined directly in 10% KOH and searched for the presence of fungal elements. In this type of preparation, the dematiaceous nature of the fungal elements can be detected. Histological study of sections stained with Gridley's or Gomori's stain will quickly reveal whether mycelium is present. Etiology of a given infection can only be determined by culturing clinical material and isolating the causative agent since tissue forms of all fungi that cause phaeohyphomycosis are basically similar. Only when the etiologic agent is isolated can the genus and species be determined.

When phaeohyphomycosis is suspected, the antifungal antibiotic cycloheximide should not be used in isolation media since the etiologic agents of this disease are sensitive to it.

Prevention and Control

Not feasible.

RHINOSPORIDIOSIS

Etiologic Agent — *Rhinosporidium seeberi*

R. seeberi has never been cultured. Therefore, its taxonomic position is uncertain. *R. seeberi* is known only in its form in infected tissue where it develops as spherical bodies that range in size from 6 to 300 μm in diameter. These represent different stages in the growth of the organism. As the spherical bodies enlarge, they develop thick refractile walls. The nucleus divides, and the cytoplasm undergoes progressing cleavage, forming numerous spores. Individual spores are lobulated, presenting a mulberry-like appearance. When the mother cell is mature, the wall ruptures and the spores are released. These gradually enlarge to become mature cells.

True and Alternate Hosts

The disease occurs in man and various lower animals including cattle, horses, mules, and dogs.[22]

Distribution

The disease is world-wide but appears to be most common in India and Sri Lanka (Ceylon).

Disease in Animals

In animals, the mucous membrane of the nose is the site most commonly affected. Lesions develop as polyps that arise directly from the mucosa or are borne on short pedicles. The polyps are soft, red, lobed, and not painful, but they may enlarge and obstruct breathing.

Disease in Man

In man, the disease is characterized by development of polyps on the mucosa of the nose and eyes and, occasionally, on the ears, larynx, and genitals. The growths are soft, red, and lobed, and they bleed readily when traumatized. They may arise directly from the mucosa or may be borne on short pedicles. The polyps are not painful but may obstruct breathing if present in the nose or larynx.[23]

General Mode of Spread

Unknown.

Epidemiology

The disease is found world-wide but appears to be most common in Asia. The source of the infection is unknown. However, the disease in man in India and Sri Lanka (Ceylon) has been associated with swimming and working in stagnant water, suggesting that *R. seeberi* has a natural habitat in water. The disease is not contagious.

Diagnosis

A diagnosis of rhinosporidiosis is dependent upon demonstration of the organism in tissue. Visual examination of the lesion may reveal the presence of the large sporangia that are white. Accurate identification can be made by the microscopic examination of direct mounts of unstained tissue or, preferably, of stained tissue sections. The etiologic agent has not been cultured.

Prevention and Control

Unknown.

CHROMOBLASTOMYCOSIS

Chromoblastomycosis is a localized chronic disease of man involving the skin and subcutaneous tissues. It is characterized by the development of nodular, verrucoid, ulcerated, and encrusted lesions that may develop on any area of exposed skin. The disease has been reported from most areas of the world; however, it is more common in tropical and subtropical areas. Infections occur after a skin wound or abrasion is contaminated with soil or vegetation containing cells of the infectious fungi.[24]

Chromoblastomycosis is caused by any one of several species of dematiaceous fungi belonging to the genera *Cladosporium, Fonsecaea,* or *Phialophora.* In nature, the fungi grow as saprophytes on wood, other vegetable matter, or in soil. The individual species of fungi can be differentiated in culture; in clinical materials, however, they are all similar. They occur in the form of thick-walled brown cells that divide by septation. These structures are called sclerotic cells. Dematiaceous, branched hyphae may also be present. The disease is not contagious. Verified cases of chromoblastomycosis in warm-blooded lower animals have yet to be recorded. Reports of chromoblastomycosis in the horse and dog have appeared. However, critical reviews of these case reports have shown that the disease was usually a eumycotic mycetoma. A disease that closely resembles chromoblastomycosis has been described in frogs and toads.[25] In most of the affected amphibians, lesions were in the subcutaneous tissue and skin; in a few cases, internal organs were affected. The tissue form of the etiologic agent resembled the one found in tissues of humans with chromoblastomycosis. However, the failure of the amphibian isolates to sporulate in culture did not permit their identification.

REFERENCES

1. **Emmons, C. W., Binford, C. H., Utz, J. P., and Kwon-Chung, K. J.**, *Medical Mycology*, 3rd ed., Lea & Febiger, Philadelphia, 1976, 406.
2. **Jungerman, P. F. and Schwartzman, R. M.**, *Veterinary Medical Mycology*, Lea & Febiger, Philadelphia, 1972, 31.
3. **Kaplan, W., Chandler, F. W., Ajello, L., Gauthier, R., Higgins, R., and Cayouette, P.**, Equine phaeophyphomycosis caused by *Drechslera spicifera*, *Can. Vet. J.*, 16, 205, 1975.
4. **Malloch, D.**, New concepts in the Microascaceae illustrated by two new species, *Mycologia*, 62, 727, 1970.
5. **Arnett, J. C. and Hatch, H. B., Jr.**, Pulmonary allescheriasis. Report of a case and review of the literature, *Arch. Intern. Med.*, 135, 1250, 1975.
6. **Bridges, C. H.**, Maduromycotic mycetomas in animals. *Curvularia geniculata* as an etiologic agent, *Am. J. Pathol.*, 33, 411, 1957.
7. **Brodey, R. S., Schryver, H. F., Deubler, M. J., Kaplan, W., and Ajello, L.**, Mycetoma in a dog, *J. Am. Vet. Med. Assoc.*, 151, 442, 1967.
8. **Jang, S. S. and Popp, J. A.**, Eumycotic mycetoma in a dog caused by *Allescheria boydii*, *J. Am. Vet. Med. Assoc.*, 157, 1071, 1970.
9. **Schiefer, B. and Mehnert, B.**, Maduromykose beim Pferd in Deutschland, *Berl. Muench. Tieraerztl. Wochenschr.*, 78, 230, 1965.
10. **Mahaffey, L. W. and Rossdale, P. D.**, An abortion due to *Allescheria boydii* and general observations concerning mycotic abortions of mares, *Vet. Rec.*, 77, 541, 1965.
11. **Pezenburg, E.**, *Allescheria boydii* Shear 1921, isoliert aus einer Hautveranderung beim Hund, *Mykosen*, 1, 172, 1958.
12. **Ajello, L.**, The isolation of *Allescheria boydii* Shear, an etiologic agent of mycetomas, from soil, *Am. J. Trop. Med. Hyg.*, 1, 227, 1952.
13. **Mahgoub, E. S. and Murray, I.**, *Mycetoma*, William Heinemann Medical Books, London, 1973.
14. **Ajello, L.**, Phaeohyphomycosis: definition and etiology, in Mycoses, Scientific Publication No. 304, Pan American Health Organization, Washington, D.C., 1975, 126.
15. **Tansey, M. R.**, *Dactylaria gallopava*, a cause of avian encephalitis in hot spring effluents, thermal soils and self-heated coal waste piles, *Nature* (London), 242, 202, 1973.
16. **Ranck, F. M., Georg, L. K., and Wallace, D. H.**, Dactylariosis — a newly recognized fungus disease of chickens, *Avian Dis.*, 18, 4, 1974.
17. **Waldrip, D. W., Padhye, A. A., Ajello, L., and Ajello, M.**, Isolation of *Dactylaria gallopava* from broiler-house litter, *Avian Dis.*, 18, 445, 1974.
18. **Mueller, G. H., Kaplan, W., Ajello, L., and Padhye, A. A.**, Phaeohyphomycosis caused by *Drechslera spicifera* in a cat, *J. Am. Vet. Med. Assoc.*, 166, 150, 1975.
19. **Kaplan, W., Chandler, F. W., Ajello, L., Gauthier, R., Higgins, R., and Cayouette, P.**, Equine phaeohyphomycosis caused by *Drechslera spicifera*, *Can. Vet. J.*, 16, 205, 1975.
20. **Forster, R. K., Rebell, G., and Wilson, L. A.**, Dematiaceous fungal keratitis. Clinical isolates and management, *Br. J. Ophthalmol.*, 59, 372, 1975.
21. **Zapatar, R. C., Albesi, E. J., and Garcia, G. H.**, Mycotic keratitis by *Drechslera spicifera*, *Sabouraudia*, 13, 195, 1975.
22. **Ainsworth, G. C. and Austwick, P. K. C.**, *Fungal Diseases of Animals*, Review Series No. 6, Commonwealth Agricultural Bureaux, Farnham Royal, Slough, England, 1973, 117.

23. **Emmons, C. W., Binford, C. H., Utz, J. P., and Kwon-Chung, K. J.,** *Medical Mycology,* 3rd ed., Lea & Febiger, Philadelphia, 1977, 419.

24. **Al-Doory, Y.,** *Chromomycosis,* Mountain Press, Missoula, Mont., 1972.

25. **Velazquez, L. F. and Restrepo, A.,** Naturally acquired chromomycosis in the toad, *Bufo marinus.* Comparison of the etiologic agent with fungi causing human chromomycosis, *Sabouraudia,* 13, 1, 1975.

SYSTEMIC MYCOSES

L. Ajello and W. Kaplan

INTRODUCTION

Systemic mycoses are generally pulmonary in origin but can involve any or all of the internal body organs, including bones. In many cases, the skin and subcutaneous tissues may also be affected. Infections may be asymptomatic or may induce signs and symptoms that vary in kind and in severity.

Subclinical infections are common and can be recognized by means of various immunodiagnostic tests, including skin tests. Their occurrence can also be recognized in some cases by the presence of healed lesions found by roentgenological examination or at autopsy after death due to other causes.

Symptomatic infections may be mild and self-limited, or the disease may be progressive with extensive tissue damage and incapacitation of the patient. Progressive infections may be fatal.

A diversity of fungi can cause systemic disease. Some are primary pathogens while others are opportunists. Most occur in the environment as saprophytes, and a few live as commensals on the skin or mucous membranes of the body. Some fungi are dimorphic and develop in two different forms, depending upon the conditions of growth.

The systemic mycoses vary in their geographic distribution. Some are cosmopolitan; others have a restricted distribution. Many affect both animals and man; others have been recognized only in man or only in animals. None are considered to be contagious.

ASPERGILLOSIS (PULMONARY) ALSO KNOWN AS BRONCHOMYCOSIS AND PNEUMOMYCOSIS

Etiologic Agents

In animals, aspergillosis is basically a pulmonary disease caused by members of the genus *Aspergillus*. Pulmonary and systemic aspergillosis are caused by members of several groups of aspergilli, the most common group encountered being *A. fumigatus*. Other pathogenic species are classified in the following groups: *A. flavus, A. nidulans,* and *A. terreus*.[1]

1. *A. fumigatus* group (description based on *A. fumigatus*) — This rapidly growing fungus forms a velvety growth on Sabouraud's dextrose agar. A colony is white initially but becomes green to bluish-green as spores are produced. Conidial heads are columnar because of the linear arrangement of the long spore chains. Echinulate, globose conidia are borne in chains from the tips of a single series of sterigmata. Sterigmata characteristically arise from the top of the flask-shaped vesicle. *A. fumigatus* grows well at 37 to 45°C.

2. *A. flavus* group (description based on *A. flavus*) — This fungus is moderately fast-growing on Sabouraud's dextrose agar. Colonies initially are yellowish-green as the conidia begin to develop. At maturity, a deeper green color develops. Conidial heads are radiate. Conidiophores are thick-walled with a distinct rough or echinulate surface. Sterigmata occur in either a single or double layer on a globose or subglobose vesicle.

3.   *A. nidulans* group (description based on *A. nidulans*) — This is a moderately fast-growing species on Sabouraud's dextrose agar. Mature colonies are dark green. If the isolates form cleistothecia, the colony assumes a light yellow color. The reverse side of the colonies are vinaceous. Conidial heads are columnar and composed of short conidial chains. Conidiophores tend to be sineous with smooth brownish walls. Their vesicles are hemispherical with primary and secondary sterigmata. Conidia are globose and have a wrinkled surface. Cleistothecia, readily formed by many isolates, are globose, 100 to 200 μm in diameter, and have a reddish brown peridium. They are generally surrounded by a yellowish layer of hulle cells.

4.   *A. terreus* group (description based on *A. terreus*) — A rapidly growing species producing velvety colonies in cinnamon to brown shades. Conidial heads are long and columnar. Conidiophores are smooth and flexuous with a dome-like vesicle. Sterigmata are in two series, giving rise to globose, smooth conidia.

True and Alternate Hosts

Man and a wide variety of animals are susceptible to respiratory and disseminated infection by various species of *Aspergillus*; however, infections are not contagious. Soil or organic material is the basic source of all infections.

Distribution

Aspergillosis has been reported from all parts of the world.

Diseases in Animals

Acute avian pulmonary aspergillosis affects a great variety of birds, both wild and domestic, that have been found to be susceptible to infections by *Aspergillus* sp.[2] Young birds are especially vulnerable to infection. Clinical signs of infection include loss of condition, rapid breathing, diarrhea, fever, and listlessness.

Chronic avian aspergillosis is a subtle form of the disease that slowly develops in older birds. Infected birds usually manifest, to a lesser degree, the symptoms of the acute form of aspergillosis. In addition, they usually become anemic.

Bronchi are the prime sites of infection in the lungs; necrotic lesions are generally found at autopsy. Mycelium and necrotized tissue are frequently present in the lumen of the bronchi. Granulomatous lesions are typically present in the lungs. Characteristically, they have a central caseous mass of mycelium. Lesions are surrounded by giant cells, epithelioid cells, lymphocytes, and fibroblasts. Blood vessels are commonly invaded by mycelial filaments.[3] The air sac system is concurrently invaded by the fungus. The serous membrane rapidly becomes lined with a layer of necrotized tissue, fibrin, inflammatory cells, and mycelium.

Dissemination by direct extension from the lungs and air sacs to other vital organs, such as the liver, kidneys, and brain, occurs in both acute and chronic cases of aspergillosis.

Mammalian aspergillosis is known to occur in many species of domestic animals: cats, cattle, dogs, horses, pigs, and sheep, etc. Wild animals have also been found to be susceptible both in captivity and in the field: American buffalo, bottle-nosed dolphins, elks, horses, monkeys, okapis, etc.

The lungs are the primary site of invasion with dissemination to vital organs throughout the body following. Clinical signs of infection are essentially similar to those described for pneumonia from other causes: coughing, sneezing, nasal discharge, and fever. Histologically, many of the features of avian aspergillosis are encountered. Multiple granulomas may be present in the lungs. In chronic lung infection, cavitation may occur.

Disease in Man

Two basic types of infectious aspergillosis occur in man: bronchopulmonary and aspergilloma. Both types are acquired through the respiratory route with dissemination throughout the body frequently taking place in the former type. Clinical signs are similar to those of respiratory infections caused by bacteria and viruses. Aspergillomas represent colonization by *Aspergillus* sp. of preexisting lung cavities caused by other diseases. Histological findings are basically similar to those described for avian and mammalian aspergillosis.

General Mode of Spread

Aspergillosis is caused by exogenous fungi, i.e., fungi that exist as free-living saprophytes in nature. Infections are not spread from person to person or from animals to man.

Epidemiology

The fungi that cause aspergillosis are abundant in the environment, living in soil as saprophytes and deriving their nourishment from dead plant and animal matter. Their spores are produced in great abundance and are readily disseminated into the air by wind currents. All the species have a cosmopolitan distribution.

Diagnosis

Definitive diagnosis of aspergillosis rests upon the demonstration of hyaline, septate mycelium (2 to 4 μm in diameter) in tissue. The mycelium frequently is in a radiating form and is dichotomously branched. The specific etiological agent involved can only be determined by isolation and study of the gross and microscopic features of the isolate. All of the pathogenic species produce the same type of mycelium in tissue. Fortunately, they give rise to distinctive colonies, conidiophores, and conidia.

In well-aerated tissue such as air sacs and cavities, conidiophores typical of the aspergilli are formed among the mycelial filaments. Serlogical tests for bronchopulmonary and aspergilloma cases in humans are of great value in diagnosis and for monitoring the effects of therapy. The most useful and highly regarded procedure is the immunodiffusion test.[4]

Prevention and Control

Use of mold-free litter and feeds would help reduce the incidence and prevalence of aspergillosis. Poorly processed and stored feed, hay, and litter are frequently heavily overgrown with *Aspergillus* sp. that sporulate heavily.

BLASTOMYCOSIS (NORTH AMERICAN BLASTOMYCOSIS, GILCHRIST'S DISEASE)

Etiologic Agent

The agent of blastomycosis is *Blastomyces dermatitidis*, a dimorphic fungus. It grows in mammalian tissues as a budding yeast and is 8 to 15 μm in diameter (occasionally reaching 20 μm or more). The yeast form can be obtained in vitro by incubating cultures at 37°C. Microscopically, yeast-form cultures are composed of large budding yeasts similar to those seen in tissue. When cultures are incubated at room temperature, they develop mycelium. Mycelial-form cultures appear as white to tan, downy to fluffy molds that bear round to oval conidia (3 to 5 μm in diameter) on the sides of the hyphae and ends of simple conidiophores.[5]

True and Alternate Hosts

The disease affects man, dogs, and occasionally cats. One case was diagnosed in a horse and one in a sea lion.

Distribution

The vast majority of reported cases have originated in the Mississippi River Valley and the southeastern U.S. The disease also occurs sporadically in eastern Canada and Africa.

Disease in Animals

The dog is the most susceptible of the lower animals. Dogs with blastomycosis display a wide range of clinical signs, depending upon the tissues or organs affected. The disease in dogs is characterized by pyrexia and debility, with cough, dyspnea, and skin lesions as the most common signs. Lungs, lymph nodes of the chest, and skin are the tissues most frequently affected. Ocular lesions, many of which lead to blindness, are not uncommon. The bones and joints may also be affected, and such infection causes pain and lameness.[6]

The disease in cats is similar to blastomycosis in dogs. Extensive pulmonary lesions have been noted along with involvement of the skin and other organs.

Disease in Man

Blastomycosis in man can be divided into two forms: systemic and cutaneous. Although both have a pulmonary inception, their clinical aspects, clinical course, and prognosis are different. The systemic form is primarily a pulmonary disease. The infection may remain confined to the lungs or may disseminate to other organs and tissues. Signs and symptoms vary depending upon the organs affected and the extent of involvement. Onset is frequently associated with respiratory signs such as cough, productive sputum, and hemoptysis. Dissemination to bones and joints is not uncommon and leads to pain, swelling, and interference with function. Dissemination to the skin leads to the formation of ulcerated or verrucous granulomatous lesions.

In cutaneous blastomycosis, the general health of the patient is not impaired and symptoms are relatively mild or may be absent. Skin lesions occur most frequently on exposed body surfaces and characteristically appear as ulcerated, verrucous granulomata with elevated serpiginous borders. The clinical course of the disease is usually chronic and marked by remissions, exacerbations, and gradual increase in size of the lesions. The incubation period is unknown.

General Mode of Spread

The disease is not transmissible from host to host. All evidence indicates that man and animals contract the infection from unknown an source in nature. The natural habitat of *B. dermatitidis* is still uncertain despite recent reports of its isolation from soils in Kentucky and Georgia. The consensus is that in the vast majority of cases the fungus enters the body via the respiratory tract and that the primary focus of infection is in the lungs. In rare cases, cutaneous blastomycosis has followed accidental direct inoculation of the fungus into skin and subcutaneous tissue.[7]

Epidemiology

All available evidence strongly suggests that *B. dermatitidis* exists in nature as a saprophyte; however, its precise ecological niche is not known. From its source in nature, the spores of this fungus enter the body of man and lower animals via the respiratory tract. In man, the disease may appear in any age group. Most cases, however, occur between the ages of 30 and 50 years, and disease is seen four times more frequently in males than females. In dogs, there appears to be no correlation of infection with age and sex. There is no evidence that the disease is transmissible from host to host.

Diagnosis

Laboratory studies are essential for a definitive diagnosis of this disease. Such a diagnosis is based upon demonstration of the fungus in clinical materials by direct microscopy and its isolation in culture. Serological tests are also useful for the presumptive diagnosis of blastomycosis. The complement-fixation (CF) and the immunodiffusion tests are useful for this purpose.

Prevention and Control
Unknown.

CANDIDIASIS (MONILIASIS, THRUSH, CANDIDOSIS)

Etiologic Agents

Candida albicans is the most frequent etiologic agent of candidiasis. Other members of the genus *Candida* may also occasionally cause this disease. Members of the genus *Candida* are yeast-like fungi. Cultures of these yeasts are white and are soft in consistency. Microscopic examination reveals yeast-like budding cells, pseudohyphae, and hyphae. When cultivated on special media, *C. albicans* also produces spherical thick-walled chlamydospores that measure 8 to 10 μm in diameter. In infected tissues, the *Candida* sp. form budding yeast-like cells, pseudohyphae, and true hyphae. Identification of the members of the genus *Candida* is based upon morphological and physiological characters that include sugar fermentation and sugar assimilation reactions.[8]

True and Alternate Hosts

The disease affects man and a great diversity of lower animals including birds (chickens, turkeys, ducks, geese, guinea fowl, pigeons, partridges) and mammals (cattle, sheep, dog, cat, hedgehog, guinea pig, mouse, various rodents, lower primates, and various wild animals).[9]

Distribution
Candidiasis is distributed world-wide.

Disease in Animals

Avian candidiasis usually involves the upper digestive tract, particularly the crop. Clinical signs are not specific. Affected birds may show unsatisfactory growth, listlessness, roughness of feathers, and loss of appetite. Gross lesions are generally confined to the crop but may be observed at other sites. Lesions in the crop vary; in acute cases, they are grayish-white, loosely adherent to the underlying mucous membrane, and may have a curd-like appearance. In chronic cases, the crop wall is thickened and the membrane is covered by a corrugated mass of yellowish-white necrotic material.

Candidiasis in mammals may involve the digestive tract, internal organs, skin, or other parts of the body. Clinical signs vary, depending upon the organs that are affected. Among mammals, candidiasis has been recognized most often in bovines and porcines. Candidiasis in calves usually involves the digestive tract. Clinical signs include watery diarrhea, melena, anorexia, dehydration, prostration, and eventually death. *Candida* sp. occasionally cause bovine mastitis. Systemic infections have been reported in feedlot cattle that were fed antibiotics. Porcine candidiasis usually involves the digestive tract and has been recognized more frequently in young animals. Clinical signs in piglets include vomition, diarrhea, and emaciation.[10,11]

Disease in Man

Candidiasis in man may appear as an acute or chronic disease which could involve mucous membranes, skin, nails, and internal organs. Clinical signs vary considerably, depending upon the organs and structures that are affected. The disease may appear as oral thrush, intertrigo, vulvovaginitis, paronychia, or onychia when the skin and mucous membranes of the mouth and vagina are affected. Systemic forms include pulmonary candidiasis, endocarditis, septicemia, and meningitis. The incubation period varies and is difficult to establish.[12]

General Mode of Spread

Candida albicans and other *Candida* spp. are common inhabitants of the mucous membranes and G.I. tract of man and lower animals. The source of infection in most cases is endogenous. Under certain circumstances, human-to-human transmission of the infection can occur. The infection may be transmitted by mother to child at birth during passage through the vagina. Balanoposthitis can result from vaginal contact. Animal-to-animal transmission has not been reported.

Epidemiology

In addition to being recovered from the mucous membranes and G.I. tract of man and animals,[13] *Candida* sp. have been isolated from soil. The occurrence of *C. albicans* in nature, however, probably represents contamination from man and animals. Various factors can predispose man and lower animals to infection and production of disease by members of the genus *Candida*. Some of these factors are prolonged broad-spectrum antibiotic and corticosteroid administration, decreased resistance due to various underlying diseases, decreased resistance due to vitamin deficiency, or general dietary deficiency. The very young and the aged are more commonly infected, probably because of reduced resistance.

Diagnosis

Laboratory studies are usually required to establish an accurate diagnosis of candidiasis. These studies include (1) microscopic examination of clinical materials to obtain evidence of tissue invasion by a *Candida* sp. and (2) culturing to determine the species involved. Serologic tests such as the immunodiffusion, latex agglutination, and indirect fluorescent antibody (FA) procedures are also very useful for the diagnosis of systemic candidiasis. The latex agglutination test is of value for monitoring the course of this disease in man.

Prevention and Control

Wherever possible and practical, factors that predispose man or animals to infection by *C. albicans* and other Candida sp. should be eliminated. This includes avoiding unnecessary prolonged broad-spectrum antibiotic and corticosteroid administration and the treatment of underlying diseases that predispose man and animals to *Candida* infections. The antibiotic nystatin is useful for the control of *Candida* sp. infections of the G.I. tract, vagina, and skin. This antibiotic can also be used for the prophylactic treatment of man and animals receiving prolonged broad-spectrum antibiotic therapy. Transmission of *Candida* sp. infections from mother to child during birth can be controlled by treatment of vaginal infections during the third trimester of pregnancy. Since

Candida sp. infections are more common in individuals who have vitamin deficiencies or an inadequate diet, correction of nutritional deficiencies is an important factor in the control of these infections.

COCCIDIOIDOMYCOSIS (VALLEY FEVER, DESERT RHEUMATISM, COCCIDIOIDAL GRANULOMA)

Etiologic Agent

The agent of coccidioidomycosis is *Coccidioides immitis,* a dimorphic fungus. Cultures on Sabouraud's dextrose agar, when incubated at room temperature or 25°C, develop as a mold composed of hyaline, septate mycelium of 2 to 4 μm in diameter. In texture, colonies are typically cottony and white. The center of the colony is frequently depressed and downy in texture. With age, the colony tends to darken.

Microscopically, most isolates are found to have produced abundant arthrospores by the close septation of mycelial filaments. These arthrospores, 2.5 to 4.0 × 3 to 6 μm in size, are generally formed in alternate cells and are discharged by disarticulation of the mycelium. The isolated arthrospores are barrel-shaped and usually have attached to both ends the remnants of the cell walls of the adjacent empty cells. Atypical isolates are not rare. They vary considerably in texture, color, growth rate, and sporulation.[14]

Inside an animal host, *C. immitis* develops in a completely different form. There the fungus is no longer filamentous but unicellular. Its tissue form is made up of spherical cells that are called spherules. They are thick-walled, smooth, and range in size from 20 to 200 μm in diameter. At maturity, the internal cytoplasm, by a process of progressive cleavage, is differentiated into small spherical spores of 2 to 5 μm in diameter. Through rupture of the wall of the spherule, the endospores are released and disseminated throughout the body by hematogenous and lymphatic routes. Each endospore has the potential to enlarge and become a spherule that forms and discharges endospores. When endospores and spherules are inoculated onto media and incubated at 25°C, the mycelial form develops anew. Special media have been developed that permit conversion of the mold form of *C. immitis* into its tissue form in vitro.[15]

True and Alternate Hosts

Man and a large variety of wild animals, captive animals, and such domesticated animals as dogs, cats, horses, swine, sheep, and cattle are infected by by *C. immitis.*

Distribution

C. immitis is only known to exist with certainty in the desert-like areas of North, Central, and South America. In the U.S., endemic areas are found in the states of Arizona, California, Nevada, New Mexico, Texas, and Utah. Fifteen of the Mexican states harbor *C. immitis,* while in Central America this fungus is only known to be found in the Montagua Valley of Guatemala and the Comayagua Valley of Honduras. In South America, endemic areas have been found in Colombia, Venezuela, Bolivia, Paraguay, and Argentina.

Disease in Animals

Among domestic animals, the dog is the most seriously affected by *C. immitis.* Canine infections are the most frequent to be brought to medical attention. Infections range from the asymptomatic to the acute and disseminated form of the disease that may terminate fatally. In clinical cases of coccidioidomycosis, dogs show signs of cough, diarrhea, poor condition, loss of weight, and fever. Radiographic studies frequently reveal pulmonary and skeletal lesions.[16] This disease in other animals is basically similar to that described in dogs.

Coccidioidomycosis in cattle may be an exception. The disease in these animals is almost invariably benign. Typically, only the bronchial and mediastinal lymph nodes are involved, and infected glands are swollen several times beyond normal size. Internally, multiple granulomas with purulent centers are present. Lung lesions are rare, and disseminated infections have not been reported.[17] The incubation period for coccidioidomycosis ranges from 7 to 21 days.

Disease in Man

Coccidioidomycosis in humans manifests itself in three basic forms: (1) pulmonary, both asymptomatic and symptomatic, (2) disseminated coccidioidomycosis, and (3) residual pulmonary coccidioidomycosis. It has been estimated that 60% of all infections are asymptomatic. The remaining 40% manifest symptoms that range from those of mild respiratory diseases to those of severe pulmonary, visceral, and meningial diseases. Early clinical symptoms in self-limited, symptomatic pulmonary coccidioidomycosis include cough, pleuritic pain, loss of appetite, malaise, and fatigue.

Patients with disseminated coccidioidomycosis continue to have the previously described symptoms, but, in addition, they may develop cutaneous and subcutaneous abscesses, as well as acute meningitis. Residual pulmonary coccidioidomycosis is usually diagnosed by the discovery of thin-walled cavities in the lungs. However, not all cases are silent. Some patients may have chest pains and cough, and they could develop hemoptysis.

General Mode of Spread

Coccidioidomycosis is an airborne disease, almost invariably acquired through the respiration of air that contains the infectious arthrospores of *C. immitis*. The disease is not contagious. Primary cutaneous infections may result from some traumatic incident that permitted the wound to become contaminated with *C. immitis* spores.

Epidemiology

The occurrence of *C. immitis* in soil as a saprophyte has been well documented. This mold is adapted to live in semi-arid climatic zones where summer mean temperatures range from 26 to 32°C and winter mean temperatures fall between 4 and 12°C. Rainfall should range from 12.5 to 50 cm/year.[7] *C. immitis* proliferates in soil during the rainy periods of the year and sporulates heavily. Then, in the ensuing dry periods, the highly infectious arthrospores are widely disseminated by air currents. There is no evidence of contagion; infections are not spread from person to person or from lower animals to man.

Diagnosis

Coccidioidomycosis is basically diagnosed by demonstration of its spherules in clinical material. This can be done by direct microscopic examination of such materials as sputum and lesion exudates. Presence of the diagnostic spherules with endospores can also be determined by appropriately stained histological sections of tissue. Gridley's stain and the methenamine silver procedure are especially effective.

Ultimate diagnosis is dependent upon isolation and identification of the etiologic agent on the basis of its gross and microscopic characteristics. Conversion of all molds suspected of being *C. immitis* is obligatory either by inoculation of mice or guinea pigs or in vitro conversion. Mice are inoculated intraperitoneally while guinea pigs are injected intratesticularly. Tissue and pus obtained 2 weeks postinoculation from these animals is examined for the presence of spherules. Since the arthrospores of *C. immitis* are highly infectious and readily airborne, all cultures suspected of being that fungus must be handled with extreme caution under a safety hood.

Serological tests have been developed for the diagnosis of coccidioidomycosis. These include the complement-fixation immunodiffusion, latex agglutination, and tube precipitin tests. Fluorescent antibody tests with specific conjugate have also been developed for the rapid detection and identification of *C. immitis* spherules in tissue.[18]

Prevention and Control

The incidence of infection may be reduced by the control of dust in endemic areas by planting grass, oiling playing fields, etc.

CRYPTOCOCCOSIS (TORULOSIS, EUROPEAN BLASTOMYCOSIS)

Etiologic Agent

The agent of disease is *Cryptococcus neoformans*, a spherical, yeast-like fungus that reproduces by budding. Cells vary in size from 5 to 20 μm in diameter and are surrounded by a mucoid polysaccharide capsule that varies considerably in thickness. So-called "dry variants" with very small capsules are not uncommon. Colonies are soft and creamy in texture or mucilaginous if considerable capsular material is present. Colonies are white or shades of cream to tan. Identification of *C. neoformans* is based upon morphological and various physiological characters including sugar assimilation and nitrate assimilation reactions.

True and Alternate Hosts

The disease affects man and a great diversity of mammals, including domestic animals, lower primates, bats, and a variety of exotic animals.[19]

Distribution

Cryptococcosis occurs world-wide, but because the disease is not reportable, accurate data on its incidence and prevalence are not available. However, most authorities agree that the disease is much more common than the reported cases would suggest. It is estimated that 200 to 300 cases of cryptococcal meningitis occur each year in the U.S., whereas 5000 to 15,000 cases of nonclinical and clinical human pulmonary cryptococcosis are estimated to occur annually in New York City alone. Data on the occurrence of cryptococcal infections in animals are not available.

Disease in Animals

With the exception of cattle, most animals known to be infected have a generalized form of the disease that terminates fatally. Many affected animals also show signs of CNS involvement. Most affected cattle have infections of mammary tissue and adjacent lymph nodes. The incubation period is unknown.

Disease in Man

The lungs are usually the primary site of infection in man. Pulmonary infections may be inapparent or may resemble tuberculosis or other pulmonary diseases. In some individuals, infection disseminates to the viscera, skin, bones, or CNS. Symptoms vary depending upon the organs that are affected. The incubation period is unknown.

General Mode of Spread

Cryptococcosis is not a contagious disease. The etiologic agent, *C. neoformans*, occurs as a saprophyte in nature. The fungus is commonly found in soil contaminated with pigeon excreta and in accumulations of pigeon excreta in old nests and under roosting sites. Such sites are the major reservoirs of this fungus. Humans and animals become infected either through inhalation of the yeast or, less commonly, by direct inoculation of the skin. Infections of the bovine mammary gland can result from introduction of the organism through the teat canal.

Epidemiology

There is no evidence that cryptococcosis is transmissible from host to host. Rather, the consensus is that man and lower animals contract the infection by exposure to sources in nature. As previously noted, *C. neoformans* is commonly found in soil contaminated with pigeon excreta and in accumulations of pigeon excreta in old nests and under roosting sites. These sources are regarded as the major reservoirs of this fungus. The association between pigeons and *C. neoformans* is considered to be indirect, as pigeons are resistant to infection by the fungus. Apparently, their excreta merely provide a suitable substrate for growth of *C. neoformans*. The multiplication of *C. neoformans* in pigeon excreta has been attributed to the fact that creatinine, which is abundant in pigeon excreta, is assimilated by *C. neoformans* but not by various other species of yeasts. Creatinine apparently provides a competitive advantage to *C. neoformans*. *C. neoformans* has been isolated from soil uncontaminated with pigeon excreta, indicating that this material per se is not essential for survival of the organism.[7]

C. neoformans can act as a primary pathogen and causes infections in apparently normal hosts. In addition, this fungus frequently is an opportunist, causing disease in compromised human hosts. Patients with hematologic malignancies, such as Hodgkin's disease, leukemia, and lymphosarcoma, patients with diabetes, and individuals being treated with steroids are particularly susceptible to infection with *C. neoformans*. Whether a similar association with a compromised state occurs naturally in lower animals remains to be determined.

Diagnosis

Laboratory studies are essential to establish a definitive diagnosis of cryptococcosis. These studies include (1) direct microscopic examination of clinical materials to detect the presence of the encapsulated yeast and (2) culturing to isolate and identify the fungus. The direct fluorescent antibody technique is also of great value for detecting and identifying *C. neoformans* in clinical material and culture. Serological tests are also of great diagnostic value. Three useful serodiagnostic tests are the latex agglutination procedure to detect soluble cryptococcal antigen and the tube agglutination and indirect fluorescent antibody procedures to detect antibodies to *C. neoformans*. For maximal serodiagnostic coverage, the three tests should be used concurrently.

Prevention and Control

Prevention and control measures should include education of the public regarding the hazard involved in exposure to an accumulation of pigeon droppings. If possible, patients with hematologic malignancies or diabetes and individuals being treated with corticosteroids should avoid contact with such material. Reduction of the pigeon population is another factor to be considered in the control of this disease. Treatment of point sources with 3% formalin solution is useful in eliminating *C. neoformans* or reducing its numbers.

HISTOPLASMOSIS

Etiologic Agent

The agent of histoplasmosis is *Histoplasma capsulatum*, a species that is not only dimorphic but exists in two different cultural varieties: *H. capsulatum* var. *capsulatum* and *H. capsulatum* var. *duboisii*. They can only be distinguished from each other on the basis of their in vivo tissue forms.[20]

In vitro on Sabouraud's dextrose agar, grown at 25°C, the two varieties are indistinguishable. Most isolates develop white fluffy colonies that tend to become tan or golden with age. The color results from the heavy production of spores. *H. capsulatum* mycelium is hyaline and septate. Spores are produced directly from the mycelium or on simple conidiophores. The most characteristic spore type produced is the macroconidium. They are large thick-walled spores that are characteristically ornamented with digitate protuberances, the so-called tubercles. Macroconidia are usually spherical and range in size from 7 to 25 μm in diameter. Pear-shaped spores are also produced. Some macroconidia may be smooth-walled. In addition to these large spores, microconidia are also formed. These range in size from 2 to 6 μm in diameter. They are usually smooth, but echinulate microconidia may also be formed.

H. capsulatum is a dimorphic fungus. At 37°C on a rich medium such as brain heart infusion agar with 5% blood, *H. capsulatum* develops as a yeast. Its colonies are soft, cream-colored, and pasty in texture. Microscopically, the colonies of both varieties are found to be composed of unicellular cells that divide by a budding process. These blastospores measure 1.5 to 3.5 μm in diameter.

In vivo, both in naturally infected animals and experimental animals, *H. capsulatum* develops as a yeast. However, in the in vivo environment, the tissue form of *H. capsulatum* var. *duboisii* attains sizes that range from 7 to 15 μm in diameter with walls 1 to 5 μm thick. In contrast, the cells of *H. capsulatum* var. *capsulatum* in tissue average 2 to 4 μm in diameter with a thin cell wall.

H. capsulatum is an imperfect fungus. However, it does undergo sexual reproduction, and the ensuing perfect form has been named *Ajellomyces capsulatus*.[22] The mating of compatible isolates of this heterothallic fungus gives rise to globose cleistothecia that measure 80 to 250 μm in diameter. Their peridium is composed of tightly coiled septate mycelial filaments. Asci are club-shaped to pyriform and bear eight globose ascospores.

True and Alternate Hosts

H. capsulatum var. *capsulatum* infects man, bats, cats, dogs, a wide variety of carnivores, marsupials, rodents, and ungulates while *H. capsulatum* var. *duboisii* affects man and the African baboon species, *Papio cyanocephalus* and *P. papio*.

Distribution

H. capsulatum var. *capsulatum* has been found on all the continents of the world. However, certain regions are more heavily infested with this fungus than others. In the U.S., the heart of the endemic area is located in Arkansas, Kentucky, Missouri, and Tennessee. The principal area of infestation covers these additional states: Alabama, Illinois, Indiana, Kansas, Louisiana, Mississippi, Ohio, Oklahoma, Texas, and West Virginia.[21] In Latin America, high areas of endemicity occur in Mexico, Guatemala, Venezuela, and Peru. Autochthonous cases of histoplasmosis have also been recorded in Asia, Australia, and Europe. Both varieties of *H. capsulatum* exist in Africa.

Disease in Animals

Among domestic animals, dogs are the most frequent victims of *H. capsulatum*. Histoplasmosis is basically a pulmonary disease, but it has a tendency to disseminate and involve all vital organs. The clinical signs of canine histoplasmosis are chronic cough, diarrhea, fever, and weight loss. In advanced stages of the disease, heptomegaly and splenomegaly may be observed. Ulcerations of the buccal and nasal mucosa may also become manifest. Similar signs also develop in the other species of animals infected by *H. capsulatum*. The natural course of histoplasmosis in such wild animals as bats and rodents has not been studied. The incubation period is generally conceded to be approximately 2 weeks.

Disease in Man

Epidemiologists have determined that approximately 90% of human infections are asymptomatic. Infection in those fortunate individuals is diagnosed on the basis of a positive reaction to the skin test antigen known as histoplasmin. Clinical signs in the 10% who develop symptoms are quite broad. Clinicians categorize the symptomatic form into three basic types: (1) acute, pulmonary histoplasmosis, (2) disseminated histoplasmosis, and (3) chronic, cavitary histoplasmosis.

In the acute form of the disease, the victim develops flu-like symptoms: nonproductive cough, chest pains, and dyspnea. In more severe forms, fever, nightsweats, weight loss, and hemoptysis may be experienced in addition to those symptoms mentioned above. Roentgenological studies reveal pulmonary infiltrates and densities. Most patients recover spontaneously from this form of the disease. Later in life, X-rays may reveal calcifications in the lungs of these recovered individuals.

In a small percentage of primary pulmonary cases, the disease may spread from the lungs to other organ systems. In disseminated cases, hepatomegaly and splenomegaly develop, and accompanying symptoms include anemia, leukopenia, and weight loss. Unless diagnosed promptly and treated adequately, disseminated histoplasmosis may prove to be fatal. Cavitary histoplasmosis is a rare consequence of pulmonary invasion. Symptoms involve a productive cough, low fever, and intermittent hemoptysis. X-rays reveal pulmonary cavitation that must be distinguished from that encountered in tuberculosis. The incubation period for histoplasmosis is approximately 2 weeks.

General Mode of Spread

Histoplasmosis does not spread by contagion. With the exception of traumatic inoculation, all infections can be traced to the inhalation of the airborne spores of *H. capsulatum*.

Epidemiology

The principle habitat of *H. capsulatum* var. *capsulatum* is soil enriched with the feces of such gregarious birds as blackbirds and chickens and, to a lesser extent, pigeons. Bat habitats, such as attics and caves where their guano has accumulated, are frequently infested with *H. capsulatum*. Old chicken coops and bell and church towers inhabitated by pigeons as well as starling roosts are frequently the point source of outbreaks of histoplasmosis. Disturbance of such sites may release clouds of the infectious spores of *H. capsulatum* var. *capsulatum*. These are disseminated by air currents, and the deadly spores are carried downwind to endanger those who inhale the spores. The natural habitat of *H. capsulatum* var. *duboisii* remains unknown.

Diagnosis

Laboratory studies are required to diagnose histoplasmosis. Since symptoms resemble those of some bacterial and viral diseases, clinical signs cannot be relied upon to arrive at a correct diagnosis. Diagnosis rests upon (1) detection of the tissue from cells of *H. capsulatum* in clinical materials and (2) isolation of this fungus. Since the yeast cells of *H. capsulatum* var. *capsulatum* are relatively small, special stains must be used to make them evident in smears of pus and sputum and in histological sections of tissue. The Giemsa and Wright stains are recommended for examination of smears. The Gridley and Gomori silver methenamine procedures are invaluable for histological studies. Fluorescent antibody procedures are highly useful for detecting *H. capsulatum* yeast cells in all types of clinical material. Highly specific fluorescein-labeled *H. capsulatum* antiglobulins can be prepared.[23]

Isolation and identification of *H. capsulatum* from a suspected case of histoplasmosis provides the most definitive basis for diagnosis. Multiple tubes (six or more) or plates of a rich medium such as blood agar base with 10% human blood are recommended for inoculation with clinical materials. The inoculated media should be incubated at room temperature or 25°C and observed for signs of growth over a 4-week period.[24]

Because of gross and microscopic variations among isolates, cultures of suspected *H. capsulatum* must be carefully studied. If tuberculate spores (7 to 25 μm in diameter) are present along with microconidia (2 to 6 μm in diameter), the fungus should only be tentatively considered to be *H. capsulatum*. Its identity can only be confirmed by conversion in vitro or in vivo to its yeast-like tissue form. Animal conversion is obligatory for the identification of *H. capsulatum* var. *duboisii*. A rapid and specific immunodiffusion procedure has been developed for the identification of cultures suspected of being *H. capsulatum*.[25] Its use obviates the need to convert cultures to their yeast form.

Serological procedures for histoplasmosis are also available as diagnostic aids. The most useful tests are those for complement-fixation and immunodiffusion.[18]

Skin tests with histoplasmin are generally of no diagnostic service since the reaction does not distinguish between a past or a current active infection.

Prevention and Control

Contacts with the classical habitats of *H. capsulatum* should be avoided or reduced to a minimum. When feasible, efforts should be made to reduce the creation of dusty aerosols that may contain the spores of *H. capsulatum*. Wetting the surface of work areas is recommended as well as the wearing of protective masks. Infested areas can be decontaminated with 3% formalin.[26]

PROTOTHECOSIS

Etiologic Agent

The disease-causing agents are all members of the genus *Prototheca*. The two species incriminated in disease processes are *P. wickerhamii* and *P. zopfii*. *Prototheca* sp. are achlorophyllous microorganisms with a life cycle morphologically similar to that of green algae in the genus *Chlorella*. *Prototheca* sp. characteristically produce thick-walled hyaline cells, termed sporangia, which divide by irregular cleavage when mature to form 2 to 20 or more endospores. After sporulation is completed, the sporangial wall ruptures and the released endospores enlarge and repeat the reproductive cycle. Colonies are soft and yeast-like in consistency and white to light tan in color depending upon the species. Although the individual *Prototheca* sp. differ morphologically, their accurate identification requires carbohydrate and alcohol assimilation tests or immunofluorescence studies.

The phylogeny and taxonomic position of the *Prototheca* sp. are in dispute. Some workers regard these organisms as achloric mutants of the genus *Chlorella* on the basis of morphology and method of reproduction. Others consider them to be fungi because they are achlorophyllous and heterotrophic.

True and Alternate Hosts

This cosmopolitan disease affects man and various lower animals including cattle, deer, dogs, and cats.

Disease in Animals

Most animal cases involved the internal organs. Occasionally, infections are localized in the skin and underlying tissue or the eye. Clinical signs vary depending upon the organs affected.

Disease in Man

Most human cases that have been observed involve the skin and subcutaneous tissue or the olecranon bursa. Lesions are slow in developing and show no tendency to heal spontaneously. An etiological relationship between protothecal infection and tropical sprue has been suggested, but this relationship has not been established. The incubation period is unknown.

General Mode of Spread

The disease is not considered to be transmissible from host to host. *Prototheca* sp. occur ubiquitously in the environment, and infections are apparently acquired by contact with sources in nature.

Epidemiology

Knowledge regarding the epidemiology of protothecosis is fragmentary. *Prototheca* sp. are widely distributed in nature, having been recovered from such diverse sites as slime flux of trees, feces of various animals, potato skin, acid stream water, and waste stabilization ponds. Undoubtedly, man and lower animals frequently come into contact with these organisms in the environment. However, routes of infection are not definitely known. It has been suggested that a change in host resistance is required before these organisms can cause disease. However, predisposing factors have yet to be established.

Diagnosis

Laboratory studies are required to establish a diagnosis of this disease. They include (1) direct microscopic examination to demonstrate the presence of *Prototheca* sp. in tissues and other clinical materials and (2) culturing to isolate and identify the etiologic agent. The fluorescent antibody procedure is useful for the detection and identification of these organisms.

Prevention and Control

Unknown.

ZYGOMYCOSIS (MUCORMYCOSIS, PHYCOMYCOSIS, ENTOMOPHTHOROMYCOSIS)

Etiologic Agents

Zygomycosis is a disease of multiple etiology. Some of the agents of this protean disease in animals are *Absidia corymbifera, Conidiobolus coronatus, Mucor pusillus, Rhizopus arrhizus, R. microsporus, R. oryzae,* and *R. rhizopodiformis.* Adequate practical keys for identification of the zygomycete species are not currently available. In general, isolates from cases of zygomycosis should be referred to taxonomic experts for authoritative identification.

Zygomycetes usually grow exuberantly and at a rapid rate on routine isolation media. Characteristically, they produce broad aseptate mycelium. Members of the genera *Absidia, Mucor,* and *Rhizopus* form loose cottony colonies that are grey to greyish-tan. Asexual spores are produced within a closed structure known as a sporangium. Sporangia are borne on long special filaments called sporangiophores. Columellae are present inside of sporangia at their base. These are vesicles that develop from the tip of sporangiophores inside of the sporangia.

Characteristics of the genera *Absidia, Mucor,* and *Rhizopus,* all members of the order Mucorales, are as follows:

1. *Absidia* — Sporangia are pear shaped, sporangiophores arise between the nodes of the stoloniferous mycelium; rhizoids are present, but they do not subtend the sporangiophores.

2. *Mucor* — Rhizoids are not formed. Sporangia are globose with a columella but no apophysis.

3. *Rhizopus* — Rhizoids are present, subtending the sporangiophores. Sporangia are globose with a columella.[28]

The genus *Conidiobolus* is classified within the order Entomophthorales. The species within this order of zygomycetes produce flat glabrous colonies that become covered with aerial mycelium as the colony matures. Sporangia are not produced, however, conidia are formed that are forcibly discharged from the conidiophores. Conidia are basically globose, and in *C. coronatus* they have a distinct papilla. Conidia in this species also have a tendency to produce numerous secondary spores. They arise all over the surface of the mother conidium, creating a corona. The surface of some conidia may be covered with hair-like filaments instead of secondary spores. Discharged conidia are found adherent to the sides of an agar slant or the top of a Petri dish.[29,30]

True and Alternate Hosts

Zygomycotic infections are not contagious. Humans as well as a wide variety of lower animals are susceptible to infection by the various pathogenic zygomycetes. Domestic animals (cats, cattle, dogs, horses, sheep, pigs, etc.) and captive and wild animals (monkeys, apes, mink, deer, okapis, harp seals, etc.) have also been found to develop zygomycosis.

Distribution

The etiologic agents of zygomycosis are common throughout the world. Cases of zygomycosis have been recorded on all seven continents.

Disease in Animals

Basically, zygomycosis is a pulmonary disease. The various pathogenic species of *Absidia, Mucor,* and *Rhizopus* induce granulomatous reactions in the host that involve the lungs and the bronchial, mediastinal, and mesenteric lymph nodes. Dissemination to the other vital organs, e.g., kidney, liver, and brain, frequently occurs.

Disease in Man

Zygomycosis is a complex of diseases that may be subdivided as follows:

1. Pulmonary zygomycosis — Frequently, this occurs as a secondary disease in compromised patients with malignant disease. Presenting signs are those of pneumonia or bronchitis. Pain and blood-streaked sputum are also signs of infection.
2. Rhinocerebral zygomycosis — This is one of the most deadly and fulminating forms of any mycosis. Almost invariably patients have an underlying, uncontrolled, acidotic diabetes. The etiologic agents (*R. arrhizus* and *R. oryzae*) invade the nasal passages and develop in the turbinates and paranasal sinuses. The fungi may then move on to the orbit and forepart of the brain and thus jeopardize the life of the patient. Presenting signs may include any of the following: orbital cellulitis, proptosis, perforation of the palate, and infarction of the brain.
3. Subcutaneous zygomycosis — This is an essentially tropical disease of the subcutaneous tissues and muscle fascia caused by *Basidiobolus haptosporus*. The infected sites (arms, legs, buttocks) greatly increase in size and become firm and palpable.
4. Rhinozygomycosis entomophthorae — This is a chronic disease that has a nasal inception. As it progresses, it involves the lower turbinates, paranasal sinuses, palate, cheek and pharynx, nasal dorsum, and upper lip. The involved tissues swell considerably, and the resulting edema disfigures the patient's face.[32]

General Mode of Spread

Zygomycosis is not a contagious disease. Infections arise from the inhalation, ingestion, or inoculation (through trauma) of infectious elements into the body.

Epidemiology

The pathogenic species of zygomycetes grow in soil and on organic matter in nature as saprophytes. Compromised hosts such as diabetic humans are victims of some of the species (*R. arrhizus, R. oryzae*). Contributing factors for infection in lower animals are unknown.

Diagnosis

Demonstration of broad (4 to 10 μm in diameter), aseptate hyphal filaments and fragments in clinical material provides a clear-cut basis for the diagnosis of zygomycosis. Since all of the etiologic agents have similar tissue forms, speciation depends upon isolation and characterization of the gross and microscopic features of the isolates.

Mycelial elements can be directly seen in wet mounts of tissues and exudates. However, use of histological stains, such as hematoxylin and eosin, Gridley's, and the Gomori methenamine silver stains are recommended for their detection and visualization. In nasal scrapings and other tissues from some cases of zygomycosis, sporangia and sporangiophores may be found. Serological reagents and procedures for the diagnosis of zygomycosis have yet to become available for routine use.

Prevention and Control

Practical methods have not been developed for preventing and reducing the incidence and prevalence of zygomycosis. Moldy hay or feed that is apt to be overgrown and contaminated by zygomycetes should not be used for the care and feeding of domesticated animals.

REFERENCES

1. **Austwick, P. K. C.,** Pathogenicity in the genus *Aspergillus,* cited in Raper, K. B. and Fennell, D. I., *The Genus Aspergillus,* Williams & Wilkins, Baltimore, 1965, 82.
2. **Ainsworth, G. C. and Austwick, P. K. C.,** *Fungal Diseases of Animals,* 2nd ed., Commonwealth Agricultural Bureaux, Farnham Royal, Slough, England, 1973, 37.
3. **Kaplan, W., Arnstein, P., Ajello, L., Chandler, F., Watts, J., and Hicklin, M.,** Fatal aspergillosis in imported parrots, *Mycopathologia,* 56, 25, 1975.
4. **Coleman, R. M. and Kaufman, L.,** Use of the immunodiffusion test in the serodiagnosis of asperigillosis, *Appl. Microbiol.,* 23, 301, 1972.
5. **Emmons, C. W., Binford, C. H., Utz, J. P., and Kwon-Chung, K. J.,** *Medical Mycology,* 3rd ed., Lea & Febiger, Philadelphia, 1977, 309.
6. **Jungerman, P. F. and Schwartzman, R. M.,** *Veterinary Medical Mycology,* Lea & Febiger, Philadelphia, 1972, 124.
7. **Ajello, L.,** Comparative ecology of respiratory mycotic disease agents, *Bacteriol. Rev.,* 31, 6, 1967.
8. **Lodder, J., Ed.,** *The Yeasts — A Taxonomic Study,* North-Holland, Amsterdam, 1970.
9. **Winner, H. I. and Hurley, R., Eds.,** *Symposium on Candida Infections,* E & S Livingstone, Edinburgh, 1966.
10. **Hurley, R.,** The pathogenic *Candida* species: a review, *Rev. Med. Vet. Mycol.,* 6, 159, 1967.
11. **Jungerman, P. F. and Schwartzman, R. M.,** *Veterinary Medical Mycology,* Lea & Febiger, Philadelphia, 1972, 61.
12. **Winner, H. I. and Hurley, R.,** *Candida albicans,* J & A Churchill, London, 1964.
13. **Van Uden, N.,** The occurrence of *Candida* and other yeasts in the intestinal tracts of animals, *Ann. N.Y. Acad. Sci.,* 89, 59, 1960.
14. **Huppert, M., Jung, H. S., and Bailey, J. W.,** Natural variability in *Coccidioides immitis,* in *Coccidioidomycosis,* Ajello, L., Ed., University of Arizona Press, Tucson, 1967, 323.
15. **Sun, S. H., Huppert, M., and Vukovich, K. R.,** Rapid in vitro conversion and identification of *Coccidioides immitis, J. Clin. Microbiol.,* 3, 186, 1976.
16. **Maddy, K. T.,** Disseminated coccidioidomycosis of the dog, *J. Am. Vet. Med. Assoc.,* 132, 483, 1958.
17. **Prchal, C. J.,** Coccidioidomycosis in Arizona cattle, in *Proc. Symp. Coccidioidomycosis,* Ferguson, M. S., Ed., Public Health Service Publication No. 575, U.S. Department of Health, Education, and Welfare, Washington, D.C., 1957, 105.
18. **Ajello, L., Georg, L. K., Kaplan, W., and Kaufman, L.,** Mycotic infections, in *Diagnostic Procedures for Bacterial, Mycotic and Parasitic Infections,* 5th ed., Bodily, H. L., Ed., American Public Health Association, NewYork, 1970, 633.
19. **Littman, M. L. and Zimmerman, L. E.,** *Cryptococcosis — Torulosis,* Greene & Stratton, New York, 1959.
20. **Kwon-Chung, K. J.,** Perfect state (*Emmonsiella capsulata*) of the fungus causing large-form African histoplasmosis, *Mycologia,* 67, 980, 1975.
21. **Ajello, L.,** Distribution of *Histoplasma capsulatum* in the United States, in *Histoplasmosis,* Ajello, L., Chick, E. W., and Furcolow, M. L., Eds., Charles C Thomas, Springfield, Ill., 1971, 103.
22. **McGinnis, M. R. and Katz, B.,** *Ajellomyces* and its synonym *Emmonsiella Mycotaxon,* 8, 157, 1979.
23. **Kaufman, L. and Kaplan, W.,** Preparation of a fluorescent antibody specific for the yeast phase of *Histoplasma capsulatum, J. Bacteriol.,* 82, 729, 1961.
24. **Larsh, H.,** Isolation and identification of *Histoplasma capsulatum,* in *Histoplasmosis,* Ajello, L., Chick, E. W., and Furcolow, M. L., Eds., Charles C Thomas, Springfield, Ill., 1971, 271.
25. **Standard, P. G. and Kaufman, L.,** Specific immunological tests for the rapid identification of members of the genus *Histoplasma, J. Clin. Microbiol.,* 3, 191, 1976.
26. **Weeks, R. J. and Tosh, F. E.,** Control of epidemic foci of *Histoplasma capsulatum,* in *Histoplasmosis,* Ajello, L., Chick, E. W., and Furcolow, M. L., Eds., Charles C Thomas, Springfield, Ill., 1971, 184.
27. **Sudman, M. S.,** Prototrichosis. A critical review, *Am. J. Clin. Pathol.,* 61, 10, 1974.
28. **Zycha, H. and Siepmann, R.,** *Mucorales,* J. Cramer, Munden, Germany, 1969.
29. **Greer, D. L.,** Fungi of phycomycosis, in *Manual of Clinical Microbiology,* 2nd ed., Lennette, E. H., Spaulding, E. H., and Truant, J. P., Eds., American Society for Microbiology, Washington, D.C., 1974, 541.
30. **Waterhouse, G. M.,** Entomophthorales, in *The Fungi,* Vol. 4B, Ainsworth, G. C., Sparrow, F. K., and Sussman, A. S., Eds., Academic Press, New York, 1973, 219.
31. **Ainsworth, G. C. and Austwick, P. K. C.,** *Fungal Diseases of Animals,* 2nd ed., Commonwealth Agricultural Bureaux, Farnham Royal, Slough, England, 1973, 53.
32. **Rippon, J. W.,** *Medical Mycology,* W. B. Saunders, Philadelphia, 1973, 268 and 430.

APPENDIX 1*

Too many patients with fungal infections of the skin receive treatment before the diagnosis has been established. Thus, when the patient returns because the condition has not improved, the physician assumes that the infection is resistant and so prescribes stronger medication that may produce a local dermatitis medicamentosa.

Three simple and inexpensive diagnostic procedures are available to help make the correct diagnosis: direct preparations, culture, and fluorescence. Of the three, only the culture takes time to produce results. Moreover, none of them takes a great deal of the physician's time.

Approach #1: Direct
Direct preparations are just that. Here are two preparations and how to use them.

Potassium Hydroxide (KOH)
For skin — Cleanse the suspicious area with an alcohol sponge or soap and water to remove any extraneous material such as medications the patient may have applied, air-borne spores, and debris. Get skin scales by scraping the edge of the lesion (the center is usually negative) or by scraping the undersurface of a bulla (such as the bulla found on the sole of the foot in tinea pedis). When scraping a dry lesion, place a drop of water on the area to be scraped; this prevents the scales from scattering and helps them adhere to the scalpel blade. Place the scales on a microscope glass slide and add one or two drops of a 15 to 20% KOH solution. Place a coverslip over the mixture and gently heat the slide. (Do not let the solution boil since the KOH may crystalize and confuse the picture.) When not using the KOH solution, keep it in a closed screw-cap container to prevent evaporation and production of confusing crystals.

First examine the slide under low power. If you see a suspicious area, use higher power for confirmation. Lower the microscope condenser so that the light reaching the slide is less intense; this helps to distinguish mycelial elements from cell-wall borders.

Figures 1, 2, and 3 are examples of fungal infections diagnosed with direct KOH skin preparations.

For hair — If you suspect tinea capitis, use forceps to collect hairs and a scalpel to collect scales from the scalp. If any scalp hairs show greenish fluorescence under a Wood's lamp, select these hairs for microscopic examination and culture. If fluorescence is negative, choose short or broken hairs for these tests.

Examine the hair after preparing a KOH slide as you do for the skin scraping. Figures 4 and 5 are examples of fungal infections diagnosed with direct KOH preparations.

For nails — Use a scalpel to get material from suspected nails. Try to get the material from areas close to the nail bed of the chalky, crumbling, or striated nails. Prepare the KOH slide as you do for skin scrapings, but allow more time for the solution to digest. Figure 6 shows a positive KOH preparation of nail debris.

Saline
Direct saline preparations are also useful if you suspect a systemic mycosis. Look for draining sinuses or microabscesses to get your specimen. Simply place the purulent material on the slide and add one or two drops of saline. Mix, place a coverslip on

---

* Jacob, P. H., Three practical approaches to diagnosing fungal disease, *Consultant,* 17(7), 90, 1977. With permission.

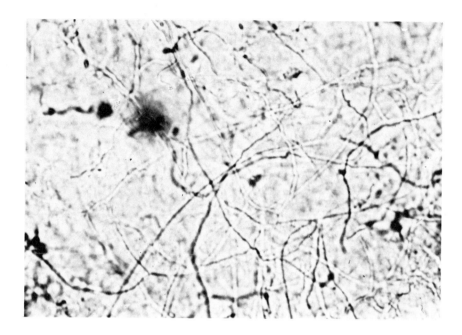

FIGURE 1.   This positive KOH indicates a fungal infection of the skin caused by a dermatophyte. Note the acute angle branching and the long mycelia.

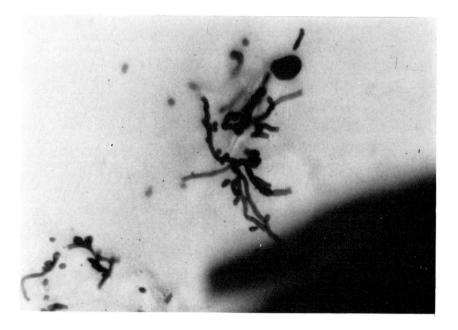

FIGURE 2.   This KOH preparation shows characteristics intermediate between a chain of
budding cells and mycelia (pseudomycelia). A budding yeast cell (blastospore) near a septa
(cross-wall) is characteristic of *Candida.*

the slide, and look for organisms. Rim the slide with petrolatum jelly and incubate
overnight at room temperature. Examine again the next day. If fungal elements are
present, you can see them ''sprouting'' under the coverslip. This is very useful in di-

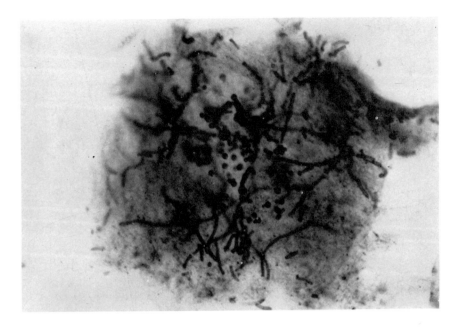

FIGURE 3.   This KOH preparation shows characteristics of tinea versicolor — short mycelia, occasional branching, and round spores of different sizes, some of which are budding.

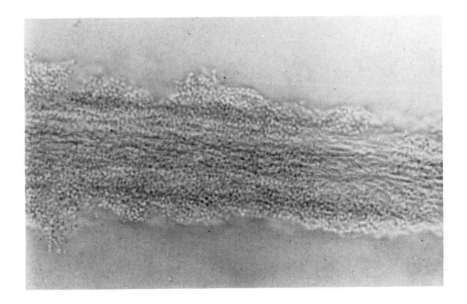

FIGURE 4.   This ectothrix hair, prepared with KOH, shows spores within the hair and also clustered in a sheath-like fashion on the outside of the hair shaft.

agnosing such diseases as disseminated coccidioidomycosis, North American blastomycosis, and other deep fungal pathogens where dissemination has produced skin lesions. Figures 7, 8, and 9 are examples of saline preparations.

Approach #2: Cultures

For years, Sabouraud's agar has been the standby for the culture of fungi. Sabour-

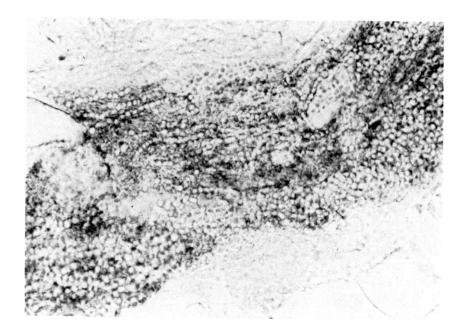

FIGURE 5.   This endothrix hair, prepared with KOH, shows that all spores are within the hair shaft.

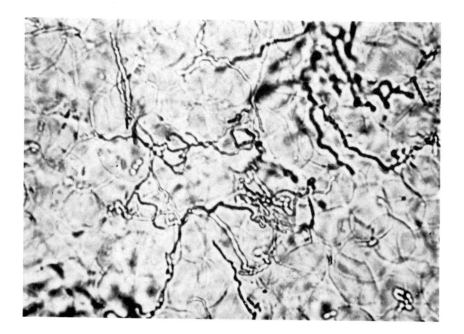

FIGURE 6.   This positive KOH preparation of nail debris indicates onychomycosis. Note the branching mycelia.

aud's agar is made even more useful by the addition of cycloheximide to inhibit many yeasts and saprophytic molds (nonpathogenic fungi) and antibiotics to inhibit bacterial saprophytes. In our laboratory we most frequently use what is essentially Sabouraud's

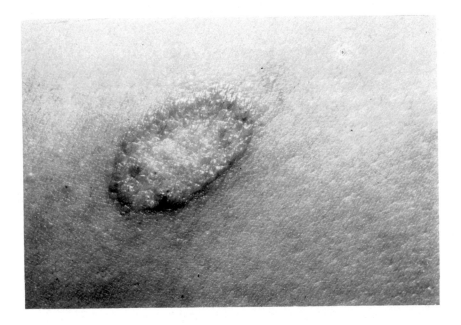

FIGURE 7.   Granulomatous lesion of coccidioidomycosis. Note the microabscesses.

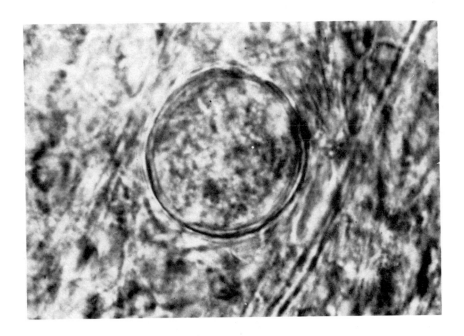

FIGURE 8.   Saline preparation of material from a microabscess reveals spherules character-istic of *Coccidioides immitis.*

agar with cycloheximide and an antibiotic. Although the cycloheximide will inhibit the growth of some yeasts, it will allow *Candida albicans* to flourish. Do not use this agar preparation if you suspect *Allescheria boydii* or *Cryptococcus neoformans* since it in-hibits both.

For growth of cultures, use a 4-oz pharmacy bottle with a screw cap. Pour the me-

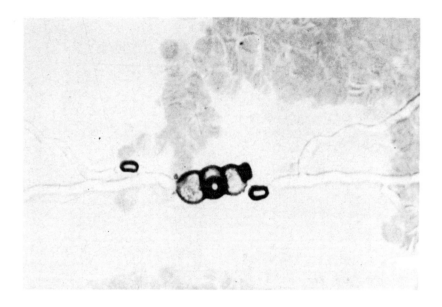

FIGURE 9.   Appearance of positive direct-saline preparation of *Coccidioides immitis* after 24 hr.

dium into the bottle at a slant and allow it to cool. After it solidifies, you can keep it for an indefinite period at room temperature. You can place skin, nail scrapings, and hairs on the medium and slice them into the surface. Be sure to keep the caps loose since fungi need a free circulation of air for growth and sporulation. Keep specimen bottles for at least 4 weeks (room temperature incubation) and check weekly for growth.

Approach #3: Fluorescence

Fluorescence is useful in the diagnosis of some superficial infections. Of course, the fluorescence is not always present. Under a Wood's lamp, for example, tinea capitis appears greenish; tinea versicolor, orange-yellow; erythrasma, coral red; and *Pseudomonas*, green. The Wood's lamp is simply ultraviolet light, filtered to give wavelengths of about 3650 A. You must use it in a totally dark room for maximum effectiveness. Fluorescence helps not only in diagnosis, but also in determining the extent of involvement.

APPENDIX 2*

Only if mycosis fungoides is treated at an early stage does the victim have any chance for normal living. Once the disease is well established, it tends to progress inexorably despite treatment. Thus, you should learn to recognize mycosis fungoides early even though early diagnosis can be very difficult.

WHAT IT IS

Mycosis fungoides *affects the skin primarily* and the visceral organs secondarily. It is thus unlike the other malignant lymphomas: lymphosarcoma, reticulum cell sarcoma, follicular lymphoma, and Hodgkin's disease, all of which affect visceral organs primarily and the skin secondarily. Mycosis fungoides is relatively rare and, like most malignancies, has no known cause. It usually occurs in adults over 40 years of age. If untreated, it produces skin lesions in all patients and visceral lesions in 40 to 50% of affected patients. The clinical course may be rapid and unrelenting over a period of months; or it may be chronic, characterized by periods of remission lasting several decades. Eventually, this disease is almost always fatal as a result of visceral lesions or infection.

The name mycosis fungoides is totally descriptive and does not suggest that this disease is in any way related to mycotic or fungal diseases, which are caused by plant parasites. It is called mycosis fungoides simply because of the mushroom-like appearance of the tumors common in its advanced stages. Mycosis fungoides is often very difficult to diagnose in its early stages, and as is to be expected, the early stages are most responsive to the treatments now available. With this in mind, let us review the diagnostic features of this disease and of several skin diseases that often precede or accompany mycosis fungoides and which may be of help in early diagnosis.

THREE STAGES OF DISEASE

Characteristically, mycosis fungoides develops in three stages, each of which is significant prognostically and therapeutically. Each may be observed singly or in combination. Each may be the first manifestation of disease. Each is characterized by a specific clinical and histologic appearance.

Stage I, the eczematous or premycotic stage, is the least malignant of the three stages. At this stage, prognosis for longevity is good, and any form of treatment is often quite successful. This stage is characterized by multiple skin eruptions that simulate many benign dermatoses (such as chronic atopic eczema, superficial fungal infections, psoriasis, seborrheic dermatitis, fixed drug eruptions, erythroderma, and exfoliative dermatitis). The patient may have red, scaling macular lesions of variable size scattered over many regions of the body; universal skin redness (Indian skin, *l'homme rouge*), loss of hair, and thick hyperkeratotic palms; or an exfoliative dermatitis.

These early lesions can persist for months or years. In most cases, this stage lasts 3 to 5 years or more and in rare cases may disappear spontaneously without treatment. The major symptom during this period is intense and unrelenting itching. The itching is so characteristic of early stage mycosis fungoides that you should suspect this disease in any patient older than 40 with chronic dermatitis and intense itching.

* McDonald, C. J., Learn to recognize mycosis fungoides early, *Consultant*, 16(11), 170, 1976. With permission.

EARLY HISTOLOGIC CHANGES

Histologically, the early stage of mycosis fungoides is difficult to diagnose, and so treatment may have to begin without a definitive diagnosis. Here are typical early findings. The epidermis may be thickened and the rete ridges elongated, simulating psoriasis. Focal spongiosis, microvesiculation, and inflammatory cells are noted in the epidermis. The stratum corneum is hyperkeratotic without parakeratosis. The dermal celular infiltrate is nonspecific, consisting of loose aggregations of lymphocytes, neutrophils, eosinophils, plasma cells, and histiocytes located perivascularly and throughout the dermis. Occasionally in this stage, but more often later in the infiltrated and tumor stages, a specific cell appears in the dermal infiltrate. This suggests mycosis fungoides. This cell, the so-called "mycosis cell," is slightly larger than a monocyte and is round with a large hyperchromatic nucleus and basophilic cytoplasm. Many pathologists consider this cell nonspecific — actually nothing more than a large, immature reticulum cell.

Stage II appears after a variable period. This is the infiltrated or plaque stage with well-defined, elevated plaques or nodules varying in color from red to brown and indurated on palpation.

At this stage, the histologic picture becomes more characteristic. In a compact zone in the subepidermal region, a cellular infiltrate appears that is somewhat similar to that in Hodgkin's disease. Many cell types appear: neutrophils, lymphocytes, eosinophils, plasma cells, and a polymorphism of histiocytes. A so-called "grenz zone" or cell-free subepidermal region may separate the infiltrate from the epidermis. It is not unusual, though, to see the infiltrate encroaching on and invading the epidermis. In the epidermis, collections of these cells form microabscesses ("Pautrier microabscesses"). These are considered pathognomonic for mycosis fungoides and must be distinguished from the spongiform eczematous dermatoses.

Stage III, the final tumor stage, develops relatively soon after the appearance of the infiltrative-plaque stage (except in the *d'emblee* type, in which the disease appears *initially* as tumors and nodules). Tumors and nodules tend to occur in previously affected skin sites or occasionally in normal-appearing skin.

Such tumors vary in size from 1 cm to several inches in diameter and are always elevated above the normal skin. Tumors and plaques often break down and form deep ulcerations. Ulcerations can also appear on apparently normal skin.

Histologically, this stage is sometimes difficult to distinguish from the plaque stage except that abnormal cells are often more prominent, and encroachment of the dermal infiltrate on the epidermis is so severe that ulcerations often occur. Occasionally, in such tumors, immature reticulum cells completely replace all other cell types, thus simulating reticulum cell sarcoma. This phenomenon may account in part for reports describing transformation of mycosis fungoides into reticulum cell sarcoma.

In untreated disease, death may occur soon after the onset of the tumor stage. Most patiets die of intercurrent infection with septicemia. Some die of visceral organ involvement or with clinical and histologic manifestations of Hodgkin's disease, reticulum cell sarcoma, lymphosarcoma, and leukemia.

VISCERAL CHANGES IN MYCOSIS

The most common clinical manifestation of visceral involvement is lymphadenopathy, also associated with liver and spleen enlargement. The spleen, lung, liver, brain, kidneys, myocardium, and G.I. tract may all show specific pathologic lesions of mycosis fungoides on histologic examination. Those cases that do not transform into leukemia or Sezary's reticulosis show a general lack of obvious peripheral blood or bone marrow involvement with mycosis fungoides. Sezary's reticulosis is generally considered a variant of mycosis fungoides. Patients with Sezary's reticulosis are marked by red skin, hair loss, and palmar and plantar hyperkeratosis. Characteristic abnormal "monocytoid" cells appear in the peripheral blood. Both mycosis fungoides and Sezary's reticulosis are thought to be diseases of T cells. In contrast, all other lymphomas are classified as diseases of B cells.

On histologic examination, a lymph node may show one of several changes *Dermatopathic lymphadenopathy* appears more commonly than specific types of infiltrates. The normal nodal architecture is obliterated by collections of immature reticulum cells, plasma cells, eosinophils, and numerous fat- and melanin-filled macrophages. This histologic finding is often mistaken for lymphomatous node involvement but is characteristic of many inflammatory skin diseases that involve large body areas. Uncommonly, a pathologic lymph node resembles one of the other malignant lymphomas. In other visceral organs, small foci of abnormal cells may closely resemble the polymorphous infiltrates found in skin diseases.

SUGGEST MYCOSIS FUNGOIDES

Several skin diseases, when they occur in middle-aged or older persons, call for studies to rule out mycosis fungoides. Patients with any of the following skin changes (even if evidence is insufficient to support a diagnosis of mycosis fungoides) need close observation for later development of this disease.

Follicular mucinosis — In 1954, Allen described mucinous changes in hair follicles in a case of mycosis fungoids. In 1957, Pinkus described a disease characterized by erythematous, scaly eczematous, coalescent papules and plaques on several body areas including the scalp. Alopecia commonly accompanied these changes, especially when lesions occurred on the scalp. Pinkus called this disease "alopecia mucinosa." Histologically, this disease was characterized by mucinous degeneration at the hair follicles. Allen believes that follicular mucinosis signals mycosis fungoides or other malignant lymphomas. Pinkus and others believe that follicular mucinosis occurs as a benign idiopathic state and as a stage in the progression of alopecia mucinosa to mycosis fungoides and other malignant lymphomas.

Parapsoriasis *en plaque* — Parapsoriasis is applied to a variety of diseases characterized by slow-developing, asymptomatic, scaling, plaque-like erythrodermas. In the *en plaque* form of the disease, well-delineated patches or plaques of varying size, shape, and color occur on the trunk and limbs. These patches vary in color from brown to red to purple and are moderately scaly. They may be elevated above the surrounding normal skin. They are persistent, and treatment to date has been ineffective.

Many observers consider the *en plaque* type of parapsoriasis either a forerunner or variant of the premycotic form of mycosis fungoides. Others feel that the various forms of parapsoriasis never develop into mycosis fungoides, and those cases described thus are early cases of misdiagnosed mycosis fungoides. In either case, the important thing is to differentiate active mycosis fungoides and parapsoriasis *en plaque*, and to closely observe patients with parapsoriasis *en plaque* since they may in fact have mycosis fungoides.

Erythroderma — This nonspecific eruption may occur in any of the malignant lymphomas. Erythroderma or red skin accounts for one fourth to one third of all skin manifestations of lymphoma. It is usually generalized and accompanied by alopecia, loss of nails, hyperpigmentation, and keratoderma of the palms and soles. Itching is its major symptom. Erythroderma associated with lymphoma usually occurs without evidence of neoplastic changes in the skin, and some consider it an indicator of good host resistance. When host resistance is overcome, infiltrates characteristic of the specific lymphomatous disease appear, and tumors begin to develop. At this time, itching usually disappears.

Poikiloderma — This rare skin condition simulates, to some degree, radiation or solar dermatitis. Clinically, it is characterized by large areas of hyperpigmentation, depigmentation, cutaneous atrophy, and telangiectasia. It may appear on any area of the body and is often symmetrical. The clinical course is characterized by slowly progressive disease ultimately accompanied by mycosis fungoides, other lymphoblastomas, collagen vascular disease (dermatomyositis), or cancer.

Sezary's reticulosis — This disease is most difficult to distinguish from mycosis fungoides both clinically and pathologically. Characteristically, it produces a generalized, erythematous, eczematous, scaling dermatitis associated with alopecia and keratoderma of the palms and soles. Very much like mycosis fungoides, Sezary's reticulosis is uniformly fatal. Histological changes in the skin are not unlike those observed in classic mycosis fungoides. An abnormal "monocytoid" cell with a cerebriform nucleus occurs in the skin and in the peripheral blood. Some offer this as evidence of difference from mycosis fungoides, which normally is not accompanied by qualitative cellular changes in the peripheral blood. Actually, the same cell has been detected in the skin of patients with mycosis fungoides as well as other benign dermatoses. Nevertheless, some studies refute this point of view.

Petechiae — Eczematous, psoriasiform, bullous, erythrodermic, and other dermatoses may precede or accompany the onset of mycosis fungoides. But I recently saw several patients with a dermatologic manifestation so far underscribed in active mycosis fungoides. These patients had petechiae as the first major manifestation of active disease. Although successful therapy has produced complete disappearance of petechiae, exacerbations of disease have been accompanied by recurrence of petechiae. Histologic changes in these areas are typical of mycosis fungoides.

PALLIATIVE TREATMENT

Like that of most malignant lymphomas, treatment of mycosis fungoides is palliative. Naturally, the treatment varies according to the clinical stage of disease. All patients, before receiving treatment, should be appropriately diagnosed as having skin and systemic disease. Topical corticosteroids, with or without occlusive dressings, and topical nitrogen mustard may successfully control skin disease. For nonresponsive skin or systemic disease, agents such as nitrogen mustard (topical and systemic) and cyclophosphamide, and antimetabolites such as actinomycin D offer varying degrees of control and should be tried. So far, the most consistent results occur in patients given cyclophosphamide, methotrexate, and streptonigrin; results are good in 50% of cases treated with any of these agents. They may evoke remissions that last from 3 to 6 months.

Most patients develop toxic drug reactions from these agents. These include leukopenia, thrombocytopenia, nausea, vomiting, hair loss, and various acute dermatoses. After repeated courses of therapy, patients do become refractory to these drugs. This factor, along with drug toxicity, limits their usefulness.

Recently, we tried the antimetabolite triacetyl-6-azauridine, high-dosage methotrexate, and leucovorin in mycosis fungoides. With azauridine alone, 6 of 13 patients with Stages II and III disease improved greatly. In five of eight patients, clinical signs and symptoms of the disease completely disappeared. And two of these patients have enjoyed complete clinical remission for more than 26 months while maintained on drug therapy. Happily, drug toxicity with this method has been minimal to date. Our experience with high-dosage methotrexate and leucovorin in more than 12 patients suggests that nearly all patients may experience a good and prolonged remission.

Radiotherapy has been an effective therapy for skin disease, producing good clinical remission in 75 to 85% of patients. However, it does not cure, and unfortunately, radiotherapy, like chemotherapeutic agents, has many serious limitations. Some of these are

1. As the number of courses is repeated, refractoriness tends to occur.
2. A certain maximum of radiation can be tolerated by the skin; beyond that, irreparable skin damage occurs.
3. There are systemic limitations to the amount of total body radiation that can be given any one patient with conventional X-ray techniques.

This limitation has been partially overcome by using electrons from linear accelerators, as described by Fromer and others. Characteristically, electrons produced this way penetrate only 3 to 6 mm of skin, thus affecting areas involved with mycosis fungoides yet not penetrating deep enough to affect visceral organs. Linear accelerators also produce X-rays capable of penetrating deeper than electrons, but they account for only a miniscule amount of the energy output of this electron apparatus and ordinarily do not produce systemic toxicity. As with other forms of radiation therapy, a limited number of electrons can be administered to a single body site without evoking irreparable skin damage. This treatment is also limited by the availability of such linear accelerators. Currently, not many medical centers (only about 30) offer such facilities in the U.S.

TO SUM UP

Mycosis fungoides is a skin lymphoma characterized by an abnormality in the T cell population. In early stages, it is localized primarily to the skin but eventually may spread to involve the internal organs. Treatment is palliative. Its selection should be based on the clinical stage of the disease and should take into account the involvement of the internal organs.

MYCOTOXICOSES

A. C. Pier

DISEASE

Mycotoxins are metabolites of fungi that grow on feeds or foods and exert undesirable biologic effects on animals or persons consuming them. The mycotoxins are important because they cause both acute and subclinical diseases (mycotoxicoses) in a broad range of animal species, including man. Because the mycotoxicoses are not infectious diseases, the format of this chapter must deviate from that of those dealing with infectious agents. The synonyms for mycotoxicoses are aflatoxicosis, alimental toxic aleukia, ergotism, fusariotoxicosis, facial eczema, leukoencephalomalacia, mycotoxic nephropathy, ochratocisosis, stachybotryotoxicosis, and uterotrophism.

ETIOLOGIC AGENTS

Mushroom poisonings were undoubtedly the first known mycotoxicoses. Later, in about 430 B.C., the first recognition of ergotism was made; epidemics of dry gangrene in both animals and man, caused by ergoted cereals, swept through Europe between the 11th and 16th centuries. A number of ergot alkaloids are mycotoxins, as are the aflatoxins, a closely related group of mycotoxins that contains highly pathogenic hepatotoxins and the most potent carcinogen known to science.

About 100 fungi that grow on standing crops or stored feeds are known to produce toxic substances. Approximately 12 of these are associated with naturally occurring mycotoxic diseases in animals or man. The majority of known toxigenic fungi belong to the genera *Aspergillus, Fusarium,* and *Penicillium.*

Toxigenic fungi are widely distributed and may occur on standing forage or stored feeds. A great portion of the mycotoxin problem in animals is associated with stored grains and other concentrate rations, particularly barley, corn, cottonseed, oats, peanut meal, and silage. The toxigenic fungi are relatively ubiquitous and can germinate, grow, and elaborate their toxins into a variety of substrates when favorable conditions of moisture, temperature, and aeration are present. There is, however, a definite proclivity for certain of these fungi to infest certain substrates. Optimal conditions for toxin production by different fungi may be quite variable; for instance, some fungi elaborate their toxin best at about 0°C while others are most effective near 25°C. Many of the mycotoxins are heat stable and survive pelleting, canning, and other processing operations. They are nonantigenic so immunity is not developed. The major sources and effects of mycotoxins associated with diseases of animals and man are presented in Table 1.

AFFECTED ANIMALS

The range of animal species affected by mycotoxins varies considerably. There are several reasons for this. First, the feeds infested by the toxigenic fungus may be peculiar to an animal species or population. Second, some animals may have protective mechanisms that inactivate the toxins (e.g., inactivation of ochratoxin A by bovine rumen flora). Third, there are considerable species, strain, and age differences in susceptibility to a given toxin. For instance, aflatoxin affects ducks and turkeys much

Table 1
MAJOR SOURCES AND EFFECTS OF MYCOTOXINS ASSOCIATED WITH DISEASES OF
ANIMALS AND MAN

Mycotoxin	Causative fungi and common feed sources	Major effects	Major animals affected
Aflatoxins (aflatoxin B₁)	*Aspergillus flavus; A. parasiticus* Corn, cotton seed, peanuts, ous cereals	Hepatotoxic, carcinogenic and teratogenic impairment of: coagulation, protein formation, production, weight gain, resistance, and immunity	Acute aflatoxicosis poultry, swine, cattle, dogs Hepatic carcinoma trout, primates, man Other associated with Reye's syndrome in human infants
Citrinin	*Penicillium citrinum; A. terreus,* et al. Wheat barley, oats	Nephrotoxic	Swine, cattle (?)
Ergot	*Claviceps purpurea* Rye, barley, oats, wheat, grasses, etc.	Vasoconstrictive and prolactin inhibition, gangrene of extremities, nervous signs, lowered reproductive efficiency	Most livestock and man
Ochratoxin (ochratoxin A)	*A. ochraceous; P. viridicatum* Corn, barley, oats, wheat	Nephrotoxic (some hepatotoxicity); enteritis, teratogenic	Swine, poultry, man: (? Balkan nephropathy)
Tremorgens	*P. palitans; P. puberulum; Claviceps paspali* Pasture, hay	Tremors, motor incoordination, convulsons	Cattle, sheep
Slaframine	*Rhizoctonia leguminicola* Clover, hay, pasture	Parasympathomimetic, salivation, lachrymation, diarrhea	Cattle
Sporidesmin	*Pithomyces chartarum* Rye grass pasture	Hepatotoxic, photosensitivity	Sheep, cattle
Stachybotryotoxin	*Stachybotrys atra* Stray, hay	Epithelionecrotic, hematopoietic depressant	Horses
T-2 toxin	*Fusarium tricinctum* et al. Corn, silage	Epithelionecrotic, hepatotoxic, hematopoietic depressant, teratogenic	Poultry, swine, cattle, man (? alimental toxic aleukia)
Zearalenone	*F. roseum* et al. Corn	Estrogenism, reduced reproductive efficiency	Swine, dogs (?), cattle (?)

Table 2
SPECIES
SUSCEPTIBILITY TO
AFLATOXIN

Subject	Approximate single oral dose LD_{50} (mg/kg body wt.)[a]
Duckling	0.4
Pig	0.6
Trout	0.8 (not oral)
Dog	1.0
Sheep	2.0
Chick	6.5
Hamster	10.2

[a] Aflatoxin B_1 activity.

more severely than it does chickens, and cattle more severely than sheep. Young animals are notably more susceptible to aflatoxin than are mature beasts. The animals most often affected by the major mycotoxins are included in Table 1. The relative susceptibility of several animals to aflatoxin B_1 is shown in Table 2.

DISTRIBUTION OF MYCOTOXINS

Some of the toxigenic fungi are distributed widely in nature. Toxigenic strains of *Aspergillus flavus* and *A. parasiticus* are found throughout the world. However, the mycotoxicoses typically exhibit both regionality and seasonality in their occurrence. Examples of regional and seasonal incidence may be found with facial eczema of sheep and cattle in New Zealand where the fungus *Pithomyces chatarum* produces toxic spores on pasture grasses during the dry periods of summer and fall. Even where the causative fungi are distributed widely, considerable regionality in the actual formation of toxin may be exhibited as in the incidence and level of aflatoxin in corn in various regions of the U.S. These variations can often be associated with local environmental conditions that favor toxin formation.

The occurrence of mycotoxins in stored feed commodities and mixed feeds that are shipped in quantity to distant and foreign markets substantially diminishes the concept of regional and seasonal exacerbations of mycotoxic disease. Some high reported levels of mycotoxins in feedstuffs are listed in Table 3.

DISEASE IN ANIMALS

The mycotoxins have considerable biologic variability. Some exert pharmacologic activities without causing detectable lesions (e.g., neurologic effects of penitrem A, histaminic effects of slaframine), some may have hormonal effects (e.g., estrogenic effects of zearalenone), others cause definitive lesions (e.g., alfatoxin and T-2 toxin), and some may exert teratogenic and carcinogenic effects (e.g., aflatoxin). Adverse effects of mycotoxins on animals may assume one of three forms:

1. Primary acute mycotoxicoses are produced when high to moderate levels of mycotoxins are consumed. Specific, overt, acute episodes of disease ensue that may

Table 3
REPORTED HIGH LEVELS OF
MYCOTOXINS IN SOME ANIMAL FEED
COMMODITIES

Toxin	Level (ppm)	Commodity
Aflatoxin[a]	320	Australian corn
	101	U.S. corn
	2.7	Thai corn
	0.25	Thai millet
	22	U.S. peanuts (damaged)
	1000	U.S. peanuts (selected kernel)
	1.5	U.S. cottonseed
	960	U.S. cottonseed (selected bowls)
Ochratoxin[b]	28	Danish barley
	27	Canadian wheat
	16	U.S. corn
	0.04	U.S. barley
T-2 toxin	2	U.S. corn
Zearalenone	2909	U.S. animal feed
	5	U.S. corn
	35.6	Yugoslav corn

[a] Part of original data reported as aflatoxin, part as aflatoxin B_1 activity.
[b] Part of original data reported as ochratoxin, part as ochratoxin A.

include such signs as hemorrhaging, acute hepatitis, nephritis, necrosis of oral and enteric epithelium, and death.

2. Primary chronic mycotoxicoses, resulting from moderate to low levels of mycotoxin intake, often cause reduced productivity in the form of lower growth rates and reduced reproductive efficiency. These effects may occur with or without the production of an overt, primary mycotoxic syndrome. Carcinogenisity and teratogenicity are produced by some mycotoxins.

3. Secondary mycotoxic diseases result from lesser levels of mycotoxin intake that do not cause an overt mycotoxicosis but effect predisposition to infectious diseases through reductions in native mechanisms of resistance and immunity. Suppression of the cellular immune system is a known sequela to low levels of aflatoxin in certain disease systems. In secondary mycotoxic disease, symptoms are those of the infectious process to which the host was predisposed.

A brief resume of the major mycotoxicoses of animals is presented below.

Aflatoxin Poisoning

Some strains of *A. flavus* and *A. parasiticus* that grow on corn, peanuts, cottonseed, and other substrates produce a potent hepatotoxin, aflatoxin B_1. Particularly susceptible are young ducklings, turkey poults, hatchery-reared trout, weanling pigs, calves, dogs, and subhuman primates. After prolonged intake, aflatoxin causes liver damage, depresses protein formation by the animal body, and causes hepatic tumors in several animal species including man (epidemiologic evidence). Teratogenic effects have been observed in laboratory animals. Acute aflatoxin poisoning causes hepatitis, necrosis of liver cells, and prolonged blood clotting time, and affected animals often die with severe hemorrhages. The single-dose oral LD_{50} of aflatoxin B_1 for several animals is presented in Table 2. Feed containing 1 ppm or more can produce acute poisoning in some animals including young poultry and swine. In subacute cases of aflatoxin poisoning, liver changes include hepatic lipidosis, portal fibrosis, and proliferation of bile-duct epithelial cells. Growth rate is depressed, but death of the animal may not occur. Chronic aflatoxin poisoning causes subtle changes that are often overlooked but are economically important since they include reduced growth rate. Resistance to infection and responsiveness to vaccination may be impaired in some species, notably poultry, swine, and calves. Teratogenic changes, tumor formation, and carcinogenesis occur in some animals after prolonged consumption of feed containing as little as 0.5 to 15 ppb of aflatoxin.

Ergotism

Ergot alkaloids are among the oldest recognized mycotoxins. They are produced by the growth of the fungus *Claviceps purpurea* in the embryo of a number of cereals including rye, barley, wheat, oats, and some grasses. Unlike several of the other mycotoxins, ergots are formed in the standing crop in the field rather than in grain stored at improper moisture levels. The most frequently recognized effects are gangrenous lesions of the fetlock, ear, and tail caused by these alkaloids. Occasionally, nervous derangement, ataxia, and an abnormal gait may be caused by ingestion of toxic quantities of ergot. In pigs, growth retardation may result, possibly as a result of reduced palatability. In the first 35 days after breeding, gilts that consumed grain containing 0.5% ergot had lower pregnancy rates than controls. Pregnant sows consuming 0.1 to 1.0% ergot during the last trimester developed agalactiae, gestation was shortened by 5 days, and pigs died shortly after birth. Agalactiae appears at least partially reversible if ergot is removed from the ration.

Ochratoxicosis

Ochratoxin and citrinin may be involved singly or in combination in causing mycotoxic nephropathy in swine and possibly in man. Ochratoxin is produced by some strains of *A. ochraceous* and *Penicillium viridicatum* growing on corn, barley, oats, and wheat. Citrinin is produced by strains of *P. citrinum* and *A. terreus* (among others) growing on wheat, barley, and oats. Porcine mycotoxic nephropathy is seen in Europe and occasionally in Canada but has not yet been reported in the U.S. Ochratoxin poisoning has been observed in poultry in the U.S. and causes inappetence, reduced growth, kidney tubular necrosis, and death. Ochratoxin is both nephrotoxic and hepatotoxic causing tubular degeneration, necrosis, and nephrosis at lower levels of intake, particularly in swine. At higher levels hepatic degeneration and necrosis are also produced in some animals as are neural effects. Inflammation of the small intestine also occurs.

Typical signs of ochratoxicosis include polyuria, polydypsia, diarrhea, and decreased growth rate. Ochratoxin is also teratogenic. Citrinin is nephrotoxic and may interact with ochratoxin in producing porcine nephrosis. Definitive information is not available on single-dose oral LD_{50} of ochratoxin, but gross lesions of the swine kidney are produced at levels of 0.04 mg/kg and microscopic lesions at 0.01 mg/kg body weight of young growing swine.

Toxic Trichothecenes (T-2 Toxin, Vomitoxin, and Feed Refusal Factor)

Fungi of the genus *Fusarium* produce a number of metabolites that exert undesirable biological activities when consumed by susceptible animals; among these substances are the toxic trichothecenes. *F. tricinctum* and certain other fungi growing on standing or stored corn, silage, and other feeds produce a trichothecene called T-2 toxin. This and other trichothecene toxins are often produced at temperatures approximating 0°C. T-2 toxin is noted for its destruction of rapidly dividing cells such as epidermis, gut epithelium, and bone marrow. It is epithelionecrotic and to a lesser degree hepatotoxic. Consumption at high levels causes necrosis of the lips or beak, ulceration of the oral and gut mucosae, hepatic degeneration, hemorrhage, thymic involution, and death in many animal species. Chronic consumption of lower levels causes reduced weight gain, hematopoietic depression, coagulation defects, and nervous effects. *In utero* fetal deaths and abortion have been observed experimentally in swine. The acute oral LD_{50} dose of T-2 toxin in swine is approximately 4 mg/kg body weight. Other trichothecenes of importance are vomitoxin (deoxynivalenol), which causes emesis, and feed refusal factor; both are associated with the consumption of moldy corn.

Estrogenism (Uterotrophism)

One of the most frequently encountered mycotoxins is zearalenone, a metabolite produced by *F. roseum* that produces estrogenic effects in young swine. Zearalenone affects reproductive efficiency resulting in weak or stillborn young and precocious swelling of the vulva and mammae of gilts. It occurs frequently in moldy corn and may be accompanied by other *Fusarium* metabolites including feed refusal factor, vomitoxin, or other toxic trichothecenes.

Facial Eczema

This is a disease primarily of cattle and sheep that grazed in New Zealand rye grass pastures infested with the fungus *Pithomyces chartarum*. This fungus sporulates on the grass during dry periods in the late summer. The spores and other fungi parts contain a potent hepatotoxin — sporidesmin — that produces an acute, obliterative cholangiohepatitis. Faulty metabolism of chlorophyll results in build-up of phyloerythrin in the blood that in turn causes photosensitivity from whence the disease gets its name. Facial eczema is an important economic disease during the appropriate seasons in New Zealand.

Stachybotryotoxicosis

The fungus *Stachybotrys atra (S. alternans)* grows on hay and straw during the winter months and has been reported to produce a potent trichothecene toxin, the effects of which closely resemble those of T-2 toxin. Horses and mules that consume the infested hay exhibit severe irritation and necrosis of the skin and mucous membranes of the upper G.I. tract, hematopoetic depression with severe leukopenia, coagulopathy, and death. In some instances of high toxin intake, death preceded detectable signs or lesions. The disease caused severe losses in Russia during World War II. Major effects of other mycotoxins on animals are summarized in Table 1.

DISEASE IN MAN

Mycotoxicoses in man span the historic effects of a number of hallucinogenic to lethal intoxications, from mushrooms and other fleshy fungi to the epidemics of gangrene and nervous derangement caused by ergot in cereal grains (i.e., "St. Anthony's Fire") that swept Europe from the 11th through the 16th centuries. Three additional mycotoxicoses of man should be mentioned.

On the basis of substantial epidemiologic evidence, aflatoxicosis in man is suspected of being responsible for the high incidence of hepatitis and hepatic carcinoma in human populations in areas of Africa, Southeast Asia, and India where foods heavily endowed with aflatoxin are substantial parts of the diet. More definitive evidence of human involvement by aflatoxin has been found in children dying of Reye's syndrome (fatty degeneration of the liver and encephalitis) in Thailand and Czechoslovakia; in these cases significant levels of aflatoxin were detected in the livers of children who died from the disease but not in the livers of children dying from other causes in the same populations.

Alimental Toxic Aleukia (ATA)

A severe disease of man that is now attributed to *Fusarium* infestation of overwintered rye was observed in Russia during World War II. Signs of the disease included irritation and necrosis of the skin and mucous membranes of the G.I. tract, hematopoetic depression with leukopenia, thrombocytopenia, coagulopathy, hemorrhage, and death. It is believed by some that ATA was caused by a toxic trichothecene.

Balkan Nephropathy

With the recognition in areas of central Europe of mycotoxic nephropathy of swine and poultry caused by ochratoxin and possibly citrinin, there came an association with a histologically similar human nephropathy in areas where the swine disease and ochratoxin in cereal grains were prevalent. To date, the association between ochratoxin and Balkan nephropathy of man appears possible, but a definitive association remains to be demonstrated.

EPIDEMIOLOGY

Occurrence of mycotoxicoses in animals or man is associated with the consumption of nutrients that are (or have been) colonized by toxigenic fungi. In most cases (e.g., aflatoxicosis, ochratoxicosis, et al.), the toxin is elaborated into the substrate when conditions of moisture, temperature, gaseous environment, etc. are suitable for mold growth and toxin elaboration; in a few cases the toxin is retained within fungal thallus or spore (e.g., ergotism, facial eczema). As mentioned previously, high incidence of a mycotoxicosis may be evident in a given location, season, and crop product when conditions favor toxin production. Development of toxins in stored crops and shipment of contaminated commodities tend to diffuse both the geographic and seasonal epidemiologic peaks.

Considerable attention has been given to the entrance of mycotoxins into the human food chain. Because of its potent carcinogenic effects, aflatoxins have been extensively studied in this regard. It is known that where intake levels in animal feeds are sufficiently high, very low levels of aflatoxin residues and metabolites have been found in selected animal tissues, milk, and eggs. When aflatoxin is consumed, part of it is metabolized to a toxic metabolite, M_1 toxin, that may be found for short periods at low levels in liver, milk, urine, and certain other body components. The differentiation of these toxins has important epidemiologic significance. In one instance when Reye's syndrome in children was suspected to have been caused by a contaminated dairy product, aflatoxin B_1 rather than M_1 was demonstrated in the powdered dairy product indicating that the toxin arose from fungal contamination of the product rather than from the cow. The source of recognized mycotoxicoses invariably has been primary contaminated crops or foods; animal-to-animal or animal-to-human transfer causing intoxication has not been reported.

DIAGNOSIS

Mycotoxicoses are diagnosed by demonstration of specific mycotoxins in the feed that are of a type and level compatible with observed clinical signs and pathologic changes. Cultural demonstration of fungi (even known toxigenic species) in the feed is not evidence of the presence of mycotoxins. These fungi are relatively ubiquitous and only some strains are toxigenic. Conditions necessary for toxin elaboration may not have occurred in a feed in which a toxigenic fungus is present, or the causative fungus may no longer be viable in feed that contains a mycotoxin. Current methods of mycotoxin detection include (1) solvent extraction of suspected feeds, (2) purification of the extract through precipitation, partitioning, or column chromatographic techniques, and (3) demonstration of a specific toxin in thin-layer chromatograms (TLC) or by gas chromatography and mass spectral analysis. In some cases (e.g., T-2 toxin and zearalenone), the use of biological tests (dermonecrotic and uterotrophic effects, respectively) are more sensitive — albeit less definitive — than current TLC methods. Literature citing specific toxin detection methods is included in the references.

PREVENTION AND CONTROL

Development of mycotoxins in field crops presents a number of substantial problems because toxin development is often weather related. Either extremely wet or dry conditions may foster the invasion and growth of toxigenic fungi as does insect damage. The latter, of course, is controllable by insecticides, to a degree.

If the source of mycotoxicosis is from stored commodities, toxin production can be minimized by proper storage (e.g., rapid drying and storage of corn at less than 15% moisture content). Preservatives such as sodium proprionate may be added to high-moisture products to prevent the growth of fungi; they do not, however, have any effect on preformed toxins.

Utilization, decontamination, and disposal of feeds containing mycotoxins present a number of enigmas and represent a large economic problem. Prevention of mycotoxin formation is the most highly recommended cure for this complex group of diseases. Detoxification methods are currently under investigation and in experimental field use. Ammoniation under heat and pressure is one of the more promising methods for inactivating aflatoxin in shelled corn.

REFERENCES

1. **Goldblat, L. A.,** *Aflatoxin,* Academic Press, London, 1969.
2. **Hesseltine, C. W.,** Natural occurrence of mycotoxins in cereals, *Mycopathol. Mycol. Appl.,* 53, 141, 1974.
3. **Krogh, P.,** Mycotoxic nephropathy, in *Advances in Veterinary Science and Comparative Medicine,* Vol. 20, Brandly, C. A., Cornelius, C. E., and Beveridge, W. I. B., Eds., Academic Press, New York, 1976, 147.
4. **Microcha, C. J. and Christensen, C. M.,** Fungus metabolites toxic to animals, *Annu. Rev. Phytopathol.,* 12, 303, 1974.

5. Pier, A. C., Cysewski, S. J., and Richard, J. L., Mycotoxicoses of Domestic Animals and their Diagnosis in Proc. 18th Annu. Meet. of the Am. Assoc. Veterinary Laboratory Diagnosticions, 1975, 419.
6. Pier, A. C. et al., Proceedings of the symposium on mycotoxicoses of domestic animals, *Am. Vet. Med. Assoc.*,163, 1259, 1973.
7. Rodericks, J. V., Ed., *Proc. Conf. on Mycotoxins in Human and Animal Health*, Pathotox, Chicago, 1977.

POISONING BY FRESH-WATER BLUE-GREEN ALGAE*

B. G. Archer

DISEASE

Disease or death caused by ingesting toxins of blue-green algae is commonly referred to as blue-green algal poisoning or algal poisoning.

ETIOLOGIC AGENTS

Species of fresh-water, blue-green algae incriminated in algal poisonings include *Anabaena flos-aquae, Microcystis aeruginosa, Aphanizomenon flos-aquae, Coelosphaerium kuetzingianum, Gloeotrichia echinulata,* and *Nodularia spumigena.* Occasional reports mention a few additional species, but *Anabaena, Microcystis,* and *Aphanizomenon* have been involved in most incidents of toxicity.[1-3] Apparently, only certain strains within each of these species produce toxins, at least in amounts great enough to be consequential. All of these species can be found wherever looked for, but they present no hazard to human or animal health until environmental conditions are conductive to rapid proliferation. When temperature, sunlight, nutrients, and competing plant and animal forms permit, these algae can multiply within a period of a few days to form large masses of thick green scums that float on or just below the surface of the water. The algal masses are sometimes swept by winds so that the scum is concentrated along the water's edge or deposited on banks. The rapidly developing, dense algal blooms invariably associated with algal poisonings need not be unialgal in composition, but the species responsible for toxin production will nearly always be predominant. Identifying which of the known toxic species is involved is easily done on the basis of microscopic, morphological characteristics of the algal cells, trichromes, or colonies.[4] The following criteria are adequate to guide a tentative identification. *Anabaena flos-aquae* grows in unbranched, moderately curved or coiling trichromes that do not form discrete colonies but are often entangled in dense masses. The cells are uniformly barrel-shaped, and heterocysts may be numerous. *Microcystis aeruginosa* forms poorly delineated and irregularly shaped colonies of densely aggregated, small spherical cells. The trichromes of *Aphanizomenon flos-aquae* are straight or slightly curved and aggregate in parallel orientation to form spindle-shaped fascicles. Dense growths of *Aphanizomenon* can appear macroscopically as finely chopped grass in the water. *Coelosphaerium kuetzingianum* usually forms spherical colonies that have a gelatinous envelope enclosing a single spherical layer of loosely distributed cells. *Nodularia spumigena* forms individual unbranched trichromes showing little tendency to coil that are distinguished by having cells broader than long. *Gloeotrichia echinulata* forms distinctive colonies in which unbranched, individually sheathed, and slowly tapering trichromes emanate radially from the center of the colony. A reference text on the taxonomy of algae should be consulted for positive classification to the level of species.

SUSCEPTIBLE SPECIES

Observations from natural occurrences of algal toxicities and experimental studies, while incomplete, support the belief that all mammalian and avian species are suscep-

* The author's work with algae has been supported by award SER77-06943 from the National Science Foundation.

tible to algal toxins.[2,3] Fish kills have also been reported, particularly with *Aphanizo-menon flos-aquae*.[5] In laboratory studies, goldfish were killed by toxins from *Anabaena flos-aquae* when injected intraperitoneally or administered intragastrically but were unaffected when placed in water containing the toxin.[6] Several reports (reviewed by Schwimmer and Schwimmer[7]) indicate the toxicity of *Microcystis* toxins to fish. The susceptibility of fish to other toxic algae has not been established. As dense algal blooms undergo decay, depletion of dissolved oxygen in the water occurs and can aggravate the effects of algal toxins or cause fish kills by itself.[8]

DISTRIBUTION

Since the first report of poisoning by blue-green algae over 100 years ago, incidents of toxicity involving blue-green algae have been noted from almost all continents and in all but the extreme latitudes.[3] Despite this world-wide distribution, information about the prevalence on a more regional level is very incomplete except in a few localities.[9] Many believe that occurrences of toxic algal blooms go unrecognized because the period during which the toxic algae or their released toxic principles exist in lethal concentrations may be very brief.[7] Also, toxic algal blooms frequently develop sporadically and may not recur in successive years even when conditions appear to be similar and nothing has been done to prevent their recurrence.[1] This sporadicity contributes to toxic algal blooms being considered uncommon and undoubtedly results in an unknown number of animal deaths being mis- or undiagnosed.[7]

DISEASE IN ANIMALS

In most natural poisonings by blue-green algae, the poisoned animals are found dead as the toxins of at least the commonly involved algal species are readily absorbed, potent, neuromuscular toxins that cause death within minutes or a few hours.[10] Nonspecific signs including abdominal distention, dysphagia, salivation, and respiratory distress have been described in surviving poisoned cattle,[1] but only rarely in natural conditions have effects of less than lethal doses been noted. Experimentally, death in laboratory species usually results within 20 min after intraperitoneal or intragastric administration of toxic *Anabaena* or *Aphanizomenon* cells or extracts and within ½ to 24 hr after *Microcystis* cells or extracts.[10-13] The significant signs are neuromuscular, beginning with restlessness and progressing to isolated spasms, convulsions, paralysis, and death. With *Anabaena*, injected mice characteristically drag one or both hind legs before paralysis becomes complete. The major toxin produced by *Anabaena* has been characterized as a depolarizing neuromuscular-blocking agent whose chemical structure has been determined to be a bicyclic secondary amine.[14-16] *Aphanizomen* toxins reversibly block the development of action potentials and have been shown to be similar in both their chemical structure and pharmacologic activity to saxitoxin, a substance produced by some members of the marine dinoflagellate genus, *Gonyaulax*.[13] The toxins produced by *Microcystis* are cyclical polypeptides that are unique among algal toxins for causing hepatocellular degeneration.[1,17-19] No significant anatomical lesions have been described for other algal toxins.

DISEASE IN MAN

Blue-green algae and their toxins have been suspected in several apparently water-supply-related epidemics of acute gastrointestinal disease when bacterial and viral agents could not be found.[7,20-22] However, positive evidence that algae were involved was also lacking. In a few isolated instances, *Anabaena, Microcystis,* and *Aphanizomenon* have caused acute gastrointestinal illness after accidental ingestion by humans while swimming or after falling into algae-containing waters.[7] The manifestations included headache, vomiting, cramps, and diarrhea in contrast to animal poisonings where neuromuscular effects and rapid death are usually observed. These differences between the clinical manifestations exhibited by poisoned animals and humans could easily be explained by the presence of multiple toxins with different pharmacological activities and different latent periods. Although the best-studied blue-green algal toxins have potent neuromuscular effects, Aziz[23] has detected a substance in cultures of *Microcystis* that induced fluid accumulation in guinea pig ligated intestinal loops. This diarrhea toxin was different from the acutely lethal polypeptides of *Microcystis* in that it was nondialyzable. Thus while the role of blue-green algae in human gastrointestinal disease is only suspected at this time, epidemiologic and laboratory data supporting this connection exist.

EPIDEMIOLOGY

The epidemiology of blue-green algae poisonings involves considerations of factors that influence the development of dense algal blooms, the production of toxins by the algae, and the consumption of toxin-containing water by animals and man. The growth of algae is affected by weather-related environmental factors, such as sunlight, temperature, and precipitation, and by perturbations of the environment of a body of water that affect its balance of flora and fauna or hasten the process of eutrophication, i.e., the addition of organic and inorganic substances to the water.[1,3] The majority of dense blooms of toxic algae occur in the summer when high sunlight intensities and long, warm days favor the multiplication of photosynthetic organisms. In many instances of blue-green algal poisoning, some change in the environment of the toxic body of water that has accelerated the process of eutrophication had also occurred. Some of the changes that have been associated with algal blooms include increases in human or animal activity (e.g., recreational use of a lake increased or animal-rearing operations expanded), the occurrence of a drought that lowered water levels significantly, or flooding that inundated vegetation causing it to decay in the water or caused water from drainage or sewage systems to contaminate water supplies. In laboratory studies toxin production was found to vary with pH, temperature, aeration, and light intensity, but the importance of these factors or others that might influence toxin production by algae in natural circumstances or favor the blooming of toxic strains are largely unknown.[1] However, observations that dense blooms in one part of a lake may be toxic while those in another, even though apparently composed of the same species may not, and that the toxicity of blooms may vary greatly within a period as brief as a few days might be explained by local differences in these environmental variables or by the local predominance of toxic or nontoxic strains.[1,9]

The toxins produced by the principal toxic species have median lethal doses lower than 1 mg/kg body weight when injected into mice.[11-13] Oral toxicities are somewhat less.[10,14] Complete data that would permit definitive statements is lacking, but extrapolations of these laboratory data to natural conditions lead one to predict that even the greatest amounts of toxins produced by the algae would no longer be fatal after dissipated by diffusion and convection to approximately 10% of maximal concentrations if most of the toxin is extracellular. If significant amounts of toxin are intracellular, the dissipating effects of diffusion and currents can be reversed by winds that increase the density of floating algal masses along shores and banks where animals drink.[12,24] Whether or not algal cells are swallowed along with water will influence the amount of toxin ingested by animals. Some birds actually peck at and eat from the algal masses; however, observations that cattle that could enter shallow water to drink beyond a wind-concentrated toxic bloom survived while sheep forced to drink at the edge of the water died indicate that at least cattle are not completely without discrimination in what they drink.[25] Thus, the likelihood that livestock would be poisoned by toxic algae in their watering sources would be lessened by the avilability of alternate water supplies.

DIAGNOSIS

When poisoning by blue-green algae is suspected, several samples of the algae and water should be collected as quickly as possible for testing since lethal amounts of toxin may persist only briefly and the toxic strain of algae may be succeeded by a nontoxic one. Direct microscopic examination of the algae to verify that a potentially toxic species is predominant in the bloom and mouse inoculations of water and cells should be done. In the most toxic blooms, sufficient toxin is present in the water that 0.5 mℓ injected intraperitoneally into a 20- to 25-g mouse will cause death with the signs and within the times described above. If toxicity cannot be demonstrated by direct injection of cells or water, algal cells can be concentrated before injection by centrifugation or lyophilization. The latter method is preferred since extracellular toxin is also concentrated, the amounts of algae injected are more easily quantified, and the process of freeze-drying disrupts the cells releasing intracellular toxins. Typical lethal intraperitoneal doses of lyophilized toxic algae are in the range 0.5 to 10 mg per mouse. Quite massive amounts of nontoxic algal cells can be injected with no, or only nonspecific, effects. A positive diagnosis is established by identifying the algae and demonstrating that it causes death with characteristic signs and latent period in mice. Since the toxins cause death quickly, no characteristic anatomical lesions, either gross or microscopic, result except in the case of *Microcystis* that causes hepatocellular changes.[17,18] The failure to demonstrate toxins by mouse inoculations cannot be reliably interpreted as eliminating algal toxicity as a diagnosis because lethal concentrations may exist for only brief periods or occur only locally, making it possible that collected samples would not contain the toxin.[26]

PREVENTION AND CONTROL

At the present time, approaches to the prevention and control of poisoning by blue-green algae involve inhibiting the growth of toxic blooms by chemical treatments, avoiding or reversing eutrophication of water supplies, and preventing humans and animals from contacting water when potentially toxic algae are present in heavy blooms. Both organic and inorganic substances have been used as algicides and may be indicated under certain circumstances. However, their use should not be considered as a substitute for correction of the eutrophication that leads to enhanced algal growth. Eutrophication is combatted by reversing the environmental changes that add nutrients to water or reducing nutrients by chemical treatment. For example, precipitation of phosphorus in eutrophic waters by treatment with aluminum or ferric ions that form insoluble phosphates may temporarily reduce the levels of phosphorus below that needed to support a dense algal bloom. Standard references on management of natural and man-made waters should be consulted for information on the use of algicides and chemical treatments of bodies of water. A more practicable control measure is preventing animal or human contact with potentially toxic blooms by surveillance and policing of recreational and drinking water sources. When potentially toxic blooms develop, safe, algae-free water must be provided until the blooms regress.

REFERENCES

1. Gorham, P. R., Toxic algae, in *Algae and Man*, Jackson, D. F., Ed., Plenum Press, New York, 1964.
2. Schwimmer, D. and Schwimmer, M., Algae and medicine, in *Algae and Man*, Jackson, D. F., Ed., Plenum Press, New York, 1964.
3. Gentile, J. H., Blue-green and green algal toxins, in *Microbial Toxins*, Vol. 7, Kadis, S., Ciegler, A., and Ajl, S. J., Eds., Academic Press, New York, 1971.
4. Smith, G. M., *The Fresh Water Algae of the United States*, McGraw-Hill, New York, 1933.
5. Gentile, J. H. and Maloney, T. E., Toxicity and environmental requirements of a strain of *Aphanizomenon flos-aquae*(L.) Ralfs, *Can. J. Microbiol.*, 15, 165, 1969.
6. Carmichael, W. W., Biggs, D. F., and Gorham, P. R., Toxicology and pharmacological action of *Anabaena flos-aquae* toxin, *Science*, 187, 542, 1975.
7. Schwimmer, D. and Schwimmer, M., Medical aspects of phycology, in *Algae, Man, and the Environment*, Jackson, D. F., Ed., Syracuse University Press, New York, 1968.
8. Mackenthun, K. M., Herman, E. F., and Bartsch, A. F., A heavy mortality of fishes resulting from the decomposition of algae in the Yahara River, Wisconsin, *Trans. Am. Fish. Soc.*, 75, 175, 1945.
9. Hammer, U. T., Toxic blue-green algae in Saskatchewan, *Can. Vet. J.*, 9, 221, 1968.
10. Carmichael, W. W., Gorham, P. R., and Biggs, D. F., Two laboratory case studies on the oral toxicity to calves of the freshwater cyanophyte (blue-green algae) *Anabaena flos-aquae* NRC-44-1, *Can. J. Comp. Med.*, 18, 71, 1977.
11. Carmichael, W. W. and Gorham, P. R., Anatoxins from clones of *Anabaena flos-aquae* isolated from lakes of western Canada, *Mitt. Int. Ver. Theor. Angew. Limnol.*, 21, 285, 1978.
12. Konst, H., McKercher, P. D., Gorham, P. R., Robertson, A., and Howell, J., Symptoms and pathology produced by toxic *Microcystis aeruginosa* NRC-1 in laboratory and domestic animals, *Can. J. Comp. Med. Vet. Sci.*, 29, 221, 1965.
13. Alam, M., Ikawa, M., Sasser, J. J., and Sawyer, P. J., Purification of *Aphanizomenon flos-aquae* toxin and its chemical and physiological properties, *Toxicon*, 11, 65, 1973.
14. Carmichael, W. W. and Biggs, D. F., Muscle sensitivity differences in two avian species to anatoxin-a produced by the fresh water cyanophyte *Anabaena flos-aquae* NRC-44-1, *Can. J. Zool.*, 56, 510, 1978.
15. Devlin, J. P., Edwards, O. E., Gorham, P. R., Hunter, N. R., Pike, R. K., and Stavric, B., Anatoxin-a, a toxic alkaloid from *Anabaena flos-aquae* NRC-44h, *Can. J. Chem.*, 55, 1367, 1977.
16. Huber, C. S., The crystal structure and absolute configuration of 2,9-diacetyl-9-azabicyclo(4,2,1)non-2,3-ene, *Acta Crystallogr.*, B28, 2577, 1972.
17. Heaney, S. I., The toxicity of *Microcystis aeruginosa Kutz* from some English reservoirs, *Water Treat. Exam.*, 20, 235, 1971.
18. Ashworth, C. T. and Mason, M. F., Observations on the pathological changes produced by a toxic substance present in blue-green algae (*Microcystis aeruginosa*), *Am. J. Path.*, 22, 369, 1946.
19. Bishop, C. T., Anet, E. F. L. J., and Gorham, P. R., Isolation and identification of the fast-death factor in *Microcystis aeruginosa* NRC-1, *Can. J. Biochem. Physiol.*, 37, 453, 1959.
20. Dean, A. G. and Jones, T. C., Seasonal gastroenteritis and malabsorption at an American military base in the Philipines. I. Clinical and epidemiologic investigations of the acute illness, *Am. J. Epidemiol.*, 95, 111, 1972.
21. Tisdale, E. S., The 1930-1931 drought and its effect upon public water supply, *Am. J. Public Health*, 21, 1203, 1931.
22. Veldee, M. V., An epidemiological study of suspected water-borne gastroenteritis, *Am. J. Public Health*, 21, 1227, 1931.
23. Aziz, K. M. S., Diarrhea toxin obtained from a waterbloom producing species, *Microcystis aeruginosa Kutzing*, *Science*, 183, 1206, 1974.
24. McBarren, E. J., Walker, R. I., Gardner, I., and Walker, K. H., Toxicity to livestock of the blue-green alga *Anabaena circinalis*, *Aust. Vet. J.*, 51, 587, 1975.
25. May, V., A toxic algae in New South Wales and its distribution, *Contrib. N. S. W. Nat. Herb.*, 4, 84, 1970.
26. Gorham, P. R., McLachlan, J., Hammer, U. T., and Kim, W. K., Isolation and culture of toxic strains of *Anabaena flos-aquae (Lyngb.) de Breb*, *Verh. Int. Ver. Theor. Angew. Limnol.*, 15, 796, 1964.

EDITORIAL COMMENT — AFLATOXIN IN CORN IN THE SOUTHEASTERN U.S.*

According to a Food and Drug Administration (FDA) news release dated October 14, 1977, aflatoxin contamination of the 1977 corn crop is unusually severe in most southeastern states. Although this region is expected to contribute only about 3% of the total U.S. corn crop in 1977, there are indications that about half of the corn crop in these states will not be marketable because of aflatoxin contamination in excess of the FDA's allowable levels (20 ppb).

One of the FDA's primary concerns is that affected corn will be milled into corn meal or other foods for human consumption. The FDA has instituted a program to examine corn products destined for human consumption that move in interstate commerce and is taking the necessary action to remove any found to contain over 20 ppb aflatoxin from the market. The FDA has also suggested similar action to the states for corn moving intrastate.

The FDA will also implement a program to sample market milk and eggs from the southeastern states to determine the aflatoxin levels in these products.

Human exposure to the aflatoxin present in the 1977 corn crop can occur in two ways. The first is through direct consumption of products made from corn. Only dry-milled products, such as corn meal or grits, are of concern since it is a well-known fact that wet-milled corn products, such as refined corn oil, fresh (sweet) corn, and cornstarch, do not contain aflatoxin even if they are prepared from contaminated raw material.

A second possible route of exposure is through consumption of meat, milk, and eggs from animals that have been fed aflatoxin-contaminated corn. Because most ingested aflatoxin is excreted by such animals, the levels of aflatoxin found in meat, milk, and eggs are generally well below the level present in the ingested feed. However, because of the importance of meat, milk, and eggs in the human diet and because young children and infants may be more susceptible to the effects of aflatoxin, there is a need to control this route of exposure by limiting the level of aflatoxin in corn used for animal feeds. About 80% of the corn harvested in the area is used for animal feeds.

Aflatoxins are a group of chemically related substances produced as a natural by-product of the growth of certain common molds. The major member of the group is aflatoxin B1, which is a highly toxic chemical. In addition to its toxic properties, aflatoxin B1 has exhibited highly potent cancer-producing properties in certain species of experimental animals. According to epidemiologic studies conducted in Southeast Asia and Africa, there is evidence that consumption of aflatoxin-containing foods is associated with cancer of the liver in humans.

For over a decade it has been known that under certain conditions aflatoxin can contaminate foods and animal feeds produced and consumed in the U.S. Because of the possible health effects of this substance, the FDA considers aflatoxin a significant public health problem and has established regulatory controls to limit exposure to this substance.

*   Center for Disease Control, Veterinary Public Health Notes, U.S. Department of Health, Education and Welfare, Public Health Service, Atlanta, October — November, 1977, 5.

New Problems

BACTERIA ASSOCIATED WITH FISH AND THEIR RELATIVE IMPORTANCE

E. B. Shotts, Jr.

Perhaps one of the most important economic aspects involved both in fish culture and in the pet fish industry is bacterial disease. Estimates indicate that fish diseases amount to 10 to 30% of the costs of production.[43] A discussion of bacterial diseases of fish should be approached with regard to those organisms usually associated with disease problems and to an expanding group of opportunistic organisms that have been associated with fish mortality, many of which are of known zoonotic potential in mammalian hosts.

The latter group of organisms appears to be increasing for a number of reasons including: (1) increasing bacterial contamination of the aquatic environment that has been prompted by (2) an increased and more intimate contact between man and the environment due to population increases and changing recreational trends and (3) the declining supplies of "red meat" have resulted in an increase in the use of fish for human consumption. Another factor contributing to the growth of this group of organisms includes infections of fish with bacterial organisms usually restricted to mammalian hosts. In such cases, these outbreaks or reports have usually resulted from a combination of environmental insults including thermal, chemical, and biological and/or toxic pollution of surface waters. This factor(s) provides the stress(es) and environmental conditions necessary for development of a wide variety of bacterial diseases in fish.

Disease conditions in fish will be considered in two groups: those classically associated with fish and those that, although they may have at sometime been reported in disease conditions of fish, are usually thought of as pathogens of mammals. Documentation for this latter group is often difficult because the literature is sketchy, and in many instances isolated reports provide the only available information.

It should be emphasized that this discussion is not necessarily limited to a restricted geographical area but is of potential world concern. With changing husbandry, species of fish involved, and the constant flux of environmental quality, some of the diseases discussed may be of less importance in the future and others, perhaps unknown at present, will be quite important.

MAJOR FISH PATHOGENS

Furunculosis — *Aeromonas salmonicida*

This disease was first noted in Germany, and in 1890 the organism was isolated there from trout.[18,19] It has been reported from a number of species of fish but is most commonly associated with fresh-water salmonids. Furunculosis is considered to be distributed world-wide except for possibly New Zealand.

In salmonids, the disease may be acute, chronic, or inapparent (potential carrier fish). Bacteriologic isolation and identification of *A. salomicida* from diseased tissue are necessary for diagnosis. Typically, this nonmotile, Gram-negative rod is characterized diagnostically by a diffusable brown pigment in older cultures, cytochrome oxidase activity (+), and temperature requirement (20 to 25°C).[20] Other diagnostic tools including several agglutination tests and fluorescent antibody are also available.[35]

Control of this disease is often complicated but must include a combination of preventative medicine and chemotherapy. Adequate sanitation is paramount, involving sanitation of eggs brought into the hatchery as well as facilities there.[3] Chemotherapeutics commonly used include sulfonamides,[62] oxytetracycline,[63] and nitrofurans.[44]

Motile Aeromonas Septicemia (MAS) — *Aeromonas hydrophila (liquefaciens) complex*

This condition, often referred to as bacterial hemorrhagic septicemia, is usually caused by *A. hydrophila* complex;[13] however, most Gram-negative rods will produce many, if not all, of the symptoms seen in this disease. The disease is common, having been noted world-wide, and affects most, if not all, fresh-water fish.

MAS is most frequently encountered in temperate and semi-tropical areas and appears to be associated with waters having a high organic content, generally following some stress or injury to the fish. The disease usually follows the course of an acute generalized septicemia. However, in lingering fish, some ulcers and/or abscesses have been noted.

Since this organism is common in surface waters, it is imperative that diagnosis be based upon isolation of the organism from a **live** diseased fish. The organ of choice for isolation is the kidney. The organism may be characterized as a motile, Gram-negative rod that is fermentative and resistant to vibriostat 0/129 and cytochrome oxidase positive.[10] Diagnostic time may be reduced to 24 hr by use of a differential medium designed to detect these organisms.[55]

To control MAS, a basic approach incorporating both chemotherapy and preventive control is imperative. A number of potential control measures, including immunization, prophylactic chemotherapy, and selection of resistant strains of fish, have been studied with varied success. Chemotherapeutic agents that have been used to treat clinical disease include oxytetracycline, penicillin-streptomycin mixtures, and Chloromycetin®.[13]

Vibriosis — *Vibrio anguillarium*

Conditions produced by members of the genus *Vibrio*, most of which are *V. anguillarium*-like organisms, are usually referred to as ulcer or boil disease and are usually seen in brackish or salt water. The disease has been reported world-wide, and some outbreaks have been noted in fresh-water fish.[51] Epidemiologic studies of the fresh-water outbreaks have not conclusively eliminated the chance of marine contamination (i.e., feedstuffs or waterbirds). This disease may manifest itself as a typical generalized bacterial septicemia; however, toward the end of an outbreak, the chronic cases usually form skin ulcers that progress into the musculature.[5,49]

When this disease occurs in a salt-water environment, bacterial diagnosis should be performed with care since this group of organisms is considered ubiquitous with this environment. For this reason, it is mandatory that cultures be obtained from moribund fish, preferably from the kidney. Care should be taken in interpretation of isolates from ulcers from fish due to the ubiquitousness of the organisms in salt or brackish environments. Classically, the organism is a motile, slightly curved Gram-negative rod that is fermentative and sensitive to vibriostat 0/129 and novobiocin and demonstrates a positive cytochrome oxidase reaction.

The classic approach to bacterial disease control should be employed, including the immunization of hatchery populations via the oral route. Chemotherapeutics such as oxytetracycline, sulfonamides, and nitrofurans have been used for both prophylactic and supportive control.

Enteric Redmouth (ERM) — "Hagerman Redmouth" Bacterium

This disease of salmonid fish that was for a number of years confined to the northwestern U.S. and Canada is caused by an ill-defined bacterium of the "enteric" group and is currently called RM bacterium.[48] The apparent spread of this disease within the salmonid population suggests that it is an emerging problem in salmonids of the U.S. ERM has not yet been reported from other parts of the world.

Clinically affected fish present typical signs of acute generalized septicemia. In chronic cases, cutaneous petechiation may be noted, particularly around the mouth and on the ventral surface. Bilateral exophthalmia is occasionally seen.

Recovery and identification of the organism from the kidney of a diseased fish is considered diagnostic. The organism is a motile, Gram-negative rod that is cytochrome oxidase negative and fermentative (without gas). Additionally, it agglutinates specific antisera.

Control of ERM requires strict sanitation at all levels in hatchery operations, and prevention of the disease is very important. Immunization is applicable and is a standard practice in many hatchery operations.[4] Chemotherapeutics used to control outbreaks include sulfonamides, oxytetracycline, and Chloromycetin®.[50]

Edwardsiella Septicemia (ES) — *Edwardsiella tarda*

This condition, often referred to by the more descriptive name of emphysematous putrefactive disease, is caused by *E. tarda*.[37] It has been observed primarily in freshwater eels, goldfish, and catfish from Southeast Asia and southern areas of the U.S.

Although this disease may produce mortality and symptoms of an acute generalized septicemia, it is most commonly noted as small cutaneous lesions that develop into abscesses of the musculature. Characteristically, necrotic tissue and a malodorous gas are associated with these abscesses.[68]

Diagnosis of the condition is dependent upon recovery and identification of the organism from diseased fish. The organism is a motile, Gram-negative rod that is cytochrome oxidase negative, fermentative, and produces indole and lysine decarboxydase.[37] Oxytetracycline and sulfonamides have been used as chemotherapeutics in conjunction with preventive sanitation measures.

Columnaris Disease — *Flexibacter (Chondrococcus) columnaris*

This disease, commonly referred to as "cotton wool disease," is a condition of freshwater fish. It is world-wide in distribution, and although the classic etiologic agent is *F. columnaris,* other members of this genus may cause similar lesions.

Clinically, severity of the disease may vary from peracute to chronic. The external lesion is often yellowish to orange because of the pigmentation of the organism. Scrapings from the lesion should contain characteristic long, thin (0.75×5 to $12\ \mu m$), Gram-negative rods. Fresh preparations should have characteristic "haystacks" or "columns" of organisms. If the lesion is cultured on Ordal's medium, the typical colony is dry, rhizoid, and has a yellow pigment following incubation for 3 to 5 days at 20°C. Motility is by a gliding flexing motion.[39,40] Suspicious colonies should be examined using a slide agglutination technique with specific antisera. Biochemical characterization is impractical because of the fastidiousness of the organism.

Control of the disease on both a prophylactic and supportive basis can be accomplished using oxytetracycline or nitrofurans. Addition of oxidizing agents such as potassium permanganate to the water or reduction of water temperature to less than 15°C are useful control measures.

MINOR FISH PATHOGENS

A number of bacterial organisms of lesser importance have been responsible for significant fish kills. These sporatic outbreaks, although infrequent, have prompted investigators and diagnosticians to consider these organisms as potential causes of fish mortality.

Hemorrhagic septicemia similar to that noted in fish that have the classic characteristics of Gram-negative bacterial septicemia may be caused by *Pseudomonas fluorescens* or a closely related *Pseudomonas* species.[12] These species that are ordinarily considered nonpathogenic may produce disease via proteolytic enzymes and/or apparent mutations that may enhance their virulence.[11,36]

Although rarely noted in recent years, an ulcerative disease caused by *Haemophilus piscium* was of significance in the late 1940s and early 1950s. Similarly, in the 1960s massive septicemic kills caused by an organism identified as *Pasteurella piscicida* were noted in white perch.[25,64]

The bacterial diseases mentioned above are all caused by Gram-negative organisms and constitute the bulk of those microbial agents responsible for fish mortality. There are, however, four Gram-positive organisms that should be mentioned as potential fish pathogens. These include members of the genera *Corynebacterium, Mycobacterium, Nocardia*, and *Streptococcus*.

Bacterial kidney disease, sometimes known as "Dee" disease, is caused by a *Corynebacterium* species.[61] The exact taxonomic description of this organism is not well defined because of cultivation difficulties. The disease has only been observed in salmonids and has been diagnosed in North America, Scotland, and Japan. It is generally observed as a chronic disease in fish of more than 6 months of age. Pathology includes liver and spleen lesions and, in older fish, turbid ascites of the abdominal and pericardial cavities. Inapparent carrier stock are important factors in the spread of this disease. Diagnostic techniques employed to detect these carriers have been important in controlling this disease in cultured salmonids.[14]

Those *Mycobacterium* spp. that produce disease in fish received a great deal of attention in the late 1950s in conjunction with feeding procedures at Pacific salmon hatcheries.[47,71] Epidemiologic studies and corrective measures have eliminated this endemic foci, but members of this genus are still occasionally isolated from aquarium and marine fish. Although the taxonomy of *Mycobacterium* is still in flux, it appears that at least three species have been involved: *M. marinum, M. fortuitum,* and *M. platypolcilis*. Pathology is observed either as isolated skin lesions or as systemic bacterial granulomas of vital organs.

The ecology and epidemiology associated with this group are unique and perhaps represent the most, if not the only, significant zoonosis associated with fish. It is reasonable to assume from environmental studies that the mycobacterial species isolated are found in surface waters and in soil.[8] The fish become infected by chance and transmit their infection primarily to aquarium fanciers who continually immerse their hands in infected tanks.[1,6] Observations indicate that "top-feeding" fish are at a greater risk of becoming infected and therefore reflect a larger potential risk to the fancier.[59] Another Gram-positive organism has been isolated from time to time from lesions similar to those of mycobacteriosis. This organism, *Nocaria asteroides,* has also been recovered from salmonids and aquarium fish.[16,17,21] It is possible that a portion of the uncultured diagnoses of mycobacteriosis may have in fact been caused by this organism that has similar cellular and morphologic characteristics.[28]

Although rare, occasional outbreaks of fish disease caused by streptococci have been reported in both fresh- and salt-water fish. It has been suggested that most of these outbreaks are the result of a contaminated environment. Thus far, Lancefield Groups B and D streptococci have been involved.[27,46] The most recent documented outbreak occurred in marine fish in a Gulf Coast bay.[41] In this case (as in those mentioned above), a possibility of zoonotic implication might exist; however, the probability is remote.

OPPORTUNISTIC ROLE OF BACTERIA IN MAN AND FISH

The implication that wild, cultured, or aquarium fish serve as a source of bacterial pathogens of human importance has been discussed.[25,65] Some of the most important of these will be discussed in light of currently available knowledge.

Classically, fish are associated with the bacterial genus *Aeromonas,* an organism that has been reported to cause human and animal disease.[54,67,70] Upon examining the literature closely, one notices a common theme of patient debility prior to aeromonad infection. Because of the current taxonomic instability with regard to *Aeromonas,* one must be careful as to the exact species reputed as the etiologic agent when reading the literature.[52,56,57] Presently, most diseases are attributed to *A. liquificans, A. punctata,* or *A. hydrophila.* Current research efforts suggest that all of these species are probably the same organism.[36]

It has been documented that *Aeromonas, Vibrio,* and *Pseudomonas* compose the bulk of the bacterial genera associated with fish.[10] The role of fish in transmitting various members of the genus *Vibrio* to man is not as important in the U.S. as it is in other areas. Workers in Japan and the U.S.S.R. implicate fish in the spread of *V. cholera* in these countries.[24,31,42] Another member of this group, *V. parahemolyticus* (a cause of human food-borne disease), has been shown to be indigenous in marine environments. Its growth and maintenance in and on fish for long periods of time are as well known as the fact that it is the leading cause of food-borne disease in Japan.[73] It has also been shown that this organism may be pathogenic for fish.[69] The difference in the importance of this organism in Far Eastern nations, as opposed to the U.S., is one of methods of food preparation.

In keeping with the zoonotic aspects of disease transmitted via fish, two other human enteric diseases — salmonellosis and shigellosis — and their relationship to fish must be considered. There is adequate documentation to assume that fish may become carriers and shedders of salmonellae if the environment is contaminated.[15,26,53] It should be pointed out, however, that a number of domestic and pet animals also become salmonellae carriers. There is information available to suggest that once established, *Salmonella* species may persist in fish for long periods.[34,66] These reports, based on laboratory studies, document infection where fish were infected with unusually large numbers of organisms often exceeding $10^5/ml.$[32] Under ordinary conditions, the concentration of salmonellae in surface waters seldom exceeds $10^2/ml$ even in highly contaminated environments. Documentation of the isolation of *Shigella* from fish is found in the literature; however, zoonotic implications were not well defined.[31]

Isolation of *Escherichia coli* from fish taken from contaminated environments has been reported, and subsequent infectivity studies have failed to produce disease in fish when known enteropathogenic strains were employed.[22]

Indirectly, both staphylococci and *Clostridium botulinum* may by chance become a part of the flora of processed fish and, if improperly handled, may result in human food-borne disease.

Other organisms reported from fish include *Leptospira* spp. While some reports suggest urine contamination of caught fish by rodents as a source of leptospires, others suggest that the organism may infect fish and can be readily recovered from internal organs.[7,33] *Erysipelothrix rhusiopathiae,* commonly considered to be an ubiquitous organism associated with fish slime, has been shown to produce "fish rose." This severe cutanous infection is an occupational disease among European fish handlers.[45]

A thorough search of the literature reveals reports implicating fish as actual or potential vectors of almost all pathogenic bacteria including such exotic ones as those that cause anthrax, plague, and tularemia.[9,38] A number of serologic studies indicate the presence of antibodies in fish sera against a variety of human pathogens.[29]

No reports regarding the isolation of either mycoplasma or rickettsia associated with human disease from fish were found in the literature. No etiologic agent belonging to either of these groups is known to be associated with fish disease. A parasite of salmonid fish may carry a neorickettsia that, when ingested by a canine, may result in a disease referred to as "salmon poisoning."

Despite literature reports that document the infection of fish with an arrray of pathogens and implications including the infection of fish under laboratory conditions, it must be noted that these infections were for the most part accomplished by injecting overwhelming doses of organisms. Only in a few situations has laboratory infection of fish been shown to occur under natural conditions. Often under natural conditions, very exacting parameters of stress, temperature, etc. must be met in order for infection to be acquired.[2,65] It is a well-accepted fact among biologists that, with the exception of one or two known obligate pathogens, some extreme stress is necessary to institute a bacterial infection in fish.

It may be noted that the environmental deterioration of our streams and waterways may produce some unique parameter of stress never before observed. Fish could become infected with some potentially pathogenic bacteria of zoonotic importance; however, this has not been the case to date.

In the U.S., more than 20 million household aquariums are maintained, accommodating an annual sale of approximately 600 million pet fish. During the last 4 years, extensive bacterial studies of aquarium fish have been carried out. The sources of these fish were the countries and areas supplying the U.S. market, including Hong Kong, Taiwan, Bangkok, Singapore, Columbia, Guyana, Peru, Brazil, and south central Florida. The results indicate that there are no unique or potentially zoonotic organisms present in fish from any of these sources.[23,58,60]

Despite the number of varied and sundry organisms and their relative pathogenicity previously discussed, to this author's knowledge there have been no documented significant outbreaks of human disease for which diseased fish were directly responsible.

REFERENCES

1. **Adams, R. M., Remington, J. S., Steinberg, J., and Siebert, J. S.,** Tropical fish aquariums: a source of *Mycobacterium marinum* infections resembling sporothriclosis, *JAMA*, 211, 457, 1970.
2. **Allen, N. and Pelczar, M. J.,** Bacteriological studies on white perch (*Roccus americanus*), *Chesapeake Sci.*, 8, 135, 1967.
3. **Amend, D. F.,** Comparative toxicity of two iodophors to rainbow trout eggs, *Trans. Am. Fish. Soc.*, 103, 73, 1974.
4. **Amend, D. F.,** personal communication, 1977.
5. **Anderson, J. I. W. and Conroy, D. A.,** Vibrio disease in marine fishes, in *A Symposium on Diseases of Fishes and Shellfishes,* Spec. Publ. No. 5, Snieszko, S. F., Ed., American Fisheries Society, Washington, D.C., 1970, 266.
6. **Black, H., Rush-Munro, F. M., and Woods, G.,** *Mycobacterium marinum* infections aquired from tropical fish tanks, *Aust. J. Dermatol.,* 13, 155, 1971.
7. **Brandt, H. J.,** Uber Berufskrankheiten in der Binnenfischerei, *Z. Fish. Deren Hilfswiss.*, 3(4), 295, 1953.

8. **Brown, J.,** personal communication, 1977.
9. **Brunner, G.,** Fische als Bazillentrager, *Vom Wasser,* 17, 9, 1949.
10. **Bullock, G. L.,** Pseudomonadales as fish pathogens, *Dev. Ind. Microbiol.,* 5, 101, 1964.
11. **Bullock, G. L.,** Characteristics and pathogenicity of a capsulated *Pseudomonas* isolated from goldfish, *Appl. Microbiol.,* 13, 89, 1965.
12. **Bullock, G. L., Snieszko, S. F., and Dunbar, C. E.,** Characteristics and identification of oxidative pseudomonads isolated from diseased fish, *J. Gen. Microbiol.,* 38, 1, 1965.
13. **Bullock, G. L., Conroy, D. A., and Snieszko, S. F.,** *Bacterial Diseases of Fish,* THF Publications, Neptune City, N.J., 1971, 21.
14. **Bullock, G. L., Stuckey, H. M., and Chen, P. K.,** Corynebacterial kidney disease of salmonids: growth and serological studies on the causative bacterium, *Appl. Microbiol.,* 28, 811, 1974.
15. **Buttiaux, R.,** Salmonella problems in the sea, in *Fish as Food,* Vol . 2, Borgstrom, G., Ed., Academic Press, New York, 1962, 503.
16. **Campbell, G. and Mackelvic, R. M.,** Infection of brook trout (*Salnelines fontinalis*) by nocardiae, *J. Fish. Res. Board Can.,* 25, 423, 1968.
17. **Conroy, D.,** Tail rot in fish, *Nature* (London), 201, 732, 1964.
18. **Emmerich, R. and Weikel, E.,** Uber eine durch bakterien verursachte Infektions krankheit der forellen, *Allg. Fisch. Ztg.,* 15, 73 and 85, 1890.
19. **Emmerich, R. and Weikel, E.,** Uber eine durch bakterien erzeugte Seuche unter den farellen, *Arch. Hyg. Bakteriol.,* 21, 1, 1894.
20. **Evelyn, T. P. T.,** An aberrant strain of the bacterial fish pathogen *Aeromonas salmonicida* isolated from a marine sablefish (*Anoplopoma fimbria*) and from two sepcies of cultured Pacific salmon, *J. Fish. Res. Board Can.,* 28, 1629, 1971.
21. **Ghittino, P. and Penna, R.,** Recherches microbiologiques sur la nocardiose de la truite arc-en-ciel, *Off. Int. Epizoot. Bull.,* 69, 1045, 1968.
22. **Glantz, P. J. and Krantz, G. E.,** *Escherichia coli* serotypes isolated from fish and their environment, *Health Lab. Sci.,* 2, 54, 1965.
23. **Gratzek, J. B., Shotts, E. B., and Blue, J. L.,** A survey of parasites, bacteria and viruses associated with tropical fish imported from Southeast Asia, *Aquatic Mammals,* 4, 1, 1976.
24. **Greig, E. D. W.,** *A System of Bacteriology,* Vol. 5, British Medical Research Council, London, 1930, 339.
25. **Griffin, P. J.,** The nature of bacteria pathogenic to fish, *Trans. Am. Fish. Soc.,* 83, 241, 1954.
26. **Guelin, A.,** Polluted waters and the contamination of fish, in *Fish as Food,* Vol. 2, Borgstrom, G., Ed., Academic Press, New York, 1962, 481.
27. **Hoshina, T., Sano, T., and Morimoto, U.,** A streptococcus pathogenic to fish, *J. Toyko Univ. Fish.,* 44, 57, 1958.
28. **Heuschmann-Brunner, G.,** Norcardioses bei Fischen des Susswasser's und des Meeres, *Tieraerztl. Wochenschr.,* 5, 94, 1965.
29. **Janssen, W. A. and Meyers, C. D.,** Fish: serologic evidence of infection with human pathogens, *Science,* 159, 547, 1968.
30. **Li, M. F. and Fleming, C.,** A proteolytic pseudomonad from skin lesions of rainbow trout. I. Characteristics of the pathogenic effects and the extracellular proteinase, *Can. J. Microbiol.,* 13, 405, 1967.
31. **Lyayman, E. M.,** *Textbook on the Diseases of Fish,* 3rd ed., Izdanja Vpshays Skkola Moscow, 1966, 115.
32. **Martin, W. T.,** personal communication, 1977.
33. **Maestrome, G. and Benjaminson, M. A.,** Leptospira infection in the goldfish, *Nature* (London), 195, 719, 1962.
34. **Martin, W. T.,** Occurrence and Survival of *Salmonella* in the Alimentary Tract of Some Freshwater Fishes, M. S. thesis, Kansas State University, Manhattan, 1966.
35. **McCarthy, D. H. and Rawle, C. T.,** The rapid serological diagnosis of fish furunculosis caused by "smooth" and "rough" strains of *Aeromonas salmonicida, J. Gen. Microbiol.,* 86, 185, 1975.
36. **McCarthy, D.,** personal communication, 1977.
37. **Meyer, F. P. and Bullock, G. L.,** *Edwardiella tarda,* a new pathogen of channel catfish (*Ictalurus punctatus*), *Appl. Microbiol.,* 25, 155, 1977.
38. **Meyer, K. F.,** *Pasteurella* and *Francisella,* in *Bacterial and Mycotic Infections of Man,* 4th ed., Dubos, R. J. and Hirsch, J. G., Eds., Lippincott, Philadelphia, 1965, 685.
39. **Pacha, R. E. and Porter, S.,** Characteristics of mycobacteria isolated from the surface of freshwater fish, *Appl. Microbiol.,* 16, 1901, 1968.

40. **Pacha, R. E. and Ordal, J. E.**, Mycobacterial diseases of salmonids, in *A Symposium on Diseases of Fishes and Shellfishes,* Spec. Publ. No. 5, Sneiszko, S. F., Ed., American Fisheries Society, Washington, D.C., 1970, 243.

41. **Plumb, J. A., Schachte, J. H., Gaines, J. L., Peltier, W., and Carroll, B.**, *Streptococcus* sp. from marine fishes along the Alabama and northwest Florida coast of the Gulf of Mexico, *Trans. Am. Fish. Soc.,* 103, 358, 1974.

42. **Pollitzer, K.**, Cholera, World Health Organization, Geneva, 1959, 174.

43. **Poppensick, G. C.**, *Aquatic Animal Health,* National Academy of Sciences, Washington, D.C., 1973, 46.

44. **Post, G.**, A preliminary report on the use of nitroguran compounds for furunculosis of trout, with special emphasis on furoxone, *Prog. Fish Cult.,* 21, 30, 1959.

45. **Reichenbach-Klinke, H. and Elkan, E.**, *The Principal Disease of Lower Vertebrates,* Academic Press, New York, 1965, 190.

46. **Robinson, J. and Meyer, F.**, Streptococcal fish pathogen, *J. Bacteriol.,* 92, 512, 1966.

47. **Ross, A. J., Earp, B. J., and Wood, J. W.**, Mycobacterial infections in adult salmon and steelhead trout returning to the Columbia River basin and other areas in 1957, in Fisheries, Spec. Sci. Rep. No. 332, United States Department of Interior, Washington, D.C., 1959,

48. **Ross, A. J., Rucker, R. R., and Ewing, W. H.**, Description of a bacterium associated with red mouth disease of rainbow trout (*Salmo gairdneri*), *Can. J. Microbiol.,* 12, 763, 1966.

49. **Ross, A. J., Martin, J. E., and Bressler, V.**, *Vibrio anguillarum* from an epizootic in rainbow trout (*Salmo gairdneri*) in the USA, *Off. Int. Epizoot. Bull.,* 69, 1139, 1968.

50. **Rucker, R. R.**, Red mouth disease of rainbow trout (*Salmo gairdneri*), *Off. Int. Epizoot, Bull.,* 65, 825, 1966.

51. **Schaperclaus, W.**, Unterschungen uber die Aalseuchen in deutschen Binnenund Kustenwassen, 1930-1933, *Z. Fisch. Deren Hilfswiss,* 32, 191, 1934.

52. **Schubert, R. H. W.**, Zur Taxonomie der anerogenen Aeromonaden, *Zentralbl. Bakteriol. Parasitenlck. Infektionskr. Hyg. Abt.1.: Orig.,* 193, 343, 1964.

53. **Shewan, J. M,** Food poisoning caused fish and fishery products, in *Fish as Food,* Vol. 2, Borgestrom, G., Ed., Academic Press, New York, 1964, 443.

54. **Shotts, E. B., Gaines, J. L., Martin, L., and Prestwood, A. K.**, Aeromonas-induced deaths among fish and reptiles in an eutrophic inland lake, *J. Am. Vet. Med. Assoc.,* 161, 603, 1972.

55. **Shotts, E. B. and Rimler, R. B.**, Medium for the isolation of *Aeromonas hydrophila,* Appl. Microbiol., 26, 550, 1973.

56. **Shotts, E. B. and Bullock, G. L.**, Bacterial diseases of fish: diagnostic procedures for gram negative pathogens, *J. Fish. Res. Board Can.,* 32, 1243, 1975.

57. **Shotts, E. B. and Bullock, G. L.**, Rapid diagnostic approaches in the identification of Gram-negative bacterial disease of fish, *Fish Pathol.,* 10, 187, 1976.

58. **Shotts, E. B., Kleckner, A. L., Gratzek, J. B., and Blue, J. L.**, Bacterial flora of aquarium fishes and their shipping waters imported from Southeast Asia, *J. Fish. Res. Board Can.,* 33, 732, 1976.

59. **Shotts, E. B. and Gratzek, J. B.**, unpublished data, 1977.

60. **Shotts, E. B., Gratzek, J. B., and Blue, J. L.**, unpublished data, 1977.

61. **Smith, I.**, The occurrence and pathology of Dee disease, *Freshwater Salmon Fish. Res.,* 34, 1, 1964.

62. **Snieszko, S. F., Gutsell, J. S., and Friddle, S. B.**, Various sulfonamides treatment of furunculosis on brook trout (*Salnelinus fontinalis*), *Trans. Am. Fish. Soc.,* 78, 181, 1950.

63. **Snieszko, S. F., Griffin, P. J., and Friddle, S. B.**, Antibiotic treatment of ulcer disease and furunculosis in trout, *Trans. North Am. Wildl. Conf.,* 17, 197, 1952.

64. **Snieszko, S. F., Bullock, G. L., Hollis, E., and Boone, J. G.**, *Pasteurella* sp. from an epizootic of white perch (*Roccus americanus*) in Chesapeake Bay tidewater areas, *J. Bacteriol.,* 88, 1814, 1964.

65. **Snieszko, S. F.**, Remarks on some facets of epizootiology of bacterial fish diseases, *Dev. Ind. Microbiol.,* 5, 97, 1964.

66. **Tung, M.**, Channel Catfish; A Potential Carrier of Salmonella, M. S. thesis, University of Georgia, Athens, 1972.

67. **Von Gravenitz, A. and Mensch, A. H.**, The genus *Aeromonas* in human bacteriology, report of 30 cases and review of literature, *N. Engl. J. Med.,* 278, 245, 1968.

68. **Wakabayashi, H. and Egusa, S.**, *Edwardsiella tarda* (*Paracolobacterium anguillimortiferum*) associated with pond-cultured eel disease, *Bull. Jpn. Soc. Sci. Fish,* 39, 931, 1973.

69. **Wang, L. R., Colwell, R., Lovelace, T. E., and Krantz, G. E.**, Isolation of *Vibrio parahemalyticus* from Chesapeake Bay, *Bacteriol. Proc.,* 1, 1969.

70. **Wohlgemuth, K., Pierce, R. L., and Kirkbride, C. A.**, Bovine abortion associated with *Aeromonas hydrophila, J. Am. Vet. Med. Assoc.,* 161, 603, 1972.

71. **Wood, J. W. and Ordal, E. J.**, Tuberculosis in Pacific salmon and steelhead trout, *Fish Commission of Oregon, Contribution* No. 25, 1958.

72. **Wood, J.**, Diseases of Pacific Salmon. Their Prevention and Treatment, State Department of Fish, Hatchery Division, Seattle, Wash., 1968.

73. **Zen-Yoji, H., Sakai, S., Terama, T., Kudo, Y., and Hitogoto, H.**, Studies on the interopathogenic halophilic bacteria. I. On the epidemiology of food poisoning due to halophilic bacteria in Toyko District during 1961, and bacteriological examination, *J. Jpn. Infect. Dis. Assoc.*, 37, 195, 1963.

ZOONOSES — AN INTERNATIONAL PROBLEM *

B. Velimirovic**

There are, of course, excellent books on zoonoses, but the dynamic of science is rapid — the world output of new books is about 1000 per day. New scientific and technical information was generated at a rate of about two million documents (six million pages) per year in 1970. American doctors handle approximately 25 million pieces of medical information monthly and there are some 30,000 to 100,000 scientific journals. In *Ulrich's International Periodical Directory*, 56,000 are listed — 220 subjects, of which more than one half concern the sciences, medicine, and technology — and this only in Latin-derived languages! Thus, it is now difficult to assess all that is new even in one's own narrowly defined speciality.

Over the last decade, there has been considerable change in the importance of certain zoonotic communicable diseases in many parts of the world, resulting from ecological changes such as urbanization, industrialization, a diminishing proportion of persons working in the so-called primary sector: agricultural production branches in developed countries. Furthermore, the new technology and public health measures such as legislation, vaccination, and antibiotic treatment have changed the nature of the risk and fear of the zoonoses that remain. This, however, does not mean that the teaching of zoonoses has lost its importance. It means only that the role of the veterinarian has changed in those countries and is moving closer to the ever more important field of food hygiene (e.g., residual antibiotics and insecticides used in livestock and found in food products), and toward comparative medicine, increased use of laboratory animals (often imported from afar), biomedical research in general, monitoring of environmental hazards, and medical ecology. We do not know with what challenges nature will confront us in the world of constant interference with ecology. Even now, when a new disease occurs, the paraphrased advice, "cherchez l'animal," is valid. Reference the various types of encephalitis, eosinophilic meningitis, capillariasis, anisakiasis, monkeypox disease in humans, Lassa fever and Marburg disease, and African and other hemorrhagic fevers, all for which an animal link has been found.

Zoonoses occur throughout the world, transcending national boundaries. Their important effect on global economy and health is well known, from the international movement of animals and importation of diseases to bans on importation of animal products and even to seemingly unrelated problems such as the obstacles confronted during construction of the Pan American Highway. Epidemiological surveillance of zoonoses is no longer solely a national problem — continental and ultimately global surveillance is now necessary. It has also become obvious that with recognition of the interrelationships between countries, the consequent internationalization of control efforts, and the realization that these efforts are becoming more and more relevant to technical, economic, and social fields, it has become easier to obtain support through the World Bank, the International Bank for Development, the United Nations Development Program, etc., particularly for control of foot-and-mouth disease, brucellosis, bovine tuberculosis, and cysticercosis. Zoonoses control is no longer marginal to international assistance, as FAO and WHO have known, of course, for a long time. Thus, control of zoonoses retains its prominent place among the activities of WHO and PAHO, according to the health and economic problems specific to each region.

* Paper presented at the Zoonoses Symposium, School of Public Health, University of Texas Health Science Center at Houston, June 20 to 22, 1977.
** The author alone is responsible for views expressed in this article.

Speaking from my own experience (more than 15 years in international health work on several continents) dealing with veterinarians, particularly in trying to win their cooperation in epidemiological endeavors, I have seen two extreme poles: (1) those mainly or almost exclusively dedicated to private practice (e.g., serving racetracks or household pets) and generally not interested in public health issues and (2) those at the other extreme, who want to demonstrate a more comprehensive role for the profession by entering positions held at some time by physicians and that, paradoxically, the medical profession has left to better equipped, nonmedically trained professional groups such as engineers, statisticians, chemists, demographers, economists, system analysts, physicists, managers, etc. This trend originated in part from the real need for indispensable research as well as from the need for socioeconomic and ecologic evaluation of zoonoses. However, between these two extremes was the largest group, interested in disease control and food and animal production.

Veterinarians have been visionaries and pioneers in mass testing and immunization, epidemiology, and vector control, all of which are useful for combating diseases of livestock and man. In so doing, they have earned full recognition from the health "team" as qualified, medically trained specialists. A profession concerned with control and prevention of zoonotic diseases of human and animal significance and fighting for the health of animals, veterinary medicine is increasingly extending its responsibility and importance. Its practitioners are in short supply. Of some 250,000 veterinarians throughout the world, more than half are in three countries: the U.S., U.S.S.R., and Japan. Even in the U.S., *Public Health Reports* (1977) states: "Veterinary medical schools must increase first-year enrollment during the next 4 years by 5%, and they must also assure that clinical training will emphasize care of food- or fiber-producing animals." If we discount Egypt and South Africa, there are only 1659 veterinarians remaining on the entire African continent, and there are no more than 17,056 in the whole of Asia.

One should perhaps also ask, is there an international "type" or are there many different types of professionals, according to particular interest, educational background and, last but not least, to the economy and prevalent zoonoses in the respective countries. There is a wide variety of curricula in teaching institutions, and in a survey conducted by PAHO, only 50.9% of students thought that veterinary schools prepare the graduating veterinarian for his or her role in community health activities, of which the general public and sometimes medical personnel are not aware, and the teaching of which, if elective, would probably not be selected by a majority of students.[3] Thus, a new type of public health-oriented worker — with global vision, interested, skeptical, questioning, and able to anticipate future problems — is very necessary if the challenges are to be met.

My contention is that veterinarians have, in addition to prevention of animal diseases transmissible to man (e.g., rabies and brucellosis) and improvement of food hygiene (particularly in respect to microbial and environmental contaminants),* another evermore important function that is easily overlooked. They have moved, together with agriculturists, to the forefront of the fight for survival, the fight against starvation. Today, malnutrition has emerged as the major "health problem" of the world, and the number of persons suffering from its clinical manifestations reach several million.

Synergistic association of nutritional deficiency with infectious diseases and child mortality is well known. Although the food gap rather than the protein gap is mainly

---

* In 1974, the Center for Disease Control reported 456 outbreaks of food-borne diseases involving 15,489 persons. Bacterial contaminants were responsible for 85 to 95% of all cases.

responsible, proteins are already scarce. A pertinent question is, will the supply keep up with the population increase? For animal products, practical increases in effective world-consumption demand projected for 1985 are (1) in meat — 56% and (2) in milk and dairy products — 43% greater than the relative increase in population. To increase animal protein and satisfy the biological needs of humanity, adequate control of animal diseases is necessary. In the Americas, the potential for increased production is greater than in many other parts of the world; hence, the importance of the veterinary profession has another dimension. Loss due to animal tuberculosis alone costs more than $1½ billion, and it is said that, in terms of dollars, this loss exceeds all of the foreign aid given to South America. It is not by chance that the "Ten-Year Plan for Health for the Americas, created by PAHO, requires reduction of protein deficiency and malnutrition through zoonoses control.

Let us turn to a field of food production in which I see another increased need for veterinarians and zoonoses control in the future. I expect that not everyone will agree. "Conventional wisdom — of both the collectivist Left and the feudal Right — is that food production, also production of animal proteins, can be best achieved by large farms as the individual peasant will end by creating a depressed peasantry, too ignorant and small-minded to apply the knowledge that is necessary if productivity is to be increased."[5] This is based on the knowledge that there are essentially only four cereal surplus-producing countries — the U.S., Canada, Australia, and Argentina — that provide 75% of the grain needs of developing countries. From an average per capita consumption of food grains of about 1 ton/year in the affluent countries, only about 70 kg are consumed directly, while the remaining 930 kg are used as animal feed to produce meat, milk, and eggs for human consumption. All four countries mentioned above use a highly mechanized style of farming. (In the U.S., there are only two workers per 100 acres.) It is true but forgotten that these countries have no acute population pressure, whereas in developing countries the situation is different. In spite of the disastrous "urban bias" in economies run by bureaucrats and politicians, who risk dependancy on foreign aid, and despite the staggering rate of migration to the cities, the rural population of the developing world almost doubled in the last 50 years, whereas acreage of agricultural land increased by only one fourth. The urban population increased even more rapidly, e.g., in Latin America, it will represent 60 to 70% of the total population. With unemployment rates of more than 15%, more and more persons are finding food (particularly animal protein) out of reach. "For employment to grow at a rate of 4.5% per year in the urban areas of the developing world would be a tremendous achievement, beyond anything that has been achieved in the past. Yet a 4.5% growth in urban jobs would provide work for an increase in the total rural and urban labor force of only 1.3%, or approximately one half of the increase anticipated."[8]

Although cities cannot usefully employ this ever-increasing number of people, nothing is done to stop the flight and forced exodus to slums and shanty towns, assuming that large farms are more productive and that there is thus nothing technically wrong with the tendency toward displacement of small farming (in terms of overall output), even if it is disastrous from human and social standpoints. For example, in one country, 64.2% of the agricultural land belongs to 3.6% of the population, while 4.2% of the land is owned by 56% of the population.[9] There are many such countries. "But it has been established — and the World Bank has accepted these findings — that the intensity of land use declines as farm size rises in developing countries. Both FAO and the World Bank found independently that a smaller average size of holding and a low concentration of ownership produced an increase in output per hectare. Fertilizer production is likely to run into even more problems, and the warning signals are already out.''[5,6] Although protein deficiency in developing countries is expected to be solved largely by vegetable sources (through an appropriate mix), animal protein will remain the main desideratum of the masses. Expectations are outstripping the socioeconomic resources in large parts of the world, and those resources are further strained by unnecessary losses due to disease-related factors.

The proof of whether any system works is whether it feeds, clothes, shelters, and provides its constituents with reasonable health services. Experience shows that the systems of developed countries score poorly in developing countries because the realities, e.g., population growth, are different. Thus, small farming is considered by many development economists to be an alternative to starvation[5] — not a return to a sort of idyllic, pastoral-type mystique, but an agricultural revolution with fair prices, available credit, and on-the-spot technical assistance and tools and including incentive goods and concentrated social effort. Where possible, this should parallel to volume industrial production. The growing social and nutritional distress of both individuals and nations may hopefully lead to a salutory reappraisal centered around actual human needs.

Development is a complex process with many determinants and cannot be simply reduced to one formula, but the food outlook is grim, and every alternative aiming to achieve self-sufficiency merits serious consideration. It is certainly absurd that, for example, milk has to be imported to a Latin American country that has the largest milk-producing capacity of any country on the continent. Self-sufficiency and total rural employment, not the increasing distribution of food to an ever larger world population, is the primary objective for the future. If this alternative is accepted, more primary protein-producing animals will have to be kept by more small farmers; thus, more control of zoonoses, i.e., wider spread of knowledge to more people over a larger area under a variety of conditions, will be needed. For (1) decreasing the risk to exposed persons and preventing disease in humans and (2) increasing production, man is the most important factor of production. However, the responsibility for production of protein belongs to predominantly rural, overpopulated, and economically and politically destitute areas. It rests on those persons most likely to be in contact with, be exposed to, or suffer from zoonoses, the same persons who are least likely to have access to adequate health services. Thus, knowledge of zoonoses control must be brought to the producer; it should not remain in the ivory towers of the universities. Inaccessible knowledge is not useful. It must be used for adequate training of all health professionals, medical and veterinary, and applied in developing regions.

In the meantime, your work will provide the basis for taking stock of present knowledge, understood as a scientific quest for truth, not simply information. Scientific achievements are not final and cannot be dogmatic; however well supported by experiment, observation, and theory, they are not exempt from further research and analysis that could make them obsolete tomorrow. Research and international cooperation is obviously necessary in problems of global magnitude. Even problems manageable on the local level look different from a regional or intercontinental perspective. The whole world is today exposed to challenges which must be met jointly. To use a quote from T. S. Eliot:

The endless cycle of idea and action,
Endless invention, endless experiment,
Brings knowledge of motion but not of stillness.
Where is the life, we have lost in living?
Where is the wisdom we have lost in knowledge?
Where is the knowledge we have lost in information?[10]

REFERENCES

1. **Anderla, G.,** Information in 1985, A Forecasting Study of Information Needs and Resources, Organization for Economic Cooperation and Development, Paris, 1973, 15.
2. **Whiteside, D. F.,** Training the nation's health manpower — the next four years, *Public Health Rep.,* 92(2), 99, 1977.
3. A competency-based curriculum for veterinary public health and preventive medicine, *Pan Am. Health Organ. Sci. Publ.,* 313, 23; 25, 1975.
4. **Hubbard, H. B.,** Impact of animal disease on protein of animal origin in Latin America, *Inter. Am. Med.,* 2(1), 13, 1977.
5. **Power, J.,** The alternative to starvation, *Encounter,* 45(5), 20; 24, 1975.
6. FAO Production Book, Food and Agricultural Organization, Rome, 1971, 10; 21; 23.
7. United Nations Monthly Bulletin of Statistics, 26(4), April 1972 and 27(11), November 1973.
8. **McNamara, R.,** *One Hundred Countries, Two Billion People,* Praeger, New York, 1973, 63.
9. **Aguirre, A.,** *Stud. Fam. Plann.,* 1(11), 1, 1966.
10. **Eliot, T. S.,** Choruses from the rock, cited by Bell, D., Teletext and technology, *Encounter,* 18(6), 9, 1977.

INTERNATIONAL COOPERATION ON ZOONOSES CONTROL IN THE AMERICAS*

F. Mulhern

Before I comment on international cooperation on zoonoses control in the Americas, I would like to discuss the situation and explain why there is a need for such control. "The world is shrinking" has become a common cliche, and although it is not physically diminishing, the rapid pace with which we and our animals move around in it, compared to a generation or two ago, does give one the feeling that it has become smaller.

Naturally, as people and animals (and their by-products) moved, they took many things with them, one of which was zoonotic disease. There was a time when we were somewhat isolationist — we will take care of our diseases and you will take care of yours. We now know that this is obsolete thinking.

Zoonoses take a heavy toll and should be of concern to all. I do not believe that, because we in the U.S. have more resources and fewer disease problems than others, we should be critical of those who are less fortunate. In fact, we should be pooling our resources — money, people, and brain power — to unravel many of the unanswered questions that plague those who work in zoonoses control in the Americas.

We know relatively little about the epidemiology of most infectious, contagious diseases whether or not they are zoonotic. We concentrate on diseases of great importance, but despite all of the literature published over the years, we often find essential data lacking to help us fight the diseases in our changing times. What worked yesterday will not necessarily work today. Even with a disease like brucellosis that we have been trying to control and eradicate for 40 years, there are many unanswered questions.

I do not know how much is known about the exchange of viral, bacterial, or parasitic diseases among persons living in close concentration in our ghettos or when there is mass movement under close confinement, as in the ships that brought my parents from Ireland. However, I do know that we in the U.S. should know a great deal more about what happens to these agents since thousands of animals are moved in and out of concentration points each day throughout our country. Likewise, we need to know much more about what is happening to them during their time in feedlots or wherever we are raising large numbers of animals under close confinement.

I am not referring only to those diseases that appear outwardly among them; I am talking about a greater understanding of what is happening to whatever host-parasite relationships are occurring simultaneously when large numbers of animals are being moved. We in the U.S. Department of Agriculture (USDA) became more involved with the concept when we were criticized for not attacking salmonellosis on a large enough scale to reduce its prevalence in livestock and poultry and thus reduce the number of human food-poisoning cases attributed to the disease.

Today, as in the past, we are dealing with these diseases in a very elementary fashion compared with the sophistication that we should have because of the emphasis placed on improved technology in recent decades. We should be able to predict what will happen with the various agents as we move animals within and between our countries.

We are often unaware of what happens to these agents when a vaccine is introduced into the population, or several strains of vaccines in some cases. Oh yes, we know

---

* Paper presented at the Zoonoses Symposium, School of Public Health, University of Texas Health Science Center at Houston, June 20 to 22, 1977.

what effects this may have on the clinical evidence of the disease for which it was administered, but what are the long-term effects on other animals in the herd or in the area?

We know what diseases do appear as we move animals into concentration points because a cadre of veterinarians and paramedics is usually in the sick bay treating or vaccinating them for certain afflictions. In raising cattle, hogs, and poultry under confinement — which we have done for years — we have resorted to antibiotics and growth promoters in the feed.

Today, we see indications that this may not continue at its present rate since the use of these additives in feed is being questioned. Here again we know that their use enabled animals and poultry to gain weight more quickly, but what was actually happening within their bodies?

Back to our shrinking world, or more specifically our shrinking hemisphere, more persons traveled in and out of U.S. ports last year than we have in the total population of this country. Our livestock and poultry owners have private planes that enable them to commute between countries to look at, buy, or sell animals. One day they are on a ranch in South America looking at cattle and the next day in their own pastures, grasslands, or feedlots.

Billions of pounds of meat and other animal by-products enter or leave through our ports legally. This figure does not include the tons of prohibited animal by-products taken from passengers' baggage annually as they come into our ports nor the smuggled products and birds that are not caught.

Markets being used by the industries involved can oftentimes be the same, thus also intertwining the relationships of the animal health officials concerned. Naturally, there is a great howl for uniformity of treatment and for keeping up with the advancement of science in the application of disease-control techniques.

There is no doubt that the need for international cooperation in controlling zoonoses and other diseases is essential and is in fact taking place — not to the degree that it should, but the fact that control is moving evermore in that direction is heartening.

Prior to World War II, there was some exchange of veterinary personnel and other scientists between the countries of North America, Central America, and Panama, but it was on a somewhat limited scale. Shortly after the war there was a broader recognition of the need for closer cooperation when Dr. Fred Soper was placed in an influential position within the Pan American Health Organization (PAHO). Just a small cadre of personnel was assigned to countries in South America and Mexico, but this was a step in the right direction.

At about this time — 1947 — foot-and-mouth disease broke out in Mexico, and the U.S. provided that country with manpower and funds in a joint eradication program. This emergency produced an atmosphere very conducive to blending the values of persons from both countries in the shortest possible time.

The objective of eradication was reached despite what many said were unsurmountable odds. The potential existing for added cooperation of this type in other programs, especially zoonosis control, became quite obvious.

Shortly after this, PAHO established regional centers, and the Zoonoses Center that was to serve all of South America was established in Argentina. Also about this time, Organization International Regional Sanidad Agropecuaria (OIRSA) was formed. It was originally established to more effectively combat plant pests such as the Mediterranean fruit fly, but the organization also had a great interest in keeping countries free of foot-and-mouth disease. The Food and Agricultural Organization (FAO) has become involved in personnel training, but I do not believe it has played as extensive a role as it has in other parts of the world. The Office of International Epizootics (OIE) has been mainly a disease-reporting organization in this hemisphere.

During the past 20 years, there has been an acceleration in the exchange of scientists among the countries of the Americas with noted improvements. Emphasis has been placed on veterinary education, training, research, and diagnostic capabilities.

Inter-American banks have recognized a major weakness in the efforts to improve zoonosis and other disease control — lack of an effective infrastructure staffed with persons of high professional competency. In recent years, they have developed 12 loans with 11 countries for a total of $107,300,000. In order for those countries to be eligible for such loans, they had to provide $293,434,000 as an indication of their commitment.

The area of chief concern is whether or not there is enough enthusiastic commitment to fulfill regulatory requirements. Unless this is recognized, much of the effort to date will have been of little value. Getting persons to commit themselves fully to regulatory responsibilities is not an easy accomplishment even in the U.S.

The USDA has encouraged participation by all international zoonosis organizations in the Americas because improvements made by any one of them will benefit all of the countries involved. It is also quite evident that the greatest risks from zoonoses probably exist between the countries of the Americas.

It is unfortunate that so little money and manpower is available for the PAHO Zoonoses Center. We who have been involved in recommending increased activities by the Center are limited in getting our recommendations accepted because of the priorities established for all projects within the PAHO.

Definite positive steps are being taken to increase cooperation among our countries. It seems that OIRSA pointed the way back in the 1950s on the need for regional projects to combat diseases of the Western Hemisphere; we have been working for years on separate programs with Mexico and Canada, and annual meetings are now being held among the three countries.

After the experience with Venezuelan equine encephalomyelitis, we have had more frequent contacts with the countries of Central America and, naturally, with OIRSA. There are more meetings and better communication among countries of the Caribbean than ever before; all recognize the effects of these interrelationships.

PAHO has done much to bring the countries together to recognize their total needs. This organization has had annual meetings at the Minister of Agriculture level for the past 10 years, providing veterinary officials of each country with an opportunity to learn about progress — or lack of it — and to plan for the future. In addition, it has done much to train personnel, improve diagnostic capabilities, and provide valuable research to meet the needs of the Americas. This organization also provides needed leadership in zoonoses control, especially for Central and South America and the Carribean countries.

Countries do not have to be told what needs to be done — that was established long ago. They do need the resources and, equally important, the will and commitment to do what is necessary to substantially reduce losses from zoonoses and other diseases. We need not be discouraged by the slow rate of progress. We do need to be *encouraged* by the progress that is being made.

There may be criticism of how funds are utilized, but like the Alaskan pipeline, one day the objective will be reached.

I believe there are good working relationships among the veterinary officials of most of our countries. I see the need to pool our total interests and resources in the control of zoonoses and other diseases, to make each other aware of what we are doing, and to establish a common direction for improving zoonoses control within the Western Hemisphere.

We are all more aware than ever of the fact that unlimited resources are not available — especially manpower and funds — for zoonoses control. However, surely diseases communicable to man and animals should have a high priority as we evaluate our nations' needs. All those in areas of influence should do everything that they can to stress and improve international cooperation for zoonoses control in the Americas as a meaningful step in improving the health status of the world.

CONTAGIOUS EQUINE METRITIS

J. S. Walker

INTRODUCTION

The information contained in this section was obtained from the references listed and personal communication with investigators, veterinarians, and horse breeders in the U.K. and Ireland during an investigative visit by a team from the U.S. in September 1977.

The parts concerning gynecological veterinary examination of mares and stud hygiene are taken directly from the David, Frank, and Powell article (Suggested Reading Number 7).

Members of the team that investigated the situation in the U.K. and Ireland included Drs. R. C. Knowles, Animal and Plant Health Inspection Service; J. Moul-throp, Animal and Plant Health Inspection Service; J. S. Walker, Plum Island Animal Disease Center, Science and Education Administration, Federal Research; and W. R. McGee, American Association Equine Practitioners.

IDENTIFICATION OF DISEASE

Definition

Contagious equine metritis (CEM), also termed contagious metritis 1977, is a highly contagious, acute venereal disease of horses that severely affects breeding operations and fertility.

Etiology

The causative organism is a bacterium, *Hemophilus equigenitals.* The nonmotile coccobacillus is Gram-negative. It is catalase and oxidase positive and is characterized by being very unreactive or completely negative on standard bacteriological differential tests commonly used. The medium used for primary isolation is chocolate agar incubated at 37°C in an atmosphere of hydrogen or air containing 5 to 10% CO_2. When Eugon agar is used as a base for the chocolate agar, the colonies can be observed after 24-hr incubation. The colonies are shiny, smooth, butyrous, and slightly gray. After prolonged incubation, (beyond 72 hr), the colonies appear white, raised, and glistening. An aid to isolation of this organism from field specimens is its resistance to streptomycin, although some strains are sensitive.

Unpublished data indicate that after about seven passages in the laboratory, the organism starts to lose virulence for the horse and dependency on CO_2 for in vitro growth. Both of these characteristics apparently can be restored by in vivo passage.

History

The disease was first officially reported in the early summer of 1977 in the U.K. where 29 thoroughbred horse stud farms around Newmarket were affected so greatly that some of them were forced to close. The British have estimated that the economic losses to the thoroughbred industry during the 1977 breeding season totaled at least $30 million. Information recently obtained revealed that CEM occurred on at least four stud farms in Ireland during both the 1976 spring breeding season and the 1976 fall breeding season. It recurred in Ireland again during the 1977 breeding season, as well as in France. Although unconfirmed, some reports indicate that CEM may have occurred in France before 1976.

Interestingly, Ireland, the U.K., and France entered into a tripartite agreement in the early 1970s by which free movement of horses was allowed among the three countries without quarantine and with minimal veterinary inspection.

CEM occurred in Australia during the 1977 breeding season. As of February 1978, CEM has been diagnosed on six stud farms in Australia in three difrerent states. All cases except three mares were directly traceable to horses imported during the last year from the three countries in Europe involved in the outbreak. This means the infected horses carried the organism for several months.

As of September 1977, the U.S. and Canada placed a ban on the importation of all equidae except geldings, weanlings, and yearlings from Ireland, the U.K., France, and Australia.

CEM was diagnosed in the U.S. during the breeding seasons of 1978 and 1979 in Kentucky and in 1979 in Missouri. The original sourse of the outbreak in Kentucky was traced to two stallions from France that were imported just before the importation ban went into effect. The disease was also reported during the 1978 breeding season in West Germany and Belgium.

SIGNS OF DISEASE

Clinical Features

To the clinician or stud owner, the first noticeable indication that anything is wrong is that suddenly each mare being covered by a particular stallion starts coming back into premature estrus and is what the horse clinicians term dirty on vaginal examination. Upon routine aerobic culture, no specific important organism is isolated during certain phases of the infection except perhaps *Proteus* sp. and other secondary invaders or opportunistic organisms. However, when special culture techniques are used, the Gram-negative coccobacillus can be isolated. The role that *Proteus* sp. and other opportunistic organisms play in the total disease picture has not yet been fully defined.

The infection is characterized by an endometritis associated with cervicitis and vaginitis. A copious mucopurulent discharge is sometimes seen coming from the vulva, smearing the buttocks, and matting the tail. However, the severity varies from mares that have an almost complete sloughing of the endometrium to mares that appear almost clinically normal on examination but are in premature estrus.

The stallion is completely normal upon examination and shows no clinical signs of disease, yet they may remain carriers and transmit the disease for extended periods of time. One stallion in Ireland contracted the disease in the spring of 1976, was treated with ampicillin during the early summer, and still infected mares during the 1976 fall breeding season. Thus, the stallion in CEM appears to play the identical role in the spread of the disease that the bull does in *Trichomonas*.

Little is known at this time about chronic asymptomatic carriers; however, there are such carriers. For example, Gram-negative coccobacillus can still be isolated from two mares in England that are 200-plus days in foal. They were infected early in 1977, treated, cleared up clinically, and conceived when rebred in the early summer. However, the Gram-negative coccobacillus has been isolated from practically every swab during the pregnancy. Another known example is a barren mare in England that had a severe case of the disease early in 1977, was treated, but was not rebred. She became completely normal on clinical examination and was negative for the organism on two consecutive estrus cycles, yet reverted to positive on the third estrus cycle.

The true incidence of abortions caused by CEM is unknown at this time. However, some mares do abort, generally within the first 60 days of pregnancy; these mares were judged in foal on 3- and 6-week examinations but came up empty on 90- and 120-day examinations.

Incubation Period

The incubation period varies from 2 to 14 days under natural conditions. Although experimental work is preliminary at this stage, appparently the average incubation period is 2 to 4 days for the appearance of exudate in the vaginal tract; inflammation of the cervix and vaginal mucosa is maximal about 5 to 10 days post-inoculation.

PATHOLOGIC CHANGES

Post-mortem Lesions

Very few mares have been examined; thus, the description given here is subject to change. The gross lesions varied from a slightly enlarged uterus containing a small amount of grayish fluid to an almost normal uterus. More extensive changes have been reported; however, they are probably the results of secondary infections. Thus, apparently, the gross pathology varies greatly, as do the clinical signs.

Microlesions

This information is based on endometrial biopsy material. Infected mares showed changes of focal luminal epithelial hyperplasia and very marked degenerative changes at sites immediately below the luminal epithelium at the junction with the stratum compactum. Some epithelial cells showed advanced cytoplasmic and nuclear degenerative change; subepithelial vacuoles containing amorphous debris sometimes gave the impression of inclusion bodies. Often, a supraepithelial amorphous layer contained polymorphonuclear leukocytes. However, the predominant cellular infiltration in the stroma was mononuclear and occurred densely in some areas. Limited examination of experimentally infected mares essentially confirms the conclusion that the lesions are minimal and confined to the endometrium.

DIAGNOSIS

In the Field

The clinical disease will appear during the breeding season, which is from February through mid-July in the northern Hemisphere. CEM is presumptively diagnosed when several mares covered by a particular stallion come back into premature estrus and appear dirty upon vaginal examination. (See Clinical Features.)

In the Laboratory
Endometrial Smear

During active infection, large numbrs of polymorphonuclear leukocytes (PMNs) can be found in uterine lumen and in vaginal exudate. If PMNs are found on the smear stained either with Leishman or the rapid trichrome stain, they indicate active uterine infection even if bacteriological swabs are negative. Gram-stained smears are also useful; but because of the presence of several types of Gram-negative organisms in the genital tract, the Gram-negative coccobacillus cannot be positively identified from a smear.

Swabs for Culture from Mares

Cervical swabs for bacteriological examination are best taken at estrus when the cervix is relaxed. Experienced clinicians of the disease have observed that even at estrus, the cervix is difficult to penetrate in infected mares. Ideally, the swab should be guarded to avoid contamination, should be rigid enough to penetrate the cervical canal, and should be easily deposited into transport medium; in addition, a urethral and clitoral swab should always be taken. The clitoral swab may may be particularly important in suspect carriers of CEM. Stuart's or Amies charcoal transport medium should be used. Of the two, Amies transport medium with charcoal is preferred. If there is over a 4-hr delay getting the sample to the laboratory, the transport medium containing the swab should be frozen at dry-ice temperatures.

Swabs for Culture from Stallions

If several mares covered by a particular stallion are affected with the clinical signs, the stallion should also be swabbed for culture. The swabs should be taken from the penile sheath, the urethral fossa, and the urethra. Of the three sites, the urethral fossa is the most important. The swabs should be handled as outlined for the mares.

Laboratory Culture

Upon arrival at the laboratory, the swabs are streaked on chocolate agar plates with and without 200 to 400 $\mu g/\ell$ of streptomycin as well as regular blood agar plates. One plate of each is incubated aerobically and one each in 5% CO_2 at 37°C for 24 hr. The coccobacillus will grow only on the chocolate agar plate in 5% CO_2; thus, both blood agar plates and the aerobic chocolate agar plates should be negative for the coccobacillus colonies. Colonies that appear typical are picked with a fine glass rod, and the oxidase test is performed. If the oxidase test is positive, a Gram stain and a catalase test are performed with other colonies that appear similar. If all three are positive, the laboratory diagnosis is positive. If any one of the three tests is negative, cooked meat medium is inoculated with a suspect colony and incubated overnight at 37°C. From this, new plates are streaked and then incubated at 37°C in 5% CO_2 for another 24 hr, and the three tests are repeated.

Serology

Two serological tests have been developed. However, it appears that specific antibodies to the causative organisms are short lived and the tests cannot be relied upon to detect carrier stallions and mares.

Differential Diagnosis

Although the clinical signs, vaginal examination, and smear examination may lead one to suspect CEM, a final diagnosis can be determined only upon isolation of the causative organism. The two most common vaginal infections in mares that can be confused with CEM are those caused by *Klebsiella* sp. and *Proteus* sp., and the latter organism may be involved in CEM as a secondary invader.

PROGNOSIS

Apparently, a stallion once infected will transmit the disease to each mare he covers. The infected mares generally will remain barren until the next breeding season because of the time required to treat them and assure that they remain negative for the organisms through a minimum of three estrus cycles. Data from Ireland indicate, however, that conception rates for the mares and breeding rates for stallions both return to normal the next breeding season if they have been cleared of the infection. Recent data indicate that a significant number of infected mares may become asymptomatic carriers of the organism between breeding seasons even following treatment as now practiced.

EPIZOOTIOLOGY

Geographical Distribution
See History.

Transmission
The disease is spread primarily by venereal transmission, but it can be spread by personnel and their equipment in the handling and examination of infected mares. Routine veterinary examination presents a particular hazard, and techniques must be rigidly aseptic during genital examination of all mares. Stud personnel who handle the genitalia of mares at teasing, those who wash up the genital area of mares and stallions in the covering yard or stalls, and those who assist at veterinary examination can also transmit the disease.

Host Range
We assume that all equidae are naturally susceptible, and several types of ponies have been experimentally infected. Experimental work in Ireland has failed to produce the disease in cattle, sheep, and swine. Laboratory animals have not been tested to date. CEM was first reported only in thoroughbreds. However, during the 1978 and 1979 breeding seasons other equidae were involved.

CONTROL AND ERADICATION

Preventive Measures
Breeding stock from affected countries should not be allowed into countries that are free of the disease. Any mares or stallions currently in a country that is free of the disease but that were used or covered in one of the affected countries should be swabbed and cultured before the next breeding season. Pregnant mares should have only a urethral and clitoral swab made.

Gynecological Veterinary Examination of Mares and Stud Hygiene
Because of the highly contagious nature of the disease, careful attention should be paid to hygiene when mares are examined.

1. Disposable gloves, one pair per mare, should be used by the veterinary surgeon and his assistant. A washable gown and boots should be kept at each large stud farm, but veterinary surgeons who examine only the occasional mare should take great care to wash all protective clothing in chlorhexidine before leaving the premises.
2. A thorough cleansing of the vulva with disposable swabs and a suitable antiseptic is a must.
3. A separate sterile speculum should be used for the examination of each mare. Instruments should be sterilized by boiling or autoclaving.
4. Separate equipment should be provided on each stud farm, particularly if an outbreak is occurring in the area. If separate equipment is not available, the veterinary surgeon must ensure that the equipment is sterile.
5. Stud farm personnel, when they handle the genitalia and tails of mares, should wear disposable gloves, one pair per mare. The attending veterinarian must emphasize the importance of hygiene to all stud personnel and explain the need for it.

PUBLIC HEALTH ASPECTS

There is no proven transmission to man at this time. However, caution should be practiced because little is known about the organism and disease, including the original source of the organism.

THERAPY

Treatment of Infected Mares

Laboratory tests indicate that the Gram-negative coccobacillus of CEM is sensitive to a wide range of antimicrobial agents. Experience obtained during the 1977 outbreak indicates that intensive parenteral treatment should be undertaken although a single course of treatment does not eliminate the disease in every case. Apparently, 2 to 4 g of ampicillin administered intramuscularly two or three times a day (total of 6 to 8 g daily) for 10 to 14 days along with intrauterine irrigation is the treatment of choice. In addition, recent work in Ireland indicates that parenteral neomycin at the dose rate of 2 g daily for 5 days along with intrauterine irrigation is also effective. Less intense therapy appears to induce a carrier state in certain mares although this conclusion is not fully supported by experimental work to date. The parenteral therapy should be supplemented by intrauterine irrigation with nitrofurazone, ampicillin, benzylpenicillin, or a combination of nitrofurazone and neomycin solution daily for 3 to 5 days; particular attention should be taken to include a thorough cleansing of the clitoral fossa.

Treatment of Infected Stallions

If the diagnosis that the stallion is transmitting the CEM organism is confirmed, then covering should cease immediately. The penis and prepuce should be thoroughly cleansed with chlorhexidine (1 oz/gal) and treated with nitrofurzaone once daily for at least 3 days or with 3 treatments over a 5-day period; particular attention should be given to the urethral fossa. In conjunction with this local treatment, oral treatment with either nitrofurantoin for 5 days or ampicillin intramuscularly for 10 days appears to be successful. Further treatment may be necessary, depending on the results of bacteriological tests and trial breeding. In any case, covering of mares should not begin until three consecutive negative samples have been obtained. Sampling should begin 1 week after treatment has ceased with an interval of not less than 7 days between samples. On each sampling, swabs should be obtained from the sheath, the urethral fossa, the urethra, and the preejaculatory fluid and submitted in transport medium. Trial breeding is a must for certification that a stallion is not a carrier of CEM.

These methods of treatment may be modified as further information becomes available and are based on empirical information from clinical data from Ireland and the U.K. Detailed experimental controlled studies have not been completed at this time.

SUGGESTED READING

1. Allen, W. E. and Newcombe, J. R., Aspects of genital infection and swabbing techniques in the mare, *Vet. Rec.,* 104, 228, 1979.
2. Atherton, J. G., Isolation of CEM organism, *Vet. Rec.,* 102, 67, 1978.
3. Atherton, J. G., Inhibition of CEM organism in mixed cultures, *Vet. Rec.,* 103, 432, 1978.
4. Benson, J. A., Dawson, F. L. M., Durrant, D. S., Edwards, P. T., and Powell, D. G., Serological response in mares affected by contagious equine metritis, *Vet Rec.,* 102, 277, 1978.

5. Crowhurst, R. C., Genital infection in mares, *Vet. Rec.*, 100, 476, 1977.
6. Crowhurst, R. C., Simpson, D. J., Greenwood, R. E. S., and Ellis, D. R., Contagious equine metritis, *Vet Rec.*, 102, 91, 1978.
7. David, J. S. E., Frank, C. J., and Powell, D. G., Contagious metritis 1977, *Vet. Rec.*, 101, 189, 1977.
8. David, J. S. E., Frank, C. J., and Powell, D. G., Additional recommendations for the control of contagious equine metritis 1977, *Vet. Rec.*, 102, 61, 1978.
9. Wingfield Digby, N. J., The technique and Clinical application of endometrial cytology in mares, *Equine Vet. J.*, 10(3), 167, 1978.
10. Fernie, D. S., Growth of the contagious equine metritis organism in a liquid medium, *Vet. Rec.*, 103, 187, 1978.
11. Newcombe, J. R. and Allen, W. E., Swabbing for contagious metritis tests, *Vet. Rec.*, 101, 351, 1977.
12. O'Driscoll, J. G., Venereal infection in thoroughbreds with bacillus *Proteus mirabilis*, *Vet. Rec.*, 100, 534, 1977.
13. O'Driscoll, J. G., Troy, P. T., and Geoghegan, F. J., An epidemic of venereal infection in thoroughbreds, *Vet. Rec.*, 101, 359, 1977.
14. O'Driscoll, J. G., Troy, P. T., and Geoghegan, F. J., Contagious equine metritis, *Vet. Rec.*, 101, 491, 1977.
15. Pierson, R. E., Sahu, S. P., Dardiri, A. H., and Wilder, F. W., Contagious equine metritis: clinical description of exerimentally induced Infection, *J. Am. Vet. Med. Assoc.*, 173(4), 402, 1978.
16. Platt, H., Atherton, J. G., Simpson, D. J., Taylor, C. E. D., Rosenthal, R. O., Brown, D. F. J., and Wreighitt, T. G., Genital infection in mares, *Vet. Rec.*, 101, 20, 1977.
17. Platt, H. and Atherton, J. G., Contagious equine metritis, *Vet. Rec.*, 101, 434, 1977.
18. Platt, H., Atherton, J. G., Dawson, F. L., and Durrant, D. S., Isolation of the CEM organism from the clitoris of the mare, *Vet. Rec.*, 102, 19, 1978.
19. Platt, H. and Atherton, J. G., The experimental infection of ponies with contagious equine metritis, *Equine Vet. J.*, 10(3), 153, 1978.
20. Powell, D. G., Contagious equine metritis, *Equine Vet. J.*, 10, 1, 1978.
21. Powell, D. G., David, J. S. E., and Frank, C. J., Contagious equine metritis: the present situation reviewed and a revised code of practice for its control, *Vet. Rec.*, 103, 399, 1978.
22. Ricketts, S. W., Rossdale, P. D., Wingfield Digby, N. J., Falk, M. M., Hopes, R., Hunt, M. D. N., and Peace, C. K., Genital infection in mares, *Vet. Rec.*, 101, 65, 1977.
23. Ricketts, S. W. and Rossdale, P. D., Endometrial biopsy studies of mares with contagious equine metritis 1977, *Equine Vet. J.*, 10(3), 160, 1978.
24. Rommel, F. A., Dardiri, A. H., Sahu, S. P., and Pierson, R. E., Serological identification of the bacterial agent of contagious equine metritis, *Vet. Rec.*, 103, 564, 1978.
25. Shreeve, J. E., Preliminary observations on X-factor growth requirement of the bacterium responsible for CEM, *Vet. Rec.*, 102, 20, 1978.
26. Simons, M. A. P. and Gibson, M. W., Contagious equine metritis, *Vet. Rec.*, 102, 43, 1978.
27. Smith, P. C., and Benson, J. A., Dawson, F. L. M., and Powell, D. G., *Vet. Rec.*, 103, 275, 1978.
28. Swaney, L. M. and Sahu, S. P., CEM: bacteriological methods, *Vet. Rec.*, 102, 43, 1978.
29. Swerczek, T. W., The first occurrence of contagious equine metritis in the United States, *J. Am. Vet. Med. Assoc.*, 173(4), 405, 1978.
30. Swerczek, T. W., Inhibiton of the CEM organism by the normal flora of the reproductive tract, *Vet. Rec.*, 103(6), 125, 1978.
31. Taylor, C. E. D. and Rosenthal, R. O., Organism of contagious equine metritis 1977 and human venereal disease, *Lancet*, 2, 1092, 1978.
32. Taylor, C. E. D., Rosenthal, R. O., and Brown, D. F. J., The causative organism of contagious equine metritis 1977: proposal for a new species to be known as *Haemophilus equigenitalis*, *Equine Vet. J.*, 10(3), 136, 1978.
33. Timoney, P. J., Ward, J., and Kelly, P., A contagious genital infection of mares, *Vet. Rec.*, 101, 103, 1977.
34. Timoney, P. J., McArdle, J., O'Reilly, P. J., and Ward, J., Contagious equine metritis, *Vet.Rec.*, 101, 103, 1977.
35. Timoney, P. J., McArdle, J., O'Reilly, P. J., and Ward, J., *P. mirabilis* and CEM, *Vet. Rec.*, 102, 20, 1978.
36. Timoney, P., CEM in Ireland, *Vet. Rec.*, 103, 475, 1978.
37. Timoney, P. J., McArdle, J. F., O'Reilly, P. J., and Ward, J., Infection patterns in pony mares challenged with the agent of contagious equine metritis 1977, *Equine Vet. J.*, 10(3), 14, 1978.
38. Timoney, P. J., O'Reilly, P. J., McArdle, J. F., Ward, J., and Harrington, A. M., Responses of mares to rechallenge with the organism of contagious equine metritis 1977, *Vet. Rec.*, 104, 264, 1979.

APPENDIX *

HISTORY OF THE BUREAU OF ANIMAL INDUSTRY

The following sketch of the history of the Bureau of Animal Industry (BAI) by W. D. Miles is presented in detail because it portrays the great amount of time and effort required to develop such an organization.

Animal diseases killed stock on American farms from the earliest days onward, but the fight against these diseases did not expand to national proportions until cattle raising became big business in the nineteenth century. From roughly the Civil War period onward, there was a continual barrage of suggestions in and out of Congress for a campaign to control diseases of domestic animals. In 1865, Congress enacted a law "to prevent the spread of foreign diseases among the cattle of the U.S." by prohibiting importation of cattle. This was only the first of such federal legislation.

In 1868, the Commissioner of Agriculture appointed a veterinarian to study Texas fever and a year later recommended that a division of veterinary surgery be formed. A decade later the Commissioner appointed agents in a number of states to report that presence of animal disease, and in 1878 he stationed a veterinarian in the Chicago stockyards to examine cattle.

Around 1880, European countries began to quarantine and otherwise restrict importation of American livestock and meat. These measures increased the pressure on Congress to bring the power of the federal government to bear on the problem.

Agriculturalists were not the only group in the U.S. concerned with animal disease. Since some of these diseases, e.g., trichinosis, could be transmitted to humans, physicians also were interested.

The American Public Health Association (APHA) scheduled papers on animal disease from the time of its first meeting, 1873, when Adoniran B. Judson, M.D., presented a "History and Course of the Epizootic among Horses upon the North American Continent in 1872-73." Other papers that subsequently appeared in the Association's *Reports and Papers* included Joseph R. Smith, M.D.'s "Disease Among Texas Cattle," G. B. White, M.D.'s "Report of the Examination of Hogs at the New Orleans Abattoir During the Summer of 1881, with Especial Reference to the Presence or Absence of Trichinae Spiralis," and Ezra M. Hunt, M.D.'s "Contagious Diseases of Domestic Animals." Early volumes of the *Reports and Papers* carried articles by James Law and an article on Texas cattle fever by Daniel E. Salmon, later the first chief of the Department of Agriculture's BAI.

State boards of health went into the area of animal diseases. In annual reports of boards may be found articles such as "Trichina Disease in Massachusetts" and "Charbon in Massachusetts." Some boards found themselves concerned indirectly with diseases of food-producing animals through state laws that required the boards to deal with adulterated or unhygienic foods. Some boards were linked directly to animal disease. This was the case with the New Jersey board that was required by a law of 1877 to "make inquiries and reports in reference to diseases affecting animals and methods of prevention."

On the national level, in at least one instance legislation was proposed to place animal diseases under a national public health organization. In 1873, Senator James Patterson presented a bill to establish a "Bureau of Sanitary Science" headed by a com-

---

* Miles, W. D., Appendix, in *Bovine Tuberculosis Control in Man and Animals*, Myers, J. A. and Steele, J. H., Eds., Warren H. Green, St. Louis, 1969. Reprinted with permission.

missioner who would have acquired information by correspondence, books, and practical and scientific experiments on subjects including "diseases of animals including cattle plague, foot rot in sheep, and cerebrospinal meningitis in horses . . . "

Patterson's bill for a national health organization was premature and did not pass, but in March 1879, chiefly as an aftermath of serious yellow fever epidemics, Congress created the National Board of Health (NBH), the first federal public health organization. The NBH was to obtain information "upon all matters affecting the public health," to make scientific investigations, to advise governmental bodies on public health, to cooperate with state and municipal health officials, and to have certain powers in quarantine. The Board did not receive a mission in animal disease, but as a health agency it had a natural involvement.

Creation of the NBH placed a competitor to the Bureau of Agriculture in the area of animal diseases. With the livestock industry badly in need of assistance, the stage was set for a struggle between congressional champions of public health and of agriculture to determine which agency would receive the authority.

The opening move was made by Senator John W. Johnston of Virginia, chairman of the Committee on Agriculture. Johnston, and possibly some other agricultural legislators, seemed to have looked upon the NBH at first as a device for involving the government in the fight against animal diseases. On March 31, less than 1 month after the Board was created, Johnston introduced a bill (S.267) authorizing the Board to investigate and report on contagious diseases of food animals and making an appropriation for the purpose. Along with the bill, Johnston submitted a letter from Army Surgeon John Shaw Billings, written in reply to a request from Johnston asking Billings' views "as to the line of inquiry and means of prevention to be adopted with regard to those diseases of animals which interfere with the supply of wholesome animal food for man, and more especially with regard to the lung plague of cattle, hog cholera, trichinosis, and measles in swine."

Billings suggested that the

. . . whole matter should be referred to the National Board of Health, with power to employ experts and inspectors, and with the direction to report fully to Congress at its next session both as to what has been done and what ought to be done.

I believe the National Board of Health, as organized, to be such an authority (referring to previous remarks), and that the subject of diseases of animals, especially of food-producing animals, should receive its special attention. Its duties under the law are "to obtain information upon all matters affecting the public health" and "to advise the several departments of the government, the executives of the several states, and the commissioners of the District of Columbia on all questions submitted by them, or whenever in the opinion of the Board such advice may tend to the preservation and improvement of the public health." This certainly includes the very important questions of wholesome food supply.

Billings further remarked that the duty of the NBH was to advance the knowledge of the cause of disease and to study the matter of quarantine, and in so doing the Board would necessarily have to study animal diseases and animal quarantine. He pointed out that the NBH would be cooperating with state and local boards, many of which were already considering animal diseases. Finally, he stated that it would be true economy to combine the investigations of diseases of man and animals.

Johnston's bill was referred to the Committee on Agriculture. There, a debate undoubtedly took place as to whether agriculturists would favor a veterinary branch in the NBH or in the Bureau of Agriculture. Those who favored the latter course apparently won, for Johnston's bill was buried by the committee.

Johnston's bill was actually introduced into Congress before the NBH had the opportunity to hold its first meeting, April 1, 1879. Billings' views were transmitted several days before he was detailed to the Board (he was detailed on March 31, 1879) and were therefore Billings' personal views, not official views of the Board. But a short time later, Billings had the opportunity to present his ideas to fellow members of the Board, and on this occasion they were adopted as the Board's official position.

On April 3, Senator Isham Harris asked the NBH to recommend amendments and modifications to Bill S.108, a bill to broaden the power of the Board, which Harris had introduced into the Senate. The Board met and decided upon certain changes, and then Billings brought up the subject of animal diseases:

Dr. J. S. Billings stated that in reference to the bill passed by the Board in the afternoon he had one more amendment to offer. He had it in his mind all along but was unable to decide until now whether it would be advisable or not to add it to the present bill. He had received a letter from Senator Johnson of Virginia inquiring what was the most practicable method of preventing contagious diseases among cattle.

The letter was instigated by a letter from the Commissioner of Agriculture requesting an appropriation of $250,000 for the purpose of making inspection at the different seaboard towns where this cattle plague existed. He stated that he recommended the matter be placed in the hands of the NBH, and also sent him the draft of a bill. Senator Johnson seemed to have approved both letter and bill and had the letter printed. He would not offer the bill as an amendment to the one passed in the afternoon, to be added to the Senate Bill No. 108 in such a way as it might be dropped in case of great opposition on the part of the Agricultural Department.

On motion of Dr. J. S. Billings, the Executive Committee was authorized to insert the amendment in its proper place in the bill and to increase the appropriation from $500,000 to $650,000, also to place it in the hands of the gentlemen who are to have charge of it in the House and Senate respectively, and to explain to them that in case of serious opposition it would be advisable that it be dropped and the appropriation reduced to $500,000.

Dr. Bemiss said he would second it if Dr. Billings would modify his motion so that it might be referred to the Executive Committee with power. Dr. Billings accepted the modification and the motion as modified was agreed to.

Billings' proposed amendments finally appeared in the following form:

Section 9 — That the National Board of Health is hereby directed to make, or cause to be made, an investigation into the contagious or infectious diseases of domestic animals in the United States, and especially such as tend to interfere with the supply of wholesome food, and into the best means of controlling or preventing such diseases, and to report the result of its investigations at the next session of Congress.

Section 10 — That the National Board of Health is also directed to cause a thorough inspection to be made of all animals arriving at, or exported from, the different shipping ports of the United States, and to cause the owners or shippers of such cattle to be promptly notified of the results of such inspections, with such recommendations as may be proper in each case. It shall also notify state and local sanitary authorities of the existence of such diseases of domestic animals as it deems proper to bring to their notice with such recommendations as may be deemed expedient in each case.

Shortly after the NBH had completed the modification of Bill S.108, the subject of diseases of food animals came up again in Congress. On April 12, there was a move to appropriate funds to the Department of the Interior to wipe out pleuropneumonia in cattle. Congressman Casey Young, a staunch supporter of the NBH, told the House that the Board was engaged in the investigation of the subject, that the Board would suggest "modes and methods of preventing the cattle disease," and that it would be preferable to confine the task to the Board rather than give it to Interior. During debate Young stated that the Board had had this subject under advisement for 10 days and had prepared a bill that Young was going to offer — apparently the House version of Bill S.108. Congressman Joseph Hawley sided with Young by proposing that the Board be instructed to report a bill on the subject. Congressman Joseph Chalmers tried to give Young an assist by suggesting that the subject be placed under cognizance of the Committee on Epidemic Diseases, the parent committee of the NBH. But Congressman George Dibrell remarked that "health physicians" did not know anything about cows, and he obtained sufficient support from agriculturists to send the matter to the Committee on Agriculture.

While Board and Agriculture backers were sparring, the Board was readying itself, on a small scale, to enter the field of animal diseases if Congress gave it cognizance over these diseases. One of the several Board committees created in the beginning was on "diseases of domestic animals." James L. Cabell, University of Virginia, president of the NBH; Tullio S. Verdi, M.D., Washington, D.C., the only homeopathic physician on the Board; and Preston H. Bailhache, M.D., Board member respresenting the Marine Hospital Service, comprised this committee.

The Secretary of the Board began collecting information by writing to the House and Senate document rooms and asking that the Board be placed on the mailing list to receive publications on animal diseases. He also wrote to the chief clerk of the State Department to inquire about foreign laws against our cattle:

> Can you give the National Board of Health any information regarding what countries have either wholly or partially interdicted the importation of American cattle?
>
> Great Britain has partially done so, but information is desired as to the exact status of Switzerland, Belgium, Holland, Spain, and Prussia.

Optimistic members of the Board apparently consulted with experts in the Washington area, one of whom, Charles V. Riley, chief of the U.S. Entomological Commission, thought so well of the Board's prospects that he applied for a job:

> At the instance of two of the members of the National Board of Health, I take the liberty of suggesting that, in the event of your being called upon by Congress to make full and thorough investigation into the various diseases affecting domestic animals, and of your wanting special work done in natural history, I shall be pleased to offer my services and do all in my power to aid you in such important work. You will doubtless have constant use for special knowledge of the lower forms of animal life, and to be able to help to such, so far as my abilities will permit, will be both a privilege and a pleasure. The experience gained in fifteen years' study of the insects affecting plants and animals will, I believe, enable me to be of some service to you, and I offer such service without hope of compensation, as I already draw salary under the Government as a member of the U.S. Entomological Commission.
>
> I have been asked to submit my views as to the best mode of carrying on such an investigation, but feel that to do so would, at the present time, be taking an unwarranted liberty.

One Doctor Gunnell of Washington at the same time offered his services, and the Board secretary replied with the following note:

> I have the honor to acknowledge the receipt of the communication regarding your appointment in connection with investigations into diseases of domestic animals, and to state that it will receive due consideration when the legislation now before Congress becomes a law.

Alexandre Liautard, head of the American Veterinary College and editor of the *American Veterinary Review* applied for appointment as Veterinarian. But while the NBH was readying itself, the congressional champions of Agriculture did not sit idly by and allow Harris, Young, and other legislators to give control of animal disease to the Board. Thomas J. Turner, Secretary of the Board, noted the struggle in a few words when he wrote, "the Agricultural Bureau and Treasury are inimical to us." Before Harris' bill S.108 — to broaden the duties of the NBH — passed Congress and was approved by President Hayes in June, all references to animal diseases disappeared.

Congress adjourned on July 1, 1879, and did not reconvene until December 1. During recess, the NBH continued its plans to take charge of animal diseases. Now, when Congress had created the NBH, it had done so in an emergency; it had considered the

Board as a more-or-less temporary organization, and it had directed the Board to present to the next session of Congress "a plan for a national public health organization." Since there had been no authority for work on animal diseases in the act creating the NBH, the Board determined to ask Congress to give such authority to the prospective permanent organization. To obtain a basis for its request to Congress, the Board set aside $1000 to aid in "collecting information and preparing a report upon diseases of domestic animals, reporting what legislation is desirable on the subject and what restrictions are imposed by foreign governments upon the exportation of food animals from this country on account of diseases among the same." The Board discussed at least four scientists — Alexander Liautard, Hosmer A. Johnson, T. C. Minor, and James Law — to draw up a report, picked Law, and then wrote the following letter to him at Cornell:

The National Board of Health is required by law to report to Congress at its next session a plan for a National Public Health organization. As a part of such plan, it seems probably that the prevention of disease in domestic animals and especially of such diseases in food-producing animals as may tend to make the food so produced liable to cause disease in man should be carefully considered.

To this end, the Board desired to obtain information from those who have given most attention to this subject, as to what can be properly undertaken by a national public health organization to prevent such diseases and as to the Congressional legislation which is desirable to attain such end.

The Board has directed its Executive Committee to obtain such information and has placed at its disposal the sum of one thousand dollars or so much thereof as may be necessary for this purpose.

In behalf of the Executive Committee, I write to ask your advice as to the best method of procedure to carry out the wishes of the Board and also to enquire whether you can undertake the direction of any part of the work required.

Law's "Report on Diseases of Domestic Animals," for which he received $150, reached the Board in December, was printed in the *Annual Report* of the Board for 1879, in the *Bulletin* of the Board, and was reprinted by the *American Veterinary Review.*

In this paper, Law discussed a number of animal diseases communicable to man, and made several suggestions regarding a possible role of the NBH in fighting these diseases. Law's philosophy toward the roles of the Board and the veterinary profession is stated near the end of his report:

The time may come when the nation will be sufficiently educated to allow the sanitation of man and animals to be controlled by a single national health board; but at present and for the exclusively animal plagues, we cannot afford to run any risks, and that method should be followed which will secure a certain and speedy result and establish the principle of the extinction of such pestilences on a sound and unassailable basis. I would therefore urge as the result of mature deliberation, in view of all aspects of the question, that the control of those animal contagia and parasites which affect man as well should be placed in the hands of a veterinary committee of the National Board of Health organized for this purpose, while the exclusively animal plagues and the parasites that affect animals only should be committed to an organization drawn from the stock owners and the veterinary profession, and not too large or unwieldy for the most prompt and effective action.

In addition to Law's report, the Board issued in the same *Annual Report* an article by Board member Tullio S. Verdi, "Cattle Disease in Relation to the Health of Man and in Political Economy."Verdi discussed the general problem, pointed out the economic loss owing to diseased animals, emphasized the relationship between diseases of man and animals, and suggested that a "National Sanitary Bureau" be empowered to control cattle disease. Since the only national sanitary bureau in the federal government was the NBH, Verdi's suggestion, if followed logically, would have led to the addition of animal diseases to the Board's responsibilities.

While Law and Verdi were drawing up their reports, the purpose of which was to help persuade legislators to give the Board jurisdiction over animal disease, an event took place which caused the Board to change its position and decide not to seek such authority.

Congress, in directing the Board to present a plan for a national public health organization, had ordered the Board to consult with the National Academy of Sciences. In December 1879, the Board and a committee from the Academy met. The Board presented a number of proposals to the Academy committee, including the following statement on animal disease:

> The National Board of Health shall be specifically directed by law to make or cause to be made an investigation into the contagious or infectious diseases of domestic animals in the United States, and especially such as tend to interfere with the supply of wholesome food, and into the best means of controlling and preventing such diseases, and to report the result of such investigation at the next session of Congress, and that for this purpose the sum of twenty-five thousand dollars ($25,000) should be appropriated.

The Academy committee agreed with the Board on all proposals except that of animal diseases. Here Joseph J. Woodward stated that:

> While the Committee had no recommendation to make yet, they thought it might not be good policy to press this matter at the present time because it was likely to raise strong opposition and might endanger the passage of the other recommendations. That this, however, was merely a suggestion of the Committee.

Since none of the members of the Academy committee were active in agriculture or veterinary medicine (although Woodward had been a member of a government committe on cattle disease a decade earlier), we can only surmise that the political climate in Washington at that time was cold toward the Board taking up animal diseases and that the committee members sensed this.

As a result of this conference, the NBH decided that it would no longer seek any authority to work on animal diseases. "We agreed," wrote James L. Cabell, "to the proposition of the committee of the National Academy of Science *not* to ask for any legislation on that subject." But this decision did not stop the NBH from financing some research in animal diseases, and it did not stop its supporters in Congress from trying to involve the Board in animal diseases.

The Board's entrance into research on animal disease may have been triggered by an inquiry from the State Department for information on the prevalence of hog cholera and trichinosis in the U.S., to enable the State Department to reply to a cablegram from the U.S. Minister in Great Britain. Cabell replied to this communication by stating that "this Board has no official or other information as to the alleged existence of hog cholera and trichinosis in the United States. It is proper to add that under existing laws, the Board has no special means of obtaining such information."

The Board had, however, a roundabout method by which it could obtain such information; that is, authority from its constituting act to undertake "special examinations and investigations." Under this authority, the Board had already financed a number of scientific projects carried on by Board scientists (George Sternberg, Charles Smart) and by outside investigators (Ira Remsen, Rudolph Hering, John W. Mallet, George Waring, and others).

The day after Cabell replied to the State Department question, the Board appropriated $1,000 for an investigation on trichinosis to be carried out under the direction of Charles H. Folsom, M.D., a public health expert of Boston. Folsom considered the Board's proposal and voiced his thoughts in the following letter:

> As to the trichina business, I think it would be well for me not to make any definite arrangements with Mr. Billings until I can confer with the Board or the exec. comm. in May or June.

If a proper and competent person can be found in Washington, I think it would be well to set him at work examining hogs for trichinae, especially if we can get hold of home-fed hogs or small drove hogs, especially from the South and near Baltimore and Philadelphia.

This might be done under the direct supervision of the Board. We might set Mr. Billings at work on some experiments in propagating trichinae, etc. but of this I have some doubt. It will be many years before we get at the origin of this disease. Three or four months in trichinae, etc. would be a mere bagatelle.

It seems from the above letter that Folsom was not ready to plunge headlong into trichinosis research. A week later, he sent another letter to the Board telling them that "we will leave the trichinae question for the present." Actually, Folsom and the Board left trichinae permanently since funds to finance the project soon ran out.

While trichinosis was the only project on animal disease sponsored by the Board, it is possible that the Board would have financed others had its funds not become depleted. There is nothing in the records to indicate that the Board rejected or would have rejected any proposals to conduct research into other animal diseases.

Although the NBH had decided, as a result of its meeting with representatives of the National Academy of Sciences, not to seek authority for work on animal diseases, legislators continued to press for such authority in Congress.

In December 1880, Senator John Williams introduced a bill (S.1908) to control diseases of domestic animals that placed research, quarantine, other matters, and an appropriation of $1 million under the NBH. Williams sought to send the bill to the Board's backer, the Committee on Epidemic Diseases, but Senator Johnston suggested that a select committee be set up to study all bills on the subject of pleuropneumonia and other contagious diseases of domestic animals. The Senate favored Johnston's plan, created the committee and sent Williams' bill to it. In the Select Committee, Williams' bill met sufficient opposition to kill it.

The following month, Senator Johnston reported a bill (S.2097) from the Select Committee to establish a Bureau of Animal Industry. This bill attempted to compromise differences between supporters of Agriculture and the Board of Health. The chief of the bureau would be a veterinary surgeon but approved by the NBH. Inspectors would also be approved by the Board. The Board would have no direct hand in operating the bureau, but the Commissioner of Agriculture could call on the NBH for aid whenever he felt it necessary. The bill did not satisfy all the senators. Amendments were suggested, one of which would have made the Commissioner of Agriculture and the National Board joint superintendents in suppression of animal disease. Finally, after considerable debate, the bill was sent back to committee.

In December 1881, Representative William Hatch introduced a bill (H.R.896) to establish a Bureau of Animal Industry. Under this bill, the Commissioner of Agriculture would organize in his department a Bureau of Animal Industry and appoint as chief a competent veterinary surgeon approved by the NBH. The commisioner was also authorized to call the NBH to his aid in investigating animal diseases and in providing means for prevention and cure. Finally, the commissioner, in connection with the NBH, was to prepare necessary regulations.

Bill H.R. 896, when debated in the House, brought a number of objections from congressmen, and some of these objections centered on the presence of the NBH in the proposed Bureau. The House eventually struck out references to the Board and kept the bill around until early 1883 before abandoning it.

Bill H.R. 896 seems to have been the last serious effort to couple animal disease to the NBH. The Board was dying, owing to successful efforts of legislators hostile to the Board for various reasons to block appropriations for the Board. Because the Board was almost moribund, or because the champions of agriculture were prevailing, or because of a combination of the two circumstances, there were no further efforts to join the Board and the Department in a war against animal diseases.

Bill H.R. 896 bore a decided resemblance to the bill (H.R. 3967) that Hatch introduced subsequently that passed in 1884 and established the BAI. Indeed, the resemblance between the two bills is so striking that it appears that the bill to establish the Bureau evolved from Bill H.R. 896 chiefly by elimination of all mention of the NBH.

It is interesting to conjecture what might have happened to the NBH if it had obtained authority to carry on work in animal diseases. It may then have gained additional supporters among agricultural legislators; these plus its public health legislators might have given it sufficient backing to remain alive. As it was, the Board had too few backers and it fell beneath the combined opposition of legislators who wanted economy, those who favored states' rights, and those who could not foresee the value of a national public health agency. Had the NBH survived, development of public health would have taken a different course.

Furthermore, if the NBH had gained a mission in animal diseases, the character of future public health research would have been different. As it was, research on animal disease thereafter was concentrated upon by the Department of Agriculture, research on human disease by the National Board's successor, the Public Health Service. But, it is worthy of note that future researchers in the Department of Agriculture and the Public Health Service were frequently to cross the line from animal to human diseases, and one may wonder if the future course of medical research might not have been accelerated if one agency had had cognizance over both animal and human diseases.

Index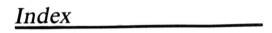

INDEX